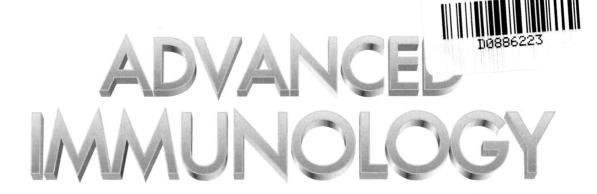

ADVANCED IMMUNOLOGY

David Male MA PhD
Senior Lecturer in Neuroimmunology
Department of Neuropathology
Institute of Psychiatry
London, UK

Anne Cooke BSc PhD
Lecturer in Immunology
Department of Pathology
Cambridge University
Cambridge, UK

Michael Owen BA PhD
Principal Research Scientist
Imperial Cancer Research Fund
London, UK

John Trowsdale PhD
Human Immunogenetics Laboratory
Imperial Cancer Research Fund
London, UK

Brian Champion BSc PhD
Department of Immunology
Glaxo Wellcome Research and Development
Stevenage, Herfordshire, UK

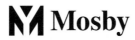 Mosby

London Baltimore Barcelona Bogotá Boston Buenos Aires Caracas Carlsbad, CA Chicago Madrid Mexico City Milan Naples, FL New York
Philadelphia St. Louis Seoul Singapore Sydney Taipei Tokyo Toronto Wiesbaden

AFZ4928

The cover illustration depicts a domain model of the interaction between an antigen-presenting cell and a CD4$^+$ T cell. The MHC class II molecules (deep blue) present antigenic peptides to the T cell receptor in which the $\alpha\beta$ dimers (red) lie around a core of CD3 polypeptides. CD4 (yellow) associated with the kinase lck (green) can phosphorylate the intracellular domains of the CD3 γ, δ, ε and ζ polypeptides.

QR.
181
A395
1996

Project Manager:	Jeremy Theobald
Development Editor:	Louise Cook
Designer:	Pete Wilder
Cover Design:	Greg Smith
Illustration:	Lee Smith
Production:	Jane Tozer
Index:	Laurence Errington
Publisher:	Dianne Zack

OLSON LIBRARY
NORTHERN MICHIGAN UNIVERSITY
MARQUETTE, MICHIGAN 49855

Copyright © 1996 Times Mirror International Publishers Limited

Published in 1996 by Mosby, an imprint of Times Mirror International Publishers Limited

Printed in Italy by Vincenzo Bona s.r.l., Turin

ISBN 0 7234 2059 9

All rights reserved. No reproduction, copy or transmission of this publication may be made without written permission.

No part of this publication may be reproduced, copied or transmitted save with written permission or in accordance with the provisions of the Copyright Act 1988, or under the terms of any licence permitting limited copying issued by the Copyright Licensing Agency, 33–34 Alfred Place, London, WC1E 7DP.

Any person who does any unauthorised act in relation to this publication may be liable to criminal prosecution and civil claims for damages.

Permission to photocopy or reproduce solely for internal or personal use is permitted for libraries or other users registered with the Copyright Clearance Center, provided that the base fee of $4.00 per chapter plus $.10 per page is paid directly to the Copyright Clearance Center, 21 Congress Street, Salem, MA 01970. This consent does not extend to other kinds of copying, such as copying for general distribution, for advertising or promotional purposes, for creating new collected works, or for resale.

For full details of all Times Mirror International Publishers Limited titles, please write to Times Mirror International Publishers Limited, Lynton House, 7–12 Tavistock Square, London WC1H 9LB, England.

A CIP catalogue record for this book is available from the British Library.

Library of Congress Cataloging-in-Publication Data applied for.

Contents

INTERACTIONS OF IMMUNOLOGICALLY ACTIVE CELLS

IMMUNOLOGICAL EFFECTOR SYSTEMS

Preface

This book has been written for people who already have a knowledge of basic immunology, and who wish to understand in greater depth how the immune system functions. We have concentrated on the central areas of immunology, namely immune recognition, the differentiation and cooperation of immunologically active cells and on immune effector systems. In order to keep the text to a manageable length we have not dwelt on basic data, which may be found elsewhere, on the assumption that readers will already be familiar with them.

This third edition has been completely rewritten to take account of the developments in molecular and cellular immunology which have occurred in the last 5 years. Some areas have faded from prominence, while other subjects which were at the leading edge of research have now found their way into basic textbooks. On the other hand, new technologies have opened up exciting areas which were previously just gaps in our understanding. Particularly notable are the advances in our knowledge of intracellular signalling and second messenger systems, together with the details of antigen-processing and presentation. The development of new transgenic strains and 'knockout' strains has given insight into the functions of particular systems and the degrees of redundancy within the immune system. The families of cytokines continue to expand and the interactive balance of T helper populations is now firmly established as a central pivot of the immune system. The definition and role of the chemokines in the control of inflammation and cell traffic is now viewed as an essential adjunct to the induction and expression of adhesion molecules. Even 'settled areas' such as the complement system continue to throw up surprises, with the description of a new lectin-mediated activation pathway.

The book is broadly divided into 5 main sections. Following the introduction, these sections deal with 1) immune recognition, 2) development of leukocytes, 3) initiation of the immune response, 4) interactions of immunologically active cells and 5) immunological effector systems. The book concludes with a totally new chapter on the ways in which this information is being used to modulate the immune system therapeutically.

As in previous editions, we have selected particular experiments from research papers to explain and illustrate specific points. We would like to acknowledge the work of the many scientists whose studies we have presented in the text and accompanying illustrations. These figures are intended to be illustrative, and many equally good studies have not been mentioned. We have included only those details of experimental designs that are essential to understand the point. Readers who wish to examine precise details of the work and see other supporting experiments are referred to the lists of additional reading at the end of each chapter. These contain the original sources for the experimental studies, together with a number of useful reviews.

David Male
Anne Cooke
Michael Owen
John Trowsdale
Brian Champion

Acknowledgments

We are most grateful to all the individuals who have contributed to this new edition, particularly Dean Madden, Don Wiley, Anton van der Merwe and Alan Ebringer who provided us with new colour illustrations, and also to J Phillips B Arnold and N Holmes. We also appreciate the enormous amount of work done by our publishers to bring this edition through quickly. Especial thanks go to Jeremy Theobald for the design and production, to Louise Cook for editorial work and to Dianne Zack and Fiona Foley who set the project in motion.

David Male
Anne Cooke
Michael Owen
John Trowsdale
Brian Champion

Permission has been obtained from the copyright holders listed below for the use of the colour figures:

Reprinted with permission of Annual Reviews Inc.
Colour fig. 2 Davie: *Ann Rev Immunol* 1986, **4**:

Reprinted with permission of Cell Press
Colour fig. 3 Madden DR: *Cell* 1993, **75**:693

Reprinted with permission of Current Biology
Colour fig. 4 van der Merwe PA: *Curr Biol* 1995, **5**:74

Reprinted with permission of AAAS
Colour fig. 5 Poljak RJ: *Science* 1986, **233**:747

Reprinted with permission of
Colour fig. 6 Wilson: *Ann Rheum Dis* 1995, **54**:216

1 The Immune System

THE IMMUNE SYSTEM

The immune system of mammals has evolved to protect individuals against pathogenic viruses, microorganisms and parasites. Immune responses depend on the ability of the system to recognize foreign molecules — antigens — on potential pathogens and then to mount an appropriate reaction to eliminate the source of the antigen. The process of immune recognition is carried out by lymphocytes and this is followed by an effector phase which may involve a variety of cell types. Immune recognition is critically important in the normal functioning of the system because the lymphocytes must recognize antigens of all potential pathogens while at the same time tolerating molecules of the body's own tissues. This presents a problem which is compounded by the enormous diversity of antigens on microorganisms and their potential for mutation. To handle this the lymphocytes in an individual diversify during development so that the population as a whole can recognize any infectious agent.

Immune responses which depend on lymphocyte mediated recognition of antigen are usually referred to as adaptive immune responses. These responses show two important characteristics, namely specificity and memory. A second or subsequent encounter with a particular antigen results in an enhanced or modified response to that antigen. The elements of the immune system which produce adaptive responses have evolved in parallel with other host defence systems, such as phagocytes and plasma enzyme systems. These are sometimes referred to as the non-adaptive or innate immune system. However, this division is too simple because extensive cooperation occurs between all the elements of the immune system.

In the initial stages of a response a group of functionally defined cells, the antigen presenting cells (APCs), take up and present antigen to lymphocytes in a form which they can recognize. The different ways in which antigens are presented to lymphocytes largely determines whether an immune response will develop and what type of response it will be. An overview of these interactions is shown in *Figure 1.1*.

In the later, effector phase of the response an amazing diversity of reactions may occur. This is related to the great variety of potential pathogens — the reactions needed to destroy a virally infected cell are quite different from those involved in the expulsion of a large parasitic worm. However, cooperation between the various elements of the immune system is again vital. In particular, IgG antibodies from B lymphocytes can opsonize immune complexes for uptake by phagocytes via their Fc receptors. IgE can modulate inflammatory responses via Fc receptors on mast cells, basophils and eosinophils and IgG can also modulate

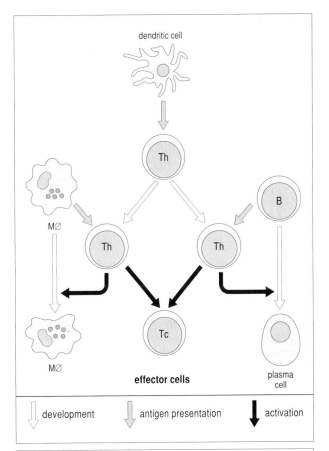

Fig. 1.1 Initiation of immune responses. Dendritic cells present antigen to naive CD4+ T helper cells (Th). Macrophages (MØ) and B cells can also present antigen to mature CD4+ T cells. Cytokines released by the T cells direct the interactions causing macrophage activation and/or driving B cells to differentiate into antibody-producing plasma cells. CD4+ T cells are also required for the generation of cytotoxic T cells (Tc). Antibodies, macrophages and cytotoxic T cells are the principal elements of the effector arm of the immune response. The balance of activity between the different groups of antigen presenting cells and CD4+ T cells determines what type of immune response will be generated.

inflammation by its action on the complement system. Cytokines released by T cells are important in controlling what types of antibodies will be produced, while others activate mononuclear phagocytes to destroy material they have endocytosed. The effector mechanisms of an immune response are summarized in *Figure 1.2*.

1.1

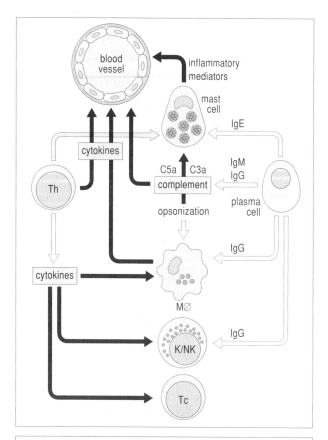

Fig. 1.2 Effector mechanisms of the immune response. The activity of effector cells and the complement system (centre) is controlled by the actions of Th cells via cytokine release (as shown) or by direct cell–cell contact and antibody. Different antibody isotypes mediate different types of response. Similarly, different T cell subsets also control different types of response. Also important are the actions of the various mediators on blood vessels, controlling inflammatory responses and the influx of leukocytes, antibodies and other serum molecules from the blood stream. (K/NK = killer/natural killer cell.)

CELLS OF THE IMMUNE SYSTEM

Immune responses are effected primarily by lymphocytes and phagocytes which are derived from bone marrow stem cells *(Fig. 1.3)*. These cells circulate through the body via the blood, tissues, lymphatics and lymphoid organs. Broadly speaking, different phases of the response occur in different areas of the body. Thus, the initial differentiation of lymphocytes occurs in primary lymphoid tissues, the thymus and bone marrow, the recognition of and initial reponse to antigen occur in the secondary lymphoid tissues and the effector phase of the response develops wherever the initiating antigen is found. As cells move between different compartments they may continue their differentiation; for example, a virgin lymphocyte will usually differ from one that has previously contacted antigen, both in its surface phenotype and in its responses. Similarly a tissue macrophage differs from the blood monocyte from which it has developed. The lineage of a cell and its stage of development can broadly be defined by the surface molecules which it expresses, referred to as 'markers'.

Markers

Different markers of haemopoietic cells are currently identified by a CD (cluster of differentiation) number. This nomenclature has been established through a series of international workshops which analysed the specificities of anti-leukocyte monoclonal antibodies submitted for analysis. Antibodies having similar patterns of reactivity with different cell populations and which immunoprecipitate the same surface molecule define a particular CD marker. Many of these markers are also defined functionally and are identified accordingly. For example, the intercellular adhesion molecule ICAM-1 is CD54 and the complement receptor CR3 is formed of an α-chain, CD11b, and a β-chain, CD18. As the CD system is defined by antibodies, molecules are distinguished according to the epitopes they express. In some cases, variant RNA splicing leads to forms of a molecule which have different epitopes. For example, CD45R is a restricted form of leukocyte common antigen

Fig. 1.3 Morphology and lineage of leukocytes and antigen presenting cells. The electron micrographs indicate the morphology of the cells involved in the immune response and the way in which they are derived from the bone marrow stem cell. T and B cells are both derived from lymphocytic stem cells following differentiation in the primary lymphoid organs. They both have large nuclei and a thin rim of cytoplasm containing relatively few mitochondria and polysomes. After activation, lymphocytes appear as blast cells (in this instance a B cell blast is shown), where the cytoplasm is expanded and contains more endoplasmic reticulum and Golgi apparatus. B cells may ultimately develop into plasma cells which are entirely devoted to antibody synthesis. Null cells have many of the attributes of lymphocytes, but appear to arise by a separate differentiation pathway. Mature null cells appear as large granular lymphocytes (LGLs). The blood monocyte typically has a horseshoe-shaped nucleus and a variety of enzyme-containing granules. After emigration from the blood stream, they mature into macrophages, with increased metabolic and phagocytic capacities. Antigen presenting cells (APCs) are also thought to be derived from bone marrow stem cells. APCs are here exemplified by the interdigitating cell (IDC) seen in the T cell area of a lymph node. This cell belongs to the dendritic cell lineage, and is seen in close contact with a number of surrounding lymphocytes. The neutrophil is a short lived phagocyte with a polymorphic nucleus and numerous cytoplasmic granules containing proteolytic enzymes. The granules of the eosinophil contain a central crystalloid core and other toxic molecules, while the large electron dense granules of the basophil contain a variety of inflammatory mediators. The eosinophil and neutrophil are actively phagocytic, whereas the basophil is not; indeed the basophil may be more closely related to the tissue mast cell, with which it shares functional similarities.

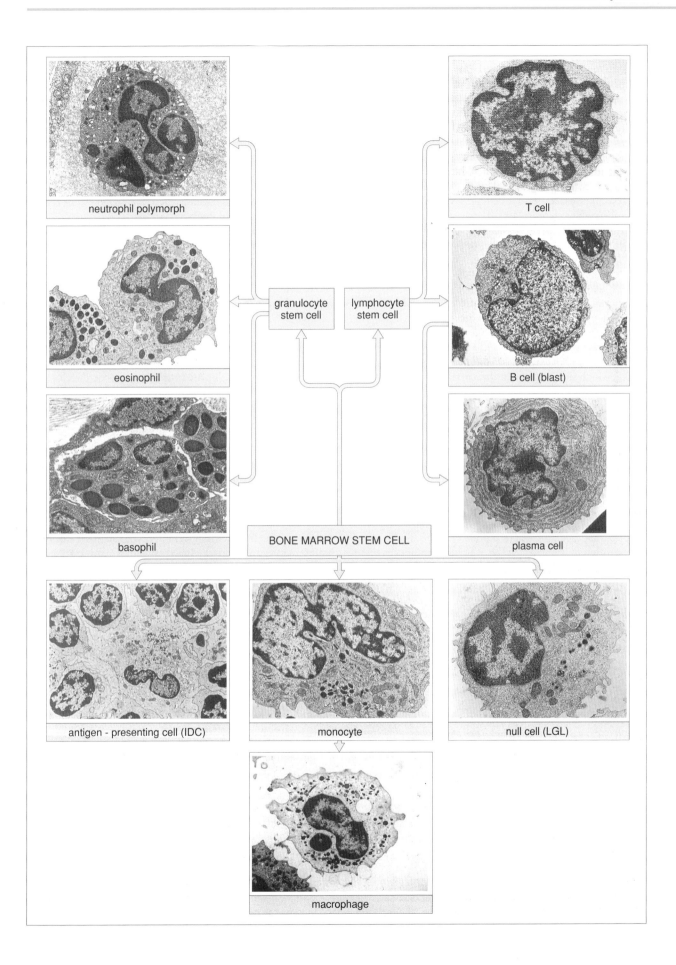

neutrophil polymorph

T cell

eosinophil

B cell (blast)

basophil

plasma cell

granulocyte stem cell

lymphocyte stem cell

BONE MARROW STEM CELL

antigen - presenting cell (IDC)

monocyte

null cell (LGL)

macrophage

(CD45), produced by variant RNA splicing, which is present on only a subpopulation of cells expressing CD45.

The CD system includes molecules which distinguish particular lineages of cells, those common to several lineages and those which appear transiently during particular stages of cellular activation. Some CD molecules also appear on non-haemopoietic cells. For example, the transferrin receptor (CD71), present on activated lymphocytes, also occurs on brain endothelium and many dividing cells. Since several clearly defined markers are not included in the CD system (surface Ig on B cells and MHC molecules, for example), a cell is defined by its overall profile of surface molecules. Nevertheless some markers are more useful than others for defining individual lineages (*Fig. 1.4*). A complete listing of the CD system is given in the Appendix.

Lymphocytes

Lymphocytes constitute about 20% of blood leukocytes and are specialized in the recognition of antigens. Lymphocytes are of two main types, namely B cells which develop in the bone marrow and which may subsequently differentiate into antibody-producing plasma cells, and T cells which differentiate in the thymus. T cell functions include helping B cells to make antibody, killing virally infected cells, regulating the level of the immune response and stimulating the microbicidal and cytotoxic activity of other immune effector cells, including macrophages. Communication between the cells is effected either by direct cell-cell contact or by cytokines and antibodies.

Each lymphocyte carries a surface receptor which is capable of recognizing a particular antigen. Although an individual lymphocyte carries only one type of receptor and therefore can recognize only one type of antigen, other lymphocytes have different receptors, each specifically recognizing different antigens. In this way the lymphocyte population as a whole can recognize a wide range of antigens. The antigen receptors are generated during lymphocyte development by processes of somatic mutation and recombination acting on a relatively small number of initial germline genes. The antigen receptors used by B cells and T cells are different. The B cells' antigen receptor is surface immunoglobulin (sIg), a membrane bound form of the antibody which it will ultimately secrete. The T cells' antigen receptor is generated from a different set of genes which encode only the cell surface receptor. T cells and B cells recognize antigen in different forms: B cells recognize an unmodified antigen molecule, either free in solution or on the surface of other cells; T cells however, recognize antigen only when it is presented to them in association with molecules encoded by the major histocompatibility complex (MHC). The functional consequence of this is that T cells recognize processed antigens present only on the surface of other cells, whereas antibodies can recognize antigens in tissue fluids.

The basis of the adaptive immune response is that of clonal recognition and response. An antigen selects the clones of cells which recognize it. Since the number of different lymphocyte specificities is very large, the number of cells available to recognize any one antigen is relatively small — perhaps only a few hundred lymphocytes in a human. As this is not sufficient to tackle an invading pathogen, the first element of a specific immune response must be rapid proliferation of the specific lymphocytes. This is followed by further differentiation of the responding cells as the effector phase of the immune response develops.

These events underlie the difference between primary and secondary immune responses. During the primary response the small number of specific cells increases and cells undergo differentiation. If the antigen is encountered again (or persists), there will be a larger population of specific cells to react and these cells will be able to respond more quickly because they have already undergone several steps along their differentiation pathway. Lymphocytes which have been stimulated by antigen (primed) and their progeny may either differentiate fully into immune effector cells or form the expanded pool of cells (memory cells) which can respond more efficiently to a secondary challenge with the same antigen.

B cells

B cells are responsible for antibody formation. They recognize antigen by endogenously synthesized cell surface immunoglobulin which is their characteristic marker. The main B cell population, designated B-2, has high levels of

	B cells	T cells	Large granular lymphocytes	Mononuclear phagocytes	Neutrophils
Whole population	**sIg** - Antigen receptor CD19 ⎤ Lineage CD20 ⎦ markers CD21 - Complement receptor-2	**CD3** - Part of T cell receptor complex **CD2** CD5 ⎤ CD6 ⎥ Lineage markers CD7 ⎦	CD56 CD57 Ly49 (Mouse) ⎤ NK Receptor NKR-P1 (Rat) ⎥ complex NKG2 (Man) ⎦ products	**CD64** - High affinity Fc receptor CD11b - Complement receptor III CD35 - Complement receptor I	**CD10** - Neutral endopeptidase CD11b ⎤ CD35 ⎥ Receptors for antibody and complement CD16 ⎦
Subsets	**CD5** ⎤ Distinguish CD116 ⎦ the B-1a subset	**CD4** - Class II restricted Th **CD8** - Class I restricted Tc	CD16 - K cell. Fc receptor	CD71 - Activated cells **CD68** - Tissue macrophages	CD66 ⎤ Lineage CD67 ⎦ markers

Fig. 1.4 Critical leukocyte markers. The table shows the more important markers and receptors of the major cell populations involved in the immune response. The markers most often used to define a particular cell type are shown in bold.

surface IgD and lacks the marker CD5. A minor population (B-1) is predominately CD5⁺ and tends to express high levels of IgM and lower IgD. The B-1 population constitutes a distinct lineage of self replenishing cells which produces much of the serum antibody, although its usage of immunoglobulin *V* genes (and therefore its diversity) is rather restricted. This group is subdivided into the majority B-1a cells which express CD5 and the B-1b subset which do not. Most B cells express MHC class II and can act as antigen presenting cells In addition, B cells carry receptors for a variety of signalling molecules, including receptors for complement (CR2), the Fc region of antibody, receptors for direct interaction with T cells (e.g. CD40) and receptors for B cell growth and differentiation factors. Many of these are only expressed following an encounter with specific antigen and Th cells.

To produce an antibody response most B cells require both antigen and help from antigen-specific T cells. Antigens which cannot induce B cells to produce antibody without T cell help are called T-dependent (T$_{dep}$) antigens. However, a number of antigens (T$_{ind}$) stimulate B cells directly. The majority of protein antigens are T-dependent while many of the T$_{ind}$ antigens are large non-protein polymeric molecules with repeated epitopes. The antibody response to T$_{dep}$ antigens generally matures during a secondary immune response, in that it consists of a greater proportion of IgG and has a higher average affinity for antigen than in the primary response. The response to T$_{ind}$ antigens does not usually mature in this way and remains predominantly IgM.

Activated B cells proliferate and mature under the influence of T cells, and ultimately differentiate into plasma cells — cells almost wholly devoted to the production of secreted immunoglobulin. In the process they lose most of their surface Ig, develop a greatly expanded cytoplasm and extensive endoplasmic reticulum.

T cells

T cells are lymphocytes which develop and differentiate in the thymus before seeding the secondary lymphoid tissues. T cells recognize antigen and MHC molecules via the T cell receptor (TCR) which is distinct from, but related to, immunoglobulin. This receptor consists of an antigen binding portion formed by two different polymorphic chains, which is associated with CD3, a complex of polypeptides involved in signalling cellular activation. The antigen binding portion may consist of an αβ heterodimer or a γδ heterodimer: the great majority of peripheral T cells have αβ. In man, the markers CD2 and CD5 are also present on all T cells, while in mouse the molecule Thy1 is a characteristic T cell marker. In some species, including man, activated T cells also carry endogenously synthesized MHC class II molecules, although these are absent from resting T cells. Activated T cells may also be induced to express CD25, which forms part of the high affinity IL-2 receptor and is important in clonal expansion. Other markers differentiate T cell subsets.

There are two main subpopulations of T cells which can be distinguished according to their expression of CD4 or CD8. These molecules act as receptors for class II and class I MHC molecules, respectively, and contribute towards both T cell immune recognition and cellular activation. Most CD4⁺ T cells recognize antigen associated with MHC class II molecules and these cells act predominantly as helper T cells (Th). CD8⁺ T cells recognize antigen associated with MHC class I molecules and are primarily responsible for cytotoxic destruction of virally infected cells.

Clones of mature CD4⁺ T cells fall into two major groups, which are functionally defined according to the cytokines they secrete. Th1 cells interact preferentially with mononuclear phagocytes, while Th2 cells tend to promote B cell division and differentiation. The balance of activity between these two subsets is related in part to how antigen is presented to the cells and it ultimately determines the type of immune response which develops.

The surface phenotypes of T cell populations change during development. In man, virgin T cells express CD45RA, while activated cells express CD45R0 and higher levels of adhesion molecules such as the β$_1$ integrins (CD29). The relationship of activated cells to resting memory T cells is still debated. The enhanced secondary response to antigen is only partly due to the increased numbers of cells available. Primed T cells also respond to antigen more efficiently than virgin T cells but, unlike B cells, this does not appear to be due to affinity maturation of the T cell receptor.

Large granular lymphocytes (LGLs)

Some lymphocytes express neither antigen receptors nor other key markers of B and T cells, while others have an ambivalent mixture of lymphocyte and macrophage surface proteins. These cells are morphologically large granular lymphocytes and are sometimes referred to as null or third population cells.

They appear to be a distinct lineage, where the cells carry some T cell markers (e.g. CD3ζ) at an early stage of differentiation and acquire the macrophage markers later. Useful markers for distinguishing these cells are the Fc receptor III (CD16), CD56 and CD57, in association with the absence of T and B cell markers. This population is particularly effective at killer (K) and natural killer (NK) activity. K cells are leukocytes which can recognize and kill target cells, coated with specific antibody, by binding and being triggered via their Fc receptors. NK cells recognize and kill some tumours and virally infected cells. NK cells recognize targets via lectin-like molecules, which presumably recognize carbohydrate groups on target cells. The presence of MHC class I molecules on the target tends to inhibit NK cell cytotoxicity. This explains why targets recognized by T cells and NK cells are generally different. Although K cell and NK cell activities are functionally distinct, they may be performed by the same cell.

Phagocytes

Phagocytic cells include the neutrophil polymorph, blood monocyte and the various cells of the mononuclear phagocyte system distributed throughout the body. Among the latter are the tissue macrophage, Kupffer cells of the liver, microglial cells of the brain and mesangial phagocytes of the kidney.

Phagocytes use an array of cell surface receptors to recognize material for endocytosis. These include receptors for carbohydrates, for activated complement components (C3b, C3bi and C3d) and for the Fc portion of IgG, which become attached to antigenic particles. By attaching to antigenic particles, IgG and complement act as opsonins to facilitate recognition and endocytosis.

Neutrophil polymorphs are short lived cells, constituting about 70% of blood leukocytes which are produced in large numbers by the bone marrow. They spend about 24 hours in the circulation before migrating out into the tissues, where they phagocytose material and ultimately die by apoptosis. Activation enables them to live slightly longer. By contrast the blood monocyte is a long lived cell which also migrates into the tissues but further differentiates into the tissue macrophage. Macrophages are more metabolically active than monocytes. They are also more strongly phagocytic due to their increased density of surface receptors and have a larger battery of lysosomal enzymes.

While many antigens are degraded in phagolysosomes within the cell, enzymes and granule contents may also be released to the outside (exocytosis) and, in association with cytokines such as tumour necrosis factor (TNF), can produce cytotoxic damage to a variety of target cells.

Some macrophages seen in lymph and the medulla of lymph nodes appear to migrate around the body, while others such as the marginal zone macrophages of spleen and lymph nodes are fixed. These populations of cells perform different functions. For example, many of the mobile macrophages can present antigen to MHC class II-restricted T cells, while marginal zone macrophages are particularly efficient at taking up T_{ind} antigens, presumably to present them to B cells.

Antigen presenting cells

Cells that can present antigen to lymphocytes in an immunogenic form are collectively termed antigen presenting cells (APCs). Since all nucleated cells normally express MHC class I molecules (although at widely varying levels), any cell can present antigen to class I-restricted $CD8^+$ T cells. Therefore the term more usually refers to class II-restricted antigen presentation (*Fig. 1.5*).

This group of cells includes several types derived from bone marrow stem cells, such as the Langerhans cell of the skin, which migrates to lymph nodes where it becomes the interdigitating cell seen in T cell areas of the node. B cells and some mononuclear phagocytes also express class II MHC molecules and play a central role in antigen presentation to T cells. In special circumstances many other cell types can be induced to express class II molecules. *In vitro*, the cytokine interferon-γ (IFNγ) is a potent inducer of MHC class II molecules on most cell types — exceptions include neurons and oligodendrocytes. However, the range of cells which express class II *in vivo* is more limited.

Broadly speaking, there are three major groups of APC:

- The dendritic cell lineage, which presents effectively to virgin T cells.
- B cells, macrophages and other cells which constitutively express class II and present antigen effectively to primed T cells.

Cell		Area of lymphoid tissue	Recirculation	Fc:C3 receptor	MHC class II	Present to
Marginal zone macrophages		Lymph node: marginal zone sinus. Spleen: marginal zone	–	+	–	B cell (T_{ind} response)
Follicular dendritic cells		Follicles and B cells	–	+	–	B cells
Langerhans cell becomes interdigitating dendritic cell		Skin → Lymph node: paracortex	+	±	+	T cells
Macrophages		Lymph node: medulla	+	+	+	T cells and B cells
Interdigitating cells		Thymus	–	–	+	Thymocytes

Fig. 1.5 Antigen presenting cells. The table indicates the location of antigen presenting cells within lymphoid tissues. Some of the cells recirculate, including the Langerhans cell which appears as the dendritic cell of lymph nodes. Fc and C3 receptors permit the cell to take up antigen in the form of immune complexes, while the presence of MHC class II molecules on the cell surface permits it to present antigen to $CD4^+$ T cells.

- A variety of other cells which may be induced to express class II and which can present antigen to T cells, but do not necessarily induce T cell proliferation. They sometimes induce T cell anergy and in other cases may even become the target for class II-restricted cytotoxicity.

The ability of a cell to present antigen depends on many factors, including how it takes up and processes antigen and subsequently expresses it at the cell surface, in association with MHC class II molecules. The production of appropriate cytokines by the APC and neighbouring cells, as well as expression of adhesion molecules, also plays an important role. Moreover, the timing of the signals is critical as to whether T cell activation or tolerance is established. *In vitro*, B cells present antigen effectively to Th2 cells while macrophages present to Th1 cells. Hence B cells and macrophages, when acting as APCs, present antigen to the T cell population which activates their own effector functions. Thus, antigen presentation by these cells is really a mutually stimulating interaction, rather than an unidirectional process.

Auxiliary cells

Many cells may become involved in an immune response, as they respond to cytokines such as IL-1, TNF and IFNγ released by cells of the immune system. However, the term 'auxiliary cell' is often used to describe the actions of mast cells, basophils, eosinophils and platelets, which are essential in the control of inflammation. Basophils and mast cells both express a high affinity IgE receptor and may become sensitized by IgE and subsequently triggered by contact with antigen to release inflammatory mediators. They are also triggered by the complement fragments C3a and C5a. Eosinophils can be activated by cytokines such as IL-5 to release a variety of mediators which can have both pro-inflammatory and anti-inflammatory effects. Platelets express an Fc receptor for IgG (FcγRIII, CD16) by which they can bind immune complexes and may be induced to release their vasoactive amines, platelet-derived growth factor (PDGF) and other mediators. All these cells can also be triggered non-immunologically.

THE LYMPHOID SYSTEM

Leukocytes and most types of auxiliary cells are derived from bone marrow stem cells. B cells mature in the bone marrow (liver in the foetus) and T cells in the thymus — these are the primary lymphoid organs. Lymphoid stem cells start to colonize the thymus in waves during late foetal life. The pre-T cells lack the majority of surface markers associated with mature cells which develop during thymic differentiation. There is considerable proliferation in the thymic cortex and cell death associated with the selection of viable and functionally useful T cell clones. The main events that occur during thymic development are as follows:

- The generation of diverse T cell antigen receptors.
- Selection of functionally active T cells which may recognize antigen associated with self MHC molecules.
- Selective deletion of autoreactive T cells.
- Differentiation of the major peripheral T cell subpopulations expressing CD4 or CD8.

In birds, B cells develop in a special organ, the bursa of Fabricius, for which there is no mammalian equivalent. In mammals B cells complete their differentiation in the bone marrow. As with T cells, the generation of a functional antigen receptor (antibody) is one of the first steps in this process. B cells initially express IgM and/or IgD as their surface receptor but this may switch to another class during development, although the antigen-binding specificity remains unchanged.

Lymphocytes from the primary lymphoid organs are released into the circulation and move to the secondary lymphoid tissues, where they may remain for considerable periods or circulate via the lymphatics back to the blood or die. In adults, the secondary lymphoid tissues may be replenished from bone marrow or thymus but there also appear to be some self-renewing populations of lymphocytes in the periphery.

Secondary lymphoid organs include the spleen and lymph nodes as well as the various accumulations of lymphoid tissue associated with mucosal surfaces, which are collectively called mucosa-associated lymphoid tissue (MALT). Within each of these organs there is an orderly arrangement of lymphocytes into distinct zones *(Fig. 1.6)*.

For example, T cells predominate in the paracortex of the lymph node while B cells are more abundant in the germinal centres of the cortex. The spatial organization of the lymphocytes is mirrored by that of the different types of antigen presenting cells.

There is a similar functional/structural relationship in the spleen, where lymphocytes are present as focal aggregations around the arterioles. These collections of cells constitute the peri-arteriolar lymphatic sheaths (PALS) or white pulp *(Fig. 1.6)*. In the Peyer's patch, the unencapsulated lymphoid tissue underlies a dome, projecting into the lumen of the gut, between the villi. The dome contains M cells which transport antigens from the gut lumen to the lymphocytes and APCs in the Peyer's patch *(Fig. 1.6)*. IgA-producing B cells, and T cells with Fcα-receptors are particularly prevalent at this site.

The lymph nodes lie along the draining lymphatic vessels, but they are particularly concentrated in the neck, axilla, groin, the mesentery and on either side of the spine. The majority of the lymphatic vessels from the trunk and lower limbs drain ultimately into the right thoracic duct which returns the lymph to the circulation *(Fig. 1.7)*. The arrangement of the lymphatic system ensures that antigen reaches regional lymph nodes, antigens in the blood are trapped by the spleen, antigens from the gut reach the Peyer's patch, and other mucosal surfaces have their own collections of unencapsulated lymphoid tissue to catch antigens from their vicinity.

In short, one of the functions of the lymphatic system is to bring antigen into contact with lymphocytes which are capable of recognizing it. Antigen may move freely in the blood and tissue fluids, or it may be transported to the lymphoid tissues by APCs. Equally important in this process is the migration of lymphocytes into and between the secondary lymphoid tissues.

Lymphocyte migration

As lymphocytes develop, they migrate throughout the body. Once they have matured in the primary lymphoid tissues, two main patterns of migration can be distinguished:

- Movement of virgin lymphocytes into secondary lymphoid tissues, where they may encounter their specific antigen, proliferate and differentiate.
- Migration of antigen-activated cells from the lymph nodes to the blood, and thence into sites of inflammation, to act as effector cells.

Lymphocytes migrate from the blood into lymphoid tissues across a specialized region of endothelium — the high endothelial venule (HEV). This endothelium is present in lymph nodes and Peyer's patches but may also develop in areas of chronic inflammation. The endothelial cells of these venules are distinctive columnar cells, expressing sulphated glycoproteins and other adhesion molecules on their luminal surface, which interact with adhesion molecules on circulating lymphocytes. Lymphocytes pass into the tissue by moving between the HEV cells and there is a high volume of cell traffic across the HEV. Lymphocytes may also reach a node from the tissues via the afferent lymphatics.

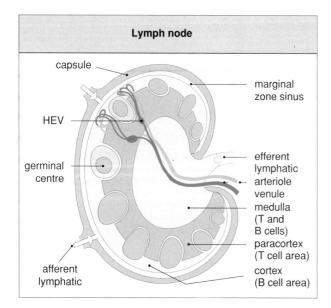

Lymph node

- capsule
- HEV
- germinal centre
- afferent lymphatic
- marginal zone sinus
- efferent lymphatic
- arteriole
- venule
- medulla (T and B cells)
- paracortex (T cell area)
- cortex (B cell area)

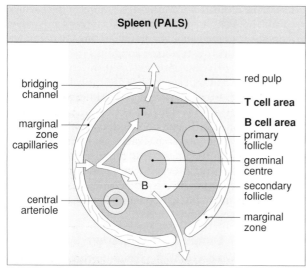

Spleen (PALS)

- bridging channel
- marginal zone capillaries
- central arteriole
- red pulp
- T cell area
- B cell area
  - primary follicle
- germinal centre
- secondary follicle
- marginal zone

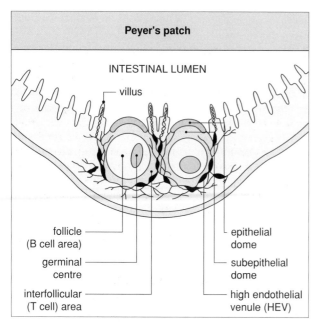

Peyer's patch

INTESTINAL LUMEN

- villus
- follicle (B cell area)
- germinal centre
- interfollicular (T cell) area
- epithelial dome
- subepithelial dome
- high endothelial venule (HEV)

Migration of activated lymphocytes to sites of inflammation is directed by adhesion molecules and controlling molecules induced on the local endothelium by cytokines. These are generally different from the molecules on HEV and include several members of the immunoglobulin supergene family. Equally important in the process is the state of lymphocyte activation; the integrins and other adhesion molecules which are induced on activated lymphocytes are critical in allowing migration to inflammatory sites.

These two routes of lymphocyte migration are not exclusive: activated lymphocytes may return to lymph nodes across the HEVs, while naive cells can migrate into inflammatory sites, particularly if chronic immune reactions are underway. The traffic pathways are summarized in *Figure 1.8*.

OVERVIEW OF THE IMMUNE RESPONSE

Immune responses are centred around the activation of clones of lymphocytes which recognize the initiating antigen. Since each lymphocyte recognizes only one antigen specifically, the ability to respond to the enormous variety of antigens depends on the generation of a large number of different antigen receptors on different lymphocytes during their development. Consequently, although there may be 10^{12} lymphocytes in a human, the number which recognize any particular antigen is relatively small. Most of these specificities will never be used in an individual's lifetime; it may seem profligate to generate so many 'unused' lymphocytes but it is essential for the system to be capable of recognizing

Fig. 1.6 Secondary lymphoid tissues. Lymph nodes, spleen and Peyer's patches are part of the secondary lymphoid tissue. Each is divided into functional areas or zones depending on the type of lymphocytes which occur there. The traffic of cells through the organs is indicated by the arrows. Lymphocytes and recirculating antigen presenting cells may enter lymph nodes via the afferent lymphatics and lymphocytes can also arrive from the blood by traversing the high endothelial venules (HEV). B cells tend to localize to the cortex and T cells to the paracortex. In most species, cells leave the lymph node via the efferent lymphatic. Lymphocytes enter the white pulp of the spleen (the peri-arteriolar lymphatic sheath — PALS) from the network of capillaries in the marginal zone. T cells traverse the PALS and re-enter the circulation by passing across bridging channels in the marginal zone before entering the red pulp. B cells may divert to the B cell areas and are particularly abundant in germinal centres. Peyer's patches are collections of lymphoid tissue found on the intestinal wall. These domed structures have a specialized epithelium containing M cells which transport antigens from the gut lumen into the patch. The B and T cell regions have structural similarities to lymph nodes. Lymphocytes enter the patch via HEV at the base and the adhesion molecules expressed on these endothelia favour accumulation of IgA producing B cells and T cells which enhance IgA production.

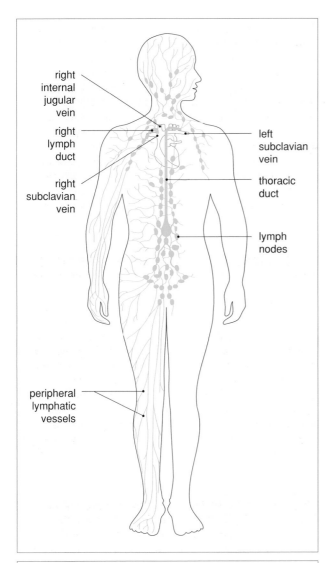

Fig. 1.7 The lymphatic system. Peripheral lymphatic vessels drain interstitial fluid and cells to lymph nodes which filter out particulate matter from the lymph. Efferent lymphatics carry lymph and recirculating lymphocytes, either directly or indirectly via further nodes back to the blood. Most of the lymphatic channels drain into the left subclavian vein via the thoracic duct. However, lymphatics of the upper right side drain via the right lymph duct at the junction between the right subclavian and right internal jugular veins.

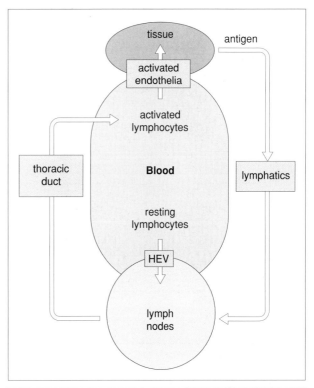

Fig. 1.8 Patterns of lymphocyte traffic. Antigen drains from tissues to reach the regional lymphatics, where it has the opportunity of encountering lymphocytes which have entered the node across high endothelial venules (HEV). Resting lymphocytes preferentially migrate into lymph nodes. Activated lymphocytes return to the blood via the thoracic duct. These cells are primed to migrate into inflammatory sites across endothelia activated by inflammatory cytokines.

any potential antigen, since pathogens are continuously mutating to evade immune recognition. Another consequence of this is that the clones of responding cells must be expanded in the initial phases of an immune response to provide sufficient cells to counter an infection. The first phase of an immune response therefore, involves recognition of the antigen and expansion of the clones of lymphocytes which can respond to it. The second phase involves further differentiation of responding cells, the recruitment and activation of effector systems — antibody production, macrophage activation, generation of cytotoxic cells, etc. —

to eliminate the initiating antigen and to resolve tissue damage caused by the infection.

Immune recognition molecules

Three sets of antigen binding molecules are involved in specific immune recognition — the B cell antigen receptor (immunoglobulin), the T cell antigen receptor and the class I and class II molecules of the major histocompatibility complex (MHC) *(Fig. 1.9)*. Lymphocyte antigen receptors are highly polymorphic and vary between clones: diversity is generated during lymphocyte development. These molecules have the function of antigen recognition. MHC molecules are highly polymorphic between different members of a population, but do not diversify within an individual. Their function is to present antigenic fragments for recognition by T cells. Class I molecules are normally expressed on all nucleated cells and platelets (although in variable amounts), while class II expression is more limited (see above).

Immunoglobulin

Immunoglobulins (Igs) are generated in two basic forms. Membrane Ig acts as the B cells' antigen receptor and is an

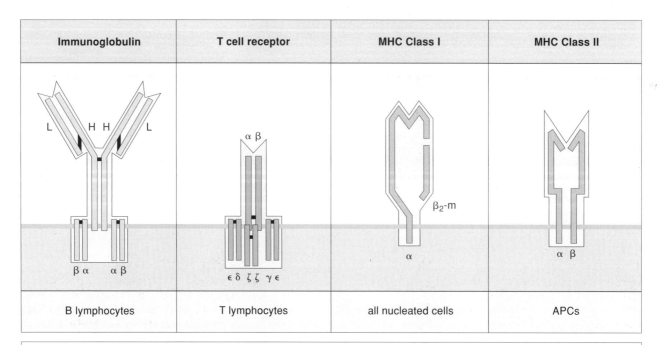

Immunoglobulin	T cell receptor	MHC Class I	MHC Class II
B lymphocytes	T lymphocytes	all nucleated cells	APCs

Fig. 1.9 Antigen binding molecules. The structures of the four principal cell surface antigen binding molecules are shown. Diversity in the antibody heavy and light chains (H and L) and the T cell receptor α and β-chains is generated by somatic recombination of germline genes. Diversity in the MHC molecules is maintained exclusively in the germline. The B cell and T cell antigen receptors are therefore clonally distinct, while expression of MHC molecules is not. The signal-transducing molecules associated with the T cell receptor (CD3γ, δ, ε, ζ and η (mouse)) and cell surface immunoglobulin (Ig-α and β) are monomorphic.

integral membrane protein. Each B cell can also produce a secreted Ig with identical antigen specificity to that of its receptor. There is enormous heterogeneity in the population of antibody molecules, although each one is constructed from a basic unit consisting of two identical heavy polypeptide chains and two identical light chains. These are crosslinked and stabilized by interchain disulphide bonds and by secondary interactions. Both heavy and light chains are folded into globular domains containing β-pleated sheets stabilized by intrachain disulphide bonds *(Fig. 1.10)*. The N-terminal domains of one heavy and one light chain together form an antigen binding site, and these domains are highly variable between different antibodies (V domains). The remaining domains are less variable (Constant — C domains) and some of these C domains are involved in interactions between antibody and receptors (Fc receptors) on other cells. Thus antibody can act as a bifunctional adapter which can crosslink antigen to cells.

Antibodies can be divided into different classes and subclasses according to the type of heavy chain they contain. In man there are nine different types of heavy chain (subclasses), each encoded by a separate gene in the heavy chain gene stack. These are IgM, IgG1, IgG2, IgG3, IgG4, IgA1, IgA2, IgD and IgE, which are grouped into the five different classes according to similarities in their overall structure. The heavy chain subclasses are isotypes, since there is a copy of each subclass in a haploid genome. There are two different classes of light chain, namely κ and λ. The individual immmunoglobulin chains are encoded by genes at three separate loci on different chromosomes. One locus encodes the heavy chain isotypes and there are separate loci for the κ and λ light chains, although a B cell only ever transcribes from one of these light chain loci (see Chapter 2).

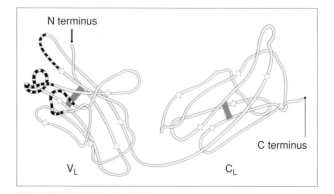

Fig. 1.10 Domain structure. The domain structure, here exemplified by an immunoglobulin light chain, is common to many molecules involved in immune recognition. Light chains contain two domains, each of which has three or four sections of β-pleated sheet, stabilized by secondary bonds and an intrachain disulphide bond (grey) — a feature conserved in domains of most members of the immunoglobulin superfamily. The hypervariable loops of the variable (V) domain responsible for antigen binding are shown hatched.

Individual B cells can change the class of antibody they produce, and may produce more than one class at the same time. Class switching occurs during the development of an immune response, and may be accompanied by mutation in the Ig genes, giving a potential increase in the affinity of the antibody. This process is under T cell control and since different classes of antibody interact with Fc receptors on different cell types, the class of antibody produced will partly determine which immunological effector systems are activated.

Membrane immunoglobulin on B cells is associated with a group of other integral membrane proteins, analogous to the C... ...transmit activatio...

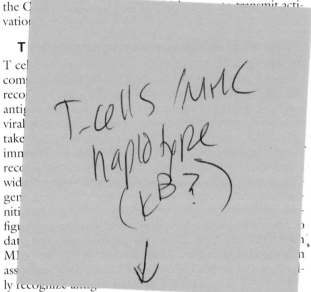

T cel...
com...
reco...
antig...
viral...
take...
imm...
reco...
wid...
gen...
niti...
figu...
dat...
MI...
ass...
ly recognize antig...

The first evidence that T cells recognized antigen presented by MHC molecules was seen in experiments which showed genetic restriction in antigen presentation to T cells. Essentially, T cells will respond strongly to an antigen only when it is presented on cells of their own MHC haplotype. The basis of this observation is that T cells are selected in the thymus by interaction with APCs; they are then stimulated on dendritic cells or other APCs in the periphery, each having the same type of MHC molecules. APCs of other MHC haplotypes cannot substitute, since they cannot present the right combination of antigenic peptide plus MHC.

It is now clear that MHC class I and II molecules have binding sites which can hold antigenic peptides. MHC binding to antigen is much less specific than that of antigen receptors, in that a particular MHC molecule can bind many different peptides and present them to T cells. The binding pocket on class I molecules can accommodate peptides of 8–9 amino acids, while that of the class II molecule accommodates larger antigen fragments. The limited number of different MHC molecules within an individual (approximately 12) must be capable of presenting nearly all the T_{dep} antigens. Consequently, MHC molecules determine which part of an antigen is presented to T cells, so it is the MHC haplotype of an individual which determines the overall pattern of T cell immune recognition. The critical consequence of this is that an individual's MHC haplotype determines susceptibility or resistance to autoimmunity, infection and hypersensitivity — any disease where immune reactions occur.

The existence of the MHC first became apparent in studies of graft rejection. Although this could not be the physiological role of the MHC, it was nevertheless important to explain how T cells educated to recognize antigen on syngeneic MHC molecules may also recognize allogeneic MHC molecules. It is now thought that a variety of different molecular processes underlie recognition of such allografts. In some cases, allogeneic MHC can resemble self MHC sufficiently for recognition, particularly as the allogeneic MHC on a graft is present at very high density. In other cases, fragments of allogeneic MHC molecules can be presented by syngeneic APCs in the conventional way.

Antigen presentation

The two classes of MHC molecules mediate two distinct types of antigen presentation, involving different processing pathways. Class I molecules capture peptide fragments of molecules which are synthesized by the cell into either the endoplasmic reticulum or the cytosol. In contrast, class II molecules generally take up material which the cell has endocytosed. The class of MHC molecule is not the only factor affecting antigen presentation. Different APCs expressing class II molecules preferentially stimulate different groups of CD4+ T cells and the outcome of these interactions can vary greatly. For example, antigen presentation may induce T cell proliferation, but in other cases cytotoxic damage to the APC results. The outcome of T cell recognition of MHC plus antigenic peptide is dependent on the co-stimulatory signals which accompany antigen presentation. These include a variety of direct cell–cell signalling interactions as well as cytokine release which ultimately determine the type of response that is initiated.

How an antigen is presented depends largely on where it enters the body because this affects which APCs will take it up and process it. For example, an antigen entering via the gut will be taken up by APCs in the Peyer's patches and be presented to the large numbers of local IgA-producing B cells and T cells which preferentially promote IgA production. Conversely, an antigen entering through the skin will be picked up by Langerhans cells and transported to regional lymph nodes where it may induce a T cell-mediated hypersensitivity reaction. Different APCs can also process antigens in different ways. For example, macrophages take up antigen by phagocytosis and partially degrade it in phagolysosomes, whereas dendritic cells are non-phagocytic, but nevertheless are extremely efficient at presenting many antigens. It is now clear that antigen presentation is the key interaction which controls immune responses.

Cellular activation

Since the function of the immune system is the elimination of antigen the majority of lymphocytes are in resting phase and must be activated and induced to proliferate in response to antigen and cytokines before they can participate in an immune response. Hence, expansion of populations of antigen-specific lymphocytes is the first essential event in an immune reponse. Activation of lymphocytes requires signals from APCs, both directly via cell–cell interaction and via cytokines. Activation pushes the responding cells into cell cycle, so that they undergo a number of rounds of division before developing their effector functions. If a lymphocyte receives an incomplete set of activation signals, it may be rendered tolerant, so that it cannot subsequently respond to a full activation stimulus. Following division, lymphocytes differentiate and develop a range of new functions. Surface adhesion molecules are changed so that the cells can reposition themselves in the body. Adhesion molecules involved in cellular interactions are synthesized or activated and sets of cytokines are secreted.

In a similar way, phagocytes and auxiliary cells all require sensitization by antibody or triggering by cytokines before they acquire their full range of effector functions. At the simplest level, each immunologically active cell can be seen as needing a series of signals for full activation: these often come from a direct cellular interaction with another cell, in which the surface molecules of one cell bind directly to receptors on another. These interactions may be purely adhesive, serving to hold the interacting cells together, or they may activate second messenger systems in one or both of the interacting cells. In either case, cytokines released by the two cells will preferentially stimulate the other, provided it carries the necessary cytokine receptors (*Fig. 1.11*).

Cell co-operation in the immune response

Although it is interesting to consider how a single cell responds to stimuli *in vitro*, the immune response *in vivo* is orchestrated by the co-operative interactions of many cell types, communicating with each other through interacting cell surface molecules and released cytokines. This is not a disordered mixture of cells in a sea of mediators — the lymphoid tissues maintain particular groups of cells together. For example, germinal centres of lymph nodes contain large numbers of B cells, small numbers of CD4+ T cells, follicular dendritic cells and some macrophages, with IgD-bearing B cells in the surrounding mantle zone. These ordered groupings of cells will largely determine which cell populations co-operate with others *in vivo*, in ways which are quite inaccessible to analysis *in vitro*.

T cells and macrophages release a number of cytokines which act as signals for other cells. This group of chemical messengers includes the interleukins (ILs), interferons (IFNs), colony stimulating factors (CSFs) and tumour necrosis factors (TNFs). The structures and functions of these molecules are set out in Chapter 10. *In vivo*, the role and specificities of cytokines are particularly difficult to investigate, since many act only as short range signalling molecules within the confines of particular areas of lymphoid organs. These microenvironmental effects and the expression of cytokine receptors are important in limiting the extent of cytokine effects to the appropriate cells. For example, receptors for TNF will act as a sink for TNF produced at an inflammatory site, limiting its range of actions. Cytokine receptors are usually cell surface molecules but some can also be produced in a secreted form to modulate cytokine effects.

Cytokines are involved in antigen presentation, the co-operation between T cells and B cells, T cells and cytotoxic cells and in macrophage activation. As noted above, different subpopulations of T cells produce different sets of cytokines. This may vary according to the lineage of a T cell and its state of activation. Since the expression of cytokine receptors on responding cells also fluctuates, this allows precise and subtle regulation of immune reactions.

Direct cellular interactions are mediated by intercellular adhesion molecules such as LFA-1 as well as by antigen-specific binding via lymphocyte antigen receptors. Several of the surface molecules of lymphocytes are coupled to, or are themselves, protein kinases or phosphatases. Many other membrane molecules have sites which become phosphorylated upon activation, allowing them to couple to various signalling systems. The crosslinking of receptors by interaction with other cells can activate a cell directly but, in addition, when cells are brought together by such interactions they are held in close proximity for effective cytokine-mediated signalling. This is particularly important where threshold levels of cytokine are required before a cell will be activated or move into cell cycle.

Regulation of immune responses

The primary function of the immune system is recognition of exogenous antigens and elimination of pathogens. Antigen is the initiator of all immune responses and the elimination of antigen is the principle brake which limits immune reactions. Additional levels of regulation are provided by leukocytes themselves. Immune responses are held in check by background levels of inhibitory cytokines, corticosteroids, enzyme inhibitors and soluble cytokine receptors. It is only when antigen breaks into this system that the conditions for activation of antigen-specific lymphocytes occur. As the immune response develops, further controls come into action. For example, the production of antibody feeds back on antigen-specific B cells via their Fc receptors to limit their further proliferation. The mode of the response is largely determined by the manner of antigen presentation and the class of T cells which become activated. Once antigen has been eliminated the negative signals normally reassert themselves and the immune response wanes.

For many years it was thought that specific subsets of T cells were responsible for regulating the actions of other T cells in antigen-specific ways. It now appears that many of the experiments which demonstrated 'suppression' were looking at shifts in the type of the immune response, or were reflections of the negative controls noted above. However, it is clear that interactions between groups of antigen-specific lymphocytes (so called idiotypic interactions) as well as neuroendocrine controls can exert some control on the strength and specificity of many immune responses. Such interactions are secondary to the primary control exerted by antigen. The different types of cooperative interaction between cells of the immune system are outlined in Chapters 10–12.

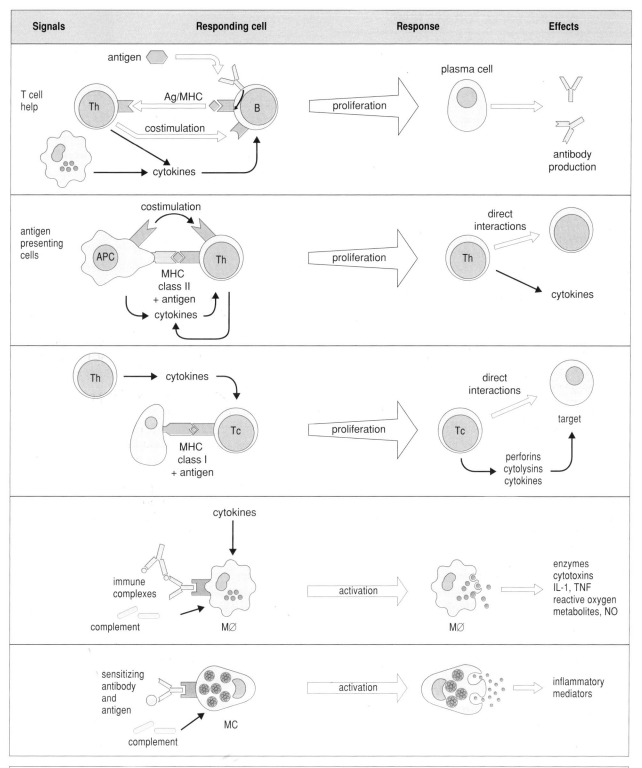

Fig. 1.11 Cellular activation steps. The responses of leukocytes may be viewed by the signals they respond to and their output or function. Lymphocytes respond to signals of antigen and cytokines by dividing and differentiating. B cells produce antibody, T helper cells (Th) cytokines, and Tc cells develop into cytotoxic lymphocytes (CTLs) which secrete molecules capable of killing other cells. Macrophages recognize antigen and immune complexes via their Fc and C3 receptors and respond to cytokines by becoming activated and secreting enzymes, oxygen metabolites and other molecules which facilitate intracellular and extracellular destruction of antigens. Auxiliary cells such as mast cells (MCs) are triggered to release inflammatory mediators by antigen binding to surface sensitizing antibody. The direct cell–cell interactions which accompany these responses are also essential to cell function.

IMMUNE EFFECTOR SYSTEMS

The recognition of antigens of invading organisms is only the first essential step in a series of reactions aimed at eliminating the source of the antigen. The principal effectors are antibody, complement, phagocytes and cytotoxic cells, with different systems being effective against different pathogens or against different phases of an infection. For example, cytotoxic T cells will eliminate cells infected with influenza virus, but antibody is required to prevent reinfection of other cells. These systems are summarized in *Figure 1.12* and discussed in detail in the final section of the book.

Inflammation

One essential element associated with many immune responses is the development of inflammation. This has three main features:

- An increased blood flow to the affected area.
- An increase in vascular permeability.
- An increase in leukocyte migration across the local endothelium.

The overall effect of these changes is to allow large serum proteins such as antibodies and serum proenzymes to reach the tissue, and to direct immune effector cells to the inflammatory site. These changes are caused by vasoactive amines, cytokines and other mediators acting on the endothelium and smooth muscle in the walls of blood vessels. Such inflammatory mediators originate from damaged tissue, serum enzymes (particularly complement), mast cells and from the infiltrating leukocytes themselves. The control of leukocyte migration is a complex process requiring interactions between adhesion molecules on the circulating cells and on the endothelium. Different classes of leukocyte use different adhesion systems and this leads to a phased arrival of different cell populations. In acute inflammatory sites, neutrophils usually appear first, with lymphocytes and monocytes migrating in later on. In chronic inflammatory lesions the lymphocytes and mononuclear phagocytes predominate. Whether an acute inflammatory response becomes chronic or not, depends on the effectiveness of the immune response and whether the antigen persists.

Intracellular and extracellular pathogens

One may make a broad distinction between those effector systems which are effective against extracellular pathogens and those active against intracellular ones and this corresponds roughly to the old description of humoral or cellular responses. Antibody and complement do not have access to intracellular antigens, unless the cell has been lysed and antigens released, but antibody can bind to free antigens in body fluids as well as to native antigens on cell surfaces. Some viruses insert their newly synthesized proteins into the host cell membrane which will ultimately become the viral envelope and such cells may then be recognized by antibody. This will occur only at a later stage of cellular infection and not all

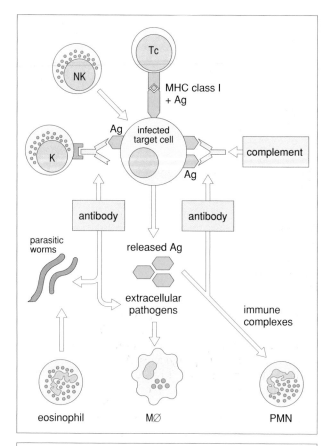

Fig. 1.12 Effector systems. The principal effector systems are directed against either intracellular pathogens (upper) or extracellular antigens or pathogens (lower). Infected cells can be recognized by presentation of antigen on MHC class I molecules to Tc cells. Antibody bound to surface antigen on the target cells can be recognized by antibody receptors, to direct complement or K cell-mediated attack. Released antigens and bacteria are taken up by macrophages and neutrophils, particularly following opsonization by antibody or complement. Some larger extracellular pathogens such as worms cannot be endocytosed but may be attacked by eosinophils, which exocytose their cytotoxic granule contents.

intracellular parasites mark their presence in this way. It is therefore necessary that the immune system can recognize cells which have become infected by viruses, or intracellular stages of microbial and parasitic infections, at an early stage. MHC molecules provide this capability. Antigenic peptides associate with MHC molecules and are passed from inside the cell to the surface, where they can be recognized by T cells and this then elicits an appropriate response.

Why does the immune system need two ways of recognizing intracellular antigens, i.e. class I and class II molecules? The answer lies in the two types of response which can be elicited, namely cytotoxicity and cytokine generation, although this distinction is not absolute. Since many cell types may become infected by virus or intracellular parasites and must then be destroyed, it is important that

MHC class I is widely distributed to ensure recognition by Tc cells. On the other hand, MHC class II is particularly associated with cells which respond to T cell cytokines, such as B cells and macrophages. In accordance with this division of function, antigens produced by a cell preferentially associate with MHC class I molecules, whereas antigen taken up by a cell becomes associated with MHC class II — provided of course the cell is capable of expressing class II. The differential use of class I and class II molecules is, therefore, a means of generating two modes of response, both of which involve recognition of antigen at the cell surface.

Antigen clearance

Antibodies bind to free antigen, forming immune complexes which can activate the complement system by binding to C1q of the classical pathway, causing activation of C3 and covalent attachment of C3b. Receptors for immunoglobulins and C3 fragments are present on mononuclear phagocytes which will take up complexes and degrade them. In primates, erythrocytes also express a C3 receptor (CR1) which allows them to take up circulating complexes and transport them to liver and spleen where they are transferred to phagocytes. Antigens in the blood are normally removed by this route but should the system become overloaded (as occurs in quartan malaria, for example), complexes may be deposited at other sites, particularly the kidney. Such immune complex deposition occurs at sites of filtration in many immune complex diseases. In addition to their role in complexing antigen, antibodies can act against the pathogens themselves. For example, they can neutralize directly some viruses by binding to receptors on the viral surface, thereby preventing attachment to cells. IgA transported across mucous membranes has a significant role in the prevention of infection and acts in the absence of complement or phagocytic cells.

Cytotoxicity

There are two distinct ways of dealing with intracellular pathogens. The infected cell may be killed by an external effector system, such as a cytotoxic cell, or activated to destroy the pathogen itself. As stated above, an intracellular pathogen may be recognized either because it expresses native molecules on the cell surface which bind antibody, or because the cell passes antigen peptides to the surface associated with MHC molecules. If antibody binds to a target cell, it may activate the classical and lytic pathways of the complement system, or it can sensitize the cell for attack by cytotoxic cells expressing Fc receptors. This antibody dependent cell-mediated cytotoxicity (ADCC) is performed by large granular lymphocytes and some activated macrophages. These cells elicit damage by releasing enzymes, cytolysins, reactive oxygen intermediates and cytokines in close proximity to the target. Mention should also be made of the cytotoxic damage caused by eosinophils to parasites such as schistosomes mediated by Fc receptors for IgG and IgE. In this case, damage is caused partly by release of the specialized proteins contained in the crystalloid core of their specific granules. Such release of enzymes and granule contents in apposition to

target organisms is the only way that the immune system can engage pathogens which are too large to phagocytose. Cytotoxic T cells are particularly important in defence against virally infected cells, although cells infected by enveloped viruses will also express antigens recognizable by antibody. The mechanisms of cytotoxic damage by Tc cells include the induction of target cell apoptosis and the release of perforin onto the target cell membrane. Perforin is homologous to C9, the lytic component of the complement pathway, and its polymerization results in holes in the target cell membrane. Clearly, if an infected cell loses its MHC molecules, it may not be recognized by Tc cells and some intracellular pathogens try to conceal themselves by suppressing MHC expression. However, such cells then become targets for NK activity by large granular lymphocytes. The actions of cytotoxic cells are discussed fully in Chapter 15.

In non-immune individuals, macrophages may take up microorganisms which they are unable to destroy, such as *Mycobacterium leprae* or *Leishmania*; these pathogens subsequently multiply within the phagocyte. They can, however, be destroyed in an immune individual. This demonstrates the importance of T cell immunity in the destruction of certain intracellular parasites. In effect, macrophages can present antigen to T cells which respond by releasing cytokines such as IFNγ ('macrophage arming factor') which in turn enable the phagocytes to deal with the pathogen themselves. Recognition of intracellular pathogens therefore results either in the destruction of the pathogen or the destruction of the infected cell before the microorganism can multiply.

NORMAL AND ABERRANT IMMUNE RESPONSES

Immunodeficiency may be inherited, such as with thymic aplasia, or may be acquired, as occurs in AIDS. It may affect any aspect of the immune system, with results ranging from profound to innocuous. For example, complement C9 deficiency does not appear to be noticeably associated with susceptibility to infection, whereas severe combined immunodeficiency due to failure of lymphoid stem cell differentiation results in impaired B cell and T cell responses and is life threatening. Other systems can compensate partially for some deficiencies but abnormalities in lymphocyte generation and phagocyte function are particularly associated with infection.

Although many lymphocytes can recognize self molecules, they do not normally react to them — the phenomenon of self-tolerance. During their development, lymphocytes pass through a stage at which they are highly susceptible to the induction of tolerance. It is much more difficult to render mature cells tolerant, particularly if they have already been primed with antigen. Since the whole immune system is immature in the earliest stages of neonatal life, a newborn animal is particularly susceptible to the induction of tolerance. The functional deletion of self-reactive clones at this early stage of life is thought to be one way of developing self-tolerance. Not all self-reactive cells are destroyed, since they can be found in the circulation of an adult animal, allowing self-tolerance to be broken by experimental manoeuvres. Although breakdown of self-tolerance occurs surprisingly frequently, it is only in a limited number of cases that these autoimmune reactions develop into autoimmune disease. Hypersensitivity reactions are more difficult to define, since the borderline between the damage and repair caused by an adaptive immune response and a hypersensitivity reaction is often unclear. For example, the T cell mediated response to *Mycobacterium tuberculosis* is essential for resisting the spread of the organism and the development of immunity. However, in some cases the damage to normal tissue produced by the immune response is out of all proportion to the amount of damage generated by the relatively small numbers of *mycobacteria*. Other cases such as pollen allergy are more clearcut. There are many cases where the response is inappropriate because it is not well suited to the elimination of a pathogen. An example of this is subacute sclerosing panencephalitis, where a large quantity of ineffective anti-measles antibody is produced, which fails to destroy infected cells in the CNS and viral spread continues with progressive destruction of neurons.

SUMMARY

This chapter has presented an overview of the important features of the immune system which will be examined in detail in later sections. It is important to remember that the key function of the immune system is as a defender against pathogens. The system may generate many interesting and indeed clincally important phenomena, such as graft rejection and autoimmunity; it may be used to target drugs to tumours, or be enlisted as a tool of many other biological sciences, but its primary function is host defence.

FURTHER READING

Kuby J. *Cells and Organs of the Immune System*. WH Freeman: New York; 1992.

Roitt IM, Brostoff J, Male DK (Eds). *Immunology*, edn 4. Mosby-Year Book: London; 1995.

Schlossman SF, Boumsell L, Gilks W, Harlan JM, Kishimoto T, Morimoto C, Ritz J, Shaw S, Silverstein RL, Springer TA, Tedder TF, Todd RF. CD Antigens 1993. *Immunol Today* 1994, **15**:98.

Zucker-Franklin D, Greaves MF, Grossi CE, Marmont AM. *Atlas of Blood Cells: Function and Pathology*. Edi Ermes: Milan and Philadelphia; 1980.

2 Antigen Receptor Molecules

There are three sets of molecules involved in immune recognition: antibodies or immunoglobulins (Ig), the T cell receptors (TCRs) and major histocompatibility complex (MHC) molecules. Of these, antibodies were the first to be identified as serum molecules which were capable of neutralizing a number of infectious organisms. Antibodies are produced by B cells in two distinct forms, either as cell surface receptors for antigen or as soluble antibodies in extracellular fluids. Elucidation of the structure of individual immunoglobulins showed them to consist of a series of globular domains, each with distinct functions. These structural motifs have since been found in a very wide range of molecules involved in immune recognition and cell–cell interaction; these constitute the immunoglobulin supergene family. Although immunoglobulins themselves are extremely diverse structurally, the essential role of secreted antibody molecules is as bifunctional molecules (adapters) which can bind to antigen via specific antigen-combining sites and then crosslink the antigen to cells of the immune system or activate complement.

ANTIBODY STRUCTURE

Domains

The basic building block of all antibodies is the four polypeptide chain unit, consisting of two identical light chains and two identical heavy chains, crosslinked by interchain disulphide bonds and stabilized by non-covalent interactions (see Chapter 1). Light chains (κ or λ) are folded into two globular domains while heavy chains comprise four or five domains, depending on the class of the antibody — IgM and IgE have five heavy chain domains and IgG, IgA and IgD have four heavy chain domains. The N-terminal domains of both light and heavy chains are highly variable between antibodies (V domains), while the remaining domains are relatively constant (C domains) although they do differ between isotypes. The domains themselves consist of a β-barrel, with seven (C domains) or nine (V domains) strands of β-sheet, stabilized by an intrachain disulphide bond. Within the V domains, the variability is clustered in three hypervariable regions, which are formed by amino acid residues 30–36, 50–65 and 93–102 (approximately). Although separated in the primary sequence, the hypervariable regions are brought together by the folding of the V domain as loops at the tip of the molecule. The association of a heavy chain V domain and a light chain V domain therefore generates a surface with six exposed hypervariable loops, three from each chain (see *Fig. 3.8*). It is this surface which forms the antibody's combining site for antigen. The precise sequence of the six hypervariable loops determines the antibody specificity, as may be demonstrated by transferring sets of hypervariable regions from one antibody to another by genetic engineering. Because of their role in forming the antigen binding site, the hypervariable regions are called complementarity determining regions (CDRs) and, conversely, the surrounding sequences, which form the β-barrel, are framework regions.

The type of heavy chain determines the antibody's class and subclass. These are the different Ig isotypes. The C-terminal domains of the heavy chains, which form the Fc region, are particularly important in determining the biological functions of the antibody. The process of antibody formation within an individual B cell allows genes for different heavy chain isotypes (*CH*) to become associated with the cell's functional heavy chain variable region gene (*VH*) gene. This means that a cell can generate antibody of a particular specificity, but with different functions, depending on which isotype(s) gene is used.

Individual Ig domains interact with their neighbours, so for example, the V_H and V_L domains interact extensively via the three-strand β-sheet layers, while Cγ1 and C_L make contacts between the four-strand layer; residues along these interacting faces are predominantly hydrophobic. The hinge region is also important in conferring segmental flexibility on the molecule and this is correlated with the length of the hinge region in different subclasses. The two forms of antibody, membrane and secreted immunoglobulin, differ only at the C-terminus where membrane Ig has transmembrane and short intracytoplasmic regions, 3–30 residues depending on the subclass.

Isotypes

In man there are nine functional heavy chain isotypes corresponding to the immunoglobulin subclasses and these may be associated with either of the two light chain isotypes κ or λ. In mouse there are eight heavy chain isotypes but 90% of the serum antibody has κ light chains. The mouse λ chain locus has only a limited capacity to generate diversity, although there are four λ isotypes.

Antibody function is largely determined by the specificity and affinity of the antigen-binding site and by the heavy chain isotype. Different subclasses vary in their ability to bind to cellular Fc receptors, complement, and transport receptors (*Fig. 2.1*). In practice, IgG, IgA and IgE antibodies have higher antigen-binding affinities than IgM but this is related to the affinity maturation which occurs concurrently with class switching in B cells. The essential characteristics of the different subclasses of serum antibodies may be summarized as follows:

	Properties					Functional interactions in humans							Human subclasses		Mouse subclasses	
	Subunits	H chain domains	Size	Serum half life (human) days	Complement fixation	Platelet binding	Mast cell and basophil sensitization	Transplacental transfer	Transepithelial transfer	Opsonization for macrophages; neutrophils, eosinophils	Sensitization for K cells	Binding to lymphocytes	Subclasses•	Serum concentration mg/ml	Subclasses	Serum concentration mg/ml
IgM	5	5	19s	5.1	++	–	–	–	(+)	–	–	T†	μ	1.5	μ	0.6–1.0•
IgG	1	4	7s	23*	+*	+	–	+*	(+)	+*	+*	T†B	γ1	9	γ1	4.6–6.5
													γ2	3	γ2a	1.0–4.2
													γ3	1	γ2b	1.2–2.0
													γ4	0.5	γ3	0.1–0.2
IgA	1,2 or more	4	7s or 11s	5.8	–	–	–	–	++	–	–	T†B†	α1	3	α	0.26–0.4
													α2	0.5		
IgD	1	4	7s	2.8	–	–	–	–	–	–	–	–	δ	0.03	δ	–‡
IgE	1	5	8s	2.3	–	–	++	–	–	–	–	T†B†	ε	0.05x10⁻³	ε	0.1 x 10⁻³

• The range of mouse subclasses varies greatly between strains and at different ages	* Some subclasses only	‡ Serum levels of mouse IgD are very low or undetectable
	† Some subsets of cells only	

Fig. 2.1 Characteristics and functions of antibody classes. The class of an antibody is determined by its heavy chain. Effector functions relate largely to the cells and other systems which interact with the Fc regions (*Fig. 2.9*).

- IgM — first to be produced in a primary response; low affinity but high avidity to multivalent antigens; complement fixing.
- IgG — the main serum antibody, particularly in secondary response; essential in protection of neonate, by transplacental transfer or in milk; has the ability to bind many cell types and to fix complement (varies with subclass).
- IgA — the main isotype secreted across mucosal surfaces.
- IgE — triggers inflammatory reactions via specific receptors on mast cells and basophils; elicits effector responses to some gut parasites.
- IgD — primarily a cell surface receptor, expression varies during B cell differentiation.

Polymeric immunoglobulins

Mammalian IgM is a pentamer or hexamer of the basic four chain immunoglobulin unit, and in most mammals (humans are an exception) the great majority of serum IgA is polymeric, consisting mostly of dimers. Polymerization of these classes is dependent on the J (joining) chain, and the abundance of J chain also determines the proportion of pentamer to hexamer IgM. The J chain consists of 137 amino acid residues in both man and mouse, encoded by four exons with 77% homology between the two sequences. One model of the J chain suggests that it consists of a single domain with a β-barrel structure similar to immunoglobulin domains, although it is not a member of the immunoglobulin supergene family.

The J chain assists polymerization by disulphide cross-linking cysteine residues in the C-terminal domains of secreted IgM and IgA, which are absent from the membrane forms. Evidence for the role of J chain in polymerization comes from somatic cell hybrids of IgG-producing myelomas (also producing J chain) fused with a B cell lymphoma producing monomeric IgM. These hybrid cells were able to assemble pentameric IgM. The actual polymerization is probably effected by a sulphhydryl oxidase, found exclusively in fully differentiated antibody forming cells. J chain is critical for facilitating IgM polymerization, although polymers lacking a J chain can still be secreted. Strangely, even cells producing IgG exclusively synthesize considerable quantities of J chain. The function in these cells, if any, is unknown and it is broken down internally.

The antigen-combining site

Crystallographic analyses of complexes between antibodies and intact protein antigens have clarified the nature of the antigen binding site. Antibody contacts large antigens over an extended area of surface shape-complementarity (about 750Å²) equivalent to about 30% of the total CDR-determined paratope surface. In these cases there are no obvious antigen binding clefts, but the opposing surfaces of the antigen and antibody are in such close proximity that water is largely excluded from the interface. In different antibodies there are 14–19 contact residues, and similar

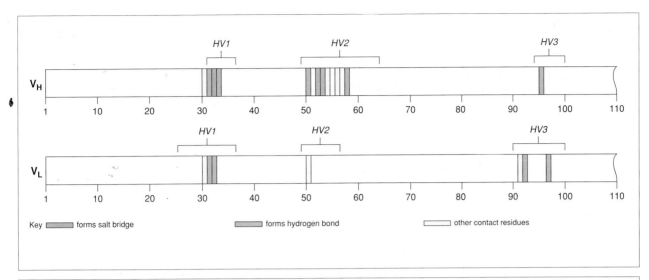

Fig. 2.2 Antigen contact residues on antibody to lysozyme. The amino acid residues from the antibody HyHEL-10 make contact with a discontinuous epitope on hen egg-white lysozyme (see *Colour figures*). Residues from both the V_H and V_L domains contact the antigen. Hydrogen bonds and van der Waals forces contribute a large part of the bond strength together with a single salt bridge. The relationship of these residues to the hypervariable regions is apparent, but note that one contact residue of V_H lies in the first framework segment. Based on data from Padlan *et al*, 1989.

numbers on the antigen (*Fig. 2.2*). In the examples studied to date, every one of the hypervariable loops made some contribution to the binding site and in some instances framework residues contribute to the binding.

Hydrogen bonds, salt bridges and van der Waals forces generate the bond, with little contribution from hydrophobic interactions. In the interaction of D1.3 with lysozyme it has been shown that four water molecules retained in the interface as well as those at the edge of contact zone contribute to a hydrogen bonding network which stabilizes the bond. The anti-lysozyme antibody, HyHEL-10, and its antigen provide a typical example of the amino acid side chain interactions involved in an antigen–antibody complex. In this case there are 14 hydrogen bonds, 11 van der Waals contacts and one salt bridge. Virtually the entire surface of an antigen is potentially antigenic (see *Colour figures*). The three antibodies which have been crystallized in complexes with lysozyme contact three epitopes with virtually no overlap covering nearly 50% of the surface of the antigen, suggesting that, with enough antibodies available, the entire surface could form epitopes. Nevertheless, some areas of antigens are more immunogenic than others, and these are often in regions of greatest molecular mobility. It is thought that these areas will tolerate more distortion as the antigen–antibody bond is formed and are therefore more able to make a complementary fit to the paratope. This distortion is termed 'induced fit' (see below).

It is particularly notable that charged residues on the antigen are frequently neutralized by oppositely charged residues on the antibody. For example, in HyHEL-5 (anti-lysozyme) there are two adjoining glutamic acid side chains lying at the base of a groove, which neutralize the charge of a pair of protruding arginine residues on lysozyme. Charge neutralization is particularly important at the centre of the binding region; around the periphery, charged residues are not always neutralized since they are partially accessible to water. In some cases, comparison of the crystallographic structures of complexed and uncomplexed molecules has shown that the interaction between antigen and antibody can induce changes in the molecular structure of either partner. Changes in the overall secondary structures are slight, however, there may be considerable alterations in the orientation of individual side chains. For example, Trp 62 in lysozyme rotates through 150° about the C2–C3 bond in order to avoid steric hindrance from a tyrosine residue on the HyHEL-10 antibody. The degree of antigen distortion allowed depends on the degree of local flexibility. Complexed antibodies sometimes also show small positional modifications of binding site residues. The relative contributions of the different CDRs to the binding site are discussed more fully in Chapter 3.

Idiotopes

Idiotopes are antigenic determinants associated with a receptor binding site. Individual antibodies (and TCRs) may be identified by their set of idiotopes, and the set of idiotopes defines a particular idiotype. Some idiotopes are detected on many different antibodies (cross-reactive, recurrent or public idiotopes) while others are apparently unique to a single clonotypic antibody (private idiotope). In some cases, anti-idiotypic antibodies could block the binding of antigen to the cognate antibody implying that the idiotope is associated with the antigen binding site (site-associated idiotope). Other anti-idiotopes appear to recognize structures outside the binding site.

Experiments in mice have shown that certain idiotypes are characteristic of the immune response to specific antigens in particular strains. For example, in C57BL/6 mice, the primary antibody response to phosphoryl choline is dominated by antibodies expressing the T15 idiotype. Evidence has accumulated to show that immunglobulin heavy and light chain haplotypes are the critical factors which determine whether one of these 'germline idiotypes' may be produced by a particular strain. Other studies have shown that antibodies from genetically different individuals, directed to the same antigen, can also share particular idiotypes. This has been described for a number of human autoantibodies. In such cases, it appears that the constraint of binding to a particular epitope leads to the generation of antibodies with similar binding sites.

The cross-reactive idiotope IdX which occurs on antibodies to dextran, in mice of the IgH^a haplotype, has been studied in some detail. The IdX-bearing antibodies can be generated by two or more related V$_H$ segments in association with a number of different D segments. The IdX idiotope appears to depend on two residues (Asn–Asn) in the second hypervariable region. Two IdX-bearing antibodies, M104 and J558, differ by only two amino acid residues in the D segment but can still be distinguished by anti-idiotypic antibodies (see *Colour figures*). The M104 private idiotope corresponds with Tyr–Asp or Ala–Asp residues in their D segments while the J558 idiotope is expressed by antibodies having Arg–Tyr at these positions. This example illustrates how very similar antibodies can express both public and private idiotopes.

Comparison of idiotopes in different strains has confirmed the association between particular haplotypes and genes. For example, the T15 idiotype, mentioned above, is expressed on a heavy chain assembled from *Vh1* of the *S107* gene family, recombined with *DhFL16.1* and *Jh1*, and associated with a κ light chain using the *Vk22* germline gene. The idiotope AB1-2 on this antibody depends on the 3rd heavy chain hypervariable loop (D region) but is absent from IgH^j strains which is correlated with an allelic form of *DhFL16.1* in IgH^j mice.

C domains

Constant domains and the hinge region are involved in the interactions of antibody with complement C1q and Fc receptors. In IgG, the two C$_H$3 domains are paired with a contact area of approximately 1000Å^2, but the C$_H$2 domains are separated, with carbohydrate units lying in the cleft between them (*Fig. 2.3*).

Complement C1q binds to a region in the C$_H$2 domain of IgG with a binding affinity (K$_a$) of approximately 10^{4}M^{-1}. The core residues are D318, K320 and K322. Complexed IgG makes a much higher avidity bond to C1q because of the multivalent interactions between the complex and C1q and not because of any conformational change in the C$_H$2 domain. Different subclasses vary in their ability to bind C1q and activate complement (Chapter 13) but binding alone is not the only factor which determines whether a subclass is active. For example, isolated Fc fragments of IgG4 bind C1q but the intact molecules do not due to steric hindrance from the Fab arms. In addition, complement C3b and C4b often bind to the C$_H$1 domains of IgG, and so activation efficiency may also depend on the availability of suitable binding sites

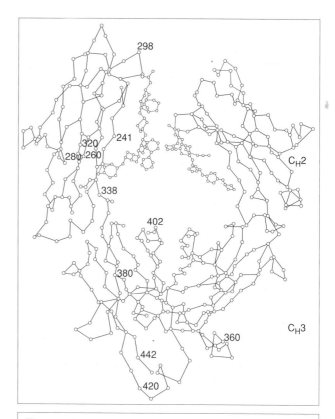

Fig. 2.3 Structure of the Fc region. This illustrates the α-carbon backbone of an IgG Fc region. The paired C$_H$3 domains are closely linked by non-covalent bonds but the C$_H$2 domains lie apart and two carbohydrate units (one from each chain) run down the cleft. The C$_H$2 domains contain the C1q binding site and this domain is also part of the binding region for most Fc receptors. The protein A binding site lies between C$_H$2 and C$_H$3.

in this domain. The situation with IgM is quite different. In this case a conformational change associated with antigen binding is thought to flex the Fab arms, leading to exposure of a site in Cμ3 analogous to that in IgG. Other Fc-dependent functions are related to the ability to bind specific Fc receptors (discussed below).

Allotypes

The immunoglobulins of individuals of a species express allotypic determinants which can be recognized by other individuals lacking the allotype. Five sets of allotypic markers have been described in humans. These are the Gm, Am and Mm systems which are determined by the heavy chain C regions, the Km (=Inv) system determined by the kappa genes, and the Hv system determined by the *Vh* genes (which could be considered a public idiotype marker). Since heavy chains of different classes may combine with κ chains the Km allotypes may occur in association with any of an individual's heavy chain allotypes on different antibodies (*Fig. 2.4*).

The Gm series of heavy chain allotypic determinants, occurring on IgG constant regions is the most numerous (at least 24 variants). The majority of the allotypic sites

Allotype system	Location	Comment
Km (=Inv)	κ chains	expressed on IgG1 and IgG3; 3 variants; requires IgG quarternary structure for expression
Hv	heavy chain V domain	one variant
Am	Fcα	two variants of IgA2
Mm	Fcμ	one variant
Gm	Fcγ and $C_H 1$	at least 24 variants 3 associated with IgG1, 1 with IgG2, 13 with IgG3 + 7 unassigned

Fig. 2.4 Allotypes of human Ig. The table lists five major systems of human Ig allotypes and their gene locations.

have been localized to the Fc region, but G1m(4) and G1m(17) are determined by the Ch1 domain. Since the anti-allotype sera recognize determinants rather than individual isotypes, a few allotypic markers, called isoallotypes, can occur on different subclasses, although most are expressed on only one subclass. To indicate this, the nomenclature includes a figure showing which subclasses each allotype is associated with. For example, G1m(4) and G1m(17) are associated with IgG1, while G3m(5) and G3m(6) occur on IgG3. An example of an isoallotype is IgG4 nG4m(a) which is also present on all IgG1 and IgG3 molecules. In some cases, if an individual haplotype carries one Gm allotype it precludes the presence of another. Sometimes, the presence of the allotype depends on just a single amino acid. For example, G1m(4) has Arg at position 214 of the g1 chain while IgG1 antibodies lacking this allotype do not. In other cases the determinant is produced by the three dimensional structure of the immunoglobulin. For example, the Km light chain determinants are only weakly expressed on free light chains or on k chains associated with g2 or g4 heavy chains.

Although Ig allotypes are of interest to population geneticists, one might wonder whether they have any functional significance. There have been reports of disease association with particular allotypes (e.g. rheumatoid arthritis) but this may reflect only a tighter linkage to V region idiotypes and the B cell repertoire. In fact, the associations are relatively weak when compared with MHC-related disease associations. However, the levels of particular isotypes within an individual are partly dependent on that individual's allotype. For example, individuals who are homozygous for G3m(5) have approximately twice the amount of serum IgG3 than individuals who lack the allotype. Heterozygotes have intermediate levels. Likewise G2m(23)+ individuals have 35% more IgG2 than those who are G2m(23)-. The haplotypes generate no apparent differences in IgM, IgE or IgA levels. Ig allotypes have been present in every animal species tested so far.

Carbohydrate units

Immunoglobulins are glycoproteins with 3–12% carbohydrate. The main units are biantennary structures based on one of about 20 different units with a mannosyl-chitobiose core. These are attached to asparagine residues in Cγ2. They confer some resistance to proteolysis and also affect the rate of catabolism *in vivo*. Although the carbohydrate does not form elements directly responsible for C1q or Fc receptor binding, it does maintain the conformation required to bind these receptors. For example, carbohydrate-deficient IgG1 and IgG3 antibodies bind with lower affinity to FcγRI and FcγRIII, although there is little conformational change in the Fc regions.

Antibodies are glycosylated in the endoplasmic reticulum (ER). Carbohydrate is also attached to the Fab units of some antibodies and occasionally affects antibody binding characteristics by limiting the access of the antigen to the antibody paratope. There is often microheterogeneity in carbohydrate units so that the molecule as a whole is not necessarily totally symmetrical.

ANTIBODY GENES

The antigen binding domains of immunoglobulins are generated during B cell ontogeny by a process of somatic recombination between different gene segments. A very similar process occurs during T cell development in the thymus. The basic principles of the recombination will be described here. The ways in which this process leads to the generation of immunoglobulin and TCR diversity are examined in detail in Chapter 3.

There are three separate loci encoding immunoglobulin chains, namely the heavy chain locus (*IGH*) and those for the κ and λ light chains. These loci undergo recombination at two separate stages during B cell development. The first stage involves the recombination of *V, D* and *J* segments to form the gene encoding the V_H and V_L domains. This takes place during differentiation of lymphoid stem cells into virgin B cells. The second type of gene recombination may occur in the *Ch* genes of differentiated B cells, and is involved in irreversible class switching by the B cell.

V, D and *J* gene segments

The heavy chain V domain gene is assembled from a *V* gene, encoding the first 94 (approximately) residues, which combines with a *D* gene segment (diversity) and a *J* gene segment (joining). The region of the *V-D-J* join forms the third hypervariable region of the V domain, while the first and second hypervariable regions are encoded within the *V* gene. There are more than 200 *V* genes in the *IGH* locus, with 10 *D* genes and four

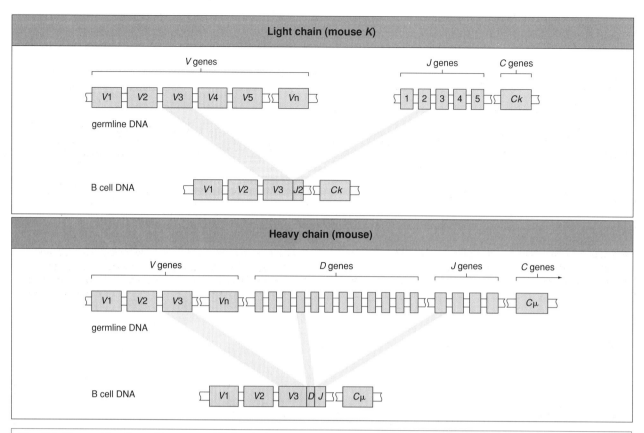

Fig. 2.5 Recombination of heavy and light chain genes. The exon encoding the V domain of a κ light chain is formed by recombination of one of many *V* genes with one of four functional *J* genes, here illustrated as recombination between *V3* and *J2*. (The third *J* gene is a non-functional pseudogene.) The exon forming the mouse heavy chain V domain is formed by the recombination at random of one of a large number of *V* genes with one of 12 *D* segments and one of four *J* genes, to produce a recombined *V-D-J* gene. The recombined genes are linked to exons encoding the C domains during mRNA splicing.

J genes. Since any of the *V* genes can recombine with any *D* gene and any *J* gene, the number of possible combinations of *V-D-J* is enormous (see Chapter 3). Light chain genes also undergo recombination, but these loci contain only *V* and *J* gene segments, so the third hypervariable region of the light chain is formed at a *VJ* junction. Recombination of either heavy or light chain genes leads to the loss of the intervening stretches of DNA, containing both introns and exons. The process is outlined in *Figure 2.5*.

Recombination takes place in a defined sequence, heavy chains first. The cell attempts to make a functional recombination from one of its chromosomes and if this fails, it turns to the other. The production of a functional μ chain is the signal for light chain gene recombination. The B cell then tries to produce a functional recombined kappa chain and if this fails it will then attempt recombination of the lambda genes. The process continues until functional *V* genes for both heavy and light chains have been generated but the process is terminated once functional polypeptides have been synthesized (see Chapter 6). One consequence of this is that individual B cells use only one heavy chain gene and one light chain gene, either maternal or paternal at random

— an example of allelic exclusion. Recombination of immunoglobulin gene segments occurs efficiently only in B cells. The process is controlled by the sequences flanking the *V*, *D* and *J* gene segments and the tissue specific operation of recombination activating genes, as described in Chapter 3.

Constant region genes

The heavy chain constant region genes lie 3' to the recombined *V-D-J* gene. Initially, B cells express only surface IgM. The *IGHM* gene is proximal to the recombined *V-D-J* and the earliest functional transcript of the heavy chain genes starts with the signal sequence 5' to the recombined *V-D-J* and extends through the *V-D-J* gene and along the intron to the *CM* gene. Each of the constant domains and transmembrane segments is encoded by a separate exon (*Fig. 2.6*). Most human *IGHGC* genes also have a single exon encoding the hinge region but in *IGHG3* there are four exons encoding the extended hinge of this subclass. The hinge region of IgA is encoded within the exon for the Cα2 domains. There are also two exons for the transmembrane segments of all the Ig isotypes; the first encodes the stretch of hydrophobic amino acids which actually traverse the membrane and the second encodes the

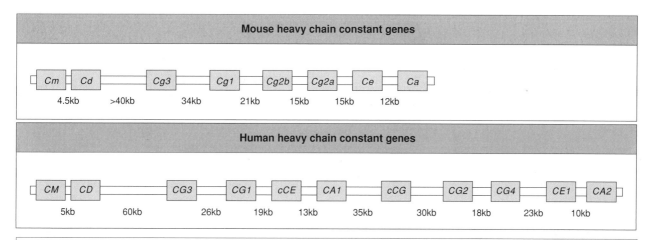

Fig. 2.6 C genes. In mouse and man the *CM* and *CD* genes are proximal to the recombined *V-D-J* gene. Each *C* gene except for *CD* is preceeded by an intronic switching sequence.

In man there are two non-functional pseudogenes (*cCE* and *cCG*) and the *C* gene stack appears to have arisen by gene duplication. Subclasses in man and mouse are not analagous.

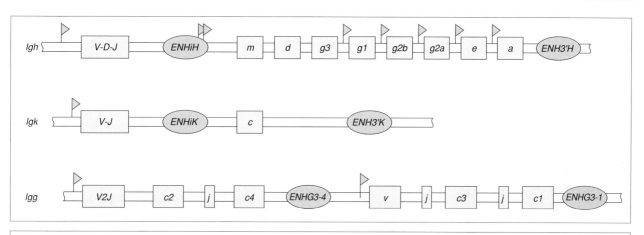

Fig. 2.7 Enhancers and promoters of Ig genes. The location of promoters (flags) and enhancers (*ENH*) in relation to the exons of the mouse immunoglobulin genes in recombined chromosomes is illustrated diagrammatically.

Additional promoters are deleted from the *V-J* intron in the *IGK* locus by the recombinational event. Such introns, and those in the middle of the *IGH* loci, may be responsible for the production of sterile transcripts.

short intracytoplasmic segment. The sequence of the transmembrane section is highly conserved among different antibody classes, which is presumably related to their interactions with the signal transducing Igα and Igβ chains. The introns between all of these exons are removed by RNA splicing during the formation of mRNA. The process of RNA splicing is also important in:

- Determining whether mRNA is produced for membrane or secreted Ig.
- Determining whether a cell will express IgM, IgD or both.
- The initial stages of class switching.

The choice between the production of membrane or secreted Ig mRNA is made when the transcript is adenylated. Poly-A is attached to the 3' end of nearly all mammalian RNA molecules which will become mRNA. This process is required for transport of the mRNA from the nucleus to the cytoplasm. The *CM* genes have two polyadenylation sites. One of them lies within the *CM4* terminal exon of secreted IgM and the second lies at the 3' end of the second membrane domain. If polyadenylation takes place at the first of these sites, then mRNA for secreted IgM will be produced, but if it occurs at the second site the RNA is spliced to remove the stop codon at the end of *CM4* and the mRNA will include the membrane exons.

Promoters and enhancers

The immunoglobulin promoter and enhancer regions consist of a collection of DNA sequence motifs which can bind to different transcription factors (*Fig. 2.7*). Of these, the octameric motifs which bind the POU-domain family of DNA-binding proteins are particularly important. Oct-1 is present in most cells, but Oct-2 is confined to B cells and a few others and is thought to determine the B cell specificity of immunoglobulin gene transcription. All Ig promoters contain the octamer motif or its inversion, which can bind Oct-2, and synthetic promoters containing just this and a TATA box are active only in lymphoid cells.

The heavy chain contains two enhancer regions, one of which lies between the *J* and *C* genes (*ENHiH*) and a second lying 3' to the *C* genes (*ENH3'H*) in rats and mice. These enhancers are cell type-specific and stage-specific. The first is a potent B cell-specific enhancer containing multiple partially redundant elements. That is to say that deletion of any one motif does not totally prevent transcription. The E-motif designated μE5 is interesting in that it is negatively regulated and acts as a silencer in non-lymphoid cells. The π-motif is active in pre-B cells only and appears to be involved in the differential regulation of *IGH* expression during B cell development. Recombination of *D-J* and subsequently *V-D-J* brings the promoters within range of this enhancer, thereby initiating transcription. In addition to the normal VDJC transcript, a variety of sterile transcripts are generated during B cell development which are not translated (e.g. DJC). It is possible that these have some regulatory function in development.

The intronic K-enhancer *ENHiK* is only active in B cells. It contains an Oct-2 site and an NF-κB site as well as a silencer which turns off NF-κB-induced activation in T cells. The E-motifs in this enhancer appear to be more important than those in the *IGH* intronic enhancer. There is a second enhancer 3' to the *C* gene, which is only weakly active in pre-B cells but is much more important than the intronic enhancer in mature cells. It also allows κ transcription in B cells which have low levels of NF-κB. There are also two enhancers in the lambda genes. Related promoters and enhancer motifs are found in the immunoglobulin-associated genes such as the J chain gene which also has elements activated by IL-2 and IL-5.

Switching sequences and class switching

Individual B cells can switch the isotype of immunoglobulin produced, while retaining the same recombined *V-D-J* gene. This process could occur by at least two mechanisms:

- B cells can generate long nuclear RNA transcripts which include V-D-J and more than one C transcript. Differential polyadenylation and RNA splicing can then generate mRNAs for different heavy chain isotypes, in an analogous way to the selection of membrane or secreted immunoglobulin and the dual production of IgM and IgD.
- A somatic gene recombination occurs in the heavy chain genes which replaces the *CM* gene with that from one of the other isotypes — the intervening sequences are excised. As a consequence of the excision, a cell which has switched isotype by this mechanism cannot switch back and there is evidence that successive downstream switches can occur.

Evidence favours the second model, in which switching occurs by looping out along the expressed chromosome and not by sister chromatid exchange. In many mature B cells which have switched their Ig class expression, there are deletions of *C* genes between *V-D-J* and the expressed *C* gene. Moreover, the long transcripts predicted by the first model have not been found. IgA-expressing B cells isolated from blood show switching deletions on both alleles, not just that with the recombined *V-D-J*, suggesting that the class switching mechanism is independent of IgH expression. Switching depends on switch sequences. All murine *C* genes except delta have a switching sequence (*S*) 5' to the first C domain exon. The sequences are of the form (GAGCT)nGGGGT, where the first element is a tandem repeat occurring one to seven times and the whole sequence is then repeated up to 150 times. This gives a region of DNA 1–10kb long which lies 1–4kb upstream of the exon. Switch recombination is not site-specific, since the switch sequences vary considerably in length and the break point does not necessarily occur in the switch region itself. The switch recombinase which directs the process has not yet been identified but it is thought that the similar *S* sequences cause the genes to be juxtaposed so that the enzyme(s) can break and reconnect the strands. The areas of recombination are usually hypomethylated, but this does not appear to be essential for the recombination. The DNA binding protein LR1 is an important regulator of class switching. In B cells, it binds to a site in the promoter of *c-myc*, and it is notable that homologous sites are found in the *IGH* region.

The specificity of class switching is determined in part by particular cytokines, as discussed in Chapters 9–11. The region 5' to the switch regions appears to be important in controlling which switch will occur. These flanking sequences become demethylated before switching. Normally, IL-4 promotes switching to *Igh-G1* in mice, but in mutant mice lacking the region 5' to the *G1* switch region, there is a 99% reduction both in the expression of IgG1 and in numbers of B cells expressing IgG1. Class switching is accompanied by somatic hypermutation of the Ig gene loci (see Chapter 3) and affinity maturation. Although these processes are usually concurrent with class switching, they may occur independently.

ANTIBODY FUNCTIONS

Antibody secretion and transcytosis

Polymeric IgA and IgM can bind to the poly-Ig receptor which is expressed on the serosal side of glandular epithelia (e.g. in the gut). This receptor is a five domain member of the immunoglobulin supergene family. Dimeric IgA binds non-covalently to the receptor via domain 1 but the IgA may subsequently form disulphide bonds with domain 5 of the receptor. The cytoplasmic portion of the receptor contains sequences that direct it to the basolateral surface and others that direct it through a transcytosis pathway to the apical surface once it has bound IgA. At the apical surface the receptor is cleaved, releasing the IgA and leaving part of the cleaved receptor to form the secretory piece. This wraps around the C-terminal domains of IgA and protects it from digestion (*Fig. 2.8*). Binding to the poly-Ig receptor is dependent on the presence of a J chain, since artificial polymers

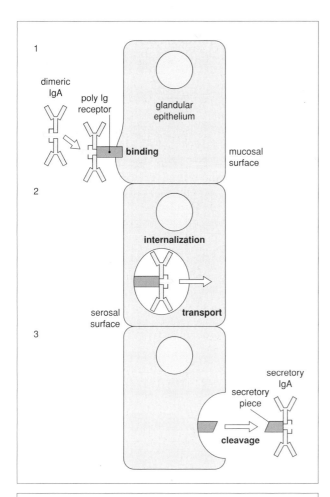

Fig. 2.8 Secretion of IgA. Dimeric IgA can link to the poly-Ig receptor exposed on the serosal side of glandular epithelia (e.g. in the gut). The IgA receptor complex is internalized and transported to the mucosal surface where it is released by proteolysis. The ligand binding portion of the receptor remains attached to the IgA dimer by disulphide bonds and is in fact the secretory piece which protects IgA from degradation in mucosal secretions.

lacking J chain bind poorly. The production of these secreted immunoglobulins is essential in the protection of mucosal surfaces.

IgG may be transported from the lumen of the gut to the basolateral surface of enterocytes. This mechanism serves to take up IgG from milk. The rat receptor has been isolated and bears a striking structural relationship to class I MHC molecules, including 50% sequence homology and the presence of β_2-microglobulin. The receptor binds IgG at pH 6 in the lumen of the gut and releases it at the basal surface at pH 7.4. Unlike the poly-Ig receptor, this IgG receptor can shuttle back and forth.

Another IgG receptor of intermediate affinity is present on syncytiotrophoblasts. This binds to the IgG isotypes with varying affinities (IgG1 and IgG3 > IgG4 > IgG2) and is essential in permitting transplacental transfer of IgG from the mother to the foetus. This is essential in protecting the unborn child from infection at a stage when its own immune system is immature and cannot mount an effective antibody response. Maternal IgG wanes over the first six months of neonatal life, by which time the child's own IgG has reached half of the adult level.

Fc receptors and effector systems

In some cases antibodies exert their principal protective action by direct neutralization of antigens. For example, antibodies which bind to a virus's cell attachment proteins can prevent host cells becoming infected. More often though, other effector systems are recruited, such as the complement system, phagocytic cells or cytotoxic cells (Chapters 13–15). As mentioned above, immune complexes activate the complement classical pathway by binding to C1q. C1q binding to monomeric IgG is relatively weak but is greatly enhanced when binding to several Ig molecules occurs, as in an immune complex. One consequence of this is that larger complexes, particularly those formed with multivalent antigens and with high affinity antibodies of the appropriate isotype, are much more effective at fixing complement than small complexes. For example, dimers bind with K_a of $10^6 M^{-1}$ and tetramers at $3 \times 10^9 M^{-1}$. In a similar way, large complexes are more effective at binding to low affinity Fc receptors, for example on phagocytic cells, than small ones. Autoantigens frequently elicit only low affinity antibodies directed to a limited number of determinants and, consequently, the small complexes so generated are less efficiently cleared from the circulation.

There are three major types of Fcγ receptor and two Fcε receptors in humans (see below). Binding affinity of monomeric IgG to FcγRI is high ($K_a = 5.5 \times 10^8 M^{-1}$) with IgG1 and IgG3 binding more strongly than IgG4, and IgG2 being inactive. The other two Fcγ receptors are of intermediate affinity ($<10^6 M^{-1}$), and therefore bind only immune complexes effectively. The binding site for FcγRI is close to the hinge in the linking region to the C_H2 domain. This was demonstrated by site-directed mutagenesis in which the affinity of a mouse IgG2b for this receptor was increased 100-fold by substituting Glu for Leu 235. The site for FcγRII appears to be in C_H2 while that for FcγRIII requires both C_H2 and C_H3.

Considerable advances have been made recently in the characterization of different Fc receptors. There are three basic types of receptor for IgG, although these have further heterogeneity due to different forms of exon usage and membrane attachment. A summary of the better characterized Fc receptors is given in *Figure 2.9*.

FcγRI (CD64) is a high affinity receptor (K_a of approximately $5 \times 10^8 M^{-1}$) of 75kDa found primarily on macrophages. Mouse FcγRI consists of a single polypeptide chain with three extracellular domains belonging to the immunoglobulin supergene family. There is a transmembrane segment and an 84 amino acid residue cytoplasmic segment. The two N-terminal domains are related to those found in FcγRII and the entire unit appears to be encoded by a single copy gene of approximately nine kilobases. Human monocytes express several tens of thousands of these receptors, but expression may be upregulated by IFNγ.

OLSON LIBRARY
NORTHERN MICHIGAN UNIVERSITY
MARQUETTE, MICHIGAN 49855

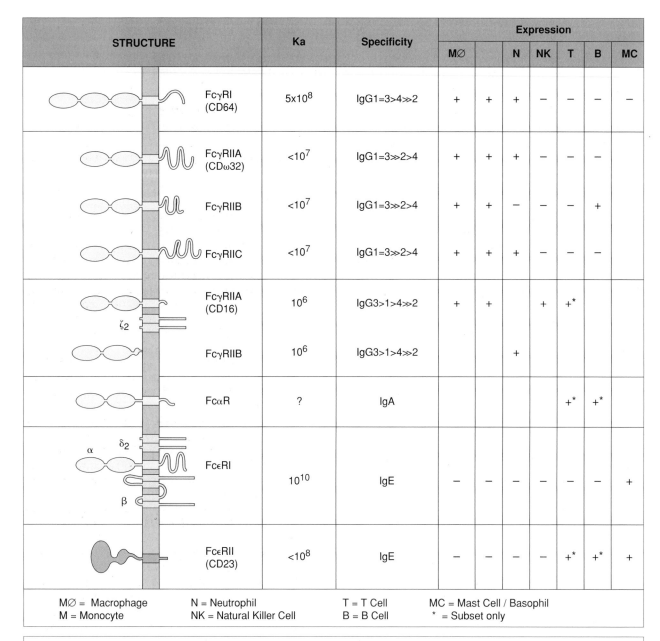

STRUCTURE	Ka	Specificity	Expression					
			MØ	N	NK	T	B	MC
FcγRI (CD64)	5×10^8	IgG1=3>4≫2	+	+	+	−	−	−	−
FcγRIIA (CDω32)	$<10^7$	IgG1=3≫2>4	+	+	+	−	−	−	
FcγRIIB	$<10^7$	IgG1=3≫2>4	+	+	−	−	−	+	
FcγRIIC	$<10^7$	IgG1=3≫2>4	+	+	+	−	−	−	
FcγRIIA (CD16)	10^6	IgG3>1>4≫2	+	+		+	+*		
FcγRIIB	10^6	IgG3>1>4≫2			+				
FcαR	?	IgA					+*	+*	
FcεRI	10^{10}	IgE	−	−	−	−	−	−	+
FcεRII (CD23)	$<10^8$	IgE	−	−	−	−	+*	+*	+

MØ = Macrophage	N = Neutrophil	T = T Cell	MC = Mast Cell / Basophil
M = Monocyte	NK = Natural Killer Cell	B = B Cell	* = Subset only

Fig. 2.9 Human Fc receptors. The diagram shows structure, properties and cellular distribution of human Fc receptors. The FcγRIII receptor on NK cells may associate with a γ or ζ dimer or a γζ heterodimer. All receptors except for the low affinity IgE receptor belong to the immunoglobulin supergene family, having 2 or 3 domain homology regions. Cell distribution: MØ = macrophage; M = monocyte; N = neutrophil; NK = natural killer cell; T = T cell; B = B cell; MC = mast cell or basophil; * = subset only; blank box = not determined.

FcγRII (CD32) is a heterogeneous low affinity receptor for IgG found on B cells, mononuclear phagocytes, granulocytes and platelets. Human FcγRII is encoded by at least three genes, designated *RIIA*, *RIIB* and *RIIC*, each of which generates a transmembrane glycoprotein belonging to the immunoglobulin supergene family and having two extracellular domains. Although the extracellular portions of these receptors are very similar, RIIA and RIIC differ considerably from RIIB in the intracytoplasmic segments. In addition, alternative splicing of RIIB can create further heterogeneity at both N- and C-termini. FcγRIIA and RIIC are preferentially expressed in phagocytic cells whereas RIIB is more prevalent in lymphocytes. In mouse there are two forms of the receptor, b1 and b2, which are related in a complex way to those in man. Transfection of the genes for the two receptors into fibroblasts indicates that b2 mediates endocytosis of complexes and their delivery to lysosomes whereas b1 does not.

FcγRIII (CD16) is a low affinity IgG receptor present on mononuclear phagocytes, granulocytes, platelets and the majority of NK cells (see Chapter 15). The form found on granulocytes (IIIB) is anchored to the membrane by a glycosyl phosphatidylinositol (GPI) link, while that on macrophages and NK cells (IIIA) is 5–7kDa larger and has a transmembrane segment. In NK cells FcγRIII is associated at the cell surface with the ζ-chain of the TCR-CD3 complex or the homologous γ-chain of the FcεRI receptor. These two forms also seem to have different functional effects, since binding of ligands to the integral membrane protein appears to signal cellular activation (see Chapter 14), whereas the GPI-anchored form on neutrophils acts as a trap for complexes.

These three Fcγ receptors, in association with the complement receptors CR1 and CR3, undoubtedly have an important role in uptake and clearance of immune complexes; the transmembrane form of FcγRIII on macrophages and NK cells is involved in triggering of cell-mediated cytotoxicity. The heterogeneity of FcγRII and its presence on B cells has lead to suggestions that it is involved in antibody-mediated control of B cell antibody secretion.

The high affinity IgE receptor, FcεRI, occurs on mast cells and basophils and is involved in binding IgE to the cell surface, where it sensitizes these effector cells for triggering by antigen. The K_a of the receptor is approximately $10^{10}M^{-1}$, which allows it to bind monomeric IgE even at the very low concentrations normally present in tissue fluids. The receptor consists of six subunits. The α1 and α2 units are exposed at the cell surface and bind to sites in the CH2 and CH3 domains of IgE. The remaining two β-chains and two disulphide-linked γ-chains are thought to be involved in signal transduction. The γ-chain has homology with the ζ-chain of the TCR–CD3 complex and can replace functionally the role of the ζ-chain in CD16 surface expression. Crosslinking of surface IgE causes an influx of Ca^{2+} which induces granule fusion with the plasma membrane and release of inflammatory mediators (see Chapter 14).

The low affinity IgE receptor, FcεRII (CD23), is found on roughly 30% of B cells and 1% of T cells. It is also present on platelets and a very small number of monocytes; a slightly different form is present on eosinophils. The receptor is a member of the family of Ca^{2+}-dependent lectins. On B cells CD23 is physically associated with CR2. Activation of B cells and macrophages by IL-4 and other cytokines causes CD23 upregulation. In transformed B cell lines, cleavage of the surface CD23 and release of a soluble form of the receptor may also occur. Soluble CD23 binds to B cells via a receptor complex formed from CD19, CD21 and CD81, which is coupled to the kinase lyn via CD19. Experimentally, soluble CD23 can modulate the proliferation of IgE producing B cells and their rate of antibody secretion. This has led to the proposal that the function of this receptor may be in controlling class switching to IgE. This suggestion is supported by an apparent increase in numbers of T cells and monocytes expressing FcεRII in individuals suffering from allergic rhinitis during the hayfever season.

A variety of less well characterized Fc receptors have been detected on subpopulations of B cells and T cells, including receptors for IgM and IgA. It is probable that these are involved in regulating the production of different antibody isotypes, although the mechanisms of action are not yet known.

T CELL RECEPTORS

Many important questions in immunology have centred around the nature of the clonally distributed receptor that mediates antigen-specific recognition by T cells. A major breakthrough occurred when the nature of the ligand for the T cell receptor (TCR) on cytotoxic T cells was defined as antigen in association with an MHC class I molecule and, soon after, MHC class II restriction was established for antigen recognition by T helper cells. However, for many years after the discovery of MHC restriction the biochemical nature of the TCR remained undefined. Early experiments claiming to demonstrate Ig-like molecules on T cell surfaces subsequently proved incorrect. As a result , two different and complementary strategies identified the genetic nature and structure of the TCR.

The initial description of the TCR at the protein level was achieved by preparing monoclonal antibodies against clonally restricted (clonotypic) determinants on human and murine T cells on the assumption that T cells should have an idiotypic part on their antigen receptors. The contention that these antibodies recognized the TCR was supported by evidence that they could inhibit, or in some cases mimic, the effect of antigen on T cells. These experiments defined immunochemically a clonally specific disulphide-linked αβ heterodimer.

Independently of these attempts to generate antibodies recognizing the TCR, putative TCR cDNA clones were isolated by subtractive or differential hybridization of cDNA libraries. Part of the predicted amino acid sequence of one such human cDNA clone was identical to the N-terminal sequence of the β-chain of the TCR purified using monoclonal antibodies. Thus, the serological and molecular approaches, whilst relying on different assumptions, had identified the same entity. Subsequently, the gene encoding the α-chain was isolated and, unexpectedly a second TCR, called γδ, was identified.

The isolation of the TCRαβ heterodimer using clonotypic antibodies capable of inhibiting or mimicking antigen, together with the demonstration that mRNA encoding these proteins is transcribed from rearranging genes, provided strong evidence that the heterodimer was responsible for antigen recognition. Conclusive proof was provided by transfection experiments in which the *TCRA* and *TRCB* genes of a T cell were shown to be sufficient to transfer the antigen/MHC recognition specificity of that T cell to other T cells.

In this chapter, the structure of the two TCRs and the organization of their genes is reviewed, and progress towards the elucidation of the function(s) and ligand(s) recognized by the TCRγδ receptor is outlined. The nature of the ligand for the TCRαβ receptor is detailed in Chapter 4.

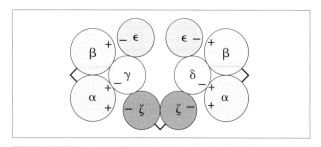

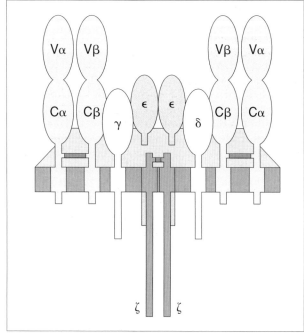

Fig. 2.10 Structure of the TCR complex. A scheme for the TCR complex is shown. The disulphide-linked αβ heterodimer, which is responsible for the specificity of each TCR, is associated with the various components of the CD3 complex (γ, δ, ε and ζ). Several lines of evidence suggest that the TCR complex exists at the T cell surface as a divalent structure. Such a stoichiometry would also neutralize the transmembrane charges of the TCR and CD3 chains. The γδ TCR complex is expected to be similar in organization to its αβ counterpart. Adapted from Terhorst *et al*, 1995.

T CELL RECEPTOR STRUCTURES

The αβ TCR

The structural features of the αβ heterodimer are presented in *Figure 2.10*. Each chain consists of two external Ig-like domains anchored into the plasma membrane by a transmembrane peptide and short cytoplasmic tail.

The structural characteristics of the Vα and Vβ regions are discussed in Chapter 3 within the context of the antigen/MHC binding site. The Ig-like constant regions comprise 87–113 amino acids and each is separated from the lipid bilayer by a short 'hinge' or connecting peptide region that contains an extra cysteine residue important in heterodimer formation. An unusual feature of both α and β-chain transmembrane regions is the presence of positively charged residues (*Fig. 2.11*). Both α and β transmembrane regions have a conserved lysine residue and the α-chain has an additional arginine and a polar asparagine residue within this region. This implies a functional significance for this region, possibly in interacting with conserved negatively charged aspartic acid and glutamic acid residues in the CD3γ, δ, ε, ζ and η transmembrane regions (*Figs. 2.10, 2.11*). Consistent with the suggestion that the TCR transmembrane regions interact with other polypeptides is the observation that this region is the most highly conserved sequence between mouse and man. The cytoplasmic tails of the TCRα and β-chains are small, comprising three to five amino acids.

The γδ TCR

An alternative form of the TCR is expressed in association with the CD3 polypeptides on some quantitatively minor populations of T cells. The overall structures of the TCRγ and δ polypeptides are similar to those of the TCRα and β-chains. Both γ and δ-chains have V and C regions with homologies to Ig domains and the transmembrane regions contain positively charged residues (two for TCRδ, one for TCRγ [*Fig. 2.11*]). Different forms of the γδ TCR exist. This is particularly evident in humans where both disulphide-linked and non-disulphide-linked forms of the receptor, which differ with respect to their γ-chain, are found. The human *TCRGC1* gene segment encodes a protein product with a cysteine residue in its connecting peptide. Hence, TCRγδ receptors with Cγ1 constant regions contain an interchain disulphide bond. In contrast, the product of the human *TCRGC2* gene lacks a cysteine residue in its connecting peptide and, consequently, γδ heterodimers with a Cγ2 region are not disulphide linked. Alleles of *TCRGC2*, which include duplication and triplication of the *TCRGC2* second exon (that encodes the connecting peptide), have been described; the use of different combinations of these exons gives rise to distinct molecular weight forms of the human γ-chain. Murine non-disulphide-linked forms of the γδ receptor have not been described, although different Cγ constant regions are encoded in the mouse genome (see below).

The CD3 polypeptides

TCRαβ and γδ heterodimers are both expressed at the cell surface in obligatory association with the CD3 polypeptides (*Fig. 2.10*). The CD3 glycoprotein is an integral part of the TCR complex, being necessary for its surface expression and function. CD3 comprises at least five polypeptide chains, termed γ, δ, ε, ζ ('zeta') and η ('eta').

The association between CD3 and the αβ or γδ clonotypic heterodimers (Ti) has been shown by co-modulation or immunoprecipitation experiments using Ti or CD3 specific antibodies. The requirement for all of the chains to be synthesized for surface expression of the functional complex in a mature T cell is evidenced by the inability of T cells lacking any one of the Ti α, β or CD3 chains to express the TCR complex; transfer of the appropriate gene

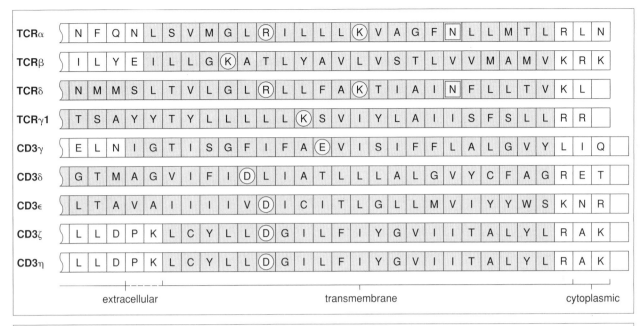

Fig. 2.11 TCR transmembrane segments. The probable transmembrane segments of the human TCR and CD3 polypeptides are shown (one letter amino acid code). For each polypeptide, the boundary between the transmembrane region and the charged cytoplasmic tail is indicated by a vertical line. TCRα, β, γ and δ-chains have short cytoplasmic tails and the C-termini are shown. CD3 chains have longer tails that are not shown. CD3ζ and its alternately spliced form, η, have the bulk of their polypeptide chains in the cytoplasm. The predicted extracytoplasmic boundary is also indicated where there is a clear cluster of hydrophilic amino acids. Charged amino acids within the bilayer are circled and the conserved asparagine residue in TCRα and TCRδ-chains is boxed.

to such cells restores surface expression. The biosynthetic details of the assembly of the chains of the TCR complex are complex and are described below.

CD3 structure

The CD3γ, δ and ε-chains are structurally related. All three chains possess an external Ig-like C domain, a transmembrane segment and cytoplasmic tail (*Fig. 2.10*). There is amino acid sequence homology among all three chains. The degree of amino acid sequence similarity between the CD3γ and δ cytoplasmic segments is particularly striking (57% identity with a further 18% conservative substitutions), although this region is very different in ε. This strong homology, and its conservation between mouse and man, suggest that the cytoplasmic domains are important in CD3 function. All three polypeptides contain a motif within their cytoplasmic domains, called a TAM (Tyrosine Activation Motif) or ARAM (Antigen Recognition Activation Motif), containing tyrosine residues that can be phosphorylated after TCR engagement. The cascade of events that ensue is detailed in Chapter 9. The evolutionary relationship between the CD3γ, δ and ε genes is supported by their genomic organization. All three genes are located within a 40kb region of chromosome 11q23 in humans and chromosome 9 in mice. This close proximity in the genome may facilitate the coordinate regulation of these genes in T cell differentiation.

An unusual feature of the CD3γ, δ and ε transmembrane peptides is the presence of a negatively charged amino acid

(*Fig. 2.11*). The location of charged amino acids within a polar transmembrane segment is generally related to the function of the protein. Several studies have shown that these residues in the CD3 chains, together with corresponding basic residues in the Ti transmembrane regions, are essential for surface expression of the TCR complex, most probably by promoting assembly of the complex. It is likely that these residues in Ti and CD3 chains form hydrogen or salt bridges within the lipid bilayer, thus stabilizing the TCR complex and permitting transport to the cell surface (*Fig. 2.12*).

The CD3ζ-chain, which is structurally unrelated to the other members of the CD3 complex, exists as a disulphide-linked homodimer. Its amino acid sequence suggests a structure distinct from those of the CD3γ, δ and ε-chains as it shows no homology to these chains nor to Ig domains. The extracellular domain is only nine amino acids long and contains a single cysteine residue responsible for ζ-chain dimerization. It is followed by a single transmembrane segment and a 113 amino acid cytoplasmic tail that contains three ARAM motifs. Like the other CD3 chains, however, the transbilayer peptide contains a single negatively charged amino acid. In a subset of αβ and γδ T cells, called intestinal epithelial lymphocytes (IEL), the FcεR1γ-chain can replace CD3ζ. The association of FcεR1γ with the remaining components of the TCR complex is probably via the transmembrane domain, which is homologous to CD3ζ.

Some murine T cells generate a CD3η-chain through alternative splicing of CD3ζ RNA. CD3η can form a disulphide-linked homodimer or with the CD3ζ-chain. A CD3η homologue has not been detected in the human.

Structure of the TCR-CD3 complex

Several lines of evidence indicate that the TCR–CD3 complex exists at the T cell surface as a higher order structure. Detailed measurements of the stoichiometry of the TCR-CD3 complex reveal that the CD3γ and δ components exist in single copies in the mature complex, whereas CD3ε is found in two copies. However, there is a 1:1 ratio of the αβ heterodimer and CD3ε molecules. Moreover, analysis of the size of the TCR complex, solubilized with non-denaturing detergents by sedimentation methods, reveals a molecular weight of about 300 000kDa. Taken together, these data point to a model for the TCR as an $(αβ)_2$, γ, δ, $ε_2$, $ζ_2$ structure. A scheme for such a structure is shown in *Figure 2.10*.

This model is consistent with the number of charged residues in the transmembrane regions of each of TCR–CD3 components. As shown in *Figure 2.10*, a divalent model for the TCR–CD3 complex would exactly match the positive and negative charges. The resulting hydrogen or salt bridges would constitute a strong force for maintaining the structure of the complex.

Biosynthesis of the TCR–CD3 complex

In mature T cells, assembly of all six polypeptides of the complex is required for efficient cell surface expression. Partial complexes fail to leave the endoplasmic reticulum and are degraded. Biosynthesis studies have revealed that CD3 complexes are initially assembled within the endoplasmic reticulum followed by addition of TCRα and β-chains in either order. CD3ζ is the last chain to assemble and dimerize prior to assembly with the αβγδε complex. It is not known where assembly of the TCR complex into a divalent structure occurs but this may also be in the endoplasmic reticulum and be rate limiting for subsequent transport through the Golgi complex to the cell surface. The details of the assembly process are summarized in *Figure 2.12*.

Incomplete cell surface TCR–CD3 complexes

Although the high level surface expression of the TCR–CD3 complex is dependent on the assembly of all six

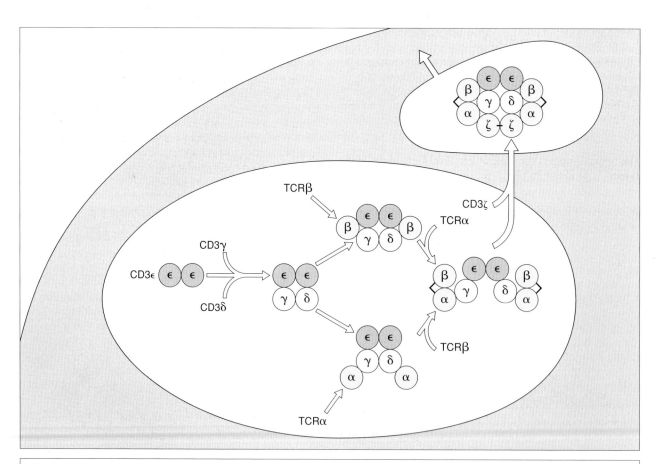

Fig. 2.12 Assembly and maturation of the TCR complex. The assembly of the components of the TCR complex occurs within the rough endoplasmic reticulum. The individual components are synthesized on membrane-bound polysomes. The CD3γ and δ polypeptides are assembled onto a CD3ε core, followed by association of TCRα and β-chains in either order. The last step in the assembly process is the assembly of CD3ζ. The whole TCR complex is transported through the Golgi cisternae, where modifications to the glycan units occur and thence to the cell surface. Partial complexes are degraded intracellularly.

components, low level expression of incomplete complexes has been observed in thymocytes at different stages of maturation. A low level of surface CD3 is expressed on prothymocytes prior to rearrangement of *TCRA* and *B* genes. Immature thymocytes expressing CD3 and TCRβ polypeptides express a pre-TCR complex comprising CD3γδε and TCRβ-chains together with an additional component called the 'surrogate α-chain' or pTα; CD3ζ is loosely associated with this complex. The existence of variant complexes on immature thymocytes but not on mature T cells presumably reflects the existence of different chaperone proteins that regulate the balance between assembly, degradation and transport of the various complexes. The physiological significance of these variant complexes for thymocyte differentiation is discussed in Chapter 6.

GENOMIC ORGANIZATION

A systematic and rational nomenclature for TCR gene segments has now been officially devised. The names for the genetic loci (*A, B, G, D*) and genetic elements (*V, D, J, C*) are self-explanatory. *S* refers to gene segments and refers to the member of a particular family. *V* regions from the *TCRA/D* locus are named *A* or *D* for gene segments used exclusively by TCRα or TCRδ chains, or *AD* when the same *V* region can be used by both α and δ. This nomenclature is used here. The chromosomal locations of the TCR loci are summarized in *Figure 2.13*.

The TCRA/TCRD locus

The organization of the murine *Tcr-A/D* locus is shown in *Figure 2.14*. This locus is unique amongst antigen receptor gene loci in that the genes encoding the TCRα and δ-chains are intermingled.

The human and murine *TCRA* loci each consist of a single *TCRAC* gene segment separated from the *AV* region by an extended cluster of *TCRAJ* gene segments. The human and murine *TCRDC-AJ-AC* region has been completely·sequenced (corresponding to about 100kb of DNA for each sequence) and shown to contain 61 human and 50 murine *TCRAJ* segments, respectively. Additional pseudo *J* gene segments were also identified. The *TCRDV* segments are interspersed with

Gene	Chromosomal location	
	human	mouse
αδ	14q11	14C-D
β	7q32	6B
γ	7p15	13A2-3

Fig. 2.13 Chromosomal location of TCR genes. The positions of the three TCR loci on human and mouse chromosomes are shown. Metaphase spreads of chromosomes can be divided into morphologically identifiable regions by staining procedures. Human chromosomes are divided into bands (11, 32, 15 etc.) on arms (p-short arm or q-long arm) either side of the centromere. Murine chromosomes, which do not have an easily identifiable centromere, are classified into bands A, B etc. Localization of genes to regions of chromosomes is carried out by *in situ* hybridization or by use of murine–human somatic cell hybrids.

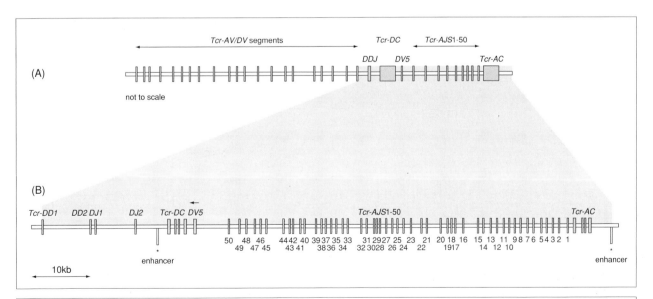

Fig. 2.14 Genomic organization of the murine *Tcr-A/D* locus. The locations of the *Tcr-A* and *D* gene segments are shown. The region between the *D* segments of the *Tcr-D* locus and the *Tcr-AC* region has been completely sequenced and the positions of the recognizable *Tcr-AJ* regions are shown. A *Tcr-A* enhancer has been located 3' of the *Tcr-AC* segment. A *Tcr-D* enhancer has been identified within the *Tcr-DJ2-DC* intron. Adapted from Gascoigne *et al*, 1995.

the *TCRAV* segments, and several *V* genes can be used by both α and δ-chains. There are probably about 100 *V* gene segments in the *TCRA/D* locus, although the exact number is not known. The majority of *TCRAV/DV* genes fall into families of several members (as defined by primary sequence similarity). The human *TCRAV/DV* locus consists of at least 30 families ranging from one to 10 members. A similar degree of complexity has also been observed for the murine *Tcr-AV/DV* locus. A genomic linkage map of the *Tcr-AV* elements from the BALB/c mouse strain has been established and has revealed that the region has arisen as a result of several rounds of gene duplication. Genomic analysis of different mouse strains has revealed significant polymorphisms with five different haplotypes being identified.

The *TCRB* locus

The genomic organization of the murine *Tcr-B* locus is shown in *Figure 2.15*. There are approximately 25 murine *Tcr-BV* genes extending over about 450kb of DNA located about 300kb upstream of the *Tcr-BD-J-C* region. One *Tcr-BV* gene, *V14*, is located downstream of *Tcr-BC2* in the opposite transcriptional orientation. The majority of murine *Tcr-BV* genes are single member families, the exception being *V5* and *V8* families which have multiple members. There are four known haplotypes of the murine *Tcr-B* locus that differ in both point mutations and the total number of *V* (and, in one case, *D-J-C*) genes.

There are about 60 known human *TCRBV* sequences that can be grouped into 25 families. About half of these families contain a single member, with the remainder being multi-membered and having probably evolved by tandem duplication. One family is located on chromosome 9, although these *V* genes are not functional (so called orphan genes). This, together with other pseudogenes within the main *TCRBV* locus, limits the functional human *TCRBV* gene repertoire to 52 genes. However, additional variability in the basic *TCRBV* repertoire derives from polymorphism of germline genes.

Comparison of the organization of the human and murine *TCRB* loci has revealed extensive similarities in this region between the two sequences. The major difference between the two loci is that the human gene complex is larger due to the repeated tandem duplication of *V* families containing multiple members.

The human and murine *TCRBD*, *J* and *C* genes are each comprised of two very similar clusters. Each *C* gene segment is associated with one *D* element and with a cluster of *TCRBJ* gene segments. The human locus contains six *TCRBJ1* and seven *TCRBJ2* genes, all potentially functional. In contrast, each murine *Tcr-BJ* cluster contains six functional segments and one pseudogene. *D* segments are 12–14bp long and *J* segments around 50bp, with particularly homologous 3' ends encoding conserved residues of structural importance within the variable domain. The coding regions of the two murine *TcrBC* genes show a remarkable degree of homology both to each other and to their human homologues. The few

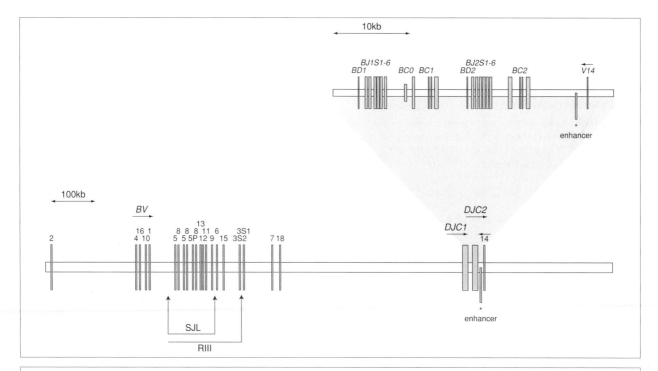

Fig. 2.15 Genomic organization of the murine *Tcr-B* locus. The positions of the various gene segments are shown. The transcriptional orientations of the *Tcr-BV* genes are indicated by arrows. The exon structure of the *Tcr-BC* gene segments is also shown. The *BCO* exon is found in some murine cDNA clones. The positions of *Tcr-BV* region deletions (▲) in the SJL and RIII mouse strains are indicated. Adapted from Gascoigne *et al*, 1995.

amino acid differences between *TCRBC1* and *BC2* genes are not conserved in position in mouse and man, suggesting that these changes are not of functional importance. In this context, no differential usage of *BC1* and *BC2* regions has been observed in different T cell subsets.

The TCRG locus

HUMAN *TCRG* GENES

The murine and human *TCRG* loci differ significantly in organization. The arrangement of the human *TCRG* genes is shown in *Figure 2.16*. The entire region has been mapped and the *V* and *C* regions linked on a 160kb DNA fragment. The locus is composed of two *C* gene segments separated by 16kb of DNA, each associated with *J* gene segments. At least 14 *TCRGV* segments are shared by the two *TCRGJ-C* clusters. No *D* segments have been found within the *TCRG* locus.

The *TCRGC* gene segments encode the Ig-like C domain, transmembrane region and cytoplasmic tail of the γ polypeptide. In some individuals the *TCRGC2* gene segment has a duplication or triplication of the second exon that encodes the peptide connecting the Ig-like C domain to the transbilayer peptide, although there is no known significance in these differences.

The *TCRGJ* gene segments encode 16–20 amino acids of the γ-chain variable domain. Five *J* segments have been identified, two associated with *TCRGC2* and three with *TCRGC1*. Each of the *J* segments can theoretically be rearranged with any of the *V* genes.

Sixteen human *TCRGV* gene segments, comprising four pseudogenes, have been identified. *TCRGV* genes can be divided into three families, called *GV1*–*GV3*. There is only about 30% homology between the different subfamilies at the protein level. Analysis of *V* usage in several TCRγδ expressing T cell lines, clones and populations has suggested some bias in *GV* gene expression (see below).

MURINE *TCR-G* GENES

The murine *Tcr-G* locus is the most completely mapped of any of the TCR loci. The *Tcr-G* locus from BALB/c mice is shown in *Figure 2.17*. It comprises four *V-J-C* clusters extending over about 205kb in an arrangement reminiscent of the Ig lambda genes.

Four *Tcr-GC* genes are present, each associated with a single *J* gene segment, and rearrangement of the *Tcr-GV* genes is limited to the *J* segments within the same cluster. The *Tcr-GC1* gene is associated with four *V* gene segments (*V2*–*V5*), which

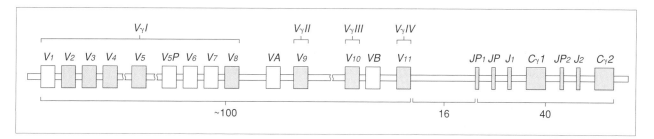

Fig. 2.16 Genomic organization of the human *TCRG* locus. The positions of the various gene segments and their genomic distances are shown. The *V* genes, some of which are pseudogenes (unshaded), are clustered over about 100kb and are divided into four subgroups. The *V10* and *V11* genes may not encode functional γ chains due to a lack of splicing of the leader intron of the signal sequence. All *V* genes are in a 5' → 3' transcriptional orientation with respect to the *C* gene segments. The exon-intron structure of the coding blocks is not shown. The nomenclature is that used by Lefranc *et al*, 1986. *JP* does <u>not</u> denote a pseudogene *J* segment but refers to three *GJ* segments identified subsequent to *J1* and *J2*.

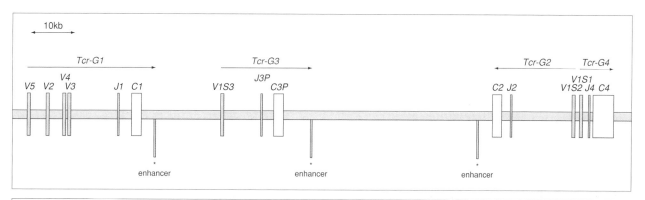

Fig. 2.17 Genomic organization of the murine *Tcr-G* locus. Four constant gene segments, and associated *V* and *J* segments have been identified. *Tcr-G3* is part of a pseudogene complex and is only present in some strains of mice. The transcriptional orientation of *Tcr-VG* genes is shown by arrows. Adapted from Gascoigne *et al*, 1995.

are expressed differentially by γδ T cells residing in different anatomical sites (see below). The *Tcr-GC3* gene is associated with a single *V* gene, although both *Tcr-GC3* and *J3* are pseudogenes, and this region is deleted from some mouse strains. The *Tcr-GC2* and *C4* clusters are each associated with one *V* gene, the *Tcr-GC2* cluster being in opposite transcriptional orientation to the rest of the *Tcr-G* locus.

REGULATION OF TCR GENE EXPRESSION

The transcription of TCR genes is controlled, in common with other eukaryotic genes, by promoter, enhancer and silencer elements. Promoters, located at transcriptional start sites, are required for the correct initiation of transcription. Enhancers, located anywhere in or around a gene, increase the level of transcription initiated from a promoter. Silencers, like enhancers, can act at a distance, but negatively affect transcription initiation from a linked promoter.

Regulatory elements associated with each of the TCR genes have been identified. Enhancer elements are located 3' of the *TCRAC*, the *BC2* and the *GC1* gene segments. The *TCRD* gene is unique in that its enhancer is located within the *J-C* intron. Promoter elements, which require the presence of the appropriate enhancers for significant transcriptional activity, have been characterized at the 5' end of the *V* gene segments. It should be emphasized, however, that additional elements that are necessary for correct temporal and tissue-specific expression *in vivo* of the TCR genes most probably exist.

Various *cis*-acting elements (segments of DNA that bind transcription factors) have been identified within the TCR gene promoters and enhancers. Protein binding sites have been located and the identities of several of the enhancer binding proteins have been established. Taken together, these studies have revealed a number of transcriptional factors that play key roles in regulating TCR gene transcription. These include the GATA, Ets and TCF-1/LEF-1 families that contain members restricted in expression to lymphoid cells. Other factors that bind to these enhancers, such as the CREB/ATF family, have a more ubiquitous pattern of expression. The specific properties of each enhancer depend on the precise combination of tissue-specific and ubiquitous transcription factors that bind and their interactions with one another and with the basal cellular transcriptional machinery. The organization of the *TCRB* gene enhancer is summarized schematically in *Figure 2.18*.

Silencer elements have been identified as part of the regulatory apparatus of the *TCRA* and *G1* genes. These elements have been most completely characterized in the *TCRA* locus where they are within the enhancer region and may be responsible for downregulation of *TCRA* gene transcription in γδ T cells. It is possible that silencer elements within TCR enhancer regions form the major level of regulation of TCR genes. The core enhancers may be equally active in all T, or possibly all lymphoid cells, and silencers may be required to restrict the expression of the TCR genes.

The regulatory elements associated with TCR genes probably control gene rearrangement (see Chapter 3) in addition to transcription, possibly by initiating transcription around the rearranging elements, thereby disrupting the nucleosomal packaging of TCR genes and allowing accessibility of these regions to the recombinase machinery. Thus, further characterization of TCR regulatory elements will allow insight into the control of both TCR transcription and rearrangement, and into the developmental switching events that establish the programme of gene activity observed in mature T cells.

DISTRIBUTION OF αβ AND γδ TCRs

The distribution of the two forms of the TCR on different T cell populations is shown in *Figure 2.19*. The TCRαβ receptor is present on the vast majority of T cells, being found on >95% of peripheral T cells and over 50% of thymocytes from adult mice. The differentiation and surface phenotypes of TCRαβ expressing thymocytes are discussed in detail in Chapter 7. Most peripheral T cells that express TCRαβ are single positive for CD4 or CD8. A small percentage, however, have a double negative phenotype. γδ T cells are usually less abundant than αβ T cells, comprising about 1–10% of T cells in the systemic circulation, spleen and lymph nodes of humans, mice and chickens. However, in sheep, γδ T cells comprise about 30% of peripheral blood T cells. The bulk of the TCRγδ subset is double negative; a small proportion expresses the CD8 antigen, and an even smaller proportion the CD4 antigen. CD8 expression is largely confined to those γδ T cells residing in the small intestine (see below). These γδ T cells are about 80–90% CD8 positive.

T cells expressing the γδ receptor often have defined anatomical locations (*Fig. 2.19*). Although γδ T cells form minor proportions of the T cells in the thymus and secondary lymphoid organs, they are abundant at various epithelia such as the epidermis (in mice but not humans), intestinal epithelium, uterus and tongue. Indeed, in the skin, essentially all the intraepithelial lymphocytes are γδ⁺.

Murine *Tcr-GV* and *DV* gene expression

The various anatomically distinct TCRγδ expressing T cell subsets can be further distinguished on the basis of their TCRs, both in *V* region expression and the degree of TCR diversity. This has been most extensively studied in mice (*Fig. 2.19*). Murine adult thymocytes express highly diverse γδ TCRs as a result of expressing multiple combinations of *Tcr-GV* and *DV* gene segments, although they preferentially utilize *V4J1* and *V7J1* *Tcr-G* genes which exhibit junctional deletions and *N* region diversity. In contrast, junctional diversity and gene segment usage are much more limited in *Tcr-GV* and *DV* genes expressed by foetal or newborn thymocyte populations. TCRγδ receptors on foetal thymocytes appear in at least two distinct waves, distinguished by *Tcr-G* and *D* gene segment usage, during development. The first wave peaks around the 15th day of gestation, and subsides by the 17th day, and expresses V5J1Cγ1 and V1DJ2Cδ chains. The second wave of γδ thymocytes starts at around foetal day 17, peaks at birth and declines thereafter, and expresses V6J1Cγ1 and V1DJ2Cδ chains.

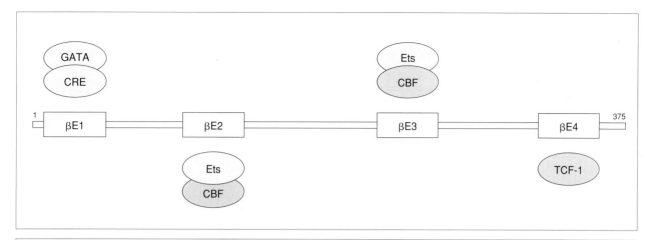

Fig. 2.18 Structure of the human TCRβ enhancer. This enhancer, located 3' to the *TCRBC2* gene segment, has been defined using reporter constructs (in which expression of a gene encoding an easily assayable product, such as chloramphenicol acetyl transferase, is driven by the regulatory elements being analysed) and transient transfection assays. At least four regions that bind to transcription factors have been identified over about 350bp. The families of transcription factors that bind to these regions and that have been shown to affect (in some cases) enhancer activity are shown.

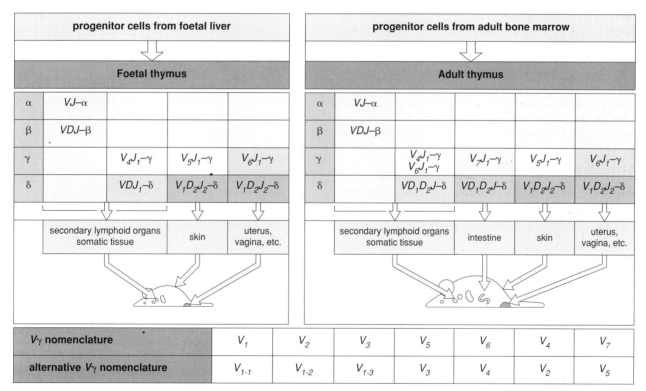

Fig. 2.19 *V* gene usage and tissue localization of murine TCRαβ and γδ receptors. Progenitor cells enter the thymus from the major sites of foetal or adult haematopoiesis. The expression of various populations of foetal and adult thymic γδ cells expressing the Cγ1 region are shown. Based on Vγ and Vδ expression, these waves probably give rise to TCRγδ cells in different anatomical locations. The split during development of the γδ and αβ T cell lineages is discussed in Chapter 6. The nomenclature used is that proposed by Tonegawa, (see, for example, Bonneville *et al*, 1988). An alternative form (Allison and Raulet, 1990), sometimes used in the literature, is shown in the lower part of the figure. This latter nomenclature corresponds to the genetic nomenclature shown in *Figure 2.17*.

The γδ T cells residing in various epithelia express γδ TCRs that are characteristic of a particular epithelium (*Fig. 2.19*). Most gut intraepithelial lymphocytes (IELs) express primarily the *V7J1GC1* gene. Although some junctional diversity is created within the *Tcr-G* gene, the main variability in the γδ TCRs of IELs is a result of the high degree of variability in the δ subunit. The genes encoding the δ subunits can use one of many *Tcr-DV* segments (although *V4, V5, V6* and *V7* predominate) and both *Tcr-DD* segments. They also utilize *Tcr-DD* gene segments in all three reading frames, exhibit *N* region diversity at most junctions and show imprecise joining of *Tcr-DV* and *J* gene segments.

In contrast to the diversity of the IEL γδ receptor, the receptors expressed by dendritic epidermal cells (DECs) and γδ expressing cells in the mucosal epithelia of uterus, vagina and tongue are remarkably homogeneous. DECs express one receptor combination (V5J1Cγ1 and V1D2J2Cδ chains). Very little N region diversity is seen and the *Tcr-DD2* segment is used alone. TCRγδ cells from reproductive tissues and tongue also express a unique receptor, although this differs from that expressed by DECs in that the same *Tcr-D* rearrangement is paired with a *Tcr-GV6-J1* rearrangement (*Fig. 2.19*).

Human *TCRGV* and *DV* gene expression

The *V* region expression of human γδ T cells has been less extensively studied. Much of the available information has been obtained using monoclonal antibodies recognizing Vγ9, Vδ1/Jδ1 or Vδ2 regions or indirectly by Southern hybridization analysis. Two main populations of peripheral blood γδ T cells can be distinguished, according to the presence of the Cγ1 or Cγ2 constant regions associated with certain V regions. Most peripheral blood γδ TCRs expressing Cγ1 have V9-JP V regions. V9-JP-Cγ1 chains are frequently expressed with Vδ2-D-Jδ1-Cδ chains. In Cγ2 expressing γδ T cells, there is no preponderance of a unique *TCRGV* gene, although those of subgroup *V1* are preferentially used. V9-J2 combinations are rarely expressed. Vδ1-D-Jδ1 chains are frequently expressed in association with V1-Jγ2 on Cγ2 expressing γδ T cells.

Only about 10% of the CD3 positive cells in the human gut epithelium are TCRγδ positive. The proportion of γδ IELs increases in patients with untreated coeliac disease and this increase is almost entirely due to γδ T cells expressing Vδ1. In contrast, γδ expressing IELs are abundant in the mouse (30–70% of IELs). This species difference is probably due to amplification of the gut αβ T cell population by antigenic stimulation in humans. In germ-free mice 95% of IELs are γδ positive, which drops to 30–50% if the mice are given a bacterial flora. A large fraction of human γδ IELs express Vδ1-D-Jδ1 chains. Interestingly, Vδ1 is the predominant V region expressed in the thymus.

TCRγδ expressing T cells are also found at unusually high levels in T cells isolated from the joint fluid of patients with juvenile rheumatoid arthritis. These cells may be involved directly in the injury process or may have been activated (because they respond to IL-2) as a result of heat shock proteins released by tissue injury (see below).

DEVELOPMENT OF γδ T CELL SUBSETS

The developmental relationships of the various γδ subsets have been most extensively studied in mice. The combination of γ and δ-chains utilized by the γδ cells in the tongue and reproductive organs is the same as that expressed in the first wave of foetal γδ thymocyte development, and γδ-expressing DECs express the same receptor as that expressed by the second wave of foetal γδ cells (*Fig. 2.19*). These identities support a precursor–product relationship between the early and late waves of foetal thymic γδ expressing T cells and the vaginal γδ TCR expressing T cells and DECs, respectively. By the same argument, IELs and γδ T cells in peripheral lymphoid organs such as spleen and lymph node may be derived from adult thymocytes which express diverse receptors with the same pattern of V, D and J gene segment usage and junctional diversity (*Fig. 2.19*). Studies with athymic (*nu/nu*) mice have suggested that there may be an extrathymic pathway of maturation for some γδ expressing T cells. Thy1 negative TCRγδ expressing T cells are present in 'nude' mice, especially in the intestine, while Thy1 positive TCRαβ expressing T cells are very uncommon.

The distinct receptor combinations of DECs and IELs suggest a mechanism for the compartmentalization of these γδ subsets: namely, that the distinct γδ receptors determine their homing specificities. Experiments using transgenic mice expressing predetermined TCRs have, however, ruled out this idea. For example, mice in which most γδ T cells express Vγ4/Vδ5 TCRs (most frequently used by adult γδ thymocytes) contain DECs and IELs expressing the Vγ4/Vδ5 receptor. Similarly, in transgenic mice expressing a Vγ5/Vδ1 receptor (expressed on most DECs) normal levels of γδ cells are present in IELs. These data demonstrate that TCRγδ receptors *per se* are not homing receptors for specific epithelia.

γδ T CELL FUNCTION

The distinct anatomical location of γδ T cell subsets has promoted the idea that these cells have an immunological function distinct from those of αβ T cells. In this context one striking observation has been the capability of γδ T cells to recognize heat shock proteins (hsps) and non-classical MHC class I genes. However, it is not yet clear that lymphoid and epithelial γδ T cells share a common function.

The epithelial location of γδ T cells has given rise to the idea that they represent a 'first line of defence' against invading pathogens. The limited TCR repertoire displayed by IELs suggests that they recognize a limited set of antigens. These may include exogenous peptides, such as *N*-formylated peptides of bacteria and autoantigens such as hsps or non-classical class I MHC antigens (for example, murine Tl or human CD1 antigens) that are expressed at high levels in epithelial sites such as the gut, epithelium or the epidermis.

The γδ T cell resident in murine skin, the dendritic epidermal T cell or DEC, is so called because it adopts a dendritic morphology that allows it to contact essentially all the epidermal melanocytes and keratinocytes. DECs, which express a single γδ TCR, can be stimulated *in vitro* to produce IL-2 by co-culture with autologous keratinocytes and this recognition is enhanced when the keratinocytes are heat shocked.

This recognition is not MHC-restricted and may involve antigen presentation by non-classical MHC class I antigens.

The junctional diversity expressed by gut γδ T cells suggests that these cells recognize multiple antigens. Clearly, the gastro-intestinal tract provides a first site of contact with an extensive array of pathogens, in particular, bacteria and one possibility is that IELs recognize predominant pathogen-derived antigens such as prokaryotic N-formylated peptides that have been shown to be presented by non-classical class I antigens. Alternatively, γδ IELs may recognize hsp proteins or hsp peptides presented on non-classical class I antigens.

A broad spectrum of specificities has been defined for lymphoid γδ T cells (i.e. those cells present in blood, spleen or lymph nodes). Thus, human lymphoid γδ T cells have been reported to recognize antigens as diverse as tetanus toxoid restricted by class II MHC, mycobacterial antigen restricted by CD1b and human hsp60 restricted by non-conventional antigens. Murine lymphoid γδ cells can respond to a peptide from mycobacterial hsp65, Tl antigens and a glutamate-tyrosine peptide restricted by Qa-1. Although there is little evidence that γδ T cells *en masse* recognize peptides presented by conventional class I or class II MHC, there does appear to be a relatively high precursor frequency towards hsp60 among murine and human γδ T cells. However, the nature of the response to hsp60 peptide is unclear, although it is not conventionally MHC restricted. For example, human hsp60-reactive γδ T cells can react to hsp60 on Daudi cells, which lack β_2-microglobulin. A key question is whether the observed hsp reactivity of lymphoid γδ cells has any relevance for protection against bacterial infection. In support of such a role, increased numbers of γδ T cells are present in the lymph nodes of areas draining sites infected with *Mycobacterium tuberculosis*, and in humans there are increased numbers of γδ T cells in *Mycobacterium*-associated lesions.

The general conclusion, in so far as one may be drawn from these extensive and diverse studies, is that γδ T cells may play a role in anti-microbial responses, although the nature of the ligands recognized by this TCR remains contentious. A major stumbling block in the analysis of this T cell population has been the difficulty in assaying γδ T cell responses against a background of αβ T cells. A real prospect that the functions of γδ T cells can soon be resolved is provided by the recent development, through gene targeting, of mice lacking either αβ or γδ T cells. For example, mice singly deficient for either αβ or γδ T cells were found to be as resistant to primary infection with *Listeria monocytogenes* (an intracellular bacterium that replicates inside mononuclear phagocytes and hepatocytes) as wild-type mice, whereas mice deficient for both αβ and γδ T cells were extremely sensitive to the disease. In secondary infections, however, αβ T cells gave considerably more protective immunity than γδ T cells. Similar experiments have shown the γδ T cells play a role in immunity against the live stages of infection with *Plasmodium yoelii* parasites, the causative agents of rodent malaria. Studies such as these should help us to understand the role of γδ T cells and the evolutionary advantage for the existence of two distinct TCRs in vertebrates.

SUMMARY

Antibodies are bifunctional molecules which bind antigen via their V domains and can interact with effector systems via their C domains. Antigen binding occurs by the formation of multiple non-covalent bonds between residues in the hypervariable regions of antibodies and those in the antigen. The antibody's binding site forms a complementary surface to that of protein antigens, in which charge neutralization and hydrogen bonding are particularly important. Small hapten antigens often bind in clefts in the binding site.

The exons for the heavy chain V domains are generated during B cell development by a process of somatic recombination between V, D and J gene segments, while light chain V domains are formed from V and J segments only. There are large numbers of V genes, but smaller numbers of D and J genes and the recombined region forms the third hypervariable loop of the V domains. The recombined V domain gene becomes linked to C domain exons during mRNA splicing. There are a number of different C genes, each one corresponding to a particular immunoglobulin isotype. At different stages of B cell development the recombined V exon can become linked to C genes for different classes. This process of class switching can be effected either by differential mRNA splicing of long primary transcripts, or by a second series of recombinations affecting the C genes.

The process of antibody formation and diversification is reflected in the diversity of antibodies found in serum and on B cells. Each antibody can be producd in a membrane or secreted form and different classes of antibodies subserve different functions in the immune response by interacting with Fc receptors on cells and/or with the complement system. IgM and most IgG isotypes activate complement. Secreted IgA is particularly important in protecting mucosal surfaces. IgG can interact with Fcγ receptors on mononuclear phagocytes and granulocytes, facilitating uptake of immune complexes and interaction of some cytotoxic cells with their targets. IgE is important in the control of inflammation, due to its ability to sensitize mast cells and basophils.

TCRs are the products of four rearranging genes, called A, B, G and D. Two forms of TCR exist. The TCR expressed on the majority of T cells comprises a disulphide-linked αβ heterodimer in non-covalent association with the CD3 antigen. The TCRγδ receptor is expressed on a minority of T cells, often associated with epithelial tissues. The TCRαβ receptor recognizes processed antigen, in the form of peptides, associated with MHC class I or class II antigens. The role of antigen processing and presentation by MHC or other molecules in recognition by the TCRγδ receptor remains to be determined. However, many γδ T cells respond to heat shock antigens and some may recognize class I-like (Tl, Qa, CD1) antigens.

The TCR genes are located at three loci: A/D, B and G. Each gene comprises V, D (for TCRB and D), J and C segments that rearrange in a somatic T cell. The TCR loci have been extensively characterized as part of the various genome mapping projects. Promoter and enhancer elements within the loci regulate both rearrangement and transcription.

FURTHER READING

Allison JP, Raulet DH. The immunobiology of γδ+ T cells. *Sem Immunol* 1990, **2**:59.

Alzari PM, Lascombe MB, Poljak RJ. Three-dimensional structure of antibodies. *Ann Rev Immunol* 1988, **6**:555.

Arden B, Clark SP, Kabelitz D, Mak TW. Human T cell receptor variable gene segment families. In *T Cell Receptor Genes*. Bell JI, Owen MJ, Simpson EL (Eds). Oxford University Press: Oxford; 1995:285

Asarnow DM, Goodman T, LeFrancois L, Allison JP. Distinct antigen receptor repertoires of two classes of murine epithelium-associated T cells. *Nature* 1989, **341**:60.

Bandeeira A, Mota-Santos T, Itohara S, Degermann S, Heussser C, Tonegawa S, Coutinho A. Localization of γδ T cells in the intestinal epithelium is independent of normal microbial colonization. *J Exp Med* 1990, **172**:239.

Bedzyk WD, Herron JN, Edmundson AB, Voss EW. Active site structure and antigen binding properties of idiotypically cross-reactive anti-fluorescein monoclonal antibodies. *J Biol Chem* 1990, **165**:133.

Bhat TN, Bentley GA, Boulot G, Greene MI, Tello D, Dall'Acqua W, Souchon H, Schwarz FP, Mariuzza RA, Poljak RJ. Bound water molecules and conformational stabilization help mediate an antigen-antibody association. *Proc Nat Acad Sci USA* 1994, **91**:1089.

Bonneville M, Itohara S, Krecko EG, Mombaerts P, Ishida I, Katsuki M, Berns JT, Farr AG, Janeway CA, Tonegawa S. Transgenic mice demonstrate that epithelial homing of γδ T cells is determined by cell lineages independent of T cell receptor specificity. *J Exp Med* 1990, **171**:1015.

Bonneville M, Janeway CA, Ito K, Haser W, Ishida, I, Nakanishi N, Tonegawa S. Intestinal intraepithelial lymphocytes are a distinct set of γδ T cells. *Nature* 1988, **336**:479.

Boulot G, Bentley GA, Karjalainen K, Msriuzza RA. Crystallization and preliminary X ray diffraction analysis of the β-chain of a T-cell antigen receptor. *J Mol Biol* 1994, **235**:795

Brenner MB, MacLean J, Dialynas DP, Strominger JL, Smith JA, Owen FL, Seidman JG, Ip S, Rosen F, Krangel MS. Identification of a putative second T cell receptor. *Nature* 1986, **332**:145.

Brooks DG, Qiu WQ, Luster AD, Ravetch JV. Structure and expression of human IgG FcRII CD32. Functional heterogeneity is encoded by the alternatively spliced products of multiple genes. *J Exp Med* 1989, **170**:1369.

Burton DR. Structure and function of antibodies. In *Molecular Genetics of Immunoglobulin*. Calabi F, Neuberger MS (Eds). Elsevier Science Publishers; 1987.

Capra JD, Tucker PW. Human immunoglobulin heavy chain genes. *J Biol Chem* 1989, **264**:12745.

Chien Y-H, Gascoigne NRJ, Kavaler J, Lee NF, Davis MM. Somatic recombination in a murine T cell receptor gene. *Nature* 1984, **309**:322.

Chien Y-H, Iwashima M, Kaplan KB, Elliot JF, Davis MM. A new T cell receptor gene located in the alpha locus and expressed early in T cell differentiation. *Nature* 1987, **327**:677.

Clevers H, Alarcon B, Wileman T, Terhorst C. The T cell receptor/CD3 complex: a dynamic protein ensemble. *Ann Rev Imm* 1988, **6**:629.

Clevers H, Oosterwegel MA, Georgopoulos K. Transcription factors in early T cell development. *Immunol Today* 1993, **14**:591.

Colman PM. Structure of antibody-antigen complexes: Implications for immune recognition. *Adv Immunol* 1988, **43**:99.

Conrad DH. FcεRII CD23: The low affinity receptor for IgE. *Ann Rev Immunol* 1990, **8**:623.

Cronkhite R, Schulze D, Cerny J. Regulation of idiotope expression. IV. Genetic linkage of two D region-dependent T15 idiotopes to the IgH allotype. *J Immunol* 1989, **142**:568.

Davie JM, Seiden MV, Greenspan NS, Lutz CT, Bartholow TL, Clevinger BL. Structural correlates of idiotopes. *Ann Rev Immunol* 1986, **4**:147.

Davies DD, Sheriff S, Padlan EA. Antibody-antigen complexes. *J Biol Chem* 1988, **263**:10541.

Davis AC, Shulman MJ. IgM — Molecular requirements for its assembly and function. *Immunol Today* 1989, **10**:118.

Dembic Z, Haas W, Weiss S, McCubrey J., Kiefer H, von Boehmer H, Steinmetz M. Transfer of specificity by murine α and β T-cell receptor genes. *Nature* 1986, **320**:232.

Duncan A R, Woof J M, Partridge L J, Burton D R, Winter G. Localization of the binding site for the human high affinity Fc receptor on IgG. *Nature* 1988, **332**:563.

Eilat D, Hochberg M, Tron F, Jacob L, Bach J-F. The *Vh* gene sequences of anti-DNA antibodies in two different strains of lupus-prone mice are highly related. *Eur J Immunol* 1989, **19**:1241.

Fudenberg HH, Pink JRL, Wang AC, Ferrara GB. The genetics of immunoglobulin molecules. In *Basic Immunogenetics,* edn 3. Oxford University Press: Oxford; 1984.

Gascoigne NRJ. Genomic organization of the T cell receptor genes in the mouse. In *T Cell Receptor Genes*. Bell JI, Owen MJ, Simpson EL (Eds). Oxford University Press: Oxford; 1995:270

Gascoigne NRJ, Chien Y-H, Becker DM, Kavaler J, Davis MM. Genomic organization and sequence of T cell receptor β-chain constant and joining region genes. *Nature* 1984, **310**:387.

Getzoff ED, Tainer JA, Lerner RA. The chemistry and mechanism of antibody binding to protein antigens. *Adv Immunol* 1988, **43**:1.

Gritzmacher CA. Molecular aspects of heavy chain class switching. *CRC Crit Rev Immunol* 1989, **9**:173.

Haas W, Pereira P, Tonegawa S. Gamma/Delta cells. *Ann Rev Immunol* 1993, **11**:637.

Happ MP, Kubo RT, Palmer E, Born WK, O'Brien RL. Limited receptor repertoire in a mycobacteria-reactive subset of γδ T lymphocytes. *Nature* 1989, **342**:696.

Haba S, Lascombe MB, Poljak RJ, Nisonoff A. Structure of idiotopes associated with anti-phenylarsonate antibodies expressing an intrastrain cross-reactive idiotype. *J Exp Med* 1989, **170**:1075.

Harriman W, Völk H, Defranoux N, Wabl M. Immunoglobulin class switch recombination. *Ann Rev Immunol* 1993, **11**:361.

Havran W, Chien Y-H, Allison JP. Recognition of self antigens by skin-derived T cells with invariant γδ antigen receptors. *Science* 1991, **252**:1430

Hay FC. The generation of diversity. In *Immunology*, edn 4. Roitt IM, Brostoff J, Male DK (Eds). Mosby Yearbook: London; 1995:6.2

Hayday AH. γδ T cell specificity and function. In *T Cell Receptor Genes*. Bell JI, Owen MJ, Simpson EL (Eds). Oxford University Press: Oxford; 1995:70.

Hedrick SM, Cohen DI, Nielsen EA, Davis MM. Isolation of cDNA clones encoding T cell specific membrane associated proteins. *Nature* 1984, **308**:149.

Holoshitz J, Koning F, Coligan JE, de Bruyn J, Strober S. Isolation of CD4 and CD8 mycobacteria-reactive T lymphocyte clones from rheumatoid arthritis synovial fluid. *Nature* 1989, **339**:226.

Honjo T, Alt FW, Rabbitts T (Eds). *Immunoglobulin Genes*. New York: Academic Press; 1989.

Itohara S, Farr AG, Lafaille JJ, Bonneville M, Takagaki Y, Haas W, Tonegawa S. Homing of a γδ thymocyte subset with homogeneous T cell receptors to mucosal epithelia. *Nature* 1990, **343**:754.

Itohara S, Mombaerts P, Ladaille J, Iacomini J, Nelson A, Clarke AR, Hooper ML, Farr A, Tonegawa S. T cell receptor delta mutant mice: independent generation of αβ T cells and programmed rearrangements of γδ T cell receptor genes. *Cell* 1993, **72**:337.

Jung S, Rajewsky K, Radbruch A. Shutdown of class switch recombination by deletion of a switch region control element. *Science* 1993, **259**:984.

Koshland ME. The coming of age of J chain. *Ann Rev Immunol* 1985, **3**:425.

Kyes S, Carew E, Cardingm SR, Janeway CA, Hayday AC. Diversity in T cell receptor γ gene usage in intestinal epithelium. *Proc Natl Acad Sci USA* 1989, **84**:5527.

Koop BF, Hood L. Striking sequence similarity over almost 100 kilobases of human and mouse T cell receptor DNA. *Nature Genet* 1994, **7**:48.

Lai E, Concannon P, Hood L. Conserved organization of the human and murine T cell receptor β gene families. *Nature* 1988, **331**:543.

Lefranc MP, Forster A, Baer R, Stinson MA, Rabbitts T. Diversity and rearrangement of the human T cell rearranging γ genes. Nine germline variable genes belonging to two subgroups. *Cell* 1986, **45**:237.

Leiden JM. Transcriptional regulation of T cell receptor genes. *Ann Rev Immunol* 1993, **11**:539.

Levy R, Assulin O, Scherf T, Levitt M, Anglister J. Probing antibody diversity by 2D NMR: comparison of amino acid sequences, predicted structures and observed antibody-antigen interactions in complexes of two anti-peptide antibodies. *Biochem* 1989, **25**:7168.

Metzger H, Alcaraz G, Hohman R, Kinet J-P, Pribluda V, Quarto R. The receptor with high affinity for immunoglobulin E. *Ann Rev Immunol* 1986, **4**:419.

Modlin RL, Pirmez C, Hofman FM, Torigan V, Uyemura K, Rea TH, Bloom BR, Brenner MB. Lymphocytes bearing antigen specific γδ T cell receptors accumulate in human infectious lesions. *Nature* 1989, **339**:544.

Mostov KE. Transepithelial transport of immunoglobulins. *Ann Revs Immunol* 1994, **12**:63.

Padlan EA, Silverton EW, Sheriff S, Cohen GH, Smith-Gill SJ, Davies DR. Structure of an antibody-antigen complex: crystal structure of of the HyHEL-10 Fab-lysozyme complex. *Proc Nat Acad Sci USA* 1989, **86**:5938.

Philpot K, Viney JL, Kay G, Rastan S, Gardiner EM, Chae S, Hayday CA, Owen MJ. Lymphoid development in mice congenitally lacking T cell receptor αβ expressing cells. *Science* 1992, **256**:1448.

Raulet DH. How γδ T cells make a living. *Curr Biol* 1994, **4**:246.

Ravetch JV, Kinet J. Fc receptors. *Ann Rev Immunol* 1991, **9**:457.

Rose DR, Strong RK, Margolies MN, Gefter ML, Petsko GA. Crystal structure of the antigen-binding fragment of the murine anti-arsonate monoclonal antibody 36-71 at 2.9A resolution. *Proc Nat Acad Sci USA* 1990, **87**:338.

Sarvas H, Rantonen N, Makela O. Allotype-associated differences in the concentration of human IgG subclasses. *J Clin Immunol* 1991, **11**:39.

Sears DW, Osman N, Tate B, McKenzie IF, Hogarth PM. Molecular cloning and expression of the mouse high affinity receptor for IgG. *J Immunol* 1990, **144**:371.

Selvaraj P, Carpen O, Hibbs ML, Springer TA. Natural killer cell and granulocyte FcγRIII CD16 differ in membrane anchor and signal transduction. *J Immunol* 1989, **143**:3283.

Sperling AI, Bluestone JA. The first line of defence? *Curr Biol* 1993, **3**:294.

Staudt LM, Lenardo MJ. Immunoglobulin gene transcription. *Ann Rev Immunol* 1991, **9**:373.

Takagaki Y, deCloux A, Bonneville M, Tonegawa S. Diversity of γδ T cell receptors on murine intestinal intra-epithelial lymphocytes. *Nature* 1989, **339**:712.

Terhorst C, Simpson S, Wang B, She J, Hall C, Huang M, Wileman T, Eichmann K, Holländer G, Levelt C, Exley M. In *T Cell Receptor Genes*. Bell JI, Owen MJ, Simpson EL (Eds). Oxford University Press: Oxford; 1995:347.

Walker MR, Lund J, Thompson KM, Jefferis R. Aglycosylation of human IgG1 and IgG3 monoclonal antibodies can eliminate recognition by human cells expressing FcγRI and FcγRIII receptors. *Biochem J* 1989, **259**:347.

Wilson RK, Koop BF, Chen C, Halloran N, Sciammis R, Hood L. Nucleotide sequence analysis of 95kb near the 3' end of the murine T cell receptor α/δ chain locus: strategy and methodology. *Genom* 1992, **13**:1198

Yancopoulos GD, Alt FW. Regulation of the assembly and expression of variable region genes. *Ann Rev Immunol* 1986, **4**:339.

3 The Generation of Diversity

A hallmark of the immune system is its ability to recognize the extensive collection of antigens to which the organism is exposed during its lifetime. The B and T cell repertoires are anticipatory; that is, appropriate receptors exist prior to encountering antigen.

The basis for the diverse repertoire of B and T cell receptor specificities resides in the organization of their genes. The variable regions of antibodies and T cell receptors (TCRs) are encoded by multiple gene segments (Chapter 2) that rearrange during B and T cell development. It is this rearrangement process that generates most of the antigen receptor diversity. The repertoires are subsequently modified according to the constraints of MHC restriction (for the TCR) and tolerance to self-antigens, as discussed in detail in Chapters 7 and 13. This chapter describes the mechanisms used to generate diversity of recognition by the immune system in terms of antigen receptor gene rearrangement and the structure of the receptor binding sites.

Most (but not all) of the genetic mechanisms for the generation of diversity are common to B and T cells. However, the relative contribution made by each mechanism varies between the two receptor systems, resulting in differences both in the extent of diversity and the location of diversity within the binding site. The extreme example of this is the variation of diversity within the different TCRγδ expressing subsets described in Chapter 2.

PROTEINS INVOLVED IN ANTIGEN RECEPTOR GENE REARRANGEMENT

The recombination activating genes, *RAG-1* and *RAG-2*

The precise mechanism of *V-D-J* recombination, although extensively studied, remains a mystery. However, several components that are involved in the process have been identified. In particular, the products of two genes, called *RAG-1* and *RAG-2*, are able to initiate rearrangement of recombination substrates in non lymphoid cells that are normally lacking in this activity.

The *RAG-1* gene was initially identified by transfection experiments in which genomic DNA was transfected into a fibroblast cell line harbouring a recombination substrate integrated into the genome. By monitoring the quantitative rearrangement during multiple rounds of transfection, a genomic clone was isolated encoding the *RAG-1* gene. A closely linked gene, *RAG-2*, was also identified within 8kb of *RAG-1*, which synergized with *RAG-1* in this assay.

Although *RAG-1* and *RAG-2* clearly fulfil a central role in *V-D-J* recombination, their function remains unknown. They may encode the lineage-specific components of the V-D-J recombinase or, alternatively, they may activate the recombinase in some way. Whatever the precise role of *RAG-1* and *RAG-2*, their coordinated expression in early B and T cells is essential for the rearrangement of antigen receptor genes. Thus, RAG-1 and RAG-2 transcripts are detected in immature lymphocytes but expression ceases in mature peripheral blood lymphocytes (PBLs) that express B or T cell receptors. More compellingly, gene disruption of either *RAG-1* or *RAG-2* genes in mice by homologous recombination prevents *V-D-J* recombination at any TCR or Ig locus.

Other proteins implicated in the recombination process

A number of other factors have been implicated in *V-D-J* recombination. The best characterized is the enzyme terminal deoxynucleotidyl transferase (TdT) that mediates *N* nucleotide addition to the coding joints (see below). Thus, mice with a disrupted *TdT* gene show no *N* region diversity in their antigen receptor genes. However, *V-D-J* recombination is unaffected by the failure to express TdT. Other activities implicated in the recombination include proteins that bind to the heptamer–nonamer recombination sequences (see below) and the factor rendered defective by the *scid* mutation. The *scid* gene product is essential for the processing of TCR and Ig gene coding junction intermediates but also has a more general role in the repair of DNA damage in addition to being part of the V-D-J recombinase machinery.

The Ku autoantigen has also been implicated in *V-D-J* recombination. This protein, which is a relatively abundant nuclear protein that associates with the DNA-dependent protein kinase, DNA-PK, is defective in a complementation class of mutant cells that are defective for both repair of X-ray-induced double-strand DNA breaks and *V-D-J* recombination. Transfection of the Ku gene restored both of these activities in these cells.

In conclusion, several proteins have been identified as playing a role in the various activities associated with the *V-D-J* recombination process. *RAG-1* and *RAG-2* clearly play a key role, although their exact function is unclear. Other factors, such as Ku, appear to link some of the components that mediate *V-D-J* recombination to the cellular machinery that responds to DNA damage.

ANTIGEN RECEPTOR GENE REARRANGEMENT

The similarity of the genetic organization of the B and T cell receptors suggests that the same rearrangement mechanism exists in each case. There is strong evidence that both TCR and Ig gene rearrangements share the same

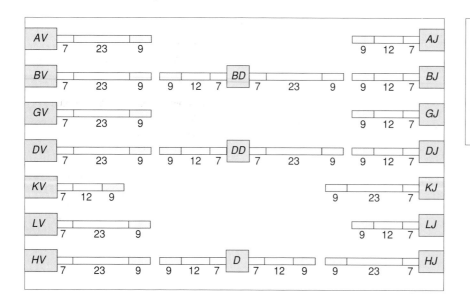

Fig. 3.1 TCR and Ig gene rearrangement recognition sequences. The arrangement of the heptamer (7bp), nonamer (9bp) and spacer sequences (12bp or 23bp) relative to the rearranging antigen receptor gene segments is shown.

enzymatic machinery. Thus, recombinant plasmids containing *BD* and *BJ* segments can rearrange as readily as *IGHD-J* elements when introduced into pre-B cell lines (in which endogenous TCR genes are not rearranged) and both TCR and Ig gene rearrangements are abolished in *RAG-1* and *RAG-2* knockout mice.

Recombination substrates

The TCR and Ig *V, D* and *J* gene segments are flanked by conserved recombination signal sequences (RSSs). The arrangement of these sequences is summarized in *Figure 3.1*. All RSSs, whether associated with Ig or TCR genes, have one of two overall consensus sequences: a heptamer and an A/T rich nonamer which are separated by a non-conserved spacer of either about 12 or 23 nucleotides. The '12–23' rule, first postulated to explain Ig gene rearrangement, also governs TCR gene recombination. Thus, RSSs with a 12bp spacer may recombine only with a 23bp spacer and vice versa.

The precise arrangements of RSSs flanking the various gene segments will determine which rearrangement combinations are possible. Thus, *IGHV* genes can recombine only with *D* segments, which in turn can recombine only with *J* segments. In contrast, the principle of the '12–23' rule allows for multiple rearrangement combinations at the *TCRB* and *D* loci. At the *TCRB* locus, *V-J*, *V-D-J* and *V-D1-D2-J* rearrangements are all formally allowed. Moreover, the *D1* segment can recombine with either *TCRBJ* cluster. At the *TCRD* locus, the same combinations as for the *TCRB* locus are formally possible. In addition, *VA* segments can recombine with *TCRDD* or *J* and *TCRDV* segments with *TCRAJ*. Although such rearrangements are allowed by the '12–23' rule, the *V* regions produced may be unable for structural reasons to associate with a partner or to form a functional combining site. However, direct *TCRBV* to *J* joining has been observed in a few cases and *TCRDV-D1-D2-J* joining is a frequent occurrence. The consequences for the generation of diversity at TCR and Ig loci are discussed below.

An additional rearrangement event has been described within the human TCRD locus. This rearrangement event joins a 5' element, called δrec, located 1kb upstream of *TCRDJ1*, to a pseudo-*TCRAJ* element about 10kb 3' of the *TCRDC* segment. This rearrangement is mediated by the Ig/TCR recombination sequences, the 5' element being associated with a 23kb spacer and the 3' element with a 12bp spacer. This recombination results in the deletion of the *TCRD* locus and may contribute to allelic exclusion in TCRαβ expressing cells (for a fuller discussion of allelic exclusion of TCRs, see Chapter 7).

Rearrangement mechanisms

The most common mechanism of gene rearrangement involves deletion of the intervening DNA segments. A plausible scheme for the steps involved in the recombination process is shown in *Figure 3.2*. It is likely that joining occurs by a two-step non-reciprocal recombination in which the first event is a precise double-stranded break between the elements to be joined and their flanking sequences. In a second step, the coding elements are joined in an imprecise event in which bases are often lost from one or both coding partners or added between the coding segments (see below). In addition to the joint formed between the various coding gene segments, circular DNA comprising the deleted intervening DNA including the two RSSs has also been isolated from thymocytes undergoing *V-D-J* recombination. The two RSSs in the DNA circles are fused in a head to head fashion at their respective heptamer sequences without any junctional variation. However, the deletion mechanism alone does not account for all rearrangements observed. For example, murine *Tcr-BV14* and *D5* gene segments are located 3' to their respective *C* genes, in the reverse orientation and are rearranged by inversion instead of deletion.

Analysis of the junctional diversity associated with *V-D-J* recombination provides insights into the process itself. The loss of nucleotides from the ends of the gene segments is presumably due to the action of exonucleases. The gain of nucleotides is due both to template-independent and

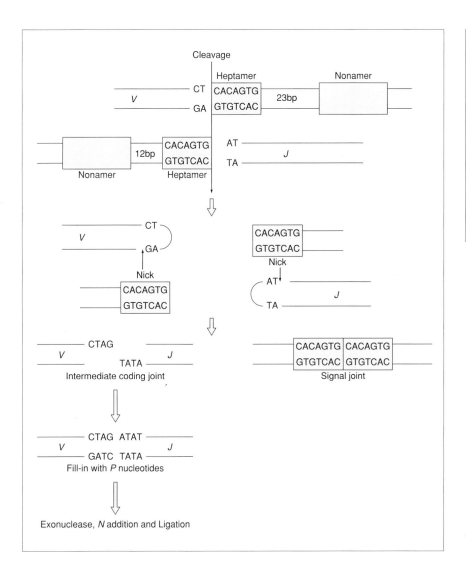

Fig. 3.2 A mechanism for antigen receptor gene recombination. After cleavage at the RSSs, hairpin loop intermediates are formed at the coding ends. After nicking and filling in, *P* nucleotides are generated. The precise length of *P* nucleotides depends upon the site of nicking. Exonuclease digestion and *N* nucleotide addition, followed by ligation, form the coding joint. Taken from Prosser and Tonegawa, 1995.

dependent mechanisms. The enzyme TdT is responsible for adding *N* nucleotides to the 3' end of the coding strands in a random pattern prior to joining. In contrast, *P* nucleotides are added in a template-dependent fashion. This form of junctional diversity was first identified in foetal thymic γδ T cells that are relatively homogeneous in TCR junctional sequences. *P* nucleotides, found at the coding joints, are complementary to the last bases of the coding end and form one half of a palindromic sequence. The existence of *P* nucleotides has led to a model for template-dependent nucleotide addition in which nucleotides are transferred from one strand to the other via intermediate hairpin loop structures which are subsequently nicked and filled in. The coding strands are then subjected to exonuclease digestion and *N* nucleotide addition prior to ligation to form the coding joint. In many cases, exonuclease digestion masks the existence of *P* nucleotides, although evidence for their existence has been found for other antigen receptor loci where no nucleotide loss has occurred.

The postulated mechanism for the recombination process involving intermediate hairpin loops is consistent with the *scid* mutation. Analysis of the coding joints from the *scid* thymus revealed the existence of DNA strands joined at the coding end in a hairpin loop structure. Thus, the *scid* mutation appears to block the processing of the coding joint intermediate structures, resulting in their accumulation within thymocytes.

GENETIC MECHANISMS FOR DIVERSITY GENERATION

The structure and organization of Ig and TCR genes have been described in Chapter 2. In a somatic B or T cell, gene rearrangements occur such that a *V* region coding block is generated from variable (*V*), diversity (*D*), for *TCRB*, and joining (*J*) gene segments. This rearrangement forms the basis of the generation of receptor diversity. The major mechanisms that produce variability in polypeptide *V* regions are listed in *Figure 3.3*. It is the interplay and relative importance of these various mechanisms that determine the extent and structural diversity of the B and T cell receptor repertoires.

Multiplicity of *V*, *D* and *J* gene segments

Clearly, the multiplicity of *V*, *D* and *J* gene segments makes an important contribution to the generation of

Mechanism		B	T
Multiple germline segments		+	+
Combinatorial association		+	+
Combinatorial joining	V–D–J	+	+
	V–J	–	+
	D–D	–	+
Somatic mutation	junction flexibility	+	+
	N–region diversity	+	+
	somatic hypermutation	+	–
	D joining in all three reading frames	–	+

Fig. 3.3 Mechanisms for the generation of antigen receptor diversity in B and T cells. The various genetic mechanisms that generate diversity are listed, with + indicating their use by *IGH* and *TCRB* genes as examples. 'Somatic mutation' is a generic heading referring to any means of introducing or removing nucleotide sequence in a somatic T or B cell.

		Ig		TcrAB		TcrGD	
		H	*K*	*A*	*B*	*G*	*D*
Germline segments	variable (*V*)	250–1000	250	100	25	5	10
	diversity (*D*)	10	0	0	2	0	2
	joining (*J*)	4	4	50	12	4	2
Variable region combinations		62 500–250 000		2500		50	
Junctional diversity	usage of different *D* and *J* segments	yes	yes	yes	yes	–	yes
	variability in 3' joining of *V* and *J*	rarely	rarely	yes	no	yes	yes
	D joining in all three reading frames	rarely	–	–	often	–	often
	N-region diversity	V-D D-J	none	V-J	V-D D-J	V-J	V-D D1-D2 D1-J
Junctional combinations		~10^{11}		~10^{15}		~10^{18}	
Total repertoire		~10^{16}		~10^{17}		~10^{19}	

Fig. 3.4 Diversity in TCR and Ig genes. The numbers of the *V*, *D* and *J* gene segments in the murine genome are given, together with estimates for the degree of variation produced by the various mechanisms for generating diversity. The estimates for diversity within the junctional region are derived from combinatorial joining of *V*, *D* and *J* regions, *N* region addition of up to six nucleotides at each junction, variability in the 3' joining position in *V* and *J* gene segments and translation of *D* regions in different reading frames. The total repertoire was calculated by multiplying the number of junctional combinations by the number of variable region combinations.

diversity. The magnitude of the contribution is a function of the numbers of these gene segments in the germline. This is shown for murine TCR and Ig *V*, *D* and *J* gene segments in *Figure 3.4*. The human *TCRAV* and *BV* repertoires are estimated to be similar to those of the mouse. However, the human *TCRGV* locus is larger than its murine equivalent, possessing 14 *TCRGV* genes (belonging to four subgroups), six of which are pseudogenes. The extent of the human *TCRDV* repertoire is unknown but at least six human genes have been described. Estimates of the TCR and Ig *V* gene repertoire were originally obtained by a combination of experimental approaches: analysis of genomic clones containing *V* or *D* gene segments, analysis of *V* gene usage in lymphocyte cDNA libraries and Southern hybridization analysis using cloned *V* gene probes at low stringency. However, these estimates are necessarily approximate. The current mapping and sequencing assault on the human and mouse genomes will eventually produce an accurate picture of the numbers of the various Ig and TCR gene segments. This has already been accomplished for the human and murine *TCRAJ* region, which has been completely sequenced and for the human *IGHV* locus. A map of this latter region, spanning about 1100kb and which accounts for almost all *VH* segments known to rearrange in B cells, has been completed. Approximately 50 functional *VH* segments have been located within the region mapped, although the exact number depends upon the haplotype.

A further complication in the measurement of *V*, *D* and *J* repertoires is the existence of pseudogenes. Relatively few *TCRV* pseudogenes have been detected. However, pseudogenes may comprise as many as 30% of *VH* genes. For example, the recently established physical map of the human *VH* locus reveals at least 29 pseudo-*VH* genes out of a total of 89. Although *V* pseudogenes cannot contribute directly to antigen receptor diversity, they may do so indirectly by providing a reservoir of diversity which can be utilized by unequal recombination or gene conversion. This has been demonstrated as the major contributor to *VH* and *VL* diversity in the chicken, where the heavy chain and λ loci both contain a single functional *V* and *J* segment. The heavy chain locus also contains about 15 *D* segments. Adjacent to both functional *V* segments are a series of pseudo *VH* and *VL* gene segments that contribute to diversity by a somatic gene conversion-like process. The heavy chain gene conversion mechanism also operates within the *D* region; all of the *VH* pseudogenes that have been analysed are fused *VD* elements. Gene conversion involving pseudogenes may also be important in the generation of new functional *V* gene segments during evolution.

V genes are classified into families on the basis of sequence homology. Six main human *VH* families (having 1–20 segments each) have been classified, with family members sharing at least 70% homology. Members of the different families are interspersed throughout the locus. *TCRV* genes are also grouped into families, with at least 25 *TCRBV* (comprising at total of 63 unique gene segments) and 28 *TCRAV* families defined. Human and murine *TCRDV* genes are interspersed with *AV* genes and in both species there is evidence for some (but not extensive) sharing of the repertoire, i.e. a few *TCRDV* genes are used in either type of receptor structure.

A number of inbred mouse strains have been found to have deletions of large portions of the *Tcr-BV* locus, some strains lacking about half the *BVs* (Chapter 2). The survival of these mice does not appear to be a consequence of the limited number of pathogens to which laboratory mice are exposed, since wild mice have also been shown to have a surprisingly uneven distribution of the TCR repertoire. Many of the wild mice analysed were homozygous for large deletions in the *Tcr-BV* locus, encompassing as many as 12 of the known *BVs*. It has been suggested that *Tcr-BV* gene deletion may confer a survival advantage. Such an advantage might operate due to the deleterious effects of some bacterial toxins that act as powerful *Tcr-BV* family-specific T cell-stimulating superantigens in mouse and man. These toxins probably exert their pathogenic effects by inducing massive cytokine release as a result of interactions with a high proportion of TCRs. Thus, failure to express *Tcr-BV* regions that recognize the superantigen would increase resistance to the toxin.

An additional contribution to the generation of diversity has been observed in some CD5 (Ly1⁺) murine pre-B cell lines and B cell lymphomas, involving the complete replacement of the functional *VH* gene by another *VH* gene. This replacement probably involves an isolated heptamer sequence (homologous to that found as part of the heptamer–nonamer motif) at the 3' end of the *VH* coding sequence. This heptamer sequence is conserved within most *VH* but not *VK* or *VL* genes. Quantitatively, this mechanism plays a minor role in the generation of antibody diversity.

The multiplicity of *D* and *J* gene segments increases diversity associated with the third hypervariable region (see below). The *TCRA* locus has a particularly large number of *J* segments and the *IGH* locus is rich in *D* regions compared to the other loci.

The *V* gene segments of the antigen receptor loci encode the first and second hypervariable regions of the binding site. The relatively limited structural diversity encoded by the functional *V* segments underscores the requirement for additional ways of generating diversity. Important among these are the various combinatorial mechanisms.

Combinatorial diversity

The ability of *V*, *D* and *J* gene segments to combine together randomly introduces a large element of combinatorial diversity into the Ig and TCR repertoires. There is some evidence, however, that functional *V* and *J* segments do not have an equal probability of contributing to the primary (that is, unselected) set of antibody specificities. Analysis of Abelson murine leukaemia virus-transformed murine pre-B cell lines, foetal liver hybridomas and adult bone marrow has shown that the more *JH*-proximal *VH* genes are used preferentially in the newly generated antibody repertoire. However, this bias is not maintained in the mature B cell population, where the relative expression of *VH* gene families correlates approximately with their size, suggesting that antigen selection is just as likely to expand clones using *JH*-distal *VH* genes as those which are more prevalent in the virgin B cell population. A comparison of the primary *Vh* repertoire with the utilization of *Vh* gene segments by polyclonally (LPS) activated mouse spleen cells has demonstrated that certain *Vh* families are heavily under-represented relative to their estimated germline gene number. These families must either have large proportions of nonfunctional genes or be influenced by regulatory mechanisms or constraints on rearrangement.

Junctional diversity

The probable mechanism of *V-D-J* joining has been discussed above. The precise point at which *V*, *D* and *J* gene segments join can vary, giving rise to local amino acid diversity at the junction. An example of the local amino acid diversity created by flexibility in *TCRBD* to *BJ* recombination is shown in *Figure 3.5*. The exact nucleotide position of joining can differ by as much as 10 residues, resulting in deletion of nucleotides from the ends of the *V*, *D* and *J* gene segments and, therefore, producing codon changes at the junctions of these segments. A consequence of this rather imprecise joining process is that on average two out of three rearrangements will be out-of-phase or non-productive because the joining has occurred in different translational reading frames. During the rearrangement process additional nucleotides not encoded by either gene segment can be added at the junction between the joined gene segments, generating *N* region diversity.

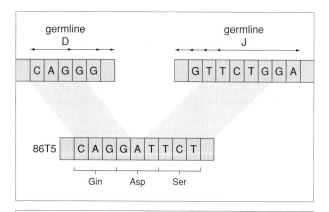

Fig. 3.5 Diversity created during recombination. The diagram illustrates the recombinational event between the *TCRBD* segment and the *BJ* segment which has occurred in T cell receptor clone 86T5, derived from the germline sequences indicated above. The GAT codon which encodes aspartate is derived from one nucleotide 3' to the *D* gene segment, one nucleotide 5' to the *J* gene segment, and from an additional nucleotide (A) inserted during the recombinational event (*N* region diversity). The arrows show positions in which rearrangements to these germline *BD* and *BJ* segments have occurred in other T cells. The same *D* and *J* gene segments may, thus, generate different amino acid sequences following recombination.

Junctional diversity of TCRs greatly exceeds that of Igs. This is true for both αβ and γδ forms of the TCR. For example, *N* region diversity has been observed in all four TCR polypeptides but only in Ig heavy chains. This is one of the most significant components of the increased junctional diversity in TCRs. Several *TCRA, G* and *DV* genes have been shown to be flexible with respect to the position of their 3' joining positions, a phenomenon that has not been seen with Igs. The variability in *D* region usage also increases the available diversity of TCRs. Because of the arrangement of the 12/23 recognition sequences surrounding the two *TCRBD* and two *DD* segments, both *D* segments can be used individually or in tandem, or they can be omitted altogether by direct *V* to *J* joining. The ability to use both *D* regions has been observed in adult T cell δ-chain cDNAs and β-chain cDNA clones with direct *V* to *J* joins have been isolated. The junctional heterogeneity in TCR β and δ-chains commonly results in the translation of *D* region sequences in all three possible reading frames. This is rare in Ig heavy chains. The contribution of junctional diversity to the murine TCRδ repertoire is shown in *Figure 3.6.*

The extensive junctional flexibility of TCR and Ig *V, D* and *J* joining concentrates variability within the CDR3-equivalent region, which comprises the *D* and/or *J* regions and the last few amino acids of the *V* region. The implications of this for models of the TCR binding site are discussed below.

Combinatorial association

In principle, any *V* region should be able to combine with its partner (i.e. *VH* with *VL*, *AV/DV* with *BV/GV*). Studies of Igs of known three dimensional structure have shown that certain amino acids are essential for association of the two *V* regions. These same amino acids are present in similar locations in all TCR and Ig *V* regions that have been sequenced. However, in at least some cases, Ig or TCR *V* regions fail to associate with sufficient affinity to mediate allelic exclusion or to reach the cell surface. For example, Igκ producers have occasionally been found to have productive *VK-JK* rearrangements on both alleles; only one of the two κ proteins produced will bind to the H chain present in the cell to form surface Ig. Although such selectivity in combinatorial association of functional *V* regions will clearly decrease the primary Ig or TCR repertoire its effect is likely to be minor, with most *V* regions able to associate with their partners.

Somatic hypermutation

The effect of somatic hypermutation on diversity appears to be specific to Igs. This mechanism is operational at a late stage in B cell development and generates single base mutations throughout the *VH* or *VL* gene segment and its flanking sequences. It thus has the effect of increasing both junctional and *VH-VL* combinatorial diversity. Somatic hypermutation is the basis of the increase in antibody affinity for an antigen which occurs during the maturation of an immune response (see Chapter 10). This can be shown most readily by studying the antibody response to haptens, in which a single *Vh-Vl* combination is often used in the primary response. The availability of hybridomas, all presumably derived from a single antibody-producing B cell clone making such antibodies, has made it possible to compare the sequences of large numbers of closely related antibodies that arise during the course of the immune response in a single animal. The diversity created by somatic hypermutation in the immune response to the hapten dinitrophenol (NP), in which the predominant germline gene utilized by C57BL/6 mice is *VH186.2*, is shown in *Figure 3.7.* Somatic hypermutation of rearranged *IGV* genes generates high affinity antibodies which, particularly under conditions of limiting antigen, enable the antibody-producing B cell to be amplified selectively within a germinal centre. Other mutations will, of course, decrease the affinity or remove reactivity altogether. However, lack of selection will delete these clones during the immune response.

Somatic hypermutation probably occurs only during a brief time in B cell differentiation. Analysis of the accumulation of mutations throughout the *V* region and its flanking sequences has led to calculations of mutation rates as high as 10^{-3} to 10^{-4} changes per base pair per cell division; this contrasts with spontaneous mutation rates of 10^{-7} or less. The molecular mechanism responsible for this high mutation rate and its regulation during B cell development is not known. A number of mechanisms have been proposed, including an error prone repair process utilizing either a specialized DNA polymerase or reverse transcription (i.e. via an RNA intermediate) and gene conversion. Identification of the mechanism will probably require the generation of cell lines that carry out somatic hypermutation *in vitro.*

Element	DV		N1	D1	N2	D2	N3		DJ
Nucleotide range			0–6	2–11	0–6	4–16	0–6		
Permutations	5		5461	55	5461	91	5461		6
Total sequence diversity				2.5×10^{16}					

Fig. 3.6 Murine *Tcr-D* gene junctional diversity. Each element that contributes to the *Tcr-D* junctional (CDR3-equivalent) region is shown. The nucleotide range shows the number of nucleotides possible for each element and the number of permutations allowed, assuming random nucleotide usage, is calculated. For example, the permutations for the *N* regions, with any combination of 0–6 of the four different nucleotides, is given by $4^0+4^1+4^2+4^3+4^4+4^5+4^6 = 5461$. The numbers under the *Tcr-DV* and *J* elements refer to the variation in the joining position for these gene segments. Data taken from Davis and Bjorkman, 1988 and references therein.

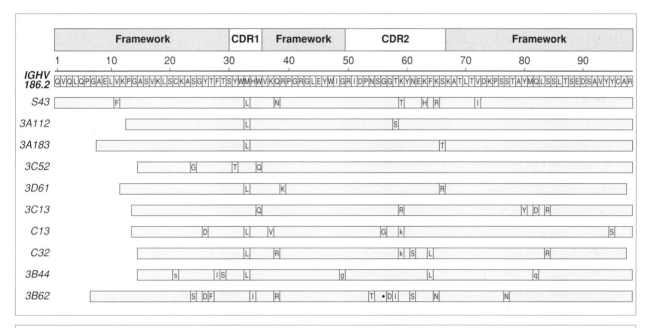

Fig. 3.7 Somatic hypermutation during the murine anti-NP immune response. The amino acid sequence encoded by the germline gene *VH186.2*, the predominant gene of the anti-NP response in C57BL/6 mice, is shown on the top line. Below are sequences of V regions encoded by hypermutated genes. Mutations are seen to cluster around the CDR1 and CDR2 regions indicated. Silent nucleotide mutations are indicated by lower case letters. A deletion at position 56 of 3B62 is indicated by a dot. Taken from Maizels, 1989.

THE SIZE OF THE PRIMARY B AND T CELL REPERTOIRES

Based on the various mechanisms for generating diversity, an estimate of the potential repertoire size can be calculated. One such calculation for murine TCR and Ig repertoire sizes is shown in *Figure 3.4*. This estimate, although only approximate, clearly shows that TCR and Ig genes are capable of generating much more diversity than could be accommodated by the total number of lymphocytes in any one mouse. However, the primary repertoire will be differentially reduced in individuals by the phenomena of MHC restriction and B and T cell tolerance. The calculation shown in *Figure 3.4* illustrates several features of the repertoire. The contribution to diversity made by the *V* gene segments, that encode the first two hypervariable regions (CDR1 and CDR2) of Igs and their equivalents in TCRs, is relatively small. In contrast, diversity within the junctional region is extensive. The estimate of the size of the junctional diversity shown in *Figure 3.4* encompasses usage of different *D* and *J* gene segments, *N* region addition of up to six nucleotides at each junction, variability in the 3' joining position in *V* and *J* gene segments and translation of *D* regions in different reading frames.

The TCRγδ repertoire forms an extreme example of the contribution of junctional diversity. Few germline Vγ Vδ combinations are possible; however, the extensive junctional combinations particularly of the *TCRD* gene generate a primary repertoire of the same order, or greater, than that of Ig or TCRαβ.

Somatic hypermutation, which increases both junctional and *VH-VL* combinatorial diversity, will further increase the Ig repertoire size. It is difficult to estimate the contribution of this mechanism but it will probably increase the B cell repertoire by at least two orders of magnitude.

STRUCTURE OF IG AND TCR BINDING SITES

The primary Ig and TCR repertoires generate a formidable amount of amino acid sequence diversity. However, the extent to which this translates into useful diversity of receptor structures depends on the nature of the TCR and Ig antigen binding sites. The three dimensional structures of a number of immunoglobulins and also of some antibody–antigen complexes, have been determined by X-ray crystallographic analysis. Therefore, the structures of Ig antigen binding sites are known at atomic resolution. The three dimensional structure of a TCR binding site has not yet been determined, although a structure for an isolated Vβ domain has been solved. In the absence of firm X-ray crystallographic data, Ig structures have been used as a basis for the modelling of the evolutionarily related TCR.

The Ig binding site

It is well established that the hypervariable loops (CDRs) of the V_H and V_L domains form the walls of the antigen binding site. When the combining site of an Ig molecule is viewed from the direction of the antigen the first and second CDRs on V_L are separate from their counterparts on V_H and the space between them is occupied by the two CDR3 regions. A schematic diagram showing the relative positions of the six loops is shown in *Figure 3.8*. Most of the residues at the V_L–J_L, V_H–D_H and D_H–J_H junctions are on the surface and in the centre of the combining site in positions to interact with a bound antigen.

Studies of a number of antigen–antibody complexes have produced a picture of the antibody–antigen interface. The quaternary structures of several lysozyme–Fab complexes have shown that little conformational change occurs to either antigen or antibody upon association. The overall picture of the antigen–antibody interface is that of two irregular, rather flat surfaces with protuberances and depressions that fit with the complementary features of the other. In the complex between the Fab fragment of the antibody D1.3 and hen egg lysozyme, 16 lysozyme residues form the conformational epitope recognized by D1.3. Seventeen amino acids from the antibody, 10 from the H chain and seven from the L chain, contact this epitope. These residues are contributed by all of the CDRs, with the exception of two that belong to framework regions. The most contacts are made by V_H CDR3 residues and the least by V_L CDR2. The antigen–antibody contacts are predominantly either hydrogen bonds or van der Waals interactions between aromatic amino acids (see Chapter 2).

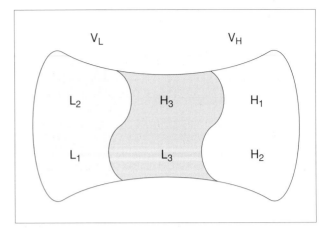

Fig. 3.8 A schematic representation of CDR loops in the antibody-combining site. The relative arrangement of the IgL (L1-3) and H (H1-3) CDRs is shown. CDR1 and CDR2 regions are separated by the CDR3 regions that are encoded by the junctions of the rearranging genes.

Analysis of the positions of the amino acids that contact lysozyme allows an evaluation of the contribution of diversity, generated by rearrangement, to antigen binding. The amino acid (Arg 96) created by imprecise joining of *VK-JK* in D1.3 is distant from the antigen, as are the *JK*-encoded residues. However, residues encoded by the *D* segment of CDR3 (Arg 99, Asp 100, Tyr 101 and Arg 102) all make very specific contacts with the antigen. In contrast, neither J_H residues nor those that originate from imprecise joining at the D_H-J_H junction contribute directly to the contacts made by D1.3 and lysozyme. A three dimensional representation of the D1.3–lysozyme complex, highlighting the important contact residues, is shown in the section of *Colour figures*.

The determination of Ig and antibody–antigen three dimensional structures makes possible knowledge-based predictions of additional antibody structures, in particular of the antibody-combining sites, based on their amino acid sequences and homology. The conformations of the hypervariable CDR loops of H and L chains are more difficult to predict accurately than the framework region. However, on the basis of comparative studies of known antibody structures and sequences there appears to be a small repertoire of main-chain conformations for at least five of the six hypervariable regions and the particular conformation adopted is apparently determined by a few key conserved residues. Analyses of IgV region sequences and structures suggest that V_H CDR1 regions have one of three different canonical structures and that V_H CDR2 regions have one of five diferent canonical structures. The different observed combinations of the V_H CDR1 and CDR2 canonical structures mean that almost all sequences have one of seven main-chain folds. The exact specificity of each of the loops will be determined by the nature of the surface residues, particularly at the centre of the combining site and sequence differences that alter the relative positions of the loops. The modelling approach based on canonical structures has been used with remarkable success to predict the structures of most hypervariable regions of a variety of different antibodies.

The TCR binding site

Although the V regions of TCRs and Ig polypeptides exhibit only low (about 25%) overall sequence similarity, several residues in TCR sequences are identical or similar at sites in Igs which are responsible for the conserved structure of the domain framework. Further residues are identical to those mainly responsible for the geometry of V_H-V_L packing in Igs. Moreover, Wu and Kabat variability analysis of TCR V region amino acid sequences has revealed areas of relatively greater variability which correspond in part to Ig hypervariable regions. Thus, it seems reasonable to assume that TCR and Ig V domains will fold in the same fashion and that the resulting combining sites of $V\alpha$–$V\beta$ and $V\gamma$–$V\delta$ will be similar to those of V_H–V_L combinations. This supposition has been confirmed by the crystallization and structure determination of a TCRβ chain.

TCR V region sequences have been modelled on the basis of known Ig coordinates. Although the positioning of the TCR CDR equivalents is problematic, the framework structure is very close to that of the Igs and the loops that form the antigen binding site are similar in size to those found in Ig binding sites. Models of the TCR–MHC–peptide ternary complex have also been generated. The basis of these models is the interaction of the CDR1- and CDR2-equivalent regions of $V\alpha$ and $V\beta$ with the side chains of the MHC at helical regions of the polymorphic α_1 and α_2 domains (Chapter 4). The centrally located CDR3-equivalent regions contact the bound peptide. An attractive feature of these models is that they position the CDR1- and CDR2-equivalent regions, which exhibit limited diversity, with the less diverse MHC molecule and allows the CDR3-equivalent region, that exhibits much greater diversity, to contact the very diverse collection of peptides which can be embedded in the MHC groove. A limitation of these models is that the orientation of the TCR relative to the MHC/peptide ligand is difficult to determine.

Modelling studies can, at best, only approximate the actual structure of a protein and there is no substitute for direct structural determination. The generation of soluble forms of the TCR should enable the crystallization and subsequent structural analysis of this receptor and eventually of the ternary complex.

Segregation of *TCRAV* and *TCRBV* sequences with antigen–MHC specificities

Numerous studies have correlated primary structures of TCRs with their fine specificities in attempts to determine whether the presence of a particular gene segment or junctional sequence in the TCR is associated with its antigen and/or MHC reactivity. The consensus from these studies is that TCRs recognizing the same antigen can sometimes express a limited repertoire of *V* and *J* gene segments and restricted junctional sequences. For example, mouse TCRs specific for the C-terminal peptide of cytochrome c preferentially use a single *AV* gene segment and among the specific TCRs that use this *AV* gene segment, a correlation has been found between *BV* usage and reactivity with different

H-2Eβ chains. Amino acid changes in the junctional regions of the TCRs from some cytochrome c-specific T cell clones alter the fine specificity of peptide recognition without affecting MHC specificity.

These data do not imply that one particular gene segment can be used in response to only one particular antigen and indeed several examples of the use of the same gene segment in different responses have been reported. However, they have implications for autoimmunity since the immune response leading to autoimmune disease might be selectively inhibited if T cells mediating the response used a limited number of TCR gene segments. In this context, an analysis of TCRs in both human and experimental autoimmune disease has, in some cases, provided evidence for restricted gene usage and, in the case of experimental autoimmune encephalomyelitis, the disease has been prevented by anti-TCR antibody therapy.

The relationship between the structure of a TCR and its functional specificity revealed by these studies is consistent with the proposed Ig-like nature of the TCR binding site. In the case of Igs the antigen specificity can be most closely associated with either the heavy chain, the light chain, or both, although both chains presumably contribute interactions with antigen in the complete binding site. A dramatic demonstration of the ability of an unassociated V_H domain to bind antigen is that of an individual recombinant V_H domain (expressed in *E. coli*) of the anti-lysozyme antibody D1.3 binding to lysozyme with high affinity (19nM versus 2nM for the parent antibody). Furthermore, lysozyme-binding single domain antibodies (dAbs) have been isolated from a cDNA library of V_H genes by selection with antigen. Thus, by analogy with Igs, T cell responses may be selected on the basis of both TCR α and β-chains or may depend mainly on the structure of one chain or the other.

SUMMARY

The diverse structures of Igs and TCRs are generated by similar genetic mechanisms. Much has been learnt about the activities involved in *V-D-J* recombination and in particular about *RAG-1* and *RAG-2*, the essential tissue-specific components of the *V-D-J* recombinase. Diversity is generated by the multiplicity of the independently assorting components (i.e. *V*, *D* and *J*) of the variable regions and the consequent combinatorial advantage, together with various somatic mutational mechanisms such as *N* region and junctional diversity. However, the relative importance of the different mechanisms varies for TCRs and Igs. For example, TCRs have a greater tendency to use *N* region diversity and frame shifts, whereas Igs have the capacity to use somatic hypermutation. This may reflect the differences between B and T cell recognition systems.

The elucidation of the way in which these genetic mechanisms for generating diversity translate to useful variations in the structures of Ig or TCR binding sites necessitates structural analysis of receptor–ligand complexes. The three dimensional structures of several antibody–antigen complexes have been determined. These studies have revealed a binding site comprising the three CDR regions with

V region determined diversity (CDR1 and 2) located on the outside and junctional diversity (CDR3) at the centre of the binding pocket. Conserved elements in the CDR sequences have defined canonical structures for V_H and V_L CDRs. In contrast, little structural information is available for TCRs. In the absence of such information, molecular models for TCR–MHC–peptide interaction have been generated that place the DJ junction (CDR3) in contact with the peptide and the CDR1 and 2 regions in contact with MHC class I or class II. These models permit the design of experiments to test which specific TCR residues affect MHC or peptide recognition.

FURTHER READING

Amit AG, Mariuzza R, Phillips SEV, Poljak RJ. Three-dimensional structure of an antigen-antibody complex at 2.8°A resolution. *Science* 1986, **233**:747.

Alt F, Blackwell TK, Yancopoulos V. Development of the primary antibody repertoire. *Science* 1987, **238**:1079.

Alzari PM, Lascombe M-B, Poljak RJ. Three-dimensional structure of antibodies. *Ann Rev Immunol* 1988, **6**:555.

Berek C, Griffiths GM, Milstein C. Molecular events during maturation of the immune response to oxazolone. *Nature* 1985, **316**:412.

Blackwell TK, Malynn BA., Pollock RR, Ferrier P, Covey LR, Fulop GM, Phillips RA, Yancopoulos GD, Alt FW. Isolation of *scid* pre-B cells that rearrange κ light chain genes: formation of normal signal and abnormal coding joints. *EMBO J* 1989, **8**:735.

Blackwell TK, Moore M, Yancopoulos G, Suh H, Lutzker S, Selsing E, Alt F. Recombination between immunoglobulin variable region gene segments is enhanced by transcription. *Nature* 1986, **324**:585.

Boulot G, Bentley GA, Karjalainen K, Mariuzza RA. Crystallization and preliminary X-ray diffraction analysis of the β-chain of a T cell antigen receptor. *J Mol Biol* 1994, **235**:795.

Carlson LM, Oettinger MA, Schatz DG, Masteller EL, Hurley EA, McCormack WT, Baltimore D, Thompson CB. Selective expression of RAG-2 in chicken B cells undergoing gene conversion. *Cell* 1991, **64**:201.

Chothia C, Boswell DR, Lesk AM. The outline structure of the T cell αβ receptor. *EMBO J* 1988, **7**:3745.

Chothia C, Les AM, Tramontano A, Levitt M, Smith-Gill SJ, Air G, Sheriff S, Padlan EA, Davies D, Tulip WR, Colman PM, Spinelli S, Alzari P M, Poljak RJ. Conformations of immunoglobulin hypervariable regions. *Nature* 1989, **342**:877.

Chothia C, Lesk AM, Gherardi E, Tomlinson IM, Walter G, Marks JD, Llewelyn MB, Winter G. Structural repertoire of the human *VH* segments. *J Mol Biol* 1992, **227**:799.

Cook GP, Tomlinson IM, Walter G, Riethman H, Carter NP, Buluwela L, Winter G, Rabbitts TH. A map of the human immunoglobulin *VH* locus completed by analysis of the telomeric region of chromosome 14q. *Nature Genet* 1994, **7**:162.

Davis MM, Bjorkman PJ. T cell antigen receptor genes and T cell recognition. *Nature* 1988, **334**:395.

Ferrier P, Covey LR, Li SC, Suh H, Malynn BA, Blackwell TK, Morrow MA, Alt FW. Normal recombination substrate *VH* to *D-J-H* rearrangements in pre-B cell lines from *scid* mice. *J Exp Med* 1990, **171**:1909.

Haqqi TM, Banerjee S, Anderson GD, David CS. An inbred mouse strain with a massive deletion of T cell receptor *BV* genes. *J Exp Med* 1989, **169**:1903.

Jorgensen JL, Esser U, Fazekas de St. Groth B, Reay PA, Davis MM. Mapping T cell receptor-peptide contacts by variant peptide immunization of single-chain transgenics. *Nature* 1992, **355**:224.

Jorgensen JL, Reay PA, Ehrich EW, Davis MM. Molecular components of T cell recognition. *Ann Rev Immunol* 1992 **10**:835.

Lafaille JJ, DeCloux A, Bonneville M, Takagaki Y, Tonegawa S. Junctional sequences of T cell receptor γδ genes: implications for γδ cell lineages and for a novel intermediate of *V-D-J* joining. *Cell* 1989, **59**:859.

Lieber MR, Hesse JE, Lewis S, Bosma GC, Rosenberg N, Mizuuchi K, Bosma MJ, Gellert M. The defect in murine severe immune deficiency: joining of signal sequence but not coding segments in *V-D-J* recombination. *Cell* 1988, **55**:7.

McCormack WT, Tjoelker LW, Thompson CB. Avian B cell development. *Ann Rev Immunol* 1991, **9**:219.

Maizels N. Might gene conversion be the mechanism of somatic hypermutation of mammalian immunoglobulin genes? *Trends Genet* 1989, **5**:4.

Malynn BA, Yancopoulos GD, Barth JE, Bona CA, Alt FW. Biased expression of *Jh*-proximal *Vh* genes occurs in the newly generated repertoire of neonatal and adult mice. *J Exp Med* 1990, **171**:843.

Mombaerts P, Iacomini J, Johnson RS, Herrup K, Tonegawa S, Papaioannou VE. RAG-1 deficient mice have no mature B and T lymphocytes. *Cell* 1992, **68**:869.

Oettinger MA, Schatz DG, Gorka C, Baltimore D. *RAG-1* and *RAG-2*, adjacent genes that synergistically activate *V-D-J* recombination. *Science* 1990, **248**:1517.

Okazaki K, Sakano H. Thymocyte circular DNA excised from T cell receptor *AD* gene complex. *EMBO J* 1988, **7**:1669.

Prosser HM, Tonegawa S. T cell receptor *V-D-J* recombination: mechanisms and developmental regulation In *T Cell Receptor Genes*. Bell JI, Owen MJ, Simpson EL (Eds). Oxford University Press: Oxford; 1995:308.

Pullen AM, Potts W, Wakeland EK, Kappler J, Marrack P. Surprisingly uneven distribution of the T cell receptor Vβ repertoire in wild mice. *J Exp Med* 1990, **171**:49.

Reth MG, Jackson S, Alt FW. *VhDJh* formation and *DJh* replacement during pre-B differentiation: non-random usage of gene segments. *EMBO J* 1986, **5**:2131.

Reynaud C-A, Dahan A, Anquez V, Weill J-C. Somatic hyperconversion diversifies the single *Vh* gene of the chicken with a high incidence in the *D* region. *Cell* 1989, **59**:171.

Schatz DG, Baltimore D. Stable expression of immunoglobulin gene V-D-J recombinase activity by gene transfer into 3T3 fibroblasts. *Cell* 1988, **53**:107.

Schatz DG, Oettinger MA, Baltimore D. The *V-D-J* recombination activating gene *RAG-1*. *Cell* 1989, **59**:1035.

Schatz DG, Oettinger MA, Schlissel MS. *V-D-J* recombination: molecular biology and regulation. *Ann Rev Immunol* 1992, **10**:359.

Schuler W, Ruetsch NR, Amsler M, Bosma MJ. Coding joint formation of endogenous T cell receptor genes in lymphoid cells from *scid* mice: unusual *P* nucleotide additions in *VJ*-coding joints. *Eur J Immunol* 1991, **21**:589.

Shinkai Y, Rathburn G, Lam K-P, Oltz EM, Stewart V, Medelsohn M, Charon J, Datta M, Young F, Stall AM, Alt FW. *RAG-1* deficient mice lack mature lymphocytes owing to inability to initiate *V-D-J* rearrangement. *Cell* 1992, **68**:855.

Smider V, Rathmell WK, Lieber MR, Chu G. Restoration of X-ray resistance and V-D-J recombination in mutant cells by Ku cDNA. *Science* 1994, **266**: 288.

Tomlinson IM, Walter G, Marks JD, Llewelyn MB, Winter G. The repertoire of human germline *Vh* sequences reveals about fifty groups of *Vh* segments with different hypervariable loops. *J Mol Biol* 1992, **227**:776.

Tonegawa S. Somatic generation of antibody diversity. *Nature* 1983, **302**:575.

Ward ES, Güssow D, Griffiths AD, Jones PT, Winter, G. Binding activities of a repertoire of single immunoglobulin variable domains secreted from *Escherichia coli*. *Nature* 1989, **341**:544.

Wraith DC, McDevitt HO, Steinman L, Acha-Orbea H. T cell recognition as the target for immune intervention in autoimmune disease. *Cell* 1989, **57**:709.

Wu TT, Kabat EA. An analysis of the sequences of the variable regions of Bence Jones proteins and myeloma light chains and their implications for antibody complementarity. *J Exp Med* 1970, **132**:211.

Yancopoulos G, Alt FW. Developmentally controlled and tissue-specific expression of unrearranged *VH* gene segments. *Cell* 1985, **40**:271.

4 Class I and II Molecules of the MHC

The ability to distinguish 'self' from 'non-self' is a protective characteristic of virtually all multicellular organisms, ensuring that defence mechanisms are directed towards invading microorganisms and other foreign molecules without causing damage to host tissues. The fundamental features are highly polymorphic cell-surface recognition structures and mechanisms for the destruction of non-self. The existence of self/non-self discrimination in mammals was first demonstrated by the ability of mice to reject grafts of foreign tissues, such as skin or tumours. This ability to reject non-self tissues was subsequently mapped to a region termed H-2 on chromosome 17 which became known as the major histocompatibility complex (MHC). The cell-surface structures involved in rejection were initially characterized by using alloantibodies, produced in one inbred strain of mice immunized with cells of other strains differing only at the MHC. Subsequently, with the use of specific antibodies to molecules encoded by small regions of the MHC and using techniques borrowed from protein chemistry and molecular biology, the characteristics of MHC genes and their products have been analyzed in great detail. Similar techniques have also been used to characterize the human MHC, known as the Human Leukocyte Antigen (HLA) region, which is located on the short arm of chromosome 6. Several diverse species ranging from cattle to chickens and amphibians have been found to have an MHC region, although the bulk of the knowledge has come from studies on the murine and human MHCs.

The main products of the MHC are the class I and class II molecules and the structures of these will be discussed before describing the genetic region encoding the genes.

STRUCTURE OF CLASS I AND CLASS II MOLECULES

Class I molecules

Class I molecules comprise a glycosylated polypeptide chain of 45kDa (heavy chain) in close, non-covalent association with beta$_2$ microglobulin (β_2m), a 12kDa polypeptide which is also found unassociated in serum.

DOMAIN STRUCTURE

Amino acid sequence analyses of both human and murine class I molecules have demonstrated that the heavy chain is divided into distinct regions: three extracellular domains, a connecting polypeptide, transmembrane region and a cytoplasmic domain (*Fig. 4.1A*).

The three main extracellular domains, designated α1 (N-terminal), α2 and α3, can be cleaved from cell surfaces with the enzyme papain. These domains each comprise about 90 amino acids. The α2 and α3 domains both have

intrachain disulphide bonds and the α3 domain also folds like an Ig constant region. Both human and mouse heavy chains have an N-glycosylated asparagine residue 86 in the α1 domain. Murine heavy chains are also N-glycosylated at residue 176 in α2 and some (D^b, K^d, L^d) have additional carbohydrate side chains at residue 256 in α3. In addition to the major papain cleavage site between α3 and the transmembrane region, there is also a minor cleavage site between the second and third domains.

The transmembrane region consists of about 25 hydrophobic uncharged residues, which probably assume an α-helical conformation and traverse the cell membrane. There is a cluster of about five basic amino acids, arginine and lysine, immediately C-terminal to the transmembrane region. Such highly charged regions are typical of membrane bound proteins and they probably help to anchor the polypeptide chain in the membrane by interacting with the negatively charged phospholipid headgroups of the inner membrane.

The hydrophilic cytoplasmic domain is about 30 (human) to 40 (mouse) residues long and consists of approximately 50% polar amino acids, particularly serine. Some of these serine residues are phosphorylated. For example, the HLA-A2 heavy chain is phosphorylated by a cyclic AMP-dependent protein kinase at two serine residues in the cytoplasmic domain. Such phosphorylation has been postulated to be involved in transmitting signals from the MHC molecule to appropriate intracytoplasmic mediators.

The class I light chain, β_2m, forms a single Ig-like domain which has strong sequence homology with Ig constant regions. Although it was initially thought that β_2m associated with the class I heavy chain primarily through interaction with the α3 domain, in the same way as inter-domain Ig interactions, subsequent X-ray crystallographic analysis has revealed a more complex mode of interaction (see following section). β_2m is encoded outside the MHC on human chromosome 15 and on mouse chromosome 2. It is a non-polymorphic protein in humans, dimorphic in mice (a single amino acid change at position 85), with a high degree of sequence homology among species implying evolutionary conservation. Association with β_2m is required for expression of class I antigens at the cell surface and for stabilization of class I structure.

X-RAY ANALYSIS

The three dimensional structure of the extracellular portion obtained by cleavage with papain of several class I structures have been elucidated (*Fig. 4.1B*). This region contains the α1, α2 and α3 domains and β_2m. The α3 and β_2m domains have Ig-folds; that is, they are each composed of two anti-parallel β-pleated sheets, one with four β-strands and one with three β-strands, connected by a disulphide bond. However, the α3 and β2m domains interact in a manner not found between pairs of constant domains in the known antibody structures.

The α1 and α2 domains have an overall structural similarity. Each consists of an anti-parallel β-pleated sheet spanned by a long α-helical region that is C-terminal to the four β-strands in the sheet. A disulphide bond in α2 connects a cysteine residue in the N-terminal β-strand to one in the α-helix. The α1 and α2 domains are paired in the HLA molecule such that the four β-strands from each domain form a single antiparallel β-sheet with eight strands. This β-sheet is topped by the helical regions from each domain. The large groove between the α-helices constitutes the binding site for processed foreign antigen in the form of peptides.

PEPTIDE BINDING SITE

T cells recognize complexes formed by class I or class II antigens and antigenic peptide fragments which will substitute for naturally processed antigen in stimulating T cells. Antigenic peptides can be demonstrated to bind directly to purified class I and class II antigens, while physiologically processed antigens eluted from MHC molecules have been sequenced and the proteins from which they were derived have been identified.

The crystallographic structure of the HLA-A2 molecule has provided a structural basis for the direct binding of peptides to class I antigen. A binding groove formed by the α1 and α2 domains of the class I heavy chain was occupied by an ill-defined electron-dense material which was interpreted as peptide(s) filling the binding site (*Fig. 4.1B and C*). Comparisons of the high resolution crystallographic structures of HLA-A2 and HLA-Aw68 has added further insights into the nature of the class I antigen binding site. The polypeptide backbones of these two class I antigens are extremely similar, the differences resulting from amino acid side chain differences at 13 positions, six of which are in α1, six in α2 and one in the α3 domain. The single α3 domain difference (at residue 245) has been shown to contribute to interactions with the CD8 glycoprotein. Ten of the α1 and α2 differences

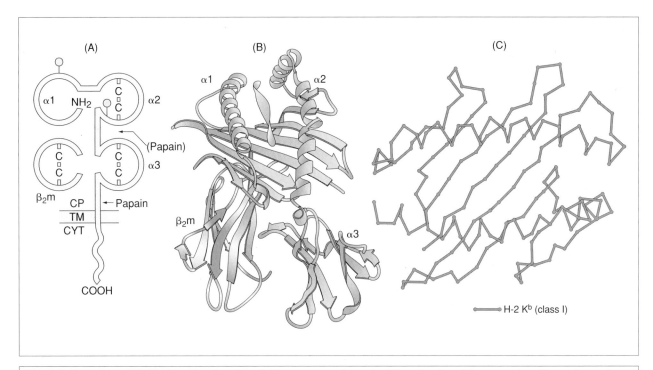

Fig. 4.1 Structure of MHC class I molecules. A. The general features of class I molecules are illustrated. The heavy chain (43kDa), coded in the MHC, is divided into six regions: three extracellular globular domains each of around 90 amino acids (α1, α2 and α3), a short connecting peptide (CP), a hydrophobic transmembrane (TM) segment and a hydrophilic cytoplasmic domain (CYT). The nonMHC encoded β2-microglobulin (β2m; 12kDa) light chain associates non-covalently with the heavy chain. Asparagine-linked glycan units are found primarily in the α1 and α2 domains of mice and the α1 domain of humans, although additional glycosylation occurs in α3 in some mouse haplotypes. Interchain disulphide bonds are found in each of the α2, α3 and β2m domains. The major and minor papain cleavage sites are also shown.
B. Three dimensional structure of the external portion of a class I molecule. Within each domain, regions of β-strands (arrows), helices (coils) and connecting loops are indicated. The putative peptide binding groove at the top of the molecule is formed by the α1 and α2 domains with α-helical sides and a β-sheet base.
C. Structure of the peptide binding site viewed from the top of the molecule, from the perspective of the T cell receptor. Compare this with the structure of a class II molecule in *Figure 4.2*. Based on Bjorkman *et al*, 1987; Brown *et al*, 1993; Stern and Wiley, 1994.

are located at positions lining the floor and side of the peptide-binding groove. The pattern of the amino acid variation between HLA-A2, Aw68 as well as other class I molecules is similar to the distribution of variable residues obtained from accumulated HLA-A, B and C sequences, which must reflect the conformations with which peptides can occupy the groove. The groove is not a smooth structure but has a number of pockets with which amino acid side chains interact.

Based on this detailed analysis of the three dimensional structures of HLA-A2 and Aw68 a picture has emerged that links the amino acid polymorphism that is such a feature of MHC proteins with limited structural changes within the peptide binding cleft, such as shape, charge distribution and local pockets. These structural changes presumably form the basis for differences in peptide binding affinity which in turn govern responsiveness versus non-responsiveness in the immune response.

Class II molecules

The products of class II genes (A and E in the mouse, DR, DQ and DP in humans) are heterodimers comprising heavy (α) and light (β) glycoprotein chains. The α-chains have molecular weights of 30–34kDa and the β-chains range

from 26–29kDa, depending on the locus involved. Amino acid sequences deduced from class II cDNA clones have complemented direct sequencing data to give the current view of the structure of α and β-chains *(Fig. 4.2)*.

DOMAIN STRUCTURE
Each chain has been shown to consist of five domains: two extracellular domains of approximately 90 amino acids each, α1 and α2 or β1 and β2, a connecting peptide and a transmembrane region of about 30 residues followed by a short cytoplasmic domain *(Fig. 4.2A)*.

The two N-terminal domains, α1 and β1, show little sequence homology with Ig, whereas the α2 and β2 domains, like α3 and β_2m of class I molecules, have the structural characteristics of a single Ig domain. The class II α2 and β2 domains are most homologous to the Cγ3 and Cγ4 Ig domains and are as similar to Ig as the various IgC domains are to each other. The β1 has cysteine residues at positions 15 and 79, which are disulphide-linked to give a 64 amino acid loop. The α1 domain lacks cysteine residues and thus cannot form disulphide bonds. Both α2 and β2 domains have disulphide loops enclosing 56 amino acids. Class II molecules are N-glycosylated at asparagine residues in α1, α2 and β1. Heterogeneity in

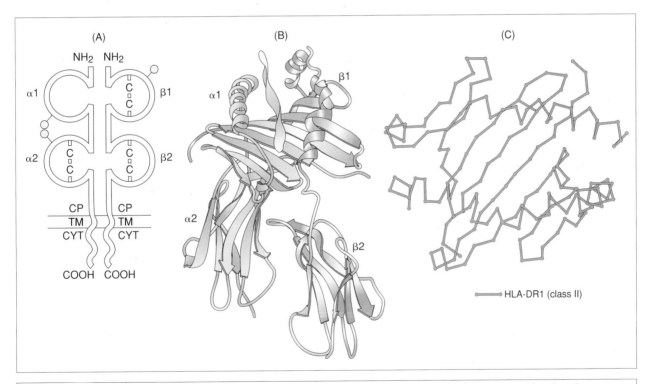

Fig. 4.2 Structure of MHC class II molecules. A. The general features of class II molecules are illustrated. Each chain contains two extracellular globular domains (α1, α2; β1, β2), short connecting peptides (CP), transmembrane regions (TM) and short hydrophilic cytoplasmic regions (CYT). Carbohydrate attachments (N-linked) account for most of the molecular weight differences between the α (34kDa) and β-chains (29kDa). The α2 and β2 domains have a strong sequence homology with Ig constant region domains.
B. Peptide backbone of the class II structure. Note how remarkably similar the structure is to that of class I molecules. This is in spite of the fact that the class II peptide binding groove is composed of two domains (α1 and β1) that are not covalently linked.
C. Structure of the class II peptide-binding groove from the top of the molecule.

carbohydrate attachments accounts for much of the difference in molecular weight of class II molecules.

The extracellular domains are connected to the transmembrane region by a short hydrophilic region, rich in glutamic acid and proline (α-chain) or serine (β-chain). The transmembrane regions of the α and β-chains form α-helices packed together and, like the class I heavy chains, they have a cluster of positively charged residues anchoring the chains in the membrane. The hydrophilic cytoplasmic regions are of variable, but generally short, length (10–15 residues).

Although the class II α1 and β1 domains show little overall sequence similarity to the polymorphic class I α1 and α2 domains, the two molecules share many structural features when their crystal structures are compared.

The class II-related molecule, DM (a heterodimer of DMα and DMβ in humans; Mα and Mβ in mice), is involved in loading antigens onto class II molecules in an intracellular compartment called MIIC. The DM molecule has a somewhat different structure from that of classical class II molecules such as DP, DQ, DR, E and A. The DM molecule contains additional di-sulphide bridges in both α1 and β1 domains and there is limited sequence identity between these domains in DM and the equivalent regions of conventional class II. DM molecules are not highly polymorphic and do not exhibit a CD4 binding site, consistent with their intracellular, rather than extracellular role.

X-RAY ANALYSIS

The crystal structure of class II molecules, DR1 for example, reveals a peptide backbone similar to that for class I (*Fig. 4.2B*). The two α-chain domains, α1 and α2, of DR superimpose quite closely onto the α1 domain and β2m subunit of class I. Similarly, the two β-chain domains of DR superimpose onto α2 and α3 domains of class I. One subtle difference is that the β2 domain of DR is off-set from its homologous region in class I, α3, by about 15°. But, the packing between the class II immunoglobulin domains still resembles the packing of class I more than the packing of a similar domain in an antibody.

PEPTIDE BINDING

The peptide binding groove of class II, like class I, is composed of eight strands of anti-parallel β-sheets, forming a floor and two anti-parallel helical regions as the sides (*Fig. 4.2C*). However, class I molecules bind primarily nonameric peptides but class II accommodates longer molecules. To fit these longer peptides, class II molecules have replaced two turns near the amino terminus of the α1 domain with a stretch of extended chain. Similarly, the carboxy-terminal end of the class II α1 helical region is more open. A number of residues that effectively close the ends of the grooves of class I molecules are not present in the class II pockets.

A DIMER OF CLASS II HETERODIMERS

A potentially interesting observation when DR was first crystallized was that the molecules formed in pairs, as a dimer of dimers. The conservation of amino acid residues at the interface between the pairs of heterodimers, in different DR allelic products, suggests there may be a biological role for the pairing, although crystallization artefacts cannot be ruled out. The capacity of DR molecules to form parallel dimers may provide part of a mechanism to initiate intracellular signalling, in T cells by crosslinking two T cell receptors and in antigen presenting cells, to induce the expression of co-stimulatory molecules. The CD4 molecule is thought to bind to the β2 domain of DR1 in a model consistent with its interaction with a class II dimer.

GENOMIC ORGANIZATION OF THE MHC

Three regions, denoted I, II and III, have been identified in the MHC of both mouse and humans (*Fig. 4.3*). At least three separate class I loci (termed *H-2K, D* and *L* in the mouse and *HLA-A, B* and *C* in humans) encoding classical transplantation antigens have been demonstrated. Other class I genes in the mouse map telomeric to the *H-2K, D* and *L* loci in regions known as *Q, T* and *M*. Products of these loci differ in tissue distribution and probably also in function. Certain Q (or Qa) antigens can be expressed by distinct T lymphocyte subpopulations. A similar cluster of class I-like genes is located telomeric to the *HLA-A* gene, although it is unclear whether any of these genes represent the human homologue of the murine *Q/T/M* genes. Class II genes, encoded in the *A* and *E* regions of the mouse MHC and the *HLA-D* region of humans, are identical to the immune response (Ir) genes known to control murine responses to different antigens. Class I products are primarily recognized by CD8+ cytotoxic T cells, whereas class II gene products (often called Ia antigens) are primarily involved in the activation of CD4+ T helper cells, although there may be exceptions to this general rule. The class III region, although originally defined as encoding four of the components of the alternate complement system, is now known to contain a rather diverse collection of genes. There is no evidence for functional or structural similarities between class III gene products and the class I and II molecules and it is not known whether class III genes reside within the MHC by accident or whether a selective advantage is enjoyed by their location. Only those MHC loci involved in antigen processing and presentation will be discussed here. The major feature of the MHC is the extreme polymorphism of some of the class I and II genes. For example, more than 50 different alleles have been demonstrated at both the *H-2K* and *D* class I loci of mice and over 100 now at some of the human loci. Class II molecules are highly polymorphic like some class I molecules, although the *Q, T* and *M* region class I genes exhibit little polymorphism. The generation and molecular basis of MHC polymorphism are discussed in subsequent sections of this chapter.

Murine class I loci

In mice, the number of class I genes in the haploid genome is around 30 but this number varies among different inbred strains. Among this multitude, the genes encoding the classical serologically defined H-2K, D and L molecules can be identified. Most of the remaining genes, which map to the

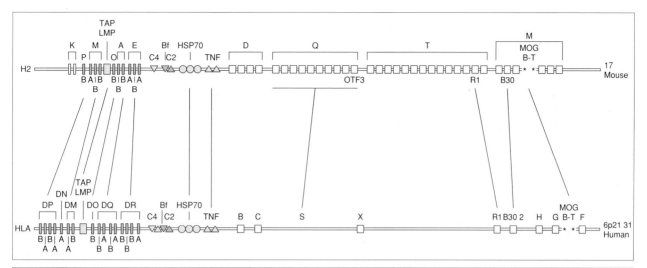

Fig. 4.3 Organization of the murine and human MHC. The locations of the major loci in the class I, class II and class III regions are shown. The maps are not completely to scale. Much of class II is conserved in linear order between the two species. The class II region is also conserved virtually gene for gene in the mouse I region and the human D region. The class I regions have undergone extensive expansion and contraction but where landmark loci have been identified they are in equivalent locations. Lines join loci thought to be equivalent in the two species. Based on information from Dr Fischer-Lindahl. In some other species, class I or class II loci can be missing. Note that the mouse class I K loci are centromeric of the class II genes. Mole rats appear to have lost *DR* (*E*)-related genes but have expanded *DP*-related genes to compensate. It seems that the MHC products can substitute for each other to some degree.

Q/T/M region, are of unknown significance. These are often referred to as class Ib or non-classical class I genes. The organization of the murine class I and class II loci are shown in *Figure 4.4*.

The organization of the H-2K region is similar in BALB/c (H-2^d), B10 (H-2^b) and AKR (H-2^k) mice. It comprises two class I genes, called *K* and *K2*, arranged in a head-to-tail configuration. The *H-2K* gene-directed expression of the appropriate H-2K antigen when assayed in gene transfection experiments. The *H-2K2* gene possesses a functional promoter but exhibits varied patterns of expression in different strains. The class II pseudogene *Pb*, related to *DPB*, is 75kb from the 5' end of the *H-2K* gene. Comparison of H-2^d and H-2^b haplotype mice reveals considerable divergence between the number of class I genes located in the *D/L* region. Five class I genes map to the *D/L* region of BALB/c H-2^d mice, two genes encoding the serologically detectable H-2D^d and H-2L^d antigens. One B10 *H-2D^b* gene has been identified. H-2D^b and H-2L^d show high sequence homology whereas H-2D^d is more divergent. Moreover, the *H-2L^d* and *H-2D^b* are each separated by about 60kb of DNA from the most proximal gene of the *Q* region.

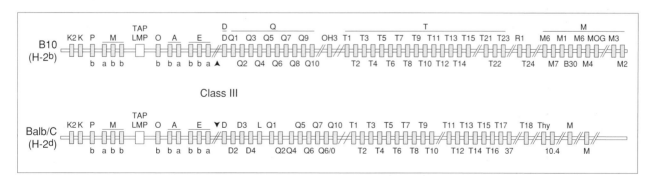

Fig. 4.4 Murine class I and class II genes. Genes of the H-2^d and H-2^b haplotypes are illustrated. Some are pseudogenes. Note that in the H-2^b haplotype (represented by the B10 mouse strain) the *Ea* gene is non-functional and therefore cannot produce cell surface E molecules (although it still produces cytoplasmic Eβ chains). The numbers of class I genes can differ markedly between different strains of mouse due to expansion and contraction. The African pigmy mouse, for example, contains thousands of class I genes. The arrows indicate the positions of class III loci which are not shown here.

The *Q* locus comprises about 200kb of DNA located distal to *H-2D/L* in BALB/c and B10 mice. This region encodes the serologically detectable specificities Qa-2, 3, 4 and 5 and contains a cluster of class I genes (eight in BALB/c and 10 in B10). The serological specificities of the products encoded by these genes have been determined by experiments involving gene transfection into L cells. For example, in B10 mice, transfected *Q6, 7, 8* and *9* genes could all be used to produce serologically detectable Qa-2 antigens. The major component of the Qa-2 products on lymphocytes is Q7-like, with a minor component being Q6-like. Interestingly, the *Q10* gene, which is non-polymorphic, is expressed specifically in mouse liver. There is an in-frame termination codon early in the transmembrane exon of this gene and the Q10 product is apparently secreted at a high rate, although its function is unknown.

The Q7 and Q9 antigens are two of an increasing number of surface antigens linked to the cell surface by a glycosyl phosphatidylinositol (GPI) tail instead of a hydrophobic protein domain. It has been shown that the GPI anchor is critical for the ability of antibodies specific for Qa-2 to activate mouse T cells.

The murine *T* locus, defined initially as *Tla*, encoding the marker antigen TL, is located distal to the *H-2K/D* locus. TL antigens are structurally related to H-2K and D molecules and are associated with β_2m but have a restricted tissue distribution, being expressed only on thymocytes, activated T cells and on some thymic leukaemias.

The murine T region contains the largest number of class I genes and the greatest gene organizational differences between the B10 and BALB/c haplotypes. In B10 mice the T region contains 13 class I genes spanning 150kb of DNA, whereas the BALB/c genome contains 18 class I genes in the *T* region. All of the B10 T class I genes have homologues in the BALB/c *T* region.

The *H2-M* region contains a cluster of related genes, at least one of which has a specialized function. The product of the most telomeric gene, *M3*, selectively binds *N*-formylated peptides of bacterial or mitochondrial origin. The M genes play a role in defence against *Listeria monocytogenes*. They are targets for T cells with receptors of the $\alpha\beta$ type. Structural studies have shown that particular residues in the peptide binding groove of the M3 molecule permit binding of the fMet group modification. Expression of M3 is TAP-dependent. The gene for myelin/oligodendrocyte glycoprotein (MOG) and the related *B-T* gene were recently found within the mouse *M* region. These genes are related to the chicken *B-G* genes, a set of polymorphic loci in the chicken MHC.

Human class I loci

The positions of the various genes within the human MHC have been mapped with precision using pulsed field gel electrophoresis (PFGE). This technique relies on restriction enzymes that cut rarely within the genome and an electrophoretic system that resolves large DNA fragments. Southern hybridization analysis using probes for MHC genes allows mapping of large regions of DNA and more recently this procedure has been facilitated by cloning of the whole of the 4Mbp of MHC DNA in yeast artificial chromosome clones, or YACs (*Fig. 4.5*).

The human class I region contains three well characterized loci, called *HLA-A, B* and *C*, encoding each of the major transplantation antigens HLA-A, B and C. The *HLA-A, B* and *C* loci reside within a class I region spanning about 2 million bases of DNA. The *HLA-A, B* and *C* genes are separated by long stretches of DNA. Analysis of these surrounding regions by cosmid cloning and hybridization with class I probes has revealed additional class I genes. These genes include *HLA-E, F* and *G*. Each of these genes can direct the synthesis of class I protein, although the functional significance of these products is unknown.

Another set of class I-related genes, the *MIC* loci, are located around the *B* and *C* loci. These genes are only weakly related to classical class I loci and they are expressed on different sets of tissues to their more well-known counterparts. *MIC* genes are inducible with increase in temperature and their promoters contain so-called 'heat shock' elements.

Several other genes of unknown function have been mapped within this region. Some of these genes were co-localized on cosmids containing class I genes, others were identified by virtue of being associated with regions of hypomethylation (called CpG islands) that are characteristic of expressed genes.

Other class I-related genes have also been detected telomeric to the *HLA-G* gene. These genes may be the human counterparts of the murine *Q/T/M* genes, although they have been insufficiently characterized as yet. The human *MOG* gene (see above) is located at the telomeric end of the human MHC, providing a landmark linking the mouse and human regions.

Murine class II region

The α and β-chains of murine class II molecules are encoded by separate genes located in the *I* region of the H-2 complex (*Fig. 4.4*). The *Ab* and *Aa* genes encode the A molecule whereas *Eb* and *Ea* genes encode the E molecule. In addition, α and β-chain genes have been cloned for which no protein product is known. One of these (*Pb*) is a pseudogene, containing a seven base pair deletion.

Related *a* and *b* genes lie close to each other and generally are orientated 3'–3'. The whole I region has been mapped as a series of overlapping cosmid clones and has been linked to the class I *H-2K* subregion.

Two sets of class II genes, more recently defined, appear to have functions unrelated to those of the classical A and E. The *H-2O* genes, *a* and *b*, are equivalent to the human *HLA-DNA* and *DOB*, respectively. Their functions are unknown but their products form a heterodimeric pair with a pattern of expression markedly different for that of A and E. The *Ma* and *Mb* genes, of which there are two *b* loci, *Mb1* and *Mb2*, also form heterodimeric molecules which are expressed in special intracellular vesicles, called MIIC vesicles, in which it is believed peptides are loaded onto class II molecules. Expression of a functional M molecule is necessary for peptide loading onto class II (see Chapter 7).

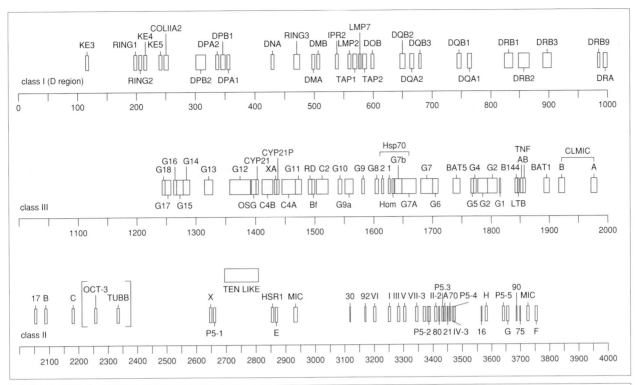

Fig. 4.5 The human MHC. A combination of pulsed field gel electrophoresis and genomic cloning and mapping has produced a detailed physical map of the ~4Mbp of the human class I, II and III regions. The class II region contains all of the class II genes, namely, the classical loci, *DP*, *DQ* and *DR* and the *DNA* and *DOB* genes whose products most likely form a heterodimeric molecule of unknown function. The other class II-related molecule, DM is involved in loading peptides onto conventional class II molecules in subcellular lysosome/endosome-like vesicles called MIICs. The processing genes for endogenous peptides destined to be loaded onto class I molecules, *LMP* and *TAP*, form a tight cluster within the class II region. The only gene in the class II region that is apparently not involved in the immune system is the *RING3* gene, which is related to a *Drosophila* locus called female sterile homeotic. The class III region encompasses a heterogeneous mixture of genes including complement components, tumour necrosis factor (*TNF*) and heat shock genes (*HSP70*-related). These heat shock products may play a chaperone role in the immune system by binding peptides. The genes are very tightly clustered in the class III region and most are not associated with the immune system. Since in some species class I and class II genes are located next to each other, without an intervening class III region, it seems possible that class III became inserted into the middle of the MHC as a late evolutionary event. The class I region contains most of the class I-related antigen presenting genes at several different loci. These include the main *A*, *B* and *C* loci as well as the non-classical (class Ib) loci, which are probably equivalent to the mouse *Q*, *T* and *M* loci. Other class I-related genes (*CD1*) are located on human chromosome 1. The *MIC* genes, distantly related to other class I sequences, comprise several members. The class I genes are interspersed with a variety of genes with many different functions. Differences in DNA content between haplotypes have been observed in the class II region, between the *DRA* and *DQA1* genes. This is reflected in a number of different *DRB* loci (from 1–4) in different haplotypes. Similarly, in the class III region the number of *C4* and flanking *CYP21* genes is known to vary and there are deletions and duplications when different haplotypes are compared over the region. Map based on Campbell and Trowsdale, 1993.

Some mice of the b, s, f and q haplotypes fail to express H-2E class II products. The b and s strains fail to make Eα chains because of a deletion of 627 base pairs in the promoter region. However, they express normal cytoplasmic levels of Eβ chains which can be utilized in hybrid H-2E molecules in F1 hybrids between b or s haplotypes and strains expressing Eα. Mice of the f and q haplotypes fail to make both Eα and Eβ chains. The Eα chain defect appears to reside at the level of RNA splicing, whereas the Eβ defect has not yet been clarified. *TAP* and *LMP* loci are situated in the mouse I region (class II) in an analogous position to their location in the human MHC, between the class II *M* and *Ob* genes. The functions of the TAPs and LMPs are discussed later and in Chapter 7.

Human class II region

Human class II genes are located in the *D* region of the HLA system. Current evidence suggests that at least six α and 10 β chains are encoded there (*Fig. 4.5*). These are organized in three different families of genes called

DR, *DQ* and *DP*. Additional genes, *DNA*, *DOB*, *DMA* and *DMB* have also been identified. The *DR* family consists of a single a gene (*DRA*) and four *DRB* genes (*DRB1–4*), although the number of *DRB* genes varies depending on the particular haplotype, whereas the *DQ* and *DP* families have two *A* and two *B* genes each. These genes are called *DQA1*, *DQA2*, *DQB1*, *DQB2* and *DPA1*, *DPA2*, *DPB1*, *DPB2*. The DR, DQ and DP α-chains associate primarily with the β-chains of their own family. *DPA1* and *DPB1* products associate to give rise to the serologically detectable HLA-DP class II molecules; similarly, *DQA1* and *DQB1* encode the HLA-DQ antigens. Within the DR locus, *DRA*, is coupled to a variable number of *B* genes (*B1*, *B3* or *B4* etc, depending on the haplotype), only some of which are expressed. Nucleotide sequence determination suggests that the *DPA2*, *DPB2*, *DVB* and *DRB2* genes are pseudogenes. The *DNA* gene appears to be intact but since it produces mostly abnormally large mRNA molecules, it is not known whether these molecules can be translated and their products expressed at the cell surface. It is likely that the DNα/DOβ heterodimer is expressed in similar situations to the mouse H-2O molecule, described above. The DM molecule has an analogous function to the mouse Mα/Mβ heterodimer in facilitating peptide loading onto classical class II molecules.

The *HLA-D* region spans about 850kb and the order of the various genes has been established in detail (*Fig. 4.5*). The order of these loci is similar to that of the homologous loci in the murine class II region, as mentioned earlier (*Fig. 4.3*) PFGE has also established a linkage map of the entire human MHC, including the class I, II and III regions, of about 4000kb.

GENETIC BASIS OF POLYMORPHISM

Most class I and II molecules are highly polymorphic structures. This polymorphism was originally defined through the use of alloantisera, alloreactive lymphocyte populations and, more recently, monoclonal antibodies and then direct DNA sequencing. The list of different HLA specificities has grown very large (*Fig. 4.6*). In some cases the location of the epitopes recognized by the antibodies or T cells used to define these specificities is known. In this section, the molecular basis of the observed polymorphism will be discussed. Mechanisms involved in generating and maintaining this variability at the genetic level will be described later.

Class I polymorphism

Amino acid sequence analysis has shown that H-2K and D and HLA-A and B molecules are highly polymorphic, whereas H-2L and HLA-C molecules appear less so. The amino acid sequence variability in class I antigens is clustered in three main (hypervariable) regions of the α1 and α2 domains (residues 62–83, 95–121, 135–177 in the mouse; 68–80, around 110 and 175 in humans). The highly variable positions line the peptide binding groove. The α3 domain appears to be much more conserved. No characteristic sequences have been identified which could classify a gene as being a product of a particular locus. That is, there is no evidence from inspection of sequences for consistent locus-specific differences, namely a 'K-ness' or 'D-ness' or an 'A-ness' or 'B-ness'.

Mutations detected by parent to offspring skin-grafting have been found most frequently in the *H-2K*^{b} locus and these are known as the 'bm' series of mutants. A number of these mutants differ in only one amino acid resulting in a single nucleic acid base substitution (for example, bm5). In other cases, two or more amino acid changes are involved and some of these require at least two base changes (for example, bm1 which has three amino acid changes and seven altered bases). Similar mutations also seem to have occurred in human class I molecules.

The determination of the three-dimensional structure of HLA-A2 has allowed the relative positions of the polymorphic amino acids to be determined. Most of the polymorphic amino acids are clustered near the top of the molecule in the peptide binding site. Most T cell epitopes are also positioned in this site.

Class II polymorphism

A high degree of polymorphism is also seen in class II molecules. Two-dimensional gel electrophoresis studies, sequence analysis and Southern hybridization analysis have

Class II								Class I		
DPB1	DPA1	DMA	DMB	DQB1	DQA1	DRB1	DRA	B	C	A
66	8	4	4	25	16	137	2	136	38	60

Fig. 4.6 Numbers of currently recognised HLA alleles and alloantigenic specificities. The numbers of alleles as distinct antigenic specificities or sequences, defined in a series of International Histocompatibility Workshops, detected at each HLA subregion are listed. Each allele is defined by the locus symbol followed by an asterisk, then a four digit number (e.g. DRB1*0101). The first two digits following the asterisks refer to the allele and the second two provide for up to 99 small variations in the allele. Data from Bodmer *et al*, 1994.

shown that most polymorphism occurs in *DRB*, *DQB* and *DPB* as well as *DQA* genes, while *DPA* genes are largely non-polymorphic and *DRA* is invariant. As with class I molecules, allelic variations are not random but occur clustered in particular regions of the molecule around the peptide groove (*Fig. 4.7*). Similarly, the DQβ-chain has three major clusters of amino acid variability residues 52–58, 70–77 and 84–90 of the β1 (N-terminal) domain.

Mechanisms

The mechanisms that generate the polymorphism of class I and II molecules continue to be debated. Clearly, random point mutations could contribute to the generation of allelic products, particularly if fixed in the population by phenotypic selection pressure. However, different class I and II alleles differ at multiple residues, unlike other allelic proteins which generally differ at single residues. Furthermore, non-allelic genes can share polymorphic sequences which differentiate alleles. Thus, mechanisms other than simple random point mutations generate the observed polymorphism.

One mechanism postulated to account for the generation of multiple nucleotide substitutions in class I and II alleles has been termed 'gene conversion' or 'copy substitution' (to distinguish it from the classical meiotic gene conversion originally described for certain fungi). Donor gene sequences present elsewhere in the genome (probably other class I and II genes) are thought to be copied and substituted in a non-reciprocal fashion onto recipient genes. Although the precise mechanism is unclear, it would probably be mediated through homologous flanking regions in the two genes and could occur following the resolution of heteroduplex hybrid DNA formed as a recombination intermediate. It has been proposed that the class I genes mapping to the *Q/T* region of the mouse MHC represent a reservoir of potential sequence variability which generates diversity of class I molecules in the H-2 region by acting as donor genes for such conversion events. For example, a donor gene *Q10* has been identified as generating the *H-2K*^{bm1} mutant allele from the *H-2K*^b gene. Similarly, the mutant bm6 appears to have incorporated a *Q4* gene

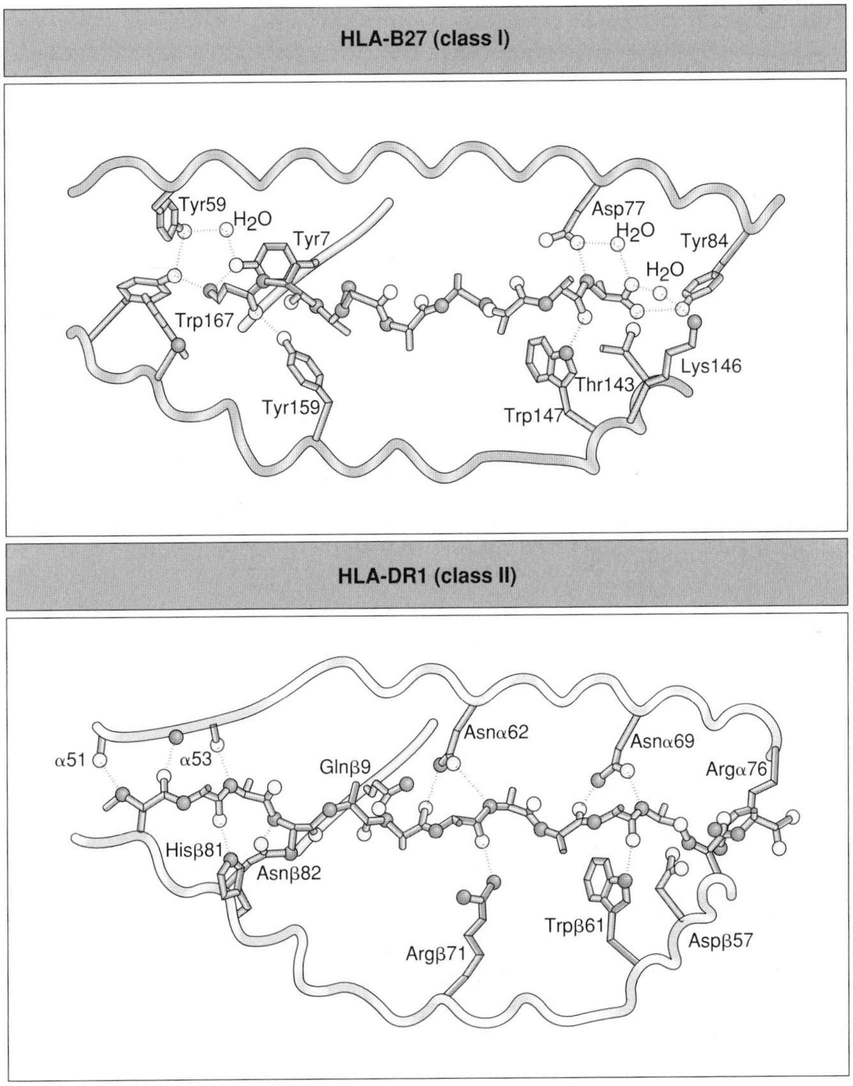

HLA-B27 (class I)

HLA-DR1 (class II)

Fig. 4.7 Interaction between peptide and MHC molecules. Two structures are shown: A, class 1 (HLA-B27); B, class II (HLA-DR1). Residues that form hydrogen bonds with atoms of the bound peptide are shown. Note how the peptide is anchored at the ends for class I and along the length of the peptide for class II. From Stern and Wiley, 1994.

segment. Nucleotide sequence comparisons of Eb^b and the Ab^{bm12} chain from the bm12 mutant have been taken as evidence that the bm12 mutation was produced by the transfer of a stretch of 14–44 nucleotides from the exon encoding the Eb^b first domain to the equivalent region in Ab^b. In contrast to class II *b* genes, *Aa* genes have shown no evidence for gene conversion, even though they have a similar clustering of regions of allelic polymorphism. These observations, together with the lower mutation rate of the D^b gene compared to the K^b gene, suggest that gene conversion does not occur with the same frequency in all class I and II genes.

Although there are a large number of alleles of the highly polymorphic class I and class II loci there is no evidence for a high mutation rate in these genes. On the contrary, MHC alleles are in some cases very old and similar allelic sequences can be found in different species. Thus, according to the 'trans-species hypothesis' new species arise with sets of many alleles from primordial species.

Some insight into the generation of novel alleles was provided by studying remote South American tribes, whose ancestors were thought to have migrated across the land bridge between Asia and North America. Certain HLA-B alleles appeared to have arisen recently (i.e. since migration) in these isolated populations, presumably selected in response to environmental pathogens. Interestingly, the alleles, although novel, were possibly derived from micro-recombination, or gene conversion, between different existing alleles.

Taking this information together with that from the bm series of mutations, it seems possible that variation in the highly polymorphic HLA genes is achieved by a variety of mechanisms, including gene conversion, recombination and mutation. At present, the relative contribution of the different mechanisms to the diversification of the MHC loci remains to be determined.

There appears to be a 'hot-spot' for recombination within a 2kb region of the intron between the first and second exons, including part of the second exon, of the E^b gene. A similar region may also exist between *DP* and *DR/DQ*, in the human *D* region, between the *TAP* genes. Other hot spots also occur in *A* and *DQ* as well as between *HLA-C* and *A*. Analysis of overlapping cosmid clones of BALB/c and AKR mouse I regions has indicated that the 'hot spot' in E^b forms a sharp boundary of polymorphism. In microorganisms, 'hot spots' often occur in regions with short palindromic sequences, which allow single DNA strands to form short loops.

BIOSYNTHESIS OF MHC CLASS I AND CLASS II MOLECULES

Assembly of protein subunits

CLASS I MOLECULES

The primary translation products of both heavy chain and β_2m mRNA have N-terminal extensions containing a signal sequence which directs the nascent polypeptide chains to the endoplasmic reticulum. The signal sequence is enzymatically removed. Glycosylation occurs concomitantly with translation. Studies with tunicamycin, which blocks N-linked

glycosylation, have demonstrated that the carbohydrate moieties are not required for membrane insertion or for transport to the membrane. Transport requires β_2m because the Daudi cell line, which does not synthesize β_2m, fails to express HLA-A and B antigens, even though class I molecules and their mRNA are present in normal amounts in the cytoplasm. Association of the heavy chain with β_2m in the endoplasmic reticulum probably occurs as the heavy chain is extended into the lumen. If association does not take place at this time, a conformational change occurs which renders the heavy chain unable to associate with β_2m. Experiments in cells lacking the *TAP* genes show that class I heavy chain molecules, β_2m and a source of peptide are all required for class I molecules to be exported to the cell surface. Following association, transport to the surface occurs via the Golgi apparatus.

An unusual category of class I mRNA molecules has recently been described; it has codons for hydrophilic amino acids as well as a termination codon in the exon normally encoding the transmembrane region. These mRNA molecules appear to be expressed in liver cells only and it is thought that they direct the synthesis of soluble class I molecules.

CLASS II MOLECULES

The biosynthesis of class II antigens is similar in many respects to that of class I molecules. Class II α and β-chains are inserted into the rough endoplasmic reticulum via their cleavable N-terminal signal sequences. Signal sequence cleavage, glycosylation and assembly of α and β-chains occur during or shortly after translation. Association of α and β-chains is obligatory for surface expression.

One peculiarity of class II antigen biosynthesis is that the $\alpha\beta$ complex is associated internally with an additional polypeptide called the invariant chain (Ii). This component is a type 2 glycoprotein and is in the opposite orientation to the class II α and β-chains with its amino-terminus exposed in the cytoplasm. At least two forms of Ii, called p31 and p41, can associate with class II antigens. These two forms are encoded by a single invariant chain gene and produced by differential splicing of a common pre-RNA. The pattern of expression of Ii chains mirrors that of class II antigens but Ii is also expressed in some other cell types that fail to express class II.

The $\alpha\beta$–Ii complex is transported to an acidic endosomal compartment where dissociation of Ii occurs. The $\alpha\beta$ complex probably spends some time in this compartment since there is a delay of 1–3 hours in transport from the *trans* Golgi to the cell surface. The Ii chain appears to have more than one role. It may facilitate loading of processed peptides onto class II antigens. It could serve this function by directing transport to an appropriate organelle, such as an endosome-like MIIC vesicle, where processing and association can occur. Invariant chain is also used to mask the peptide binding site and consequently prevent association of self-peptides in the cell. These aspects are discussed more fully in Chapter 7.

Intracellular traffic of MHC antigens and peptide binding

The intracellular traffic routes intersected by class I and class II antigens are important in considering the mechanisms by which they acquire processed antigen. In general, class I molecules are not internalized and do not recycle. There is limited internalization of class II antigens and some may recycle to the cell surface. The observation that for the large part neither class I nor class II antigens recycle dictates that they must interact with foreign antigen during the course of biosynthesis and transport. The intersection of class II antigens with the endocytic pathway prior to arrival at the cell surface provides a mechanism for association with processed peptide. Class I and class II antigens interact with processed antigen at distinct sites within the cell. Details of these processes are to be found in Chapter 7.

Peptide binding

In class I molecules, clusters of conserved residues form hydrogen bonds with the amino and carboxyl termini of bound peptide (*Fig. 4.7*). These bonds involve conserved residues in the class I structure, particularly tyrosines at the N-terminus of the peptide and a conserved lysine, as well as other residues at the C-terminus. Peptides of eight to ten residues can apparently be accommodated by maintaining hydrogen bonds at these anchor positions and by bulging out at the centre. Peptides can therefore have different conformations at their centres with ends buried in the same pockets.

As mentioned earlier, peptides bound to class II molecules extend out of the ends of the groove and the bonds tethering the peptide are not concentrated at anchor positions but are distributed. Variations in residues lining the pockets account for their different specificities.

These structures have gone a long way to explaining the high affinity/low specificity peptide binding reaction characteristic of MHC molecules.

Sources of peptide

Considerable data have now been collected on peptides sequenced from class I and class II grooves. Rammensee, 1994, pioneered the technique of purifying MHC molecules and eluting the bound peptides with acid. The initial attempts to identify peptides worked since conserved, in register, anchor residues could be identified in the mixtures of peptides which were predominantly nine amino acids long. Since these early experiments, elution and identification of peptides in smaller and smaller quantities have been made possible by advances in the application of tandem mass spectrometry.

The many peptide sequences now obtained serve to illustrate the point that the optimum size for class I peptides is nine amino acids. Class II peptides, on the other hand, tend to be longer, at over 15 residues. Once sufficient sequences have been analyzed the anchor residues for class I peptides, from different allelic products, are clearly identifiable since they lie at fixed points (e.g. position 2 and position 9). The conserved residues on class II-associated peptides are more difficult to spot because of the ragged ends and because with class II there does not seem to be such an absolute preference for anchor residues.

By searching protein databases it is possible to determine the origins of the eluted peptides and here there are some surprises. Peptides from class I molecules have been estimated to number over 10 000 different sequences. Comparisons of different cell types, such as B cells and melanoma, shows that over 90% of the prominent peptides

are shared between the two tissues. Many of the peptides eluted from HLA-A2.1 and HLA-B7 turned out to be derived from signal sequences.

Peptides eluted from class II molecules were expected to be derived from exogenous sources but more than 85% of eluted peptides were in fact from endogenous proteins that intersect the endocytic/class II pathway. The predominant endogenous peptides were derived from self MHC-related molecules, including class I, class II and invariant chain, and only a few were derived from exogenous bovine serum proteins in which the cells were grown (*Fig. 4.8*). Some of the peptides had characteristics to mark them as originating from lysosomes.

The predominance of self MHC-related peptides suggests that they may play a role as immunomodulators to which the host individual is tolerant.

EXPRESSION OF CLASS I AND II MOLECULES

Tissue distribution

Since it is now known that class I molecules principally play the role of alerting the immune system to kill infected cells, it is no surprise that many cells express class I molecules. Red blood cells are class I negative and this is understandable as they are not nucleated and are incapable of supporting viral infections. It is not always appreciated that the levels of class I molecule expression vary extremely widely between tissues. Moreover, expression of class I genes is induced by interferons so that although many tissues display a low level of constitutive class I, when the tissue is infected class I levels may be dramatically upregulated. Expression of molecules involved in processing antigens for presentation on class I, the TAPs and LMPs for example, is also upregulated by interferon. In general, cells of the immune system express particularly high levels of class I antigens (*Fig. 4.9*).

Class II antigens are generally thought to be expressed predominantly on B cells and antigen-presenting cells of the immune system. This is consistent with their role of alerting other cells of the immune system to extracellular antigens. Class II molecules on B cells are used to activate appropriate Th cells which in turn stimulate the B cell to produce antibody. Similarly, class II molecules on macrophages recruit help from T cells in order to become activated to destroy intracellular pathogens.

Other cell types can also express class II antigens, under either physiological or pathological conditions and upon induction by interferon and other inflammatory cytokines. Endothelial cells and lymphatics in most tissues normally express class II molecules and activation of human T cells also leads to class II expression. In addition, epithelial cells in a number of different organs may carry class II antigens. Interestingly, capillaries in the human brain and placenta do not appear to express class II antigens; this is an observation which might relate to the fact that both of these tissues are relatively immunologically privileged. A number of tissues have been shown to bear class II antigens under pathological conditions. For example, thyroid epithelial cells of some patients with Graves' disease and Hashimoto's thyroiditis express class II molecules. The *in vivo* function of class II

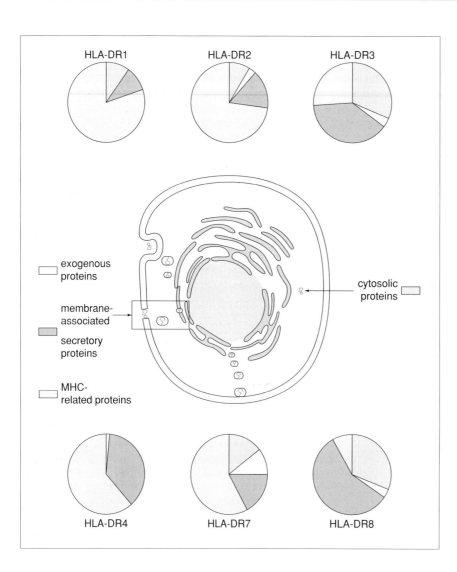

HLA-DR1   HLA-DR2   HLA-DR3

exogenous
proteins

membrane-
associated

secretory
proteins

MHC-
related proteins

cytosolic
proteins

HLA-DR4   HLA-DR7   HLA-DR8

Fig. 4.8 Origins of peptides in the grooves of class II molecules. The pie diagrams show the relative frequency and source of peptide bound to six different HLA-DR allelic products. Source proteins have been divided into: exogenous serum proteins, endogenous membrane-associated/cytosolic proteins and endogenous cytosolic proteins. The number of identified peptides for each allele has been plotted. Note the high level of MHC-related peptides. Figure from Chicz *et al*, 1993.

Tissue	MHC class I	MHC class II
Cells of the immune system		
B Cells	+++	+++
T Cells	+++	− (+ve when activated)
Macrophages	+++	++ (variable)
Dendritic cells	+++	+++
Other tissues		
Kidney	+	+/−
Hepatocytes	+/−	−
Brain	+	−
Red blood cells	−	−
Placenta	−	−

Fig. 4.9 Distribution of MHC class I and class II molecules on human tissues. The distribution of class I and class II antigens in various tissues and on different cell types shown here is based on data obtained using a sensitive immunoperoxidase method as well as other techniques. Class I molecules are expressed widely but their levels can vary considerably from tissue to tissue. Class II molecules are generally confined to cells of the immune system but appear on other tissues after induction with interferon γ.

antigens on tissues of non-lymphoid origin is unclear. However, it is reasonable to speculate that these class II antigen-bearing cells could present foreign antigen to T cells. Indeed, class II-positive thyroid epithelial cells have been shown to present peptide antigens to cloned human T helper cells.

Regulation of class I and class II gene expression

A major level of regulation of class I and class II gene expression occurs at the transcriptional stage. For both sets of genes *cis*-acting DNA elements (that is, promoters and enhancers) and *trans*-acting factors that bind to these DNA elements have been identified revealing a complex series of positive and negative regulatory events. Another way of controlling class I protein expression on the cell surface is by regulating the supply of peptides, so that low *TAP* gene expression will result in most of the class I molecules remaining in the endoplasmic reticulum, as in T2 or RMA-S mutant cells. Loss of class I expression is a feature of many tumours in order to escape immune recognition and this can take place by loss of expression of class I genes, or, more frequently, loss of β_2m or of TAP expression. Tumour cells can also switch off class I expression by failing to express the factors KBF1 and NF-κB, which bind to an upstream enhancer element. Regulation of expression of both class I and class II is highly complex, reflecting their central role.

CLASS I GENE TRANSCRIPTION

For class I genes, the region approximately -200 to -150bp upstream contains the so-called enhancer A and the interferon response element (IRE). Other regulatory sequences occur either side. As expected, the β_2m gene contains similar regulatory motifs. Some of the regulatory regions of class I genes are shown in *Figure 4.10*. It can be shown that this upstream region is not occupied by DNA binding proteins in class I-negative brain tissue.

Repression of class I gene expression is likely to take place along with downregulating immune responses and this is thought to occur in response to hormones. This may explain why hormone treatments are sometimes effective in autoimmune diseases such as rheumatoid arthritis. Hormone repression may be mediated by cAMP interacting with a DNA target within 135bp of the transcription initiation site.

CLASS II GENE REGULATION

The features involved in the regulation of class II gene transcription are known in detail. The restricted tissue distribution and inducibility of class II genes has made them popular models for studying gene regulation. Two conserved sequences, a 10bp X box and a 14bp Y box, have been identified in class II *A* and *B* genes (*Fig. 4.10B*). These sequences are separated by A and B-specific sequences of about 19bp. Deletion analysis identified the class II X and Y boxes as strong positive control elements and also pinpointed other positive and negative regulatory elements. Analysis of B cell nuclear extracts revealed the presence of numerous factors that bind to upstream regions of class II genes. These include factors that bind specifically to the W, X and Y boxes and a factor that binds to an octamer motif nearly identical to the Ig octamer motif.

Interferon γ is one of the most potent inducers of class II expression and its activity is directed through the S, X1 and Y elements (*Fig. 4.10*). TNFα, TGFβ, IFNα and β also modulate class II expression although their actions cannot be easily generalized and are dependent on the tissue and its state of differentiation.

The importance of the various class II regulatory elements *in vivo* has been underscored by establishing transgenic mouse lines harbouring class II genes deleted in these elements. Deletion of either the X or Y box results in reduced levels of transcription and, in the case of the Y box, abolition of class II expression in macrophages. These transgenic lines have been used in experiments, described in Chapter 6, to determine which cell types mediate selection in the thymus. Congenital mutations resulting in loss of expression of one or other regulatory element can also result in a severe combined immunodeficiency disease (SCID) in some patients with the bare lymphocyte syndrome (BLS).

SUMMARY

Class I and II molecules of the MHC are highly polymorphic cell-surface recognition structures that enable the immune system to distinguish self from non-self and to respond appropriately. Class I molecules consist of a membrane-associated glycoprotein chain, encoded within the MHC, in non-covalent association with β_2m, which is encoded on a different chromosome. Both class I and class II molecules bind processed antigen, the complex interacting with TCRs on cytotoxic and helper T cells, respectively. The solution of the three-dimensional structure of class I and class II molecules has provided a structural basis for peptide binding to class I antigens by defining the antigen binding cleft around which most of the amino acid polymorphism is clustered.

Class I genes can be divided into two categories: genes that encode classical transplantation antigens (mouse *H-2K, D, L* and human *HLA-A, B, C* genes) and genes that map close by but also have other functions. Some of the non-classical genes provide a pool of genetic information which is used in the generation of polymorphism of class I molecules, at least in the mouse. Other class I loci, such as *M*, are responsible for presenting bacterial peptides which are preceded by formyl methionine at their N-termini. Some novel class II genes (*DMA* and *DMB* in humans; *Ma* and *Mb* in mouse) are involved in peptide loading onto conventional class II molecules. The other class II locus, *H-2O (DNA* and *DOB* in humans), is, to date, of unknown function. Other loci in the class II region (*TAP* and *LMP*) are involved in processing antigens in order to provide peptides for class I molecules.

Class I and class II molecules obtain peptides from different sources and many peptides eluted from class II molecules are from proteins of the immune system. The different known functions of class I and class II molecules reflect their expression patterns. Class I molecules are expressed rather ubiquitously but class II is restricted to tissues of the immune system, except under the influence of immune modulators such as IFNγ. Regulation of expression of both class I and class II by transcription is complex.

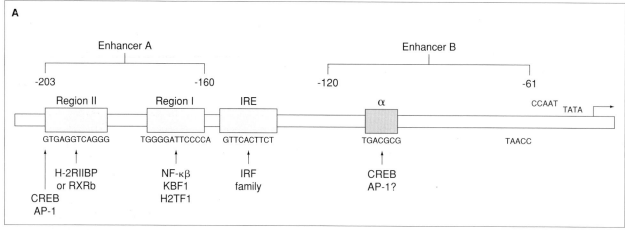

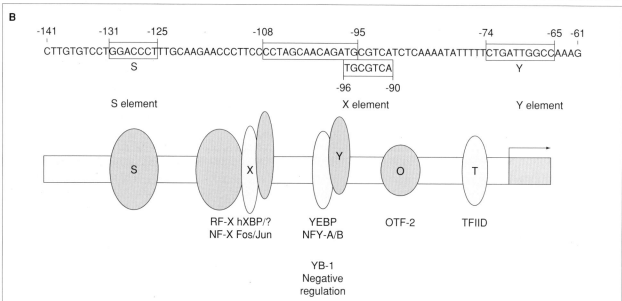

Fig. 4.10 Upstream control elements of class I and class II genes. A. Map of the 5' flanking DNA of the H-2K^b class I gene. Some of the main regulatory DNA elements are shown along with some of the proteins that bind to them. AP, activator protein. CREB, cAMP-response element binding factor. IRF, interferon regulatory factor. Note that one of the RXRβ proteins is encoded near the *DP* genes in the MHC. This is a member of the nuclear hormone receptor family that heterodimerizes with thyroid hormone and retinoic acid receptors. Also note that levels of NF-κB in the nucleus are regulated by controlling the levels of IκB, to which it binds in the cytoplasm. IκB breakdown is achieved by the proteasome. B. Transcription regulatory region of a class II gene, showing the main DNA target sequences and some of the proteins that complex with the region. hXBP binds X2,

RF-X binds X1. NFY-A, NFY-B and YEBP bind the Y element. YB-1 expression can inhibit IFNγ-induced class II expression. OTF-2 binds to the octamer (o) element. The molecular interactions involved in this complex control are subject to intensive research. It is interesting to note that some of the binding proteins may interact with each other to coordinate regulation. This is suggested by the conserved spatial arrangements between the S, X and Y region. For example, the spacing between S and X is generally 15–17bp. The addition of half a helical turn between these two abrogates constitutive as well as IFNγ inducible expression. The spacing between X and Y is similarly set at 18–21bp presumably to allow protein: protein interaction at the same side of the DNA helix. Taken from Ting and Baldwin, 1993.

FURTHER READING

Bjorkman PJ, Saper MA, Samraoui B, Bennett WS, Strominger J, Wiley D. The foreign antigen binding site and T cell recognition regions of class I histocompatibility antigens. *Nature* 1987a, **329**:512.

Bjorkman PJ, Saper MA, Samraoui B, Bennett WS, Strominger JL, Wiley DC. Structure of the human class I histocompatibility antigen, HLA-A2. *Nature* 1987b, **329**:506.

Bodmer JG, Marsh SGF, Parham *et al.* Nomenclature for factors of the HLA system. *Tissue Antigens* 1994, **44**:1.

Brown JH, Jardetzky TS, Gorga JC, Stern LG, Urban RG, Strominger JL, Wiley DC. Three-dimensional structure of the human class II histocompatibility antigen HLA-DR1. *Nature* 1993, **364**:33.

Campbell RD, Trowsdale J. Map of the human MHC. *Immunol Today* 1993, **14**:349.

Chicz RM, Urban RG, Gorga JC, Vignali AA, Lane WS, Strominger JL. Specificity and promiscuity among naturally processed peptides bound to HLA-DR alleles. *J Exp Med* 1993, **178**:27.

Daar AS, Fuggle SV, Fabre JW, Ting A, Morris PJ. The detailed distribution of HLA-A, -B and -C antigens in normal human organs. *Transplant* 1984, **38**:287.

Davidson HW, Reid PA, Lazavecchia A, Watts C. Processed antigen binds to newly synthesized MHC class II molecules in antigen specific B lymphocytes. *Cell* 1991, **67**:105.

Degen E, Williams DB. Participation of a novel 88kDa protein in the biogenesis of murine class I histocompatibility molecules. *J Cell Biol* 1991, **112**:1099.

Dunham I, Sargent CA, Trowsdale J, Campbell RD. Molecular mapping of the human major histocompatibility complex by pulsed-field gel electrophoresis. *Proc Natl Acad Sci USA* 1987, **84**:7237.

Englehard VH. Structure of peptides associated with MHC class I molecules. *Curr Opin Immunol* 1994, **6**:13.

Erlich HA, Gyllesten UB. Shared epitopes among HLA class II alleles: gene conversion, common ancestry and balancing selection. *Immunol Today* 1991, **12**:441.

Falk K, Rotzschke O, Stevanovic S, Jung G, Rammensee H. Allele-specific motifs revealed by sequencing of self-peptides eluted from MHC molecules. *Nature* 1991, **351**:290.

Fremont DH, Matsumura M, Stura EA, Peterson PA, Wilson IA. Crystal structures of two viral peptides in complex with murine MHC class I H-2K^b. *Science* 1992, **257**:919.

Garrett TP, Saper MA, Bjorkman PJ, Strominger JL, Wiley DC. Specificity pockets for the side chains of peptide antigens in HLA-Aw68. *Nature* 1989, **342**:692.

Goldberg AL, Rock KL. Proteolysis, proteasomes and antigen presentation. *Nature* 1992, **357**:375.

Guillet JG, Lai MZ, Briner TJ, Gefter ML. Interaction of peptide antigens and class II major histocompatibility complex antigens. *Nature* 1986, **324**:260.

Guo HC, Jardetsky TS, Garrett TPJ, Lane WS, Strominger JL, Wiley DC. Different length peptides bind to HLA-Aw68 similarly at their ends but bulge out in the middle. *Nature* 1992, **360**:364.

Hammer J, Nagy Z, A Sinigaglia, F. *Rules governing peptide-class II MHC molecule interactions.* Die Medizinische Verlagsgesellschaft mbH: Marburg; 1994

Hunt DF, Henderson RA, Shabanowitz J, Sakaguchi K, Michel H, Sevilir N, Cox AL, Appella E, Engelhard VH. Characterization of peptides bound to the class I MHC molecule HLA-A2.1 by mass spectrometry. *Science* 1992, **255**:1261.

Janeway CA. The T-cell receptor as a multicomponent signalling machine: CD4/CD8 coreceptors and CD45 in T-cell activation. *Ann Rev Immunol* 1992 **10**:645.

Klein J. *Natural History of the Major Histocompatibility Complex.* John Wiley and Sons. New York, 1986.

Klein J, Satta Y, OhUigin C. The molecular descent of the major histocompatibility complex. *Ann Rev Immunol* 1993, **11**:269.

Koch N, Lipp JJ, Pessara U, Schenk K, Wraight C, Dobberstein B. MHC class II invariant chains in antigen processing and presentation. *Trends Biochem Sci* 1989, **14**:383.

Li Z, Srivastava PK. *A critical contemplation on the role of heat shock proteins in transfer of antigenic peptides during antigen presentation.* Die Medizinische Verlagsgesellschaft mbH: Marburg; 1994.

Long EO. Intracellular traffic and antigen processing. *Immunol Today* 1989, **10**:232.

Madden DR, Garboczi DN, Wiley DC. The antigenic identity of peptide-MHC complexes: a comparison of the conformations of five viral peptides presented by HLA-A2. *Cell* 1993, **75**:693.

Madden DR, Gorga JC, Strominger JL, Wiley DC. The three dimensional structure of HLA-B27 at 2.1Å resolution suggests a general mechanism for tight peptide binding to MHC. *Cell* 1992, **70**:1035.

Mathis D, Benoist C. Control of transcription of class II MHC. *Ann Rev Immunol* 1990, **8**:681.

Mellor AL. Molecular genetics of class I genes in the mammalian major histocompatibility complex. In *Oxford Surveys on Eukaryotic Genes.* Rigby P (Ed). Oxford University Press: Oxford; 1986.

Mellor AL, Weiss EH, Ramachandran K, Flavell RA. A potential donor gene for the *bm1* gene conversion event in the C57BL mouse. *Nature* 1983, **306**:792.

Momburg F, Roelse J, Neefjes J, Hammerling GJ. *Peptide transporters and antigen processing.* Die Medizinische Verlagsgesellschaft mbH: Marburg; 1994.

Monaco J. A molecular model of MHC class I-restricted antigen processing. *Immunol Today* 1992, **13**:173.

Neefjes JJ, Momberg F. Cell biology of antigen presentation. *Curr Opin Immunol* 1993, **5**:27.

Parham P, Benjamin RJ, Chen BP, Clayberger C, Ennis PD, Krensky AM, Lawlor DA, Littman DR, Norment AM, Orr HT, Salter RT, Zemmour J. Diversity of class I HLA molecules: functional and evolutionary interactions with T cells. *Cold Spring Harb Symp Quant Biol* 1989, **1**:529.

Pease LR, Schulze DH, Pfaffenbach GM, Nathenson SG. Spontaneous H-2 mutants provide evidence that a copy mechanism analogous to gene conversion generates polymorphism in the major histocompatibility complex. *Proc Natl Acad Sci USA* 1983, **80**:242.

Peters PJ, Neefjes JJ, Oorschot V, Ploegh HL, Geuze HJ. Segregation of MHC class II molecules from MHC class I molecules in the Golgi complex for transport to lysosomal compartments. *Nature* 1991, **349**:669.

Powis SH, Trowsdale J. *Human major histocompatibility complex genes.* Die Medizinische Verlagsgesellschaft mbH: Marburg; 1994.

Rammensee H-G. *How the quest to identify minor histocompatibility complex antigens led to something more important.* Die Medizinische Verlagsgesellschaft mbH: Marburg; 1994.

Rammensee H-G, Friede T, Stevanovic S. MHC ligands and peptide motifs: first listing. *Immunogenetics* 1995, **41**:178.

Roche PA, Cresswell P. Invariant chain association with DR molecules inhibits immunogenic peptide binding. *Nature* 1990, **345**:615.

Roche PA, Marks MS, Cresswell P. Formation of a nine subunit complex by HLA class II glycoproteins and the invariant chain. *Nature* 1991, **345**:392.

Rotzschke O, Falk K. Origin, structure and motifs of naturally processed MHC class II ligands. *Curr Opin Immunol* 1994, **6**:45.

Ruppert J, Kubo RT, Sidney J, Grey HM, Sette A. *Class I MHC-peptide interaction: structural and functional aspects.* Die Medizinische Verlagsgesellschaft mbH: Marburg; 1994.

Santos-Aguado J, Crimmins MA, Mentzer SJ, Burakoff SJ, Strominger JL. Alloreactivity studied with mutants of HLA-A2. *Proc Natl Acad Sci USA* 1989, **86**:8936.

Seeman GHA, Rein RS, Brown CS, Ploegh HL. Gene conversion-like mechanisms may generate polymorphism in human class I genes. *EMBO J* 1986, **5**:547.

Shee JX, Boehme SA, Wang TW, Bonhomme F, Wakeland EK. Amplification of major histocompatibility complex class II gene diversity by intraexonic recombination. *Proc Natl Acad Sci USA* 1991, **88**:453.

Stern LJ, Wiley DC. *Antigenic peptide binding by Class I and Class II histocompatibility proteins.* Die Medizinische Verlagsgesellschaft mbH: Marburg; 1994.

Stern. LJ, Wiley DC. Antigenic peptide binding by class I and class II histocompatibility proteins. *Structure* 1994b, **2**:245.

Stroynowski I, Soloski M, Low MG, Hood L. A single gene encodes soluble and membrane-bound forms of the major histocompatibility Qa-2 antigen: anchoring of the product by a phospholipid tail. *Cell* 1987, **50**:759.

Ting JP-Y, Baldwin AS. Regulation of MHC gene expression. *Curr Opin Immunol* 1993, **5**:8.

Travers P, Blundell TL, Sternberg MJE, Bodmer W. Structural and evolutionary analysis of HLA-D region products. *Nature* 1984, **310**:235.

Trowsdale J. "Both man, bird, beast": comparative organization of MHC genes. *Immunogenet* 1994, **41**:1.

Vignali DAA. *The interaction between CD4 and MHC Class II molecules and its effect on T cell function.* Die Medizinische Verlagsgesellschaft mbH: Marburg; 1994.

Wang CR, Lindahl KF. Organization and structure of the *H-2M4–M8* class I genes in the mouse major histocompatibility complex. *Immunogenet* 1993, **38**:258.

5 Leukocyte Surface Molecules

The production of antibodies that recognize molecules on the surface of the various cells of the immune system has been of immense importance for defining leukocyte subsets and developmental relationships, for functional studies and for biochemical characterization of the antigens. Initially, heteroantisera or alloantisera were used; however, the advent of monoclonal antibody technology resulted in a plethora of new antibodies, many of which defined additional leukocyte surface molecules. Biennial workshops have analysed these monoclonal antibodies according to a variety of criteria, such as patterns of reactivity, their functional effects and molecular weight of the molecule(s) recognized. On the basis of this analysis, monoclonal antibodies have been clustered into CD (cluster of differentiation) groups. The CD nomenclature is used to define the antigen rather than the monoclonal antibody. Although the antibodies analysed in the workshops detect human surface molecules, many CD groups have clear counterparts in other species. The Leukocyte Typing Workshops have characterized an increasing number of CD antigens. For example, the first workshop (1982) identified CD1–10, the 1984 workshop, CD11–25, the 1986 workshop, CD26–45, the 1989 workshop, CD46–78 and the 1993 workshop, 79–130 (see Appendix).

cDNA cloning techniques have resulted in the determination of the complete primary structures of many leukocyte surface molecules. One successful strategy has utilized oligonucleotides, deduced from partial protein sequence analysis, to screen cDNA libraries. More recently, prokaryotic and eukaryotic expression systems have been widely employed. The most successful expression cloning system utilizes transient expression in the monkey Cos7 cell line followed by antibody selection. This strategy, which is outlined in *Figure 5.1*, has been used successfully for cloning genes encoding both surface molecules and growth factors. For some of these molecules DNA-mediated gene transfer combined with *in vitro* mutagenesis has permitted an analysis of the functional importance of different structural domains.

It is beyond the scope of this chapter to provide exhaustive details of the structure and function of all the leukocyte cell surface molecules that have been characterized. Rather, the general principles that have been established from the biochemical and structural analyses of these molecules will be discussed, in particular the simplifying notion that they can be grouped into superfamilies based on structural similarity.

LINEAGE FIDELITY

It is apparent from a detailed analysis of tissue distribution that the overwhelming majority of leukocyte surface molecules, although confined to the haematopoietic system, are not lineage specific. This may reflect early expression on a common progenitor or expression by different committed cell types. The implications of the expression of

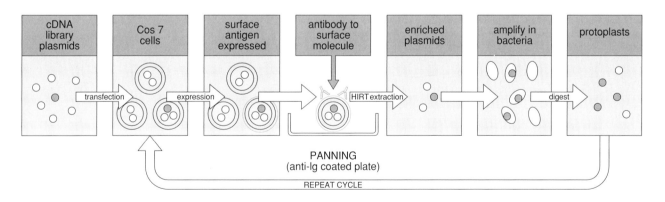

Fig. 5.1 Transient expression strategy for cloning of leukocyte antigen genes. A cDNA library, constructed in an expression vector containing a cytomegalovirus promoter is transfected using the DEAE-Dextran method into recipient Cos7 cells. After incubation to allow transient expression, cells expressing the surface antigen are separated by 'panning' using a specific antibody and anti-Ig coated plates. Plasmids harboured by Cos cells adhering to the antibody-coated plates are isolated (Hirt extraction), amplified in bacteria and reintroduced into Cos cells by protoplast fusion. Multiple rounds result in the isolation of cDNA clones encoding the surface antigen. This method has been extensively used to clone genes encoding leukocyte surface molecules Seed and Aruffo, 1987.

a surface molecule on different committed cell types for its proposed function are often unclear. The pattern of expression of a leukocyte surface molecule among cells of various haematopoietic lineages, or at different developmental stages within a lineage, can also vary between species. For example, the CD2 antigen is expressed on T cells and NK cells in the human but in mice is also found on a subset of B cells.

The lineage promiscuity and species variability of the expression of individual leukocyte surface molecules raises interesting questions concerning the tissue-specific regulation of gene expression and for the function of these molecules, in particular whether they may play different roles at different stages of development. However, it complicates the use of surface phenotypes to chart lineages and lineage relationships. Combinations of monoclonal antibodies have, nevertheless, been used to assign a cell to a particular lineage and often to a particular developmental stage within a lineage. Perhaps the most successful example of this has been the use of a battery of phenotypic markers to dissect the developmental stages in B and T cell development (Chapter 6).

THE LEUKOCYTE CELL SURFACE

It is likely that the hundred or more major CD antigens so far identified represent most of the different moderate-high abundance proteins present at leukocyte cell surfaces. Several lines of reasoning support this conclusion. For example, the major staining bands on SDS gels of leukocyte membrane preparations can be accounted for by known molecules. Furthermore, it is becoming increasingly difficult to generate monoclonal antibodies with novel specificities by immunization with leukocytes, suggesting that the major antigens have already been identified. Thus, it is likely that most of the key surface molecules involved in leukocyte function are known.

Transmembrane proteins

The amino acid sequences of leukocyte surface antigens reveal a great diversity of structures and modes of interaction with the plasma membrane (*Fig. 5.2*). Most surface antigens are transmembrane glycoproteins. However, the orientation of the polypeptide chain and the number of times that the polypeptide traverses the lipid bilayer can vary. Type I single pass transmembrane proteins form the

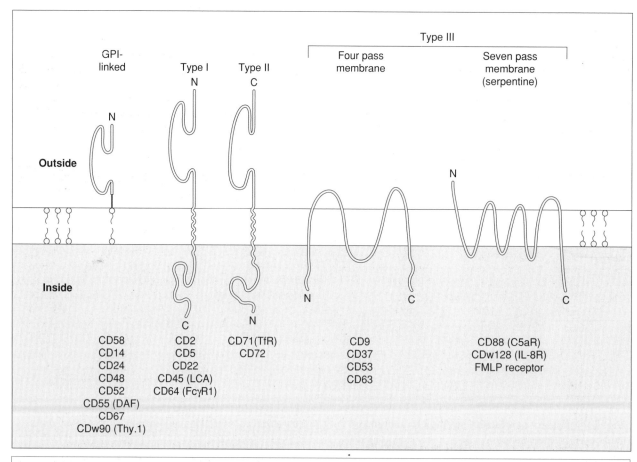

Fig. 5.2 Classes of leukocyte surface antigens. Surface proteins are classified according to the orientation of the polypeptide chain within the plasma membrane and on the basis of the number of times the protein traverses the lipid bilayer. One class of leukocyte antigens is not transmembrane, but instead is anchored via a glycosyl phosphatidylinositol (GPI) linkage. Some examples of each class of protein are given.

majority of CD proteins and are oriented with their N-terminus on the exterior face of the plasma membrane and their C-terminus in the cytoplasm. Typically, the bulk of the polypeptide chain is located outside the cell, although this is not always the case. For example, the CD3ζ-chain has only nine amino acids outside of the cell whereas its cytoplasmic tail comprises 112 residues. The transmembrane segment of type I transmembrane proteins comprises about 25 normally apolar amino acids which, if arranged in an α-helical conformation, span the 40Å lipid bilayer. This segment is usually followed by a sequence of basic amino acids, referred to as a stop-transfer sequence, that is thought to anchor the protein by binding to phospholipid headgroups at the inner face of the membrane. The cytoplasmic tail can vary in length from three amino acids (e.g. IgM heavy chains) to several hundred as in the case of CD45.

Type I membrane proteins are synthesized with a cleavable N-terminal signal sequence of about 15–30 amino acids. This sequence directs the nascent polypeptide to the rough endoplasmic reticulum (RER) and initiates translocation through the lipid bilayer. It is cleaved from the primary translation product by a signal sequence endopeptidase to generate the mature polypeptide chain.

Type II single pass transmembrane proteins have the opposite orientation to type I molecules, the N-terminus being located in the cytoplasm. An example of this type of molecule is the transferrin receptor (CD71) that has an N-terminal cytoplasmic tail of 61 amino acids, a transmembrane segment of 29 residues and a 671 residue external domain. Type II proteins are also thought to be translocated through the RER via a signal sequence, although this sequence is an internal sequence that is not cleaved. In some cases the transmembrane sequence has been shown also to act as a signal sequence.

Some leukocyte surface molecules (Type III) span the lipid bilayer multiple times. Within this class, two major categories are the seven transmembrane (or serpentine) receptors and the four transmembrane family. The serpentine family are G-protein-linked receptors that include chemokine receptors such as the IL-8 receptor (IL-8R). The four transmembrane family all have both their N- and C-termini inside the cell and members possess clear sequence similarities.

Some surface molecules are not transmembrane molecules but instead are anchored through a glycosyl phosphatidylinositol (GPI) moiety attached to the C-terminal residue of the protein (*Fig. 5.2*). This type of structure was first shown for the variant-specific glycoprotein of the *Trypanosoma brucei* parasite. The first leukocyte antigen shown to be anchored by a GPI anchor was Thy-1. A specific sequence at the C-terminus of this class of surface proteins directs the addition of the GPI anchor. This signal sequence is cleaved off shortly after biosynthesis in the RER and replaced by the GPI anchor. Some proteins, CD16, for example, can exist as either a GPI-linked or transmembrane form depending on the cell type.

Carbohydrate structures

Most leukocyte surface antigens are glycoproteins, although the levels of glycosylation can vary considerably between different molecules and the same molecule on different leukocyte populations. This is particularly striking in the case of O-linked glycosylation (see below) where simple structures are found on resting T cells (*Fig. 5.3*, structure A), whereas more complex forms occur on activated T cells and neutrophils (*Fig. 5.3*, structures B and C), presumably

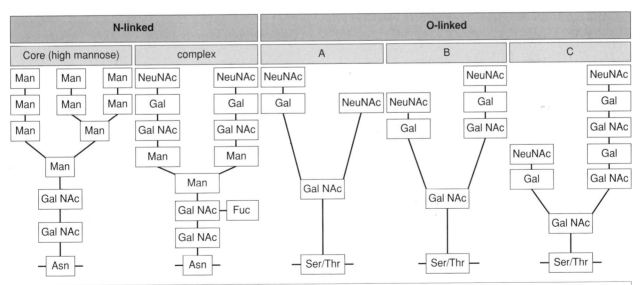

Fig. 5.3 Glycan units associated with leukocyte surface antigens. Carbohydrate moieties of leukocyte surface molecules can be broadly divided into those that are linked to asparagine (N) or serine/threonine (O) residues within the protein. N-linked glycan units are added as a core structure which is processed during transport through the Golgi complex during which various terminal sugars are added. One example of such a structure is shown. O-linked glycan units are heterogeneous and vary on different leukocytes. Some examples of structures that have been found on leukocyte surfaces are shown.

reflecting the different complement of glycosylation enzymes in these cell types. Since many leukocyte surface molecules that are extensively O-glycosylated, such as CD43, are rod-like structures, these cell type differences in the structures of the glycan units may be of functional significance in, for example, regulation of the adhesive properties of cells.

Two major classes of glycan unit are found linked to proteins at the leukocyte cell surface (*Fig. 5.3*). N-linked glycosylation occurs on asparagine residues within the consensus sequence Asn-X-Ser/Thr (where X is any amino acid except proline). N-linked glycan side chains are added to the nascent polypeptide chain within the lumen of the RER as a core, high-mannose structure. This addition is inhibited by the fungal metabolite tunicamycin. As transport to the cell surface proceeds, the core structure is modified in the Golgi complex to generate the complex sialylated forms found in the mature glycoprotein. O-linked glycosylation occurs on Ser or Thr residues. Although there is no single consensus sequence as in the case of N-linked glycosylation, a preponderance of Ser, Thr and Pro occurs within O-glycosylated regions of glycoproteins.

The functions of the carbohydrate moieties of glycoproteins are often unclear. They may perform general functions such as decreasing the susceptibility of surface glycoproteins to cleavage by serum proteases by masking sensitive sites, contributing to the net charge at the cell surface, thus preventing non-specific aggregation of leukocytes and clearance of cells from the blood by recognition of asialoglycoproteins by the Ashwell receptor in the liver. Specific functions include mediating cellular adhesion. For example, P-selectin (CD62P) interacts with Lewis-like carbohydrate structures on neutrophils. This association is discussed more fully in Chapter 14.

Dimensions of cell surface glycoproteins

The sizes and shapes of cell surface glycoproteins can vary widely. Extensively glycosylated molecules are often rod-like structures as visualized after suitable preparation by electron microscopy. Using this technique, the length of the extracellular domain of CD43 (leukosialin) was estimated to be 450Å. Other leukocyte molecules, such as the Ig superfamily members, are more compact globular proteins. In some cases, such as MHC class I and class II molecules, CD2 and CD4 the three dimensional structures are known and in other cases, such as CD48, plausible models have been constructed. Taken together, these studies suggest that interactions such as TCR-MHC class I or II and CD2-CD48 span about 135Å. A structural model for these interactions is shown in the *Colour figure* section.

The interaction of pairs of molecules such as TCR–MHC class I and II on opposing cell membranes in the presence of much larger molecules such as CD45 suggests that either discrete domains of the plasma membrane exist where specific molecules are excluded or, more likely, that some redistribution of membrane proteins occurs, for example, after initial adhesion molecule interactions between a T cell and APC. These considerations underscore the importance of the dynamic nature of the plasma membrane for leukocyte function.

PROTEIN SUPERFAMILIES

Leukocyte surface proteins can be divided into families and superfamilies. The term 'family' refers to proteins with more than 50% identity, whereas 'superfamily' describes proteins with less than 50% sequence similarity.

What does the superfamily classification signify for leukocyte surface molecules? Membership of a particular superfamily may imply a common function. It also suggests a similar three dimensional structure. Although the overall primary sequence similarity between superfamily members can be as little as 15–25% (i.e. on the borderline of statistical significance) the conservation of key residues involved in the maintenance of the tertiary structure (where such structures are known) suggests that they form a common domain or structural unit. In other words, a common general structure will dictate a unique sequence pattern that can be identified using appropriate statistical programmes.

The concept of the superfamily has arisen from extensive sequence analysis of many leukocyte membrane molecules. These studies show that many of these molecules contain domains with similarities to domains in other, apparently unrelated, molecules. The eukaryotic genome includes a number of superfamilies. Members of a superfamily are often related functionally, exhibit a common structural unit and are assumed to have arisen by gene duplication from a primordial ancestor. Genes within an ancient superfamily are generally dispersed among the different chromosomes unless a tight linkage confers a selective advantage, such as coordinate regulation of expression. Examples of the major superfamilies in the immune system are shown in *Figure 5.4*. Each of these superfamilies contains members expressed both within and outside the immune system. Presumably, a general and ancient function, such as proteolysis or adhesion, has been subverted by various systems during evolution. Some proteins comprise domains from more than one superfamily. For example, the Mel-14 or L-selectin homing receptor, CD62L, contains an N-terminal lectin C-type domain contiguous with a single epidermal growth factor-like repeat and two identical complement control protein repeats. The use of different combinations of superfamily domains provides a powerful and versatile evolutionary mechanism for generating different functional molecules.

Leukocyte surface molecule superfamilies

More than 20 different superfamilies are found in leukocyte molecules. The structural features of many of these superfamilies, which are summarized in *Figure 5.4*, are discussed in other chapters within the context of the functions of the individual superfamily members. For example, the integrin and lectin C-type superfamilies are described in Chapter 14, the cytokine receptor superfamily in Chapter 10 and the MHC superfamily (i.e. the α1 and α2 domains of MHC class I heavy chains and the α1 and β1 domains of class II α and β-chains) in Chapter 4. In order to illuminate the principles of the superfamily concept, two superfamilies, one extensively and one infrequently represented within leukocyte surface molecules are described in detail.

Superfamily domain	Examples	Common functions in immune system
Complement control protein	CD21, CD35, P-selectin (CD62P)	control of complement cascade
Cytokine receptor	IL-2Rβ (CD122), IL-6R (CDw126)	growth factor receptors
Epidermal growth factor	L-selectin (CD62L), P-selectin (CD62P)	cell surface/soluble ligand binding
Fibronectin type II	Mannose receptor	multiple functions
Fibronectin type III	Integrin β4 chain (CD104), IL-7R CDw127)	multiple functions
Immunoglobulin V set	IgV, TCRV, Thy-1 (CDw90)	adhesion; recognition
Immunoglobulin C1 set	β₂M, MHC class Iα3 domain	adhesion; recognition
Immunoglobulin C2 set	CD2 domain 2, CD3ε	adhesion; recognition
Integrin	CD11/CD18, CD49	adhesion
Lectin C-type	Mannose receptor, CD23, L-selectin (CD62L)	carbohydrate binding
Lectin S-type	Mac-2	carbohydrate binding
Leucine-rich glycoprotein (LRG) repeats	CD42a, CD42b	protein–protein or protein–lipid interactions
Link	CD44	hyaluronic acid/chrondroitin sulphate binding site
Low density lipoprotein receptor	LDL receptor	lipoprotein binding; unknown functions
Ly-6	CD59	not known
MHC	class I α1, α2 domains, class II α1, β1 domains	recognition
Nerve growth factor receptor	CD27, CD40	unknown
Rhodopsin (serpentine receptor)	IL-8R (CDw128), C5aR, fMLPR, CD5, CD6	G-protein coupled receptors
Somatomedin	PC-1 (plasma cell surface antigen)	unknown
Transmembrane 4 pass (TM4)	CD9, CD37, CD53	unknown
Phosphotyrosine phosphatase	CD45	signal transduction
Tyrosine kinase	M-CSFR, lck, flk-2, c-kit (CD117)	signal transduction

Fig. 5.4 Leukocyte antigen superfamilies. The major superfamily domains found in leukocyte membrane proteins are listed, together with some examples of proteins in which they are present. In some cases, a leukocyte antigen will comprise more than one superfamily domain (see, for example, P-selectin that contains both CCP and EGF domains). Common functions of a superfamily domain are also listed where possible. This does not imply, however, that all molecules that contain a particular domain will have such a function. Data abstracted from Barclay et al, 1993.

The Ig superfamily

The immunoglobulin superfamily (IgSF) forms the largest superfamily of leukocyte antigens and comprises proteins involved in cell recognition principally (but not exclusively) in the immune and nervous systems. About 40% of leukocyte surface molecules contain IgSF domains. The main criteria for inclusion into the Ig superfamily are that a sequence should be about the same size as, share significant homology with, and the key structural features of, an Ig domain.

The basic features of the Ig fold have been elucidated from X-ray analysis. The domain comprises two β-sheets each consisting of five to 10 amino acid stretches of antiparallel β strands (*Fig. 5.5*). The β-sheets are stabilized by interactions of hydrophobic amino acids and by an intrachain disulphide bond. IgV and C domains differ in the number of amino acids between the disulphide bond and in the number of β strands forming each β-sheet (*Fig. 5.5*). The Ig-related domains of members of the Ig superfamily can be classified as being V or C-like according to whether the pattern of β strands most resembles a V or C domain (*Fig. 5.5*). There can, however, be some deviation in the length of the β strands in Ig-related domains as well as an absence of the conserved Ig disulphide bond. Interestingly, a functional antibody has been found that has a tyrosine substituted for one of the cysteines of the V$_H$ domain, demonstrating that other interactions can replace the stabilizing force of disulphide bond formation.

IgSF C domains can be subdivided based on specific sequence patterns. IgC-type domains found in Ig, TCR and MHC antigens share the same type of sequence pattern and are referred to as the C1 set. Other IgSF members have subtly different sequence patterns, showing similarities to both V and C1 domains and are termed the C2 set. Thus, domain 2 of CD2 exhibits C2-set sequences, as do domains 2 and 4 of CD4 (*Fig. 5.5*).

The structural proof for an Ig-fold has been obtained for several of the leukocyte surface molecules, including the α3 and β$_2$-microglobulin domains of MHC class I molecules, the α2 and β2 domains of MHC class II molecules, the IgV and C domains and the CD2, CD4 and CD8α extracellular domains. In each case, the Ig-fold, consisting of a sandwich of two β-sheets, has been identified. These structural studies have also emphasized the importance of the sequence similarities of IgSF molecules for the maintenance of the tertiary structure — conserved residues generally point inwards making key contacts within the β-barrel structure, whereas sequence differences are either at the loops or pointing out and solvent-exposed.

The significance of the classification of a protein into the Ig superfamily is both functional and evolutionary. On the functional side, a prediction from the sequence homology between IgV and C regions and an Ig-related protein is that the protein folds into a β-barrel structure and that this structure is important for its function in an aspect of cell recognition.

Homology of β-strands along V and C domains	Folding pattern

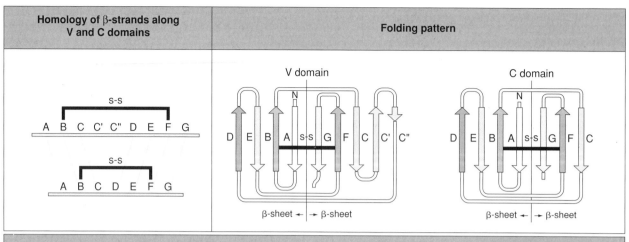

Three dimensional structure

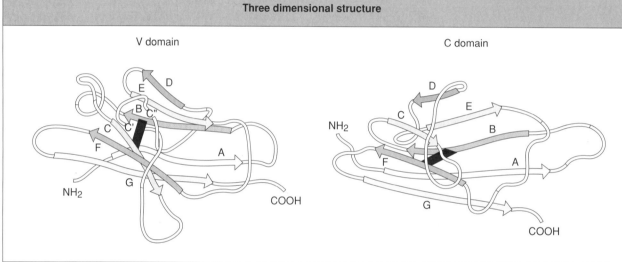

Schematic representation of immunoglobulin superfamily

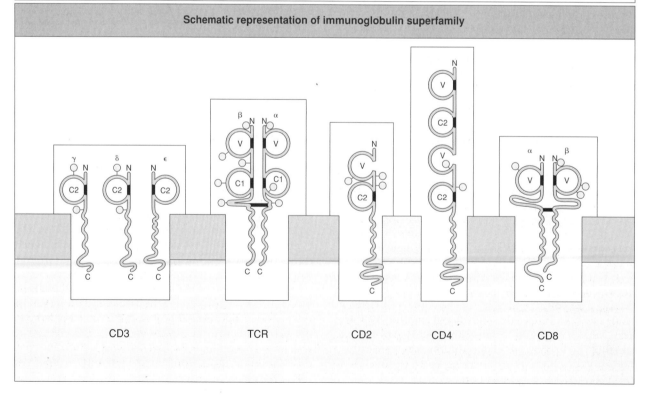

CD3   TCR   CD2   CD4   CD8

Fig. 5.5 Immunoglobulin variable (V) and constant (C) domains and the structures of some Ig superfamily members. The three-dimensional structures of immunoglobulin V and C domains, as determined by X-ray crystallographic analysis of a V_L and C_L domain, are given. The anti-parallel β-strands of the Ig fold (shown by arrows) are connected by loops of amino acids; the labelling of the β-strands along the V and C domains together with a schematic view of the fold are shown. In the schematic representation of the immunoglobulin superfamily members discussed in this chapter, domains are classified as V or C depending on whether they most resemble an immunoglobulin V or C domain. C1 and C2 are subclassifications of C-like domains. The positions of *N*-linked glycan units are shown by grey circles. Adapted from Williams and Barclay, 1988, from which a comprehensive list of Ig superfamily members can be found.

Detailed analysis of the Ig-related domains and the genes of Ig superfamily members has given rise to speculations on the evolution both of the superfamily and of recognition in the immune system. The only molecules expressing single domains, such as Thy-1, are V-like, suggesting that the V domain is the most ancient. Furthermore, although most Ig-like domains are encoded within one exon, an intron splits the domain in some instances (for example, the *CD4* gene). The primordial domain may, therefore, have been a half-domain comprising one β-sheet. Analysis of the *CD8* α and β genes has suggested a means by which antigen receptors may have evolved. The CD8β J-like segment is encoded within the same exon as the V-like domain. Thus, the CD8 αβ heterodimer may resemble the structure that gave rise to the rearranging T cell receptors and immunoglobulins by insertion of an intron and the acquisition of rearrangement machinery.

The subdivision of the Ig superfamily into groups that resemble one another most closely reveals some interesting patterns. The CD2-LFA3 receptor-ligand pair, whose genes are located close to each other on the p13 band of chromosome 1 in humans, show a relatively high overall structural similarity. The *CD3*γ, δ and ε genes also show greater than average similarity and are tightly linked on chromosome 11q23 in humans together with *Thy-1* and *NCAM*. These gene clusters of multiple Ig superfamily members might represent sites where original duplication events took place prior to dispersal of this ancient superfamily throughout the genome.

The phosphotyrosine phosphatase (PTPase) superfamily

The only member of the PTPase superfamily of integral membrane proteins expressed on leukocytes is the CD45 antigen, although other superfamily members have been identified outside of the immune system. The CD45 antigen is a major cell surface glycoprotein confined to the lymphoid and myeloid lineages. The structure of CD45 is shown schematically in *Figure 5.6*. The large globular cytoplasmic domain of about 700 amino acids is highly conserved between species with an 85% overall identity between mouse, rat and man and comprises two subdomains of internal homology of about 300 amino acids. These two homology units have been matched to the sequence of a placental cytoplasmic PTPase. PTPase activity has been shown for the membrane proximal CD45 cytoplasmic domain. The potential importance of this PTPase activity for the regulation of the PTK p56[lck] during T cell activation is discussed in Chapter 8.

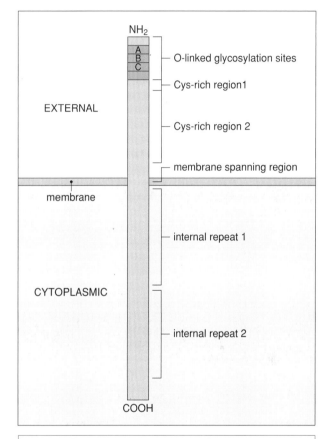

Fig. 5.6 CD45 structure. A scheme for the largest form of CD45, containing all three alternate exons (A, B and C) is shown. The positions of putative structural subdomains are indicated.

The extracellular domain of the CD45 antigen shows no homology to any known superfamily. It is divided into at least two domains. The N-terminal Ser/Thr/Pro-rich region has multiple O-linked carbohydrate. The remainder of the extracellular domain contains 16 cysteine residues that are largely conserved between man, mouse and rat. Electron microscopic studies have demonstrated that rat thymocyte CD45 consists of a rod-like structure of 180Å, comprising the external domain and membrane spanning region and a globular cytoplasmic domain of 120Å.

The extracellular domain of CD45 varies in length from 391–552 amino acids depending on the haematopoietic

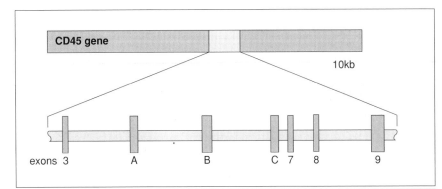

Protein	Exon usage			cDNA isolated	Glycoprotein Mω (kD)	Expression pattern of CD45				
	A	B	C			B	Thy	CD4	CD8	MØ
CD45ABC	+	+	+	h,m,r	230–240	+				
CD45AB	+	+		h	210–220			+	+	
CD45AC	+		+	—	(210–220)			?	?	
CD45BC		+	+	h,m	210–220			+	+	
CD45A	+			—	(190–200)			?	?	?
CD45B		+		hr	190–200			+	+	?
CD45C			+	m,r	190–200			+	+	?
CD45				h,m,r	170–180		+	+		+

Fig. 5.7 Differential exon usage for CD45 mRNA in humans (h), mice (m) and rats (r). The genomic organization is based on the mouse gene. The enlarged portion represents the area of the gene encoding the variable exons; each exon (indicated by a rectangle) is drawn proportional to its size, A, B and C being the three variable exons. mRNA splicing events give rise to alternate exon usage as indicated by the CD45 subscript and the variable exon(s) included in each mRNA are shown. cDNAs have not been isolated from every form (non-isolated by —). Expression of the different CD45 isoforms on B cells, thymocytes, CD4+ and CD8+ T cells and macrophages (MØ) is indicated. Data from Thomas, 1989.

lineage. This is reflected in a variation in molecular weight from 180–240kDa on SDS-polyacrylamide gels and by the existence of both common and restricted epitopes on the polypeptide chain. Six forms of the CD45 antigen have been isolated as cDNAs from human, rat and murine libraries and the expression of these various isoforms is controlled in a cell type-specific manner (*Fig. 5.7*). For example, B cells express the highest molecular weight form whereas immature thymocytes express the lowest. Mature T cells have a more complex pattern of expression with at least four different molecular weight forms depending on the subset and differentiation state of the cell. The pattern of expression also changes during activation of T cells.

The structural and genetic basis for these different forms of CD45 has been determined by cDNA and genomic cloning studies. The predicted amino acid sequences reveal extensive variability at the N-terminal end. The CD45 gene is single copy and at least 120kb long, containing 34 exons. The N-terminal seven amino acids of the mature protein are encoded in a discrete exon and are common to all members. The differential splicing events that give rise to the various CD45 isoforms involve three exons, A, B and C (*Fig. 5.7*). Differential splicing of these three exons can generate eight possible mRNAs, as shown in *Figure 5.7*, six of which have been identified from cDNAs. The predicted molecular weights of the alternatively spliced forms correlate with the CD45 species detected by gel electrophoresis.

The variable exons are expressed in a cell type-specific manner. Thus, B cells, which express the highest molecular weight form, use all three variable exons whereas immature thymocytes splice out exons A, B and C, giving rise to the lowest molecular weight form. Peripheral T cells use a number of combinations. The precise control of the differential splicing events is complex and incompletely understood but involves both tissue-specific *trans* acting factors and *cis* elements within the alternatively spliced exons and the flanking intron sequences.

The differential splicing events at the N-terminal end of the CD45 antigen clearly give rise to amino acid sequence diversity in this region that forms a structural basis both for the different molecular weight isoforms and for the existence of antibodies that recognize epitopes (called CD45R) restricted to some forms only. CD45R antibodies are further classified according to which alternately spliced exon encodes the epitope recognized by the antibody. Correlation of antibody reactivity with exon usage has in some cases permitted an assignment of an epitope to a particular exon (*Fig. 5.8*). Examples of this are the antibodies 2H4 (a CD45RA antibody), which most probably recognizes an epitope on exon A and UCHL1 (a CD45RO antibody), which recognizes a 180kDa molecular weight form of CD45, binding a determinant created by differential glycosylation within exon 7 in the completely spliced out form. Some CD45R antibodies are functionally useful in splitting T cell subsets.

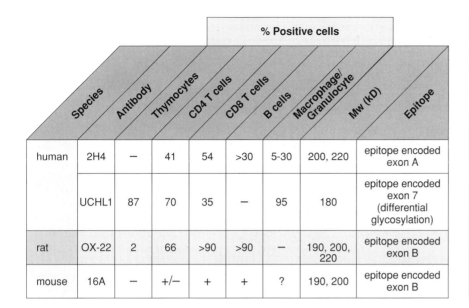

Species	Antibody	Thymocytes	CD4 T cells	CD8 T cells	B cells	Macrophage/ Granulocyte	Mw (kD)	Epitope
human	2H4	–	41	54	>30	5-30	200, 220	epitope encoded exon A
	UCHL1	87	70	35	–	95	180	epitope encoded exon 7 (differential glycosylation)
rat	OX-22	2	66	>90	>90	–	190, 200, 220	epitope encoded exon B
mouse	16A	–	+/–	+	+	?	190, 200	epitope encoded exon B

% Positive cells

Fig. 5.8 Antibodies that recognize restricted CD45 epitopes. The recognition characteristics of antibodies which were used to examine CD45 family member expression are shown. 2H4 is an example of the CD45RA class, OX-22 and 16A of the CD45RB class, and UCHL1 forms the CD45RO class of CD45 monoclonal antibodies. The reactivity of these antibodies with some leukocyte subsets expressed as the % of cells in the various tissues that react, and the CD45 molecular weight forms recognized are shown. The data on 16A subset reactivity are not quantitative, but qualitatively resemble OX-22.

For example, UCHL1 and 2H4 identify reciprocal populations of CD4-positive T cells, UCHL1 being associated with activated cells and the memory cell pool of both CD4 and CD8-positive T cells. Differentiation of a naive T cell to a CD4-positive memory cell is associated with loss of the 2H4 and gain of the UCHL1 determinant. The 2H4 antibody has counterparts in rat (called OX-22) and mouse (called 16A) that define distinct subsets of CD4-positive T cells (*Fig. 5.8*).

The protein sequence encoded by these alternate CD45 exons occurs within the Ser/Thr/Pro-rich O-glycosylated region of the extracellular domain. The resulting differential O-glycosylation that is a consequence of variable exon usage may contribute to CD45R epitopes and may be functionally important in different cell types, such as in determining specific cell–cell interactions. In this context, it has proved difficult to identify ligands for CD45, although CD45RO has been shown to bind to the B cell surface molecule CD22.

SUMMARY

The recent advances in molecular cloning techniques have led to a detailed knowledge of the amino acid sequences of numerous leukocyte antigens. These include receptors and accessory molecules, as well as molecules with unknown function but which are selectively expressed within the haematopoietic lineage. Although leukocyte surface molecules exhibit a wide variety of structures, they can be classified into families on the basis of common structural properties or sequence similarities. Thus, they are divided into families based on whether or not they are transmembrane proteins, the orientation of the polypeptide within the lipid bilayer and the number of times that the polypeptide traverses the membrane. Leukocyte antigens are also divided into superfamilies comprising members with sequence homologies which, although statistically

significant, are 50% or less. There are at least 20 known superfamilies of leukocyte surface antigens.

The superfamily concept has a number of profound implications. The sequence similarities, particularly of key regions of the sequence, implies that members of a superfamily adopt a common structural fold. Thus, if the three dimensional structure of a superfamily member is known, tertiary structural models of other superfamily members can be generated from knowledge of the primary sequence. Furthermore, a common structural unit may imply a common function, for example, in cell adhesion, membrane transport or recognition of soluble factors. However, this is by no means always true. Many superfamilies are evolutionarily ancient and different members have diverged to fulfil distinct functional roles. Moreover, leukocyte surface molecules commonly comprise domains of different superfamilies.

The IgSF represents a paradigm for the superfamily concept. It is the largest superfamily of cell surface proteins in general and for leukocyte surface molecules in particular, comprising about 35% of known leukocyte antigens. The three dimensional structures of several members of this superfamily are known, providing a structural basis for the observed primary sequence homology that defines the IgSF.

In contrast to the common occurrence of the IgSF in the immune system, other superfamilies are represented only rarely amongst leukocyte surface molecules. For example, the PTPase SF is found only in the cytoplasmic domain of CD45, where it is thought to fulfil an essential function in T cell activation. The extracellular domain of CD45 shows no sequence homology to any other protein. However, CD45 is an example of a class of leukocyte antigens, the structure of which can vary due to differential usage of alternatively spliced exons. Thus, the sequence of the external domain of CD45 varies according to which combination of three alternate exons are used. The implications, if any, for CD45 function are unknown.

FURTHER READING

Arulanandam ARN, Kister A, McGregor MJ, Wyss DF, Wagner G, Reinherz EL. Interaction between human CD2, CD58 involves the major β-sheet surface of their respective adhesion domains. *J Exp Med* 1994, **180**:1861.

Barclay AN, Jackson DI, Willis AC, Williams AF. Lymphocyte specific heterogeneity in the rat leukocyte common antigen T200 is due to differences in polypeptide sequences near the NH$_2$ terminus. *EMBO J* 1987, **6**:1259.

Barclay AN, Birkeland ML, Brown MH, Beyers AD, Davis SJ, Somoza C, Williams AF. *The Leukocyte Antigens*. Academic Press Ltd: London; 1993.

Bierer BE, Barbosa J, Herrmann S, Burakoff SJ. The interaction of CD2 with its ligand, LFA-3, in human T cell proliferation. *J Immunol* 1988, **140**:3358.

Bjorkman PJ, Saper MA, Samraoui B, Bennett WS, Strominger JL, Wiley DC. Structure of the human class I histocompatibility antigen HLA-A2. *Nature* 1987, **329**:506.

Bodian DL, Jones EY, Stuart DI, Harlos KH, Davies EA, Davis SJ. Crystal structure of the extracellular region of the human cell adhesion molecule CD2 at 2.5 Å resolution. *Structure* 1994, **2**:755.

Brady RL, Dodson EJ, Dodson GG, Lange G, Davis SJ, Williams AF, Barclay AN. Crystal structure of domains 3 and 4 rat CD4: relation to the NH$_2$ terminal domains. *Science* 1993, **260**:979.

Brown JH, Jardetsky TS, Gorga JC, Stern LJ, Urban RG, Strominger JL, Wiley DC. Three-dimensional structure of the human class II histocompatibility antigen HLA-DR1. *Nature* 1993, **364**:33.

Chothia C, Boswell DR, Lesk AM. The outline structure of the T cell αβ receptor. *EMBO J* 1988, **7**:3745.

Cyster JG, Shotton DM, Williams AF. The dimensions of the T lymphocyte glycoprotein leukosialin and identification of linear protein epitopes that can be modified by glycosylation. *EMBO J* 1991, **10**:893.

Driscoll PC, Cyster JG, Campbell ID, Williams AF. Structure of domain 1 of rat T lymphocyte CD2 antigen. *Nature* 1991, **353**:762.

Hahn WC, Menu E, Bothwell ALM, Sims PJ, Bierer BE. Overlap-ping but non-identical binding sites on CD2 for CD58 and a second ligand CD59. *Science* 1992, **256**:1805.

Johnson P, Williams AF. Striking similarities between antigen receptor J pieces and sequence in the second chain of the murine CD8 antigen. *Nature* 1986, **323**:74.

Jones EY, Davis SJ, Williams AF, Harlos K, Stuart DA. Crystal structure of a soluble form of the cell adhesion molecule. *Nature* 1992, **360**:232.

Kato K, Koyanagi M, Okada H, Takanashi T, Wong YW, Williams AF, Okumura K, Yagita H. CD48 is a counter-receptor for mouse CD2 and is involved in T cell activation. *J Exp Med* 1992, **176**:1241.

Kingsmore SF, Watons ML, Moseley WS, Seldin MF. Physical linkage of genes encoding the lymphocyte adhesion molecules CD2 and its ligand LFA-3. *Immunogenet* 1989, **30**:123.

Konig R, Huang L-Y, Germain RN. MHC class II interaction with CD4 mediated by a region analogous to the MHC class I binding site for CD8. *Nature* 1992, **356**:796.

Leahy DJ, Axel R, Hendrickson WA. Crystal structure of a soluble form of the human T cell co-receptor CD8 at 2.6 Å resolution. *Cell* 1992, **68**:1145.

Matsui K, Boniface JJ, Reay PA, Schild H, Fazekas de St. Groth B, Davis MM. Low affinity interaction of peptide-MHC complexes with T cell receptors. *Science* 1991, **254**:1788.

McCall MN, Shotton DM, Barclay AN. Expression of soluble isoforms of rat CD45. Analysis by electron microscopy and use in epitope mapping of anti-CD45R monoclonal antibodies. *Immunol* 1992, **76**:310.

Ryu S, Kwong PD, Truneh A, Porter TG, Arthos J, Rosenberg M, Dai X, Xuong N-H, Axel R, Sweet RW, Hendrickson WA. Crystal structure of an HIV-binding recombinant fragment of human CD4. *Nature* 1990, **348**:419.

Schlossman SF, Boumsell L, Gilks W, Harlan JM, Kishimoto T, Morimoto C, Ritz J, Shaw S, Siverstein RL, Springer TA, Tedder TF, Todd RF (Eds). *Leukocyte Typing V.* Oxford University Press: Oxford; in press.

Seed B, Aruffo A. Molecular cloning of the CD2 antigen, the T cell erythrocyte receptor, by a rapid immunoselection procedure. *Proc Natl Acad Sci USA* 1987, **84**:3365.

Somoza C, Driscoll P C, Cyster J G, Williams A F. Mutational analysis of the CD2/CD58 interaction: the binding site for CD58 lies on one face of the first domain of human CD2. *J Exp Med* 1993, **178**:549.

Staunton DE, Fisher RC, LeBeau MM, Lawrence JB, Barton DE, Franke U, Dustin M, Thorley-Lawson DA. Blast-1 possesses a gly-cosyl phosphatidylinositol GP1 membrane anchor, is related to LFA-3 and OX-45 and maps to chromosome 1q21-23. *J Exp Med* 1989, **169**:1087.

Stern LJ, Brown JH, Jardetsky TS, Gorga JC, Urban RG, Strominger JL, Wiley DC. Crystal structure of the human class II MHC protein HLA-DR1 complexed with an influenza virus peptide. *Nature* 1994, **368**:215.

Thomas M. The leukocyte common antigen family. *Ann Rev Immunol* 1989, **7**:339.

Tonks NK, Charbonneau H, Diltz CD, Fischer EH, Walsh KA. Demonstration that the leukocyte common antigen CD45 is a protein tyrosine phosphatase. *Biochemistry* 1988, **27**:8696.

Trowbridge IS. CD45: An emerging role as a protein tyrosine phosphatase required for lymphocyte activation and development. *Ann Rev Immunol* 1994, **12**:85.

van der Merwe PA, Barclay AN. Transient intercellular adhesion: the importance of weak protein-protein interactions. *Trends Biochem Sci* 1994, **19**:354.

van der Merwe PA, Brown MH, Davis SJ, Barclay AN. Affinity and kinetic analysis of the interaction of the cell adhesion molecules rat CD2 and CD48. *EMBO J* 1993, **12**:4945.

van der Merwe PA, McNamee PN, Davies EA, Barclay AN, Davis SJ. Topology of the CD2-CD48 cell-adhesion molecule complex: implications for antigen recognition by T cells. *Curr Biol* 1995, **5**:74.

Wang J, Yan Y, Garrett TPJ, Liu J, Rodgers DW, Garlick RL, Tarr GE, Husain Y, Reinherz EL, Harrison SC. Atomic structure of a fragment of human CD4 containing two immunoglobulin-like domains. *Nature* 1990, **348**:411.

Williams AF, Barclay AN. The immunoglobulin superfamily — domains for cell surface recognition. *Ann Rev Immunol* 1988, **6**:381.

Wong YW, Williams AF, Kingsmore SF, Seldin MF. Structure, expression and genetic linkage of the mouse BCM1 OX45 or Blast-1 antigen. Evidence for genetic duplication giving rise to the BCM1 region on mouse chromosome 1 and the CD2/LFA3 region on mouse chromosome 3. *J Exp Med* 1990, **171**:2115.

6 Leukocyte Development

The major types of blood cells, erythrocytes, lymphocytes, granulocytes, monocytes and platelets differ dramatically in morphology and function and have highly diverse patterns of gene expression. In addition, the number and life span of cells within each of these terminally differentiated populations vary considerably. To maintain homeostasis, each cell type must be generated at an appropriate rate. Remarkably, they all originate from long term repopulating pluripotential stem cells located at specific sites of haematopoiesis. These sites vary during the lifetime of the organism: haematopoiesis initially occurs in the yolk sac (until about day 16 in the mouse and day 60 in humans), transfers to the foetal liver (days 12–20 in mouse, days 50–150 in man) and finally moves to the foetal bone marrow (from day 17 in mouse and day 79 in humans). Other organs, such as the spleen, lymph nodes and kidney, can also support some foetal haematopoietic development. Stem cells generate committed progenitor cells which further differentiate to generate morphologically identifiable immature (precursor) cells from which mature cells are produced. Each major stage of differentiation is associated with cell proliferation; thus, a large pool of mature cells is produced from a small stem cell pool. The relative numbers of the different cell types are regulated both by haematopoietic growth factors and by interactions with stromal cells. Thus, the particular microenvironment and combination and concentrations of different growth factors sampled by a cell during its development will determine its pathway of differentiation.

THE PLURIPOTENT STEM CELL

During embryonic development, blood-borne pluripotential stem cells colonize various sites of haematopoiesis, such as the bone marrow, spleen and liver. The stem cell is thought to have the capacity for unlimited self-renewal, extending throughout the life span of the organism, although there is no evidence for this notion. The presence of pluripotential haematopoietic stem cells in the bone marrow was first demonstrated by experiments in which unirradiated bone marrow cells were injected into lethally irradiated recipient mice. Cells from the donor bone marrow colonized the irradiated recipient and reconstituted the haematopoietic tissues with all the differentiated blood cell types. Analysis of appropriate genetic markers revealed that the new haematopoietic cells were of donor origin. This reconstitution assay remains the only reliable one for identifying stem cells. Experiments using low numbers of donor cells produced colonies in the spleen and bone marrow. The precursor cell responsible for these colonies is referred to as a colony forming unit (CFU). Some of the colonies contained both myeloid and erythroid cells, suggesting that these CFUs were early progenitors. Karyotypic analysis, using markers induced by radiation or retroviral integration, has subsequently indicated that lymphoid cells can also originate from the same clone. The most likely origin of the spleen colonies detected by this assay is a multipotential, non-renewing progenitor cell.

It has proved impossible to identify unequivocally the haematopoietic stem cell. Initial attempts were based on cell separation by size, buoyant density or lectin binding properties. The most successful recent strategy has been the use of cell separation based on surface markers combined with the spleen colony forming bioassay. Putative 'stem' cells do not appear to express markers characteristic of mature cells. Thus, negative selection using antibodies to surface markers characteristic of B cells, T cells, macrophages and granulocytes (the resulting population is referred to as Lin⁻) produces a population, expressing low levels of Thy-1, enriched in progenitors for spleen (CFU-S) and thymic (CFU-T) colonies (cells are injected into the thymus and develop as T cell colonies) and which is active in long term B cell cultures established from bone marrow. Progenitors within this population have been enriched further by positive selection for a surface antigen, designated Sca-1 (stem cell antigen 1), which is a member of the Ly-6 family. The resulting cells are active in CFU-S assays and can generate both myeloid and lymphoid populations (*Fig. 6.1*) On the basis of these observations, coupled with calculations of the proportion of bone marrow cells able to reconstitute an irradiated mouse, it has been suggested that Sca-1⁺, Thy-1ˡᵒ, Lin⁻ cells, which represent only around 0.05% of whole bone marrow, are highly enriched for long term reconstituting haematopoietic stem cells. This population of cells expresses c-kit, the receptor tyrosine kinase that binds to its ligand, 'steel factor' or stem cell factor.

In humans, the CD34 antigen identifies 1–4% of bone marrow cells that include most of the early haematopoietic progenitor cells detected by *in vitro* assays. Moreover, baboon CD34 positive cells can reconstitute, at least in the short term, the bone marrow of irradiated hosts. However, although CD34 antibodies clearly recognize early cells, it is not known whether they define the earliest pluripotential stem cell. Whether or not CD34 is expressed by stem cells, it is not unique to this cell type, being expressed also on endothelium from blood vessels, foetal fibroblasts, some brain cells and stromal cells.

Recently, it has proved possible to obtain some haematopoietic differentiation from the best characterized pluripotential stem cell, the embryonic stem (ES) cell. In the presence of appropriate stromal cells and growth factors, erythroid, myeloid and B cell lineage cells were obtained. Using another ES cell clone, cells with rearranged *IGH* and *L* and *TCRG* and *D* gene rearrangements were observed. However, *TCRA* and *B* gene rearrangements were not detectable. These exciting observations should greatly facilitate analysis of the molecular mechanisms of haematopoietic development.

HAEMATOPOIETIC PROGENITOR CELLS

Pluripotential stem cells can undergo asymmetric cell division to generate progenitor cells that are irreversibly committed to one or other of the haematopoietic lineages (*Fig. 6.1*). This is likely to occur in a number of stages of increasing lineage commitment. The initial step is probably the generation of multipotential progenitor cells that have lost the capacity for long term repopulation but can give rise to all the haematopoietic lineages. Successive cell divisions would produce increasing commitment resulting in progenitor cells committed to one or other of the haematopoietic lineages and eventually to lineage-restricted clones that mature into specialized cells (*Fig. 6.1*). The amplification achieved by this process produces large numbers of differentiated blood cells from a very small number of pluripotential stem cells. Progenitor cells are distinguished from stem cells primarily by the inability of the former to undergo long term repopulation. Rather, the number of rounds of division that a progenitor cell can undergo is restricted before further differentiation occurs.

HAEMATOPOIETIC GROWTH FACTORS

The process of stem cell renewal and the production of differentiated progeny must be tightly regulated in order to meet the varying requirements of the body for mature effector cells. Much of the control of haematopoiesis is mediated by haematopoietic growth factors. It is not clear, however, whether growth factors can force haematopoietic progenitors to become committed to one lineage or if they allow survival of the cells once commitment occurs in a stochastic manner. These are referred to as the 'deterministic' and the 'stochastic' theories of haematopoietic differentiation.

Some haematopoietic growth factors have been identified by their ability to support the growth of CFU precursor cells, resulting in the formation of colonies, in semisolid culture, containing colony-forming cells (CFCs). Five distinct growth factors, collectively called colony stimulating factors (CSFs), can stimulate colony formation in this assay. The properties and actions of the various CSFs are shown in *Figure 6.2*. There are many additional haematopoietic growth factors which are also required for haematopoietic cell survival, differentiation and proliferation. These include interleukins 1, 2, 4, 5 and 7 (Chapter 10). These factors do not themselves possess CSF activity although IL-1 can act cooperatively with CSFs in colony forming assays to influence the nature of the cell types found in the colonies. Human IL-5 has been shown to stimulate eosinophil formation in a colony forming assay but its murine counterpart is active only in liquid culture. The haematopoietic growth factors act at various levels in the differentiation pathway and have different target cells; some act on multiple lineages while others are restricted to a single lineage. The CSFs derive their names from the type of progenitor cell on which they act. Thus, GM-CSF at low concentrations stimulates first macrophage then granulocyte–macrophage precursors and, at progressively higher concentrations, granulocyte, eosinophil, megakaryocytic and multipotential progenitors. G-CSF produces neutrophil colonies but can also act on very early progenitors. M-CSF generates monocytic precursors and, together with IL-1 and multi-CSF, is necessary for stimulating the growth of high proliferative potential CFCs — that is, CFU-S and cells with marrow repopulating ability. Multi-CSF (or interleukin 3) produces neutrophil, eosinophil, monocyte, megakaryocytic, mast cell and erythroid colonies and interleukin 6 supports the proliferation of granulocyte–macrophage progenitors directly and acts synergistically with multi-CSF in supporting the proliferation of multipotential progenitors in culture.

Although the actions of haematopoietic growth factors are complex, their modes of action are consistent with the existence of a hierarchy of haematopoietic precursor cells being stimulated by factors in the order: IL-1, IL-3, IL-6, GM-CSF, G-CSF. Combinations of factors are often required for maximal proliferation. Because of the difficulty in identifying stem cells, as opposed to early progenitors, the factors that act on this cell type have been less well defined. However, a factor called stem cell factor (SCF) has been identified that interacts with its receptor c-kit expressed on haematopoietic stem cells. This interaction is crucial for the development of these stem cells. SCF also has a wide range of other activities with direct effects on myeloid and lymphoid development and powerful synergistic effects with other growth factors such as GM-CSF, IL-3 and erythropoietin.

The genes encoding each of the haematopoietic growth factors, including CSFs, have been cloned. The predicted amino acid sequences show that the various CSFs are unrelated proteins. They are all relatively small glycoproteins and, with the exception of M-CSF which is comprised of two identical, disulphide-linked subunits, are single subunit proteins. M-CSF is unique amongst the CSFs in that two distinct molecular forms of the factor, produced by alternative mRNA splicing, are expressed. Both forms are synthesized as transmembrane precursors which are probably proteolytically cleaved to generate a secreted form. The biochemical characteristics of the CSFs are shown in *Figure 6.2*.

In addition to their proliferative role, CSFs carry out several other actions:

- Enhance survival of precursors and mature cells.
- Mediate the irreversible induction of cellular maturation.
- Stimulate functional activity (for example, phagocytosis) of mature cells.

The particular response elicited depends on the nature of the responding cell and which CSF receptors are expressed at the cell surface.

According to the deterministic theory of haematopoiesis the type and concentration of CSF will affect the probability

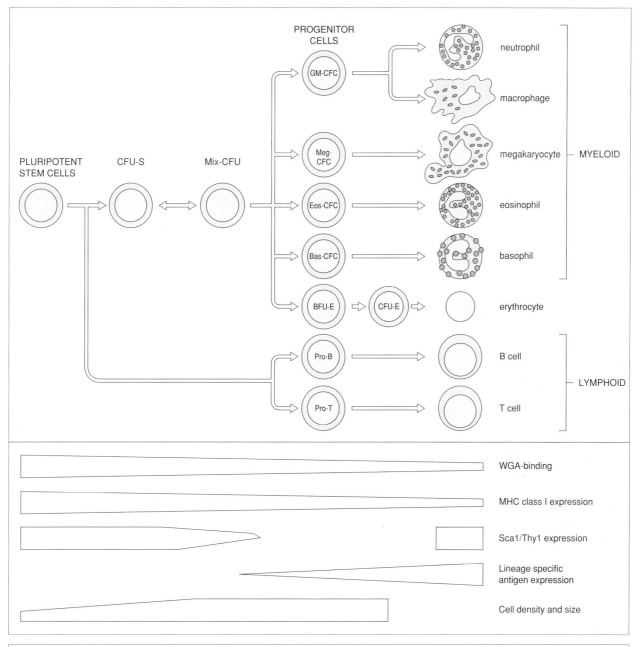

Fig. 6.1 Haemopoiesis. The most primitive haemopoietic stem cell in the bone marrow generates the CFU-S cell, the early precursor cell defined by the spleen colony-forming assay. Mix-CFU refers to multipotential cells that can form colonies in soft agar. The progenitor cells are: GM-CFC, granulocyte-macrophage colony-forming cells; Meg-CFC, megakaryocyte colony-forming cells; Eos-CFC, eosinophil colony-forming cells; Bas-CFC, basophil colony-forming cells; BFU-E, burst forming units-erythroid (primitive erythroid progenitors); CFU-E, colony forming units-erythroid (more mature erythroid progenitors). The pathway of differentiation between the pluripotent stem cell and pro-B/pro-T cells is ill-defined. There may, for example, be a committed lymphoid progenitor that can generate both B and T lineage cells. The relative capacity to bind wheat germ agglutinin (WGA) and the relative expression of MHC class I and Sca1/Thy1 antigens at different stages is shown. This scheme does not imply that precursor cells are homogeneous with respect to expression of these antigens. Lineage specific antigens are generally expressed on more differentiated cells. Different subpopulations of bone marrow cells can also be separated on the basis of their size and bouyant density. The lower half of the figure is redrawn from Spangrude, 1988.

Factor	Abbreviation	Species	No. of subunits	Mature protein M_r (kD) (N)	Glycosylated M_r (kD)	Chromosomal location of gene	Target cells
Granulocyte–macrophage colony stimulating factor	GM-CSF	murine	1	14.4 (124)	18–25	11	M, G, eo, meg, multi
		human	1	14.7 (127)	18–30	5q21-q31	
Granulocyte colony stimulating factor	G-CSF	murine	1	19.1 (178)	25	11	G, M
		human	1	18.6 (174)	20	17q21-q22	
Macrophage colony stimulating factor	M-CSF (CSF-1)	murine	2	21 (189), 18 (158)	70–90, 45–50	– 5q33.1	M, G
		human	2	21 (189), 18 (158)	70–90, 45–50		
Multipotential colony stimulating factor	Multi-CSF (IL-3)	murine	1	16.2 (140)	18–30	11	G, M, meg, mast, multi, stem
		human	1	15.4 (133)	18–30	5q21-q31	
Interleukin-6	IL-6	murine	1	21.7 (187)	22–29	8	B, T, G, multi
		human	1	20.8 (184)	19–21	7p15	

Fig. 6.2 Characteristics of the colony stimulating factors. Haemopoietic growth factors that have colony-stimulating activity are listed. All of these factors are glycoproteins containing N- and/or O-linked carbohydrates. cDNA clones encoding each of the murine and human CSFs have been sequenced and the number of amino acids in the mature protein (with the signal sequence omitted) is given (N). The apparent molecular weights of the CSFs (from SDS-polyacrylamide gel electrophoresis) are given and are in general in good agreement with the predicted M_rs (after taking into account glycosylation) with the exception of M-CSF, which is composed of two almost identical, disulphide-linked subunits. All the other CSFs are single subunit proteins. At least two different forms of M-CSF are produced from a single gene by alternative mRNA splicing. Target cells are listed: B, B lymphocytes; T, T lymphocytes; S, 'stem' cells; M, macrophage; G, granulocyte; eo, eosinophil; meg, megakaryocyte; multi, all lineages. Where they are known, the chromosomal locations of the CSF genes are given. Other factors, particularly interleukins, act as growth factors for haemopoietic cells and are important in development but do not act as CSFs. Data taken from Nicola, 1989; Metcalfe, 1989 and references therein.

of commitment to a particular lineage and competitive interactions between various CSFs will maintain the correct balance between various differentiated cell types and between stem cells, progenitors and terminally differentiated cells. The mechanism of this interaction between CSFs is unclear but it is not due to competitive binding since each factor has a distinct receptor. One possibility is that downmodulation of other CSF receptors can occur following binding of one type of CSF to its receptor. This aspect is discussed more fully in the following section. Early progenitor cells appear to have receptors for most CSFs but selective losses take place as their progeny become committed progenitors. However, more complex levels of regulation probably also exist in order to vary the relative amounts of the different progenitor cells to meet changing needs. The architecture of the bone marrow and other haematopoietic tissues, in particular the organization of stromal cells, is likely to have a strong influence in controlling self-renewal of stem cells and differentiation commitment.

Stromal cells can produce some CSFs, especially in response to various growth regulators such as IFNγ, IL-1 and TNFα, and most probably also participate in cell to cell contacts with haematopoietic precursors. Haematopoietic stem and progenitor cells are in intimate contact with stromal cells in the bone marrow. The production of CSFs by stromal cells should not be viewed simply as secretion into the extracellular fluid. Rather, they can be sequestered within the immediate environment of the stromal cell that produces them. Growth factors can be concentrated by the stroma in three ways. Firstly, they can bind to receptors on stromal cells; for example, M-CSF binds to M-CSF receptors on macrophages in bone marrow stromal layers. Secondly, they may have transmembrane forms; for example, M-CSF. Thirdly, they bind to the extracellular matrix. In long term cultures of bone marrow, the feeder layer of stromal cells can be replaced by a combination of extracellular matrix protein and growth factors. It has been shown that some CSFs are selectively retained by stromal cells by binding to glycosaminoglycans of their extracellular matrix. Moreover, growth factors can regulate production of extracellular matrix components. Terminal differentiation of haemato-poietic progenitor cells is preceded by a reduction in cell-extracellular matrix adhesiveness. Such selective compartmentalization of CSFs, combined with specific recognition and adhesion, has important regulatory implications. The specific architecture of the bone marrow may form another level of regulation; the distribution of different subpopulations of cells is not random and the resulting compartmentalization may affect the types and concentrations of CSFs experienced by a stem or progenitor cell.

Receptor	Subunits	Superfamily domains	Dissociation constant (M)
GM-CSFR	$\alpha\beta$	CK and F3 for both α and β subunits	α: 3×10^{-9} β: none $\alpha\beta$: 1.2×10^{-10}
G-CSFR	1	Ig, CK, F3	$1-5 \times 10^{-10}$
M-CSFR	1	Ig, TK	4×10^{-11}
IL-3R	$\alpha\beta$	CK and F3 for both α and β subunits	α: 5×10^{-8} β: none $\alpha\beta$: 10^{-10}
IL-6R	$\alpha\beta$	Ig, CK, F3 for both α and β subunits	α: 10^{-9} β: none $\alpha\beta$: 10^{-11}

Fig. 6.3 The subunit composition, domain structures and dissociation constants of the human colony stimulating factor receptors are shown. The superfamily domains are as follows: CK, cytokine receptor; F3, fibronectin type III; Ig, immunoglobulin; TK, tyrosine kinase. The IL-3R β-chain is common to the GM-CSF and IL-5 receptor. This chain associates with a unique low affinity α-chain to form the high affinity binding site.

RECEPTORS FOR HAEMATOPOIETIC GROWTH FACTORS

Specific, high affinity receptors have been characterized for most haematopoietic growth factors. Analysis of their primary structures has enabled many of them to be classified into superfamilies (see Chapters 5 and 10). The properties of the CSF receptors are summarized in *Figure 6.3* (see also *Figs. 10.2* and *10.3*). The main superfamily domains that comprise the CSF receptors are the cytokine receptor, Ig and fibronectin type III superfamilies. The IL-3 and GM-CSF receptors are both $\alpha\beta$ heterodimers that share a common β-chain. This chain associates with the unique low affinity receptors to form the high affinity binding site.

The CSF receptors can vary in number on different cell types but are generally expressed at low levels (about 100–4500 molecules/positive bone marrow cell). The cellular distribution of these receptors correlates with the biological specificities of each growth factor. For example, M-CSF receptors are essentially restricted to cells of the monocyte–macrophage lineage, whereas G-CSF receptors are expressed primarily on cells of the neutrophilic granulocyte lineage. In contrast, GM-CSF and multi-CSF are more widely distributed amongst precursor cell types.

Binding studies reveal that CSF–CSF-receptor interactions are of high affinity with K_ds in the subnanomolar range. Association leads to internalization of the CSF–receptor complex and ultimately to CSF degradation. Each CSF receptor also has a unique pattern of non-cognate ligands, such as other CSFs, that can cause down-regulation via interaction with their own receptors. The mechanism of this receptor 'crosstalk' is unknown but presumably occurs by intracellular second messenger systems such as phosphorylation.

The study of the molecular mechanisms that regulate the developmental signals communicated by CSF–receptor interactions represents one of the most important areas of biology. Current models suggest that developmental signals lead to the activation of a small number of 'master' genes that in turn control a regulatory cascade, resulting in the overall pattern of gene expression characteristic of a given cell type. Several transcription factors that play important regulatory roles in haematopoiesis have been identified. For example, the Ikaros transcription factor is required for development of the lymphoid lineage but not for any other haematopoietic lineage. It is likely that Ikaros promotes the differentiation of a multipotent progenitor into a common lymphoid progenitor. The PU.1 transcription factor is essential for development of the granulocytic, monocytic and lymphoid lineages but not for megakaryocytes or erythrocytes. Other transcription factors are important later in development. For example, E2A and Pax-5 play essential roles in B cell development at the pre-B cell stage, whereas Tcf-1 regulates T cell development at the step leading to CD4$^+$8$^+$ (double positive) thymocytes.

A considerable degree of commitment and differentiation clearly occurs within the bone marrow. Although further maturation, particularly of T lymphoid precursors, occurs at remote sites, most cells leaving the bone marrow are out of cell cycle (with the exception of some stem cells which circulate in the blood and are usually in cycle) and are often morphologically or phenotypically identifiable as belonging to a particular lineage. The maturing blood cells exit the bone marrow through specialized thin-walled blood vessels (high endothelial venules) and migrate to various sites in the periphery. The homing receptors that regulate this traffic are discussed in Chapter 14.

PHAGOCYTE DEVELOPMENT

In mammals, there are two classes of white blood cell that act as phagocytes: macrophages, which are widely distributed in tissues as well as blood, and neutrophilic granulocytes, also called neutrophils or polymorphonuclear leukocytes. Macrophages comprise diverse types generated from monocyte precursors on leaving the bloodstream and entering the tissues. It is easy to recognize polymorpho-nuclear leukocyte precursors in the bone marrow by their characteristic nuclear morphology, numerous lysosomes and secretory granules.

Neutrophilic granulocytes and macrophages derive from the same precursor, which is committed in the sense that it can give rise to no other cell type than these two and has a limited capacity to divide (*Fig. 6.4*). The survival of this progenitor cell is absolutely dependent on GM-CSF. Its bipotential nature has been established by elegant single cell manipulation experiments. Bone marrow cells cultured in the presence of GM-CSF develop colonies containing only granulocytes and monocytes. When single precursor cells are cultured with GM-CSF, clones can consist of either monocytes or granulocytes, or a mixture of both. These experiments have been extended to show that commitment to one or other lineage is also directed by GM-CSF. When the two undifferentiated daughter cells from a single dividing progenitor cell are cultured separately with high or low concentrations of GM-CSF, the colony growing in a high GM-CSF concentration consists of granulocytes while the colony in the low concentration consists of monocytes. Thus, further commitment of the common granulocyte–macrophage progenitor is influenced in these experiments by the available concentration of GM-CSF.

Further differentiation along the monocytic or neutrophilic lineages is also directed by M-CSF and G-CSF, respectively. It is likely that the pool of progenitors stimulated by GM-CSF also responds to G-CSF and M-CSF, although not every progenitor cell will necessarily be competent to respond to all three factors. It is probable, therefore, that both the range of growth factor receptors expressed and the relative concentrations of factor determine the degree of proliferation and/or maturation of the various cell types. Thus, the bipotential progenitor cell can be committed irreversibly to monocyte formation if the initial cell divisions are stimulated by M-CSF. However, if a mixture of M-CSF and GM-CSF is used, there is both enhancement of cell proliferation and competition for differentiation, often resulting in the generation of granulocyte and monocyte clones within the same colony. The development of the neutrophilic and monocytic lineages from the bipotential progenitor is shown in *Figure 6.4*.

Neutrophilic granulocytes leave the bone marrow and circulate in the blood for only a few hours before migrating into the connective tissues, where they remain for a few days before dying. Monocytes, in contrast, can differentiate into macrophages outside the bloodstream where they can persist for months or even years. Little is known about the differentiation of monocytes to macrophages or about maturation of the various macrophage types in the tissues. Monocytes cultured with M-CSF or IFNγ can differentiate to a macrophage cell type; however, other undefined signals generated on entering the tissues are also thought to be important for full maturation.

Antigens expressed during myeloid differentiation

Although several antigens have been used as markers for monocytes/macrophages and granulocytes, the relationship of these markers to stages of differentiation and to morphological descriptions is less clear cut than for the lymphoid markers. Several CD clusters, including CD14, CD33 and CD34, are useful markers for the myeloid lineage (see the CD Table in the Appendix and *Fig. 6.4*). The antigens defined by some of these clusters are well defined functionally. For example, the CD11b (Mac-1) antigen is the iC3b receptor that mediates phagocytosis by activated macrophages and is expressed by monocytes, macrophages and granulocytes. The CD64 cluster defines the high affinity IgG-Fc receptor, FcγR1, on monocytic cells. Other important markers for this lineage are the growth factor receptors that recognize the various CSFs which drive maturation of these lineages. The identification of additional specific markers will greatly enhance studies on both lineage relationships and the mechanisms that determine commitment.

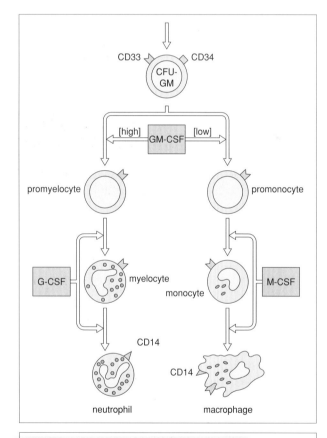

Fig. 6.4 Scheme for neutrophil/macrophage development. The branched pathway from the CFU-GM bipotential progenitor cell stage to fully differentiated cell types is shown, together with its dependence on CSFs. The pathway of maturation can be manipulated by the relative CSF concentrations, particularly that of GM-CSF. CD14, CD33 and CD34 are informative surface markers for neutrophil/macrophage development.

B CELL DEVELOPMENT

B lymphopoiesis in mammals occurs throughout life in the bone marrow. B lymphocytes are generated from a bipotential progenitor cell capable of producing both B and T cells.

A battery of intracellular and surface markers has been used to identify different stages of B cell development within the bone marrow (*Fig. 6.5*). Three major groups of developing B cell are defined on the basis of Ig expression. Pro-B cells fail to express IgH or L chains, pre-B cells express IgH chains only and B cells express both IgH and L chains on the cell surface. The earliest stage of committed B cell in which IgH gene rearrangement occurs is termed pro-B/pre-B-I. These cells express the CD45R isoform B220 (as do all other stages of B cell development with the exception of terminally differentiated plasma cells), the tyrosine kinase receptor c-kit, CD43, TdT and the products of the recombination activating genes, RAG-1 and RAG-2. Upon productive *IGH* gene rearrangement, these cells generate large pre-B-II cells that are a c-kit⁻, CD25⁺ population that has downregulated expression of TdT and *RAG* genes. In this population at least one *IGH* locus is rearranged but the *IGL* loci are in germline conformation. Large cycling pre-B-II cells give rise to resting small pre-B-II cells that have upregulated *RAG* genes. It is in this population that *IGL*

gene rearrangement occurs. Productive rearrangement at one of the *IGL* loci results in transition to short lived immature B cells expressing surface IgM.

The immature B cell repertoire is shaped by an editing mechanism. B cells expressing antigen receptors reactive with autoantigens expressed in the primary lymphoid organs have a chance to survive by undergoing secondary *IGL* gene rearrangements in an attempt to escape tolerance (see Chapter 12). Remaining autoreactive cells are negatively selected by mechanisms such as deletion and anergy, further modifying the final repertoire of mature B cells which exit into the periphery and now express surface IgM and IgD. This last stage of differentiation (that is, IgM⁺ to IgM⁺D⁺ cells) most probably occurs in the spleen.

Most newly produced virgin B cells, which express membrane-associated IgM and IgD on the cell surface, have a half life of only 3–4 days in the periphery since in order to survive they must encounter antigen. The mechanism involved in antigen presentation to and activation of B cells and the consequences of antigen selection are discussed in Chapters 9–12. Although the majority of virgin B cells produced by the bone marrow are short lived, a randomly selected proportion enter a relatively stable peripheral B cell pool and recirculate via the secondary lymphoid organs. These cells have a life span of about a month.

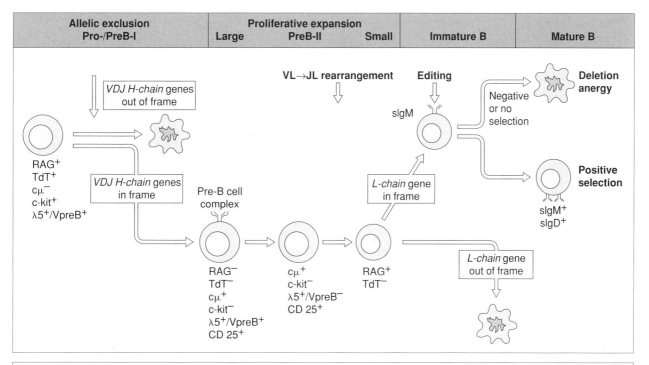

Fig. 6.5 Scheme for B cell development. *IGH* gene rearrangement occurs in large, cycling pro-B/pre-B-I cells. The IgH chain is expressed at the cell surface of large pre-B-II cells as the pre-B cell receptor in a complex with surrogate L chain. Cells progressing through this transition form the small pre-B-II compartment where *IGL* gene rearrangement occurs. Productive *IGL* gene rearrangement results in transition to immature B cells expressing IgM. These cells are subject to both positive and negative selection to generate the final repertoire of B cells. The markers that define the various subpopulations are shown. Scheme adapted from Melchers *et al*, 1995.

The surrogate light chain and B cell development

Pro/pre-B-I and large pre-B-II cells express the surrogate light chain marker which is encoded by the $VpreB/\lambda5$ locus. Pro/pre-B-I cells express V_{preB}/λ_5 at the cell surface in association with additional, as yet uncharacterized, glycoproteins. Large pre-B-II cells express a pre-B cell receptor complex comprising IgHCμ chain and surrogate light chain. The expression of the $VpreB/\lambda5$ locus is downregulated in subsequent developmental stages.

The surrogate light chain appears to function to regulate the developmental transition between the pro- and pre-B cell populations. Thus, targeted disruption of the $\lambda5$ gene results in a 10–20-fold reduction in the number of pre-B-II cells. In contrast, the size of the pro/pre-B-I pool is unaffected. Mature B cells in these mice express surface Ig and have been subject to allelic exclusion (see below). These experiments suggest that the surrogate light chain is important for cellular proliferation to generate normal numbers of large and small pre-B cells. The pre-B cell receptor also signals allelic exclusion, although the IgH chain appears to be capable of performing this function in the absence of the surrogate light chain.

Allelic exclusion

During their development, B cells become committed to the expression of only one IgH/L combination. This is the principle of allelic exclusion. Consequently, any one B cell expresses only one antigen specificity. The molecular details of the Ig rearrangement events that result in allelic exclusion are discussed in detail in Chapter 3. The sequential rearrangement of Ig genes during the maturation of pro-B cells to virgin B cells is controlled by a series of feedback regulation events. At the earliest pro-B/pre-B-I stage, the recombination machinery rearranges initially DH to JH, then VH to DH-JH segments. Ig heavy chain rearrangement continues until a contiguous VH-DH-JH block capable of generating a V_H region is formed. Translation of the corresponding mRNA produces intracellular membrane-associated μ heavy chain which, as discussed above, plays a dual role in signalling both the cessation of heavy chain rearrangement and further development as part of a complex with surrogate light chain. The experimental introduction by gene transfection of membrane-associated and secreted forms of μ heavy chains into pre-B cells harbouring either unproductive VH-DH-JH rearrangements or two DH-JH alleles showed that expression of only the membrane form and not the secreted form of μ protein resulted in activation of rearrangement of the IGK locus.

Vk-Jk assembly occurs in small pre-B-II cells, rearrangement proceeding on both alleles until a productive IGK rearrangement is generated. Assembly with heavy chains to form complete Ig molecules leads to cessation of L chain gene rearrangement. The κ polypeptide alone is insufficient to prevent further rearrangement. Failure to produce a κ polypeptide that associates with an H chain leads to rearrangement at the IGL locus. Thus, κ producers rarely have IGL gene rearrangements whereas λ producers (about 5% of murine B cells) almost always have rearrangements of both IGK genes. In rare cases, cells rearrange IGL genes because some κ polypeptides produced from productive IGK gene rearrangements fail for some reason to bind to H chains. In λ producers, one or both IGK loci are inactivated by a rearrangement that joins Vk-Jk to a heptamer sequence, called the RS element, downstream of the Ck gene, thus deleting Ck and its intronic enhancer, ENHiκ (see *Fig. 2.7*). This rearrangement event may be involved in activating Vl-Jl joining, although rearrangements to the RS element on both IGK loci are not required for initiation of IGL rearrangement.

Although the mechanism of allelic exclusion is unknown, it must involve the regulation of RAG-1 and RAG-2 activity, the lineage-specific components of the recombination machinery. In addition to the RAG genes, components of the general machinery for double-strand break repair, such as the catalytic subunit of a DNA-dependent protein kinase (the *scid* mutation) and the Ku autoantigen that binds to and regulates the activity of this protein kinase, play a key role in the recombination process. Double-stranded DNA repair occurs prior to progression from the G1 to S phase of the cell cycle, suggesting that recombination may be linked to the cell cycle. Moreover, it has been shown that RAG-2 is phosphorylated at a key threonine residue *in vitro* by the mitotic cyclin-dependent kinase, p34^{cdc2}, and that the phosphorylation event dramatically decreases the half life of RAG-2. Taken together, these observations have given rise to a model in which $IGHV$-D-J rearrangement is postulated to occur in a cell arrested in the G1 phase of the cell cycle. Successful rearrangement signals a proliferative response via the pre-B cell receptor, decreasing the length of G1 and resulting in downregulation of RAG-2 levels, thus preventing further rearrangement. Although this model is speculative, it provides a conceptual framework for a mechanistic understanding of this important process.

The CD5 (Ly-1) B cell lineage

The CD5 antigen, expressed on most thymocytes and essentially all T cells, also defines a B cell subset (usually called Ly-1$^+$ B cells in the mouse). These cells also express classical B cell markers, such as IgM, IgD and MHC class II antigens, and do not express other T cell markers. Despite much research, many aspects of this subset, in particular their function and lineage relationship to the main B cell compartment, remain unclear. Murine Ly-1$^+$ B cells reside primarily in the peritoneal cavity, comprising nearly half the lymphocytes there. Human CD5$^+$ B cells are also found in the spleens and peripheral blood of healthy individuals.

CD5$^+$ B cells have been associated with the pathology of autoimmune disease production. They are elevated in some autoimmune individuals and produce many of the IgM autoantibodies in most patients. Moreover, Ly-1$^+$ B cells are the predominant B cell subset in autoimmune NZB mice. These aspects of CD5$^+$ B cells are discussed more fully in Chapter 12.

CD5$^+$ B cells may have a distinct ontogeny and precursor origin and, therefore, represent a separate lineage of B cells. These cells appear early in ontogeny and predominate among early B cells. For example, they are the major

B cell type in the human foetal spleen and cord blood but are relatively rare in adult humans. Transplantation of murine bone marrow cells into irradiated recipients failed to regenerate the Ly-1$^+$ B cell subset. However, these cells could be transferred by grafting cells of the murine foetal omentum (connective tissue between folds of the gut), suggesting that the Ly-1$^+$ B cell lineage is capable of self-regeneration in recipient mice. CD5$^+$ B cells are, however, the earliest cells to repopulate the host after human bone marrow transplantation, suggesting that precursor cells capable of generating this subset reside in the bone marrow as well as the gut. The difference between the results of human and murine bone marrow grafting may reflect the developmental age of the donor bone marrow. *V* gene usage of CD5$^+$ B cells also differs markedly from other B cells in utilizing a limited number of germline *VH* gene segments, again suggesting separate lineages. However, these experiments do not provide an unambiguous answer to whether CD5$^+$ B cells represent a separate lineage or an early maturational stage in B lymphopoiesis; this question remains unsolved. In this context both CD5$^+$ and CD5$^-$ B cells are affected in mice with a targeted disruption of the $\lambda 5$ gene, suggesting that the pre-B cell receptor plays an important role in the development of both subsets.

T CELL DEVELOPMENT

The thymus is essential for the production of most T cells, as shown by the almost total failure to develop functional populations of peripheral T cells in neonatally thymectomized or nude mice which lack a lymphoid thymus. The thymus is a complex organ containing a variety of stromal cell types that provide the growth factors and cellular interactions that are necessary for efficient thymocyte differentiation (*Fig. 6.6*). However, it is important to note that extrathymic sites of T cell differentiation exist, most notably the gut mucosa. Other sites that may support differentiation include the liver and skin.

The origin of cells entering the thymus is the embryonic foetal liver and later the bone marrow. Thus, reconstitution of irradiated mice with bone marrow or foetal liver cells carrying an appropriate distinguishing genetic marker results in repopulation of the thymus. A more compelling observation is that foetal liver cells introduced directly into explanted embryonic thymus lobes, pre-treated with deoxyguanosine to destroy endogenous lymphoid progenitor cells, generate lymphocytes after organ culture.

Blood-borne precursor cells enter the thymus by traversing the walls of blood vessels supplying the connective tissue surrounding the thymus and migrating through the mesenchyme into the thymic epithelial rudiment. This is clearly an active and directed process. Thus, precursor cells from the foetal liver will migrate across a Millipore filter to enter a thymic lobe emptied of endogenous lymphoid cells. Moreover, the thymus is receptive to stem cells only at defined stages in ontogeny. It is likely that this movement of precursor cells involves chemotactic factors secreted by the embryonic thymic epithelium and probably also interactions of homing receptors with cell bound ligands. The use of migration assays, in which the ability of cells to move along diffusion gradients is measured, has enabled various chemotactic peptides produced by the thymic epithelium to be purified, although it has not been established that these peptides are involved *in vivo* in thymic stem cell recruitment. One such factor, called thymotoxin, purified from a rat thymic epithelial cell line has been shown to be identical to β_2-microglobulin.

In common with other haematopoietic progenitor cells, the low numbers of T lineage precursors complicate studies on their nature and colonizing potential. Cells with thymic colonizing potential are estimated to represent 0.03–0.1% of adult bone marrow cells and are about 10 times less frequent in foetal liver. These cells do not express common T cell markers prior to their entry into the thymus. A number of markers are, however, present on foetal thymocytes and on a proportion of pre-thymic haematopoietic cells. These include murine cold insoluble globulin, asialo-GM1 and Pgp-1 (CD44), as well as the human surface marker CD7, which has been identified on cells in the peri-thymic mesenchyme of the developing athymic rudiment and in the foetal liver. None of these markers are unique to cells committed to the T cell lineage. For example, the CD44 molecule is also expressed on

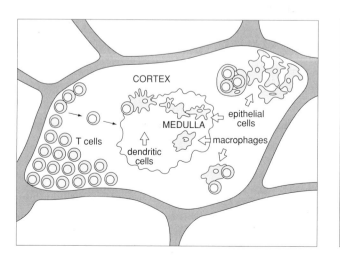

CORTEX

MEDULLA

T cells

dendritic cells

epithelial cells

macrophages

Fig. 6.6 Stromal cell-lymphocyte interactions during thymocyte development. Macrophages, dendritic cells and epithelial cells are the main MHC class I and class II-expressing cells in the thymus. Some thymocytes also express class I antigens. Macrophages and epithelial cells are present throughout the cortex and medulla, whereas dendritic cells are limited to medulla. Extensive cell–cell interactions are evident during thymocyte maturation. For example, epithelial cells envelop developing thymocytes with a network of cytoplasmic processes (nurse cells). It is thought that these interactions are involved in selection. Thin arrows represent movement of developing thymocytes through the cortex into the medulla. Thick arrows identify stromal cells which may mediate positive and negative selection during thymocyte maturation.

macrophages and granulocytes (hence the alternative name Pgp-1 or phagocytic glycoprotein 1) and on some B cells. Although there are no unique markers, selection for a combination of the surface markers mentioned above may prove useful in enriching T cell precursors, which could then be subjected to cloning or immortalization procedures to allow assay of their developmental potential.

T cell precursors show considerable proliferative potential once within the thymus. The total turnover time of 5–7 days for the entire T cell population of the adult thymus, coupled with the relatively slow rate of entry of new immigrants, suggests a high proliferative rate for cells colonizing the thymus. More direct studies using the thymus organ culture system, in which development can be studied in the absence of continuing stem cell input, have suggested that as few as one to ten cells may be able to recolonize an entire thymic lobe. The developmental capacity of an individual T cell precursor has been assessed by introducing a single micromanipulated thymic stem cell, isolated from a 13–14 day thymic rudiment, into another empty thymus lobe. Under these conditions the initial cell is capable of giving rise to up to 10^5 differentiated T cell progeny over a 14 day period.

Although these studies indicate that intrathymic precursors have a high rate of cell division the precursors are not stem cell-like in the sense of being capable of indefinite self-renewal. Reconstitution of irradiated mice with thymocyte subpopulations only results in transient repopulation of the thymus. Immigration of new cells from haematopoietic tissues is required to maintain a replete thymus.

Thymocyte subpopulations

Two surface markers have proved especially informative in classifying thymocyte subsets. Expression of CD4 and CD8 antigens divides the adult thymus into four major subpopulations. The double negative (CD4⁻8⁻) subset represents 2–4%, the double positive (CD4⁺8⁺) subset about 80% and the single positive (CD4⁺8⁻ or CD4⁻8⁺) subsets each represent 5–10% of total thymocytes. These subsets can be further divided on the basis of other surface markers, anatomical location within the thymus and functional competence. Broadly speaking, there is close resemblance between studies in mice, humans and rats. The mouse thymus has been most extensively studied and will be described in detail. A scheme for murine thymocyte development based on expression of CD4 and CD8 is shown in *Figure 6.7*.

THYMOCYTE PROGENITORS

The identity of the earliest thymocyte progenitor that colonizes the thymus has not been unambiguously established. A rare cell population, comprising about 0.05% of total adult thymocytes and expressing low levels of CD4 (called CD4ˡᵒ cells), has been identified. This population, which also expresses c-kit, is capable of reconstituting both the αβ and γδ T cell lineages and can also generate mature B cell progeny after intravenous transfer into recipient mice. However, there is no direct evidence that this cell is a committed common lymphoid progenitor cell since the

CD4ˡᵒ thymocyte population also contains a low level of myeloid precursor potential. Therefore, CD4ˡᵒ, c-kit⁺ thymocytes are best considered as recent thymic immigrants with multipotential activity.

THE DOUBLE NEGATIVE SUBSET

Double negative (DN) thymocytes can be subdivided on the basis of expression of several additional markers including the CD44 and CD25 antigens. The earliest DN thymocytes are CD44⁺, CD25⁻ and are large cycling cells. This population generates the CD44⁻, CD25⁺ DN thymocyte subset that comprises mainly non-cycling cells. The most mature DN subset lacks expression of both CD44 and CD25. It is this subset that generates double positive (DP) thymocytes, developing via an immature single positive (ISP) subset that expresses either CD8 or (less frequently) CD4. Late DN and ISP thymocytes are highly proliferating populations that generate the 100-fold expansion in cell numbers between the DN and DP thymocyte subsets.

THE DOUBLE POSITIVE SUBSET

The double positive subset is heterogeneous with respect to relative levels of CD4 and CD8 cell size, cell cycle status and surface phenotype. Early double positive cells are blasts that are in cycle and lack expression of the αβ TCR. More mature DP cells express the TCR at varying levels and many are resting cells. The most mature DP thymocytes (post-positive selection; see below) express the CD69 activation marker and high levels of the αβ TCR.

SINGLE POSITIVE THYMOCYTES

Selection processes at the DP thymocyte stage generate the mature thymocyte population of either CD4⁺8⁻ or CD4⁻8⁺ single positive (SP) thymocytes. These cells express high levels of TCRαβ, possess functional activity and represent the endpoint of the differentiation process.

Control points in thymocyte development

As for all developmental processes, thymocyte development is tightly regulated. Gene targeting technology has had a major impact in dissecting the checkpoints involved in regulating the numbers and specificities of T cells. The effect of different targeted gene disruptions on thymocyte development is shown in *Figure 6.7*.

Proliferation of immature thymocytes

An early phase of thymocyte expansion occurs when CD4ˡᵒ progenitor thymocytes proliferate to generate CD25⁺, CD44⁻ DN thymocytes. Early thymocytes are responsive to a variety of cytokines including IL-1, IL-2, IL-3, IL-6, IL-7 and SCF the ligand for c-kit. Gene targeting experiments have established that the IL-7R/IL-7 interaction is essential for the proliferation of immature thymocytes. Thus, disruption of genes for either IL-7 or IL-7R results in a drastic reduction of T (and B) cells and an abnormally small thymus which nonetheless contains all of the thymocyte subsets. It is likely that, *in vivo*, IL-7 acts in concert with other growth and survival factors to regulate this stage of development.

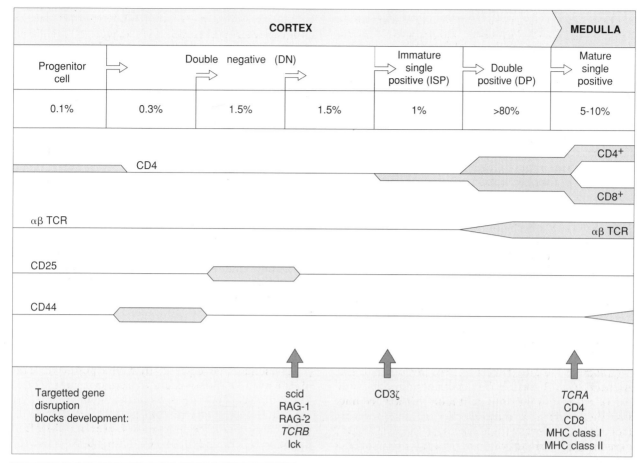

	CORTEX						MEDULLA
Progenitor cell	Double negative (DN)			Immature single positive (ISP)	Double positive (DP)	Mature single positive	
0.1%	0.3%	1.5%	1.5%	1%	>80%	5-10%	

Fig. 6.7 Scheme for thymocyte development. A scheme based on the expression of the CD4 and CD8 antigens is depicted. Not all subsets are shown. For example, the DP thymocyte subset can be subdivided based on cell size and level of expression of the αβ TCR. Populations of cycling cells are indicated by green shading. All of the immature subsets reside in the cortex (*Fig. 6.6*). Mature

SP thymocytes are found in the medulla. Mutations that arrest thymocyte development are shown below. The stages at which various mutations arrest thymocyte development are indicated. TCRβ and lck mutations fail to block development completely at the CD25⁺ DN thymocytes stage; about 10% of normal DP thymocytes are present in these mice.

Generation of CD4⁺8⁺ cortical thymocytes

Progression of DN thymocytes to the DP stage is regulated by the TCRβ-chain. *TCRB* gene rearrangement occurs within the DN thymocyte subset, *V-D-J* rearrangement being first detected in CD25⁺ DN thymocytes. TCRβ is expressed at the surface of CD25⁺ DN thymocytes as part of a pre-T cell receptor complex in association with CD3 and a 33kDa transmembrane glycoprotein called the pTα polypeptide. This molecule is analogous to the pre-B cell receptor and in both cases formation of the complex serves to select a productive rearrangement and to rescue cells from apoptotic death through proliferation. Like its B cell counterpart, the pre-T cell receptor is also thought to mediate allelic exclusion at the *TCRB* locus. A similar mechanism for allelic exclusion to that described for IgH (see above) can be envisaged. Thus, CD25⁺ DN thymocytes are out of cycle, most probably arrested at the G1 phase and contain high levels of RAG-2 protein. Late DN thymocytes are proliferating cells that contain low RAG-2 levels. The proliferative

signal induced by the pre-T cell receptor may, therefore, result in phosphorylation and degradation of RAG-2, preventing further *TCRB* rearrangement.

Thymocytes that have been selected to progress through the CD25⁺ DN checkpoint proliferate through the late DN and ISP thymocyte stages to generate DP thymocytes.

Generation of mature thymocytes

Just as the TCRβ-chain regulates the DN to DP thymocyte transition, progression through the DP thymocyte checkpoint is controlled by the TCRα-chain. *TCRA* gene rearrangement occurs at the ISP and DP thymocyte stage of development and the αβ TCR is first expressed at low levels on DP thymocytes. During the thymic selection process, interactions occur between the αβ TCR on DP thymocytes and MHC molecules expressed on thymic stromal cells. These interactions have two consequences. Associations that are able to recognize self-MHC molecules promote the survival of DP thymocytes and their differentiation (without cellular proliferation) to mature

SP thymocytes. This process is called positive selection. In contrast, thymocytes expressing self-reactive TCRs are eliminated by a deletional mechanism. This process is called negative selection. Thymocytes expressing TCRs with no affinity for self-MHC molecules fail to receive survival signals and consequently die. This process has been referred to as 'death by neglect'.

Although the evidence is not unequivocal, most studies suggest that thymic epithelium mediates positive selection; that is, these interactions promote the differentiation of DP thymocytes to mature SP thymocytes. Several phenotypic changes accompany progression through this checkpoint. Thus, the surface levels of TCRαβ increase and either CD4 or CD8 is downregulated (see below). The activation marker CD69 is also transiently expressed. Mature SP thymocytes are immunocompetent resting cells and exit the thymus to populate the secondary lymphoid organs.

Negative selection is mediated, at least in part, by bone marrow derived cells such as dendritic cells. Negatively selected cells undergo clonal deletion by apoptosis, a rapid process that involves nuclear fragmentation and membrane changes followed by engulfment by surrounding phagocytic cells.

It is important to emphasize that although thymic epithelial cells are particularly efficient at promoting positive selection and dendritic cells at promoting negative selection, there is not an absolute specialization for these functions. The exact cell type that mediates selection may depend on the route of entry of the antigen into the thymus. For example, dendritic cells are largely confined to the medulla; thus, antigens that have access to the cortex may tolerize T cells via presentation by epithelial cells. In this context virtually any cell type has the ability to induce negative selection under *in vitro* conditions.

Mechanisms of selection

Positive selection of TCRαβ⁺ DP thymocytes regulates allelic exclusion at the *TCRA* locus. From the kinetics of T cell development, it has been calculated that the average life span of a TCRβ⁺ DP thymocyte that is rearranging its *TCRA* genes is 3.5 days. During this window, thymocytes express TCRαβ which is sampled for reactivity with MHC antigens. Rearrangement can continue until a TCR capable of positive selection is generated, at which time further *TCRA* gene rearrangement ceases. Thymocytes that have failed to express a suitable TCR after this time period die. This model for functional *TCRA* gene allelic exclusion predicts that T cells with two TCRs (comprising one β-chain and two different α-chains) exist in the periphery and such cells have recently been identified.

Recent studies have established a key role for peptide in positive and negative selection. These experiments have employed foetal thymic organ culture using thymic lobes from mice with disrupted *TAP* (transporter associated with antigen processing) or β₂-microglobulin genes. In each case the thymus fails to express MHC class I antigens; consequently, thymocyte development of CD8⁺ cells is arrested. However, development of these cells could be restored by addition of some peptides but not others, although all peptides used were capable of stabilizing class I expression. These experiments have been extended by using organ cultures from TCR transgenic mice that are deficient in class I expression. Using peptides that have agonist, partial agonist or antagonist activity, it has been demonstrated that positive selection of CD8⁺ cells can be induced by small amounts of agonist peptides or moderate amounts of antagonist peptides. Higher concentrations of agonist peptides and certain antagonist peptides induced negative selection.

Since the difference between agonist and antagonist peptides is the affinity with which they bind to the TCR, these results can be interpreted in terms of an affinity/avidity model of thymic selection in which weak signalling of T cells results in positive selection whereas strong signalling causes negative selection. In this context, certain self-antigens, such as those encoded by endogenous mouse mammary tumour viruses, bind to all thymocytes bearing particular Vβ antigens and eliminate these cells at the CD3^lo to CD3^hi DP thymocyte stage. These endogenous superantigens bridge MHC class II antigens on stromal cells and Vβ regions of the αβ TCR, presumably resulting in a strong deletional signal to the developing thymocyte.

Signalling via the TCR on immature thymocytes leads to either cell survival or death. What mechanisms dictate which of these opposite consequences will prevail? The spectrum of accessory molecules, such as CD4, CD8, CD28 and other second signals, will play a major role in determining the overall avidity of interaction and the intracellular signalling pathways that are engaged. Experiments in which dominant negative mutants of the MAP kinase pathway have been overexpressed in thymocytes in transgenic mice have demonstrated that positive selection is dependent upon the activation of this signalling pathway. In contrast, negative selection was unaffected in these mice, suggesting either that additional pathways operate to transduce negative selection pathways or that the strength of the signal for negative selection activates the MAP kinase pathway to such a degree that the dominant negative transgene is unable to inhibit fully the pathway.

In addition to the positive selection events that shape the TCR repertoire for antigen recognition, selection via the pre-T cell receptor ensures the expansion of immature thymocytes with productively rearranged *TCRB* genes. Studies using constitutively active or dominant negative p56^lck transgenes or with p56^lck deficient mice have shown that this tyrosine kinase is essential for thymocytes to traverse the DN thymocyte checkpoint. Thus, p56^lck deficient mice or mice expressing a dominant negative transgene exhibit an early block in T cell development whereas expression of constitutively active p56^lck suppresses endogenous *TCRB* rearrangement. Thus, this tyrosine kinase appears to be an essential element in the signalling cascade of the pre-TCR complex.

CD4/CD8 lineage commitment

Positive selection results in the generation of mature CD8⁺ T cells with TCR specificity for class I antigens or

CD4+ T cells with TCR specificity for class II antigens. Two models for this CD4/CD8 lineage commitment have been proposed (*Fig. 6.8*). The instruction model proposes that the MHC molecule on the stromal cell instructs the lineage choice made by the DP thymocyte. Thus, binding of a MHC class I specific TCR with the CD8 co-receptor generates signals that result in the downregulation of CD4, whereas binding of a class II-restricted TCR with CD4 downregulates CD8. The stochastic model stipulates that a DP thymocyte downregulates CD4 or CD8 independently of the MHC specificity of its TCR, effectively committing itself to one or other lineage. Those thymocytes whose co-receptor and TCR recognize the same class of MHC progress through the DP to SP thymocyte checkpoint.

Both of these models make predictions that are in principle testable experimentally. For example, the stochastic model predicts that cells that have downregulated the wrong coreceptor should be rescued from cell death by the constitutive expression of a transgene encoding the co-receptor fitting the TCR. Experiments to test this prediction have yielded rather conflicting results but have broadly supported the stochastic model, although the population rescued by the transgenic co-receptor in these experiments was small. The existence of a subset of CD4^{hi}8^{lo} thymocytes in MHC class II knockout mice and an equivalent CD4^{lo}8^{hi} subset in class I-deficient mice is also consistent with the stochastic model. On the basis of these experiments a revised stochastic model was proposed in which an initial TCR–MHC engagement stimulates differentiation at random into CD4^{hi} CD8^{lo} or CD4^{lo} CD8^{hi} cells and a second TCR–MHC engagement in the presence of an appropriate co-receptor drives full differentiation into CD4 or CD8 SP thymocytes. Thus, according to this model, positive selection is a two-step process. However, it is important to emphasize that currently there is no experiment that formally excludes any model.

THE γδ T CELL LINEAGE

The subdivision of T cells into αβ and γδ populations is conserved throughout vertebrate development. The properties of γδ T cells have been discussed in detail in Chapter 2. Although some γδ T cell subpopulations are extrathymically derived, most develop within the thymus.

A major question is what is the developmental relationship between γδ and αβ T cells? It is clear that both populations arise from a common thymic progenitor cell since a single micromanipulated embryonic day 14 thymocyte can give rise to both populations in thymic organ culture. Recent data suggest that the lineage split can occur from a late common progenitor along the thymocyte developmental pathway.

A plausible model for the choice of a developing thymocyte between the γδ and αβ lineages is based on the concept that thymocytes first attempt to rearrange *TCRG* and *TCRD* genes and, if successful, are committed to the γδ lineage. Thymocytes that have failed to become

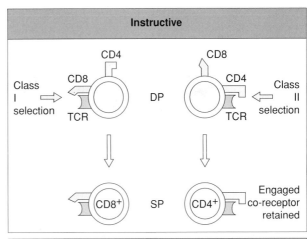

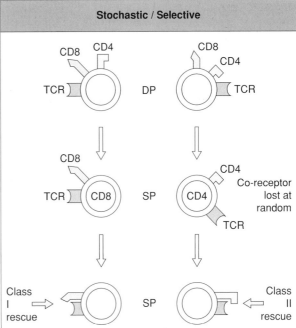

Fig. 6.8 Stochastic versus instructional models of CD4/8 lineage commitment. The instructive model proposes that the co-receptor is engaged together with the TCR during positive selection, signalling the downregulation of either CD4 or CD8 depending on the specificity of the TCR. The stochastic model proposes that developing DP thymocytes randomly downregulate CD4 or CD8 expression and then can be positively selected using only the remaining co-receptor, if this coreceptor is appropriate for the TCR specificity. In the instructional model, non-selected cells die by apoptosis. In the stochastic model, single positive cells must be rescued by interaction with the correct class of MHC molecules.

γδ T cells, because of non-productive rearrangements at these loci, can become αβ T cells; that is, αβ T cells can be failed γδ T cells. This model is presented in *Figure 6.9*. It is likely that the αβ/γδ T cell lineage split can occur up to the DP stage of development. Thus, the selection for *TCRB* rearrangement at the CD25+ DN thymocyte stage

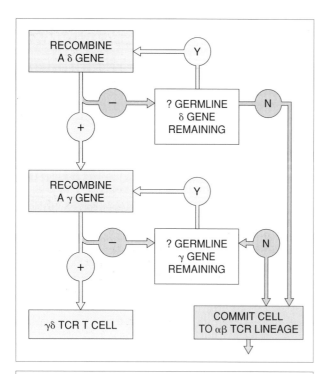

Fig. 6.9 γδ and αβ T cell lineage commitment. The model is based on the premise that precursor thymocytes rearrange their *TCRG* and *TCRD* genes first. Successful rearrangement of *TCRG* and *TCRD* generates a γδ T cell. Failure to rearrange either locus productively results in commitment to the αβ lineage. At each stage the cell can make two attempts at a productive rearrangement — one from the maternal and one from the paternal chromosome. Productive rearrangement, +; non-productive rearrangement, −. Y = Yes. N = No.

does not act as a switch for commitment to the αβ lineage but, instead, expands the pool of common precursors. In this context, peripheral γδ T cells have been shown to contain a high proportion of in-frame TCRB rearrangements. The completion of the lineage commitment most probably depends on the developmentally regulated activation of the *TCRA* enhancer that coincides with transition to the DP thymocyte stage. Subsequent *TCRA* rearrangement would delete the *TCRD* locus (see Chapter 2) thus removing any opportunity to become a γδ T cell.

SUMMARY

Haematopoiesis involves a complex series of events involving cell survival and death, clonal proliferation, differentiation and lineage commitment in order to generate a mature cell from a pluripotential stem cell. The decisions made among these choices by a developing haematopoietic cell determine the numbers, types and turnover rates of haematopoietic cells produced by the body. The pluripotential haematopoietic stem cell is defined as a cell that gives rise to complete repopulation of all haematopoietic cell compartments *in vivo* over an extended period of time. A candidate cell with these properties has been isolated based on the absence of a battery of lineage markers and the presence of the Sca-1 antigen. Development of the pluripotential stem cell involves a series of proliferation and commitment events. Each round of proliferation involves increasing commitment to a particular lineage. Regulation of the balance between proliferation and commitment determines the relative numbers of the various haematopoietic cell types. Both proliferation and differentiation signals are delivered by soluble factors (CSFs) and by interactions with stromal cells. The decisions on proliferation and lineage commitment are not fully understood but probably depend on the spectrum of growth factors that interact with a precursor cell and on the stage of differentiation of that cell. This in turn depends on the growth factor receptors expressed by that cell. Thus, cellular signalling via the same CSF-receptor interaction can result in a proliferative signal in a progenitor cell but functional differentiation in a later, more committed cell.

Most cells leaving the bone marrow are post-mitotic cells with functional activity. A notable exception to this is the progenitor T cell which undergoes further commitment and extensive proliferation and differentiation within the thymus. T cell development has many parallels with B cell development. In both cases, two distinct phases of development are involved. The first phase is driven by expression of a pre-T or pre-B cell receptor comprising a rearranged IgH or TCRβ-chain together with an additional chain called a surrogate light or α-chain. This receptor selects cells with productive in-frame rearrangements for survival and proliferation. The expanded population of cells is subjected to the second phase of lymphocyte development where rearrangement of the second receptor chain is followed by selection on the basis of the specificity of the mature antigen receptor complex. These signals can be either positive (survival) or negative (death) and shape and refine the mature B or T cell repertoire.

FURTHER READING

Abraham KM, Levin SD, Marth JD, Forbush KA, Perlmutter RM. Delayed thymocyte development induced by augmented expression of p56[lck]. *J Exp Med* 1991, **173**:1421.

Abramson S, Miller RG, Philips RA. The identification in adult bone marrow of pluripotent and restricted stem cells of the myeloid and lymphoid stems. *J Exp Med* 1977, **145**:1567.

Allen PM. Peptides in positive and negative selection: a delicate balance. *Cell* 1994, **76**:593.

Anderson G, Owen JJ, Moore NC, Jenkinson EJ. Thymic epithelial cells provide unique signals for positive selection of CD4+ CD8+

thymocytes *in vitro. J Exp Med* 1994, **179**:2027.

Anderson SJ, Levin SD, Perlmutter RM. Protein tyrosine kinase p56[lck] controls allelic exclusion of T cell receptor β-chain genes. *Nature* 1993, **365**:552.

Ardavin C, Wu L, Li C-L, Shortman K. Thymic dendritic cells and T cells develop simultaneously in the thymus from a common precursor population. *Nature* 1993, **362**:761.

Ashton-Rickardt PG, Bandeira A, Delaney JR, van Kaer L, Pircher HP, Zinkernagel RM, Tonegawa S. Evidence for a differential avidity model of T cell selection in the thymus. *Cell* 1994, **76**:651.

Ashton-Rickardt PG, Tonegawa S. A differential-avidity model for T cell selection. *Immunol Today* 1994, **15**:362.

Callard R, Gearing A (Eds). *The Cytokine Facts Book*. Academic Press: London; 1994.

Chan SH, Cosgrove D, Waltzinger C, Benoist C, Mathis D. Another view of the selective model of thymocyte selection. *Cell* 1993, **73**:225.

Clarke SC, Kamen R. The human haematopoietic colony-stimulating factors. *Science* 1987, **236**:1229.

Dudley EC, Mirardi M, Owen MJ, Hayday AC. αβ and γδ T cells can share a late common precursor. *Curr Biol* 1995 **5**:659.

Finkel TH, Cambier JC, Kubo RT, Born WK, Marrack P, Kappler JW. The thymus has two functionally distinct populations of immature αβ+ T cells: one population is deleted by ligation of αβ TCR. *Cell* 1989, **58**:1047.

Fowlkes BJ, Schweighoffer E. Positive selection of T cells. *Curr Biol* 1995, **7**:188.

Georgopoulos K, Bigby M, Wang J-H, Molnar A, Wu P, Winandy S, Sharpe A. The Ikaros gene is required for the development of all lymphoid lineages. *Cell* 1994, **79**: 43.

Godfrey DI, Zlotnik A. Control points in early T cell development. *Immunol Today* 1993, **14**:547.

Gordon MY, Riley P, Watt SM, Greaves MF. Compartmentalization of a haematopoietic growth factor GM-CSF by glycosaminoglycans in the bone marrow microenvironment. *Nature* 1987, **326**:403.

Guy-Grand D, Rocha B, Mintz P, Malassis-Seris M, Selz F, Malissen B, Vassalli P. Different use of T cell receptor transducing modules in two populations of gut intraepithelial lymphocytes are related to distinct pathways of T cell differentiation. *J Exp Med* 1994, **180**:673.

Hogquist KA, Jameson SC, Heath WR, Howard JL, Bevan MJ, Carbone FR. T cell receptor antagonist peptides induce positive selection. *Cell* 1994, **76**:17.

Ikuta K, Weissman IL. Evidence that hematopoietic stem cells express mouse c-kit but do not depend on steel factor for their generation. *Proc Natl Acad Sci USA* 1992, **89**:1502.

Jameson SC, Hogquist KA, Bevan MJ. Positive selection of thymocytes. *Annu Rev Immunol* 1995, **13**:93.

Janeway CA. Thymic selection: two pathways to life and two to death. *Immunity* 1994, **1**:3.

Jenkinson EJ, Owen MJ, Owen JJ. Thymus and T cell ontogeny: molecular and cellular. In *T cells*. Feldmann M, Lamb J, Owen M (Eds). New York: John Wiley and Sons Inc; 17:1989.

Jenkinson EJ, Anderson G. Fetal thymic organ cultures. *Curr Opin Immunol* 1994, **6**:293.

Jordon CT, McKearn JP, Lemischka IR. Cellular and developmental properties of foetal hematopoietic stem cells. *Cell* 1990, **61**:953.

Kincade PW, Lee G, Pietrangeli CE, Hayashi S-I, Gimble JM. Cells and molecules that regulate B lymphopoiesis in bone marrow. *Ann Rev Immunol* 1989, **7**:11.

Lin W-C, Desiderio S. VDJ recombination and the cell cycle. *Immunol Today* 1995, **16**:279.

MacDonald HR, Schneider R, Lees RK, Howe RC, Acha-Orbea H, Festenstein H, Zinkernagel RM, Hengartner H. T cell receptor Vβ use predicts reactivity and tolerance to Mlsª-encoded antigens. *Nature* 1988, **332**:40.

Malissen M, Trucy J, Jouvin-Marche E, Cazenave P-A, Scollay R, Malissen B. Regulation of TCR α and β gene allelic exclusion during T cell development. *Immunol Today* 1992, **13**:315.

Melchers F, Haasner D, Grawunder U, Kalberer C, Karasuyama H, Winkler T, Rolink A G. Roles of IgH and L chains and of surrogate H and L chains in the development of cells of the B lymphocyte lineage. *Ann Rev Immunol* 1994, **12**:209.

Melchers F, Rolink A, Grawunder U, Winkler TH, Karasuyama H, Ghia P, Andersson J. Positive and negative selection event during B lymphopoiesis. *Curr Biol* 1995, **7**:214.

Metcalfe D. Clonal analysis of paired daughter cells: action of GM-CSF on granulocyte-macrophage precursors. *Proc Natl Acad Sci USA* 1980, **77**:5327.

Metcalfe D. The molecular control of cell division, differentiation commitment and maturation in haemopoietic cells. *Nature* 1989, **339**:27.

Morrison SJ, Weissman IL. The long-term repopulating subset of hematopoietic stem cells is deterministic and isolatable by phenotype. *Immunity* 1994, **1**:661.

Nakano T, Kodama H, Honjo T. Generation of lymphohematopoietic cells from embryonic stem cells in culture. *Science* 1994, **265**:1098.

Nicola NA. Hemopoietic cell growth factors and their receptors. *Ann Rev Biochem* 1989, **58**:45.

Nossal GJV. Negative selection of lymphocytes. *Cell* 1994, **76**:229.

Peschon JJ, Morrissey PJ, Grabstein KH, Ramsdell FJ, Maraskovsky E, Gliniak BC, Park LS, Siegler SF, Williams DE, Ware CB *et al.* Early lymphocyte expansion is severely impaired in interleukin 7 receptor-deficient mice. *J Exp Med* 1994, **180**:1955.

Pfeffer K, Mak TW. Lymphocyte ontogeny and activation in gene targeted mutant mice. *Annu Rev Immunol* 1994, **12**:367.

Potocnik AJ, Nielsen PJ, Eichmann K. *In vitro* generation of lymphoid precursors from embryonic stem cells. *EMBO J* 1994, **13**:5274.

Poussier P, Julius M. Thymus independent T cell development and selection in the intestinal epithelium. *Ann Rev Immunol* 1994, **12**:521.

Reth M, Petrac E, Wiese P, Lobel L, Alt FW. Activation of Vκ gene rearrangement in pre-B cells follows the expression of membrane-bound immunoglobulin heavy chains. *EMBO J* 1987, **6**:3299.

Rocha B, Guy-Grand D, Vassalli P. Extrathymic T cell differentiation. *Curr Biol* 1995, **7**:235.

Rodewald H-R. Pathways from hematopoietic stem cells to thymocytes. *Curr Biol* 1995, **7**:176.

Rolink A, Melchers F. Molecular and cellular origins of B lymphocyte diversity. *Cell* 1991, **66**:1081.

Saint-Ruf C, Ungewiss K, Groettrup M, Bruno L, Fehling HJ, von Boehmer H. Analysis and expression of a cloned pre-T cell receptor gene. *Science* 1994, **266**:1208.

Smith CA, Williams GT, Kingston R, Jenkinson EJ, Owen JT. Antibodies to CD3/T cell receptor complex induce death by apoptosis in immature T cells in thymic cultures. *Nature* 1989, **337**:181.

Spangrude GJ, Heimfeld S, Weissman IL. Purification and characterization of mouse hematopoietic stem cells. *Science* 1988, **242**:58.

Spangrude GJ. Enrichment of murine haematopoietic stem cells: diverging roads. *Immunol Today* 1988, **10**:344.

Sprent J, Webb SR. Intrathymic and extrathymic clonal deletion of T cells. *Curr Biol* 1995, **7**:196.

Surh CD, Sprent J. T cell apoptosis detected *in situ* during positive and negative selection in the thymus. *Nature* 1994, **372**:100.

von Boehmer H, Kisielow P. Lymphocyte lineage commitment: instruction versus selection. *Cell* 1993, **73**:207.

von Boehmer H. Positive selection of lymphocytes. *Cell* 1994, **76**:219.

Weissman I L. Developmental switches in the immune system. *Cell* 1994, **76**:207.

Whitlock CA, Witte ON. Long-term culture of murine bone marrow precursors of B lymphocytes. *Methods Enzymol* 1987, **150**:275.

Wolf NS, Koné A, Priestley GV, Bartelmez SH. *In vivo* and *in vitro* characterization of long-term repopulating primitive hematopoietic cells isolated by sequential Hoechst 33342-rhodamine 123 FACS selection. *Exp Hematol* 1993, **21**:614.

7 Antigen Processing and Presentation

It has long been known that B cells can recognize soluble antigens directly but T cells require the presence of accessory cells in order to be activated by antigens. The classical studies by Rosenthal and Shevach, 1973, showed that the accessory cell population presents antigen in a manner requiring histocompatibility between the presenting cell and the responding T cell. We now know that T cells generally recognize antigen associated with self MHC molecules on the surface of cells and that this involves processed antigen binding in a groove on the MHC molecule (see Chapters 2 and 4). In most cases, CD8+ T cells recognize antigen on class I molecules, while CD4+ T cells see antigen associated with MHC class II molecules. This restriction, which governs effector functions of the mature cell, is established during T cell development in the thymus (see Chapter 6).

This chapter focuses primarily on the mechanisms involved in processing antigenic material for presentation to specific T cells. Molecular details of the tripartite interaction between processed antigen, MHC and the T cell receptor have been covered in detail in Chapters 2 and 4 and features important for the subsequent activation of T cells are addressed in Chapter 8.

ANTIGEN PROCESSING

The studies of Gell and Benacerraf in 1959 were the first to show that whilst B cells primarily recognize determinants on native antigenic molecules, T cells can recognize both native and denatured forms. This was subsequently confirmed by many other workers using a variety of protein antigens but it was only in 1980 that it was demonstrated that the T cells responding to native antigen were the same cells which responded to the denatured antigen. It later became clear that most antigens require some form of processing before they can be presented to either class I or class II MHC-restricted T cells.

The first evidence that an active processing step was required before antigen could be recognized by T cells came from studies of Ziegler and Unanué on macrophage presentation of *Listeria monocytogenes* antigens to polyclonal class II-restricted T cells. They found that there was a lag period between the binding of antigen to the macrophages and detection of antigen recognition by T cells (*Fig. 7.1*). Macrophages rendered metabolically inactive by fixation with paraformaldehyde immediately after pulsing with

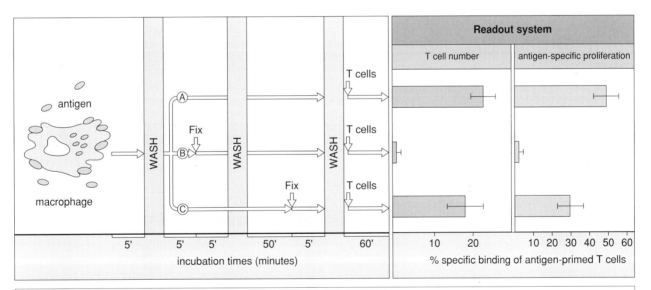

Fig. 7.1 Effect of fixation on antigen presentation by macrophages. Mouse macrophages were incubated with antigen (*Listeria monocytogenes*) for 5 minutes and, following extensive washing, were treated in three different ways (A–C) before the addition of specific antigen-primed T cells. The macrophages in A were left untreated, while those in B and C were fixed with paraformaldehyde after 5 and 60 minutes' incubation at 37°C, respectively. T cells were then allowed to interact with the antigen-pulsed macrophages for 1 hour. After this time, non-adherent cells were removed, counted and tested for antigen-specific responses (in this case, results obtained from proliferation assays are shown). The specific binding of T cells was then determined in each case from the decrease in number of T cells recovered and from the reduction in proliferative responses. These historic experiments demonstrated that T cells recognize antigen at the surface membrane of macrophages, but only after a lag period of antigen handling by these antigen presenting cells (APCs). Based on data of Ziegler and Unanué, 1981.

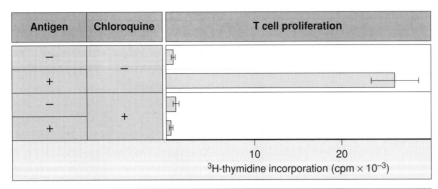

Antigen	Chloroquine	T cell proliferation
–	–	
+		
–	+	
+		

^{3}H-thymidine incorporation (cpm $\times$ 10^{-3})

Fig. 7.2 Chloroquine inhibits antigen presentation to T cells. Murine splenic macrophages were used as APCs in a proliferation assay using a T cell line specific for the bacterium *Corynebacterium parvum*. APCs were pulsed with *C. parvum* (+) or with medium only (–) for 2 hours at 37°C. Where indicated, optimal concentrations of chloroquine (0.3–0.5 mM) were added for the antigen pulsing period, and then removed by extensive washing. After 5 days of co-culture with these antigen-pulsed APCs, proliferation of the specific T cell line was measured by the incorporation of ^{3}H-thymidine. The T cell response to the *C. parvum* was completely abolished by the presence of chloroquine during the 2 hour antigen processing step. Based on data of Guidos *et al*, 1984.

antigen were not recognized by the T cells but were able to present *L. monocytogenes* antigens to specific T cells if fixed after a lag period of 45–60 minutes (depending on antigen concentration and temperature). Similar results were subsequently obtained by other investigators using soluble protein rather than particulate bacterial antigens.

Processing entails fragmentation of proteins into peptides

Different experimental approaches soon indicated that antigen processing, mediated by antigen presenting cells (APCs), for recognition by class II-restricted T cells involved proteolysis of the antigen. Macrophages treated with chloroquine which blocks protein degradation in lysosomes by raising the lysosomal pH, were found to be unable to present protein or bacterial antigens (*Fig. 7.2*). This effect was clearly specific for antigen processing rather than recognition of antigen by the T cell, since chloroquine had no effect if added after a lag period allowing processing to occur. Such observations were interpreted to mean that antigen processing (for class II presentation) involves proteolysis in lysosomes. However, vesicular acidification by agents such as chloroquine can also affect intracellular traffic. As will be discussed later, degradation of most exogenous antigens may take place in endosomal compartments.

Some of the first direct evidence that the processed antigenic moiety recognized by T cells is a proteolytic fragment of the antigen came from studies of ovalbumin (OVA)-specific T cell hybridomas by Shimonkevitz and colleagues in 1983. These cells all recognized OVA presented by untreated APCs but failed to respond when the APCs were fixed. If, however, OVA peptides (prepared either by digestion with trypsin or by cleavage at methionine residues with cyanogen bromide) were used, most of the hybridomas responded whether the APCs were fixed or not (*Fig. 7.3*).

Thus, cell-free proteolysis had completely replaced the active metabolic events involved in antigen processing by the APCs. The various cleavage procedures clearly led to the production of antigenic determinants recognizable by different T cells, suggesting that different processing mechanisms in APCs might influence which of the potential epitopes are presented to the T cell population.

Direct evidence supporting a role for protease-mediated cleavage in antigen processing by APCs rather than in cell-free systems has come from studies investigating the effect of specific protease inhibitors on antigen presentation. This approach, following for example sperm whale myoglobin recognition by various T cell clones, has led to the suggestion that proteases play a central role in processing of many antigens. Similar studies with other proteins, such as lysozyme or ovalbumin, have indicated that other proteases are important. It seems likely that proteolysis is involved in processing of most antigens before binding to class II molecules but the enzymes involved remain unknown. They may in fact vary from one peptide to the next.

Epitope structure

Technical advances for isolating class I-bound peptides and sequencing by tandem mass spectroscopy, mostly championed by Ramensee's laboratory, have been recently introduced. These techniques, coupled with detailed structural information from crystals, have revealed how MHC molecules are peptide receptors of 'peculiar specificity'. In other words they are able to accommodate millions of different peptides, provided they share certain features. These breakthroughs have gone hand in hand with the ease of producing synthetic peptides of defined sequence, facilitating detailed analyses of the epitopes recognized by many different clonal T cell populations specific for antigens of known primary sequence. An example of this is shown in

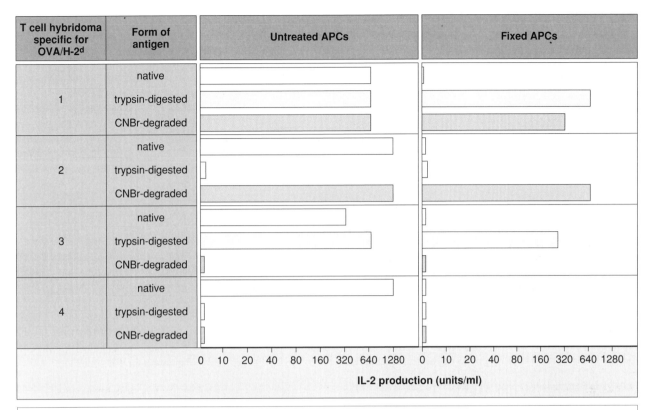

T cell hybridoma specific for OVA/H-2^d	Form of antigen	Untreated APCs	Fixed APCs
1	native		
	trypsin-digested		
	CNBr-degraded		
2	native		
	trypsin-digested		
	CNBr-degraded		
3	native		
	trypsin-digested		
	CNBr-degraded		
4	native		
	trypsin-digested		
	CNBr-degraded		

IL-2 production (units/ml)

Fig. 7.3 Effect of fixation on the recognition of native or degraded antigens by OVA-specific T cell hybridomas. Macrophage APCs were fixed or left untreated before testing their ability to present different forms of ovalbumin (OVA) to a variety of T cell hybridomas all restricted through H-2^d class II MHC molecules. The response of the hybridomas was assessed by measuring the release of IL-2. Results of representative hybridomas are shown to illustrate the four patterns of reactivity (1–4) observed with native, trypsin-digested and cyanogen bromide (CNBr)-degraded OVA. These four hybridomas all had different epitopic specificities. In all cases, fixed APCs failed to present native OVA. However, most hybridomas (1–3) could respond to a degraded form of the antigen, whether the APCs were fixed or not. In some cases (2 and 3) only one of the degraded forms of OVA were stimulatory. Thus, different modes of antigen degradation can either preserve or destroy different epitopes. Based on data of Shimonkevitz *et al*, 1983.

Figure 7.4 for pigeon cytochrome c-reactive T cells in B10.A (H-2^a) mice, where most T cells recognize an epitope centred around Lys 99 at the C-terminal portion of the molecule.

Since the mammalian genome encodes around 5×10^7 amino acids in its expressed proteins it may be calculated that peptides over eight to nine amino acids long must be displayed to ensure specificity. It is no surprise that nature has come up with this size of peptide to be bound by the grooves of class I molecules, although in some situations much longer peptides are bound (*Fig. 7.5* and *Colour figures*). The peptide is an integral part of the class I structure. Both N- and C-termini are tightly bound by hydrogen bonds to conserved residues in the class I groove. In addition, two side chains in the peptide, one at the extreme C-terminus usually position 9 and the other often at position 2, hold the peptide in allele-specific pockets. Contrary to some early ideas, peptides are stretched out and are not in a helical configuration. As well as the main anchor positions for peptide binding, in some cases more subtle auxiliary anchors may be observed. Armed with this kind of information for a particular class I allelic product it is possible to predict natural

T cell epitopes from a protein sequence with some degree of accuracy. Those positions in the peptide not essential for binding should then be available for contact with the T cell receptor. The numbers of class I ligands now identified is growing exponentially and the list contains a number of peptides from pathogens as well as self peptides. It was expected that APC would be unable to distinguish self from non-self proteins and this view has been confirmed. Self and non-self proteins seem to be processed and presented indiscriminately, calling for sophisticated mechanisms of review on the cell surface and appropriate tolerance systems discussed elsewhere in this book.

Motifs for binding to the grooves of class II molecules have also been defined. However, peptides contained within class II molecules apparently can extend from the binding groove at their N- or C-terminus. The peptides bound can vary between 12 and 25 residues but the central core is probably similar to the length bound by class I. It was no surprise that peptides from class II grooves were predominantly derived from proteins localizing to intracellular compartments bounded by membranes, such as endosomes and lysosomes. What was surprising was the large number of self

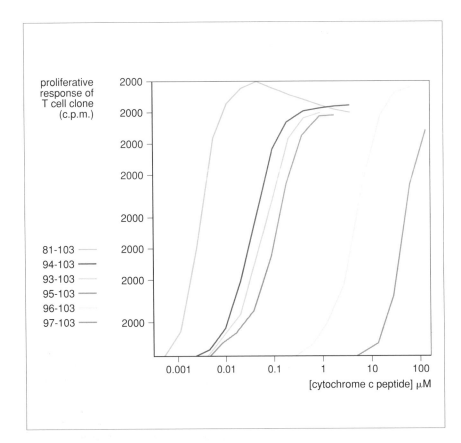

proliferative
response of
T cell clone
(c.p.m.)

2000
2000
2000
2000
2000
2000
2000
2000

81-103 ——
94-103 ——
93-103 ——
95-103 ——
96-103 ——
97-103 ——

0.001　0.01　0.1　1　10　100

[cytochrome c peptide] μM

Amino acid sequence of peptide	Relative potency
81　83　85　87　89　91　93　95　97　99　101　103 (V)(F)(A)(G)(L)(K)(K)(A)(N)(E)(R)(A)(D)(L)(I)(A)(Y)(L)(K)(Q)(A)(T)(K)	1
98-103　(L)(K)(Q)(A)(T)(K)	N.R.
97-103　(Y)(L)(K)(Q)(A)(T)(K)	9500
96-103　(A)(Y)(L)(K)(Q)(A)(T)(K)	1400
95-103　(I)(A)(Y)(L)(K)(Q)(A)(T)(K)	26
94-103　(L)(I)(A)(Y)(L)(K)(Q)(A)(T)(K)	7
93-103　(D)(L)(I)(A)(Y)(L)(K)(Q)(A)(T)(K)	20
95V-103　(V)(A)(Y)(L)(K)(Q)(A)(T)(K)	23
95F-103　(F)(A)(Y)(L)(K)(Q)(A)(T)(K)	65
95M-103　(M)(A)(Y)(L)(K)(Q)(A)(T)(K)	338
95Q-103　(Q)(A)(Y)(L)(K)(Q)(A)(T)(K)	172
95E-103　(E)(A)(Y)(L)(K)(Q)(A)(T)(K)	1508
95K-103　(K)(A)(Y)(L)(K)(Q)(A)(T)(K)	7150

Fig. 7.4 Amino acid requirements for an epitope recognized by a pigeon cytochrome c specific T cell clone. Specific peptides of different lengths (shown in one-letter code) representing part of the C-terminal region of pigeon cytochrome c were used to stimulate a specific MHC class II-restricted T cell clone from a B10.A (H-2^a) mouse. The T cell proliferative responses to the different peptides are shown as dose-response curves (upper panel) and summarized (lower panel) as the potency relative to the longest peptide (81–103). This value (relative potency) was calculated as the ratio of the peptide concentrations required to give a response of 100 000cpm. The lysine (K) residue is known to be critical for this epitope to interact with the T cell receptor of this clone. Peptide 98–103 was not recognized (NR) by the clone at any concentration tested, the shortest peptide stimulating the clone being seven amino acids long (97–103). However, the addition of two amino acids to the N-terminal region (peptide 95–103) led to a marked increase in potency. Changing the N-terminal isoleucine (I) of peptide 95–103 to different amino acids (shown only in the lower panel) had a variable effect on the potency of the peptide. Large uncharged residues, such as valine (V) and phenylalanine (F), had little effect, whereas charged amino acids such as glutamic acid (E) and lysine (K) markedly reduced the potency of the peptide. Since residue 95 is clearly not essential for activity (peptide 97–103 is still active, albeit at high concentration), it is thought to increase the efficiency of presentation by stabilizing the peptide in a suitable conformation for interaction with the MHC class II molecule and perhaps the T cell receptor as well. Based on data of Schwartz *et al*, 1985.

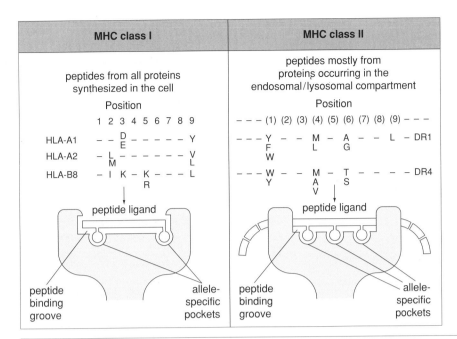

Fig. 7.5 Simplified view of MHC class I and II molecules as peptide vectors. Class I molecules hold peptides of 8–11, but mostly 9, amino acids with both amino and carboxyl termini tightly fixed in the groove. Two side chains of anchor residues of the peptide protrude into complementary allele-specific pockets of the groove. A few HLA allele-specific peptide consensus sequences are indicated above the diagram. Some of the exceptions are not considered here. Class II ligands, consisting of 12–25 residues, in contrast to the situation with class I, are not fixed by their ends in the groove but are allowed to hang out at the ends. The peptides are held in the groove by interactions with the peptide backbone as well as with some side chains. Note that, unlike class I, there is no strongly conserved -COOH terminal peptide anchor. Modified from Ramensee *et al*, 1993 and Hammer *et al*, 1992.

proteins bound. These included fragments of other MHC class I and class II proteins. New techniques, such as genetic engineering of peptide motifs produced as randomly generated expressed sequences on bacteriophage M13 pili (phage display libraries) coupled with structural determinations of class II molecules, are starting to reveal precise requirements for peptides to be accommodated in the grooves of class II molecules. The rules governing interaction with class II grooves may be more subtle than those of class I, involving interactions with the peptide backbone as well as anchor residues which are often not at the peptide ends. Nevertheless, it is now possible to construct algorithms capable of precise quantitative epitope prediction for class II peptides. Data suggest that for both class I and class II, peptides are an integral part of the molecule expressed on the cell surface and contribute to its stability.

PROCESSING FOR CLASS I-RESTRICTED RECOGNITION — ENDOGENOUS ANTIGENS

Although presentation of processed antigen to T cells appears to be similar for both class I and class II MHC molecules, involving binding of peptides in the groove, the intracellular events leading to the formation of these two types of MHC–peptide complex appear to be very different in most cases. Perhaps the first indication of this came from Morrison and colleagues who compared the processing requirements for antigen recognition by class I and II-restricted influenza virus-specific cytotoxic T cell (Tc) clones (*Fig. 7.6*). They demonstrated that class II-restricted Tc cells recognized only exogenously added viral polypeptides that required processing since recognition was blocked if the target cells were treated with chloroquine. In contrast, class I-restricted Tc recognizing the same viral polypeptides required *de novo* synthesis of viral proteins within the target cell, being unable to recognize exogenously added antigen; their recognition of newly synthesized antigen was unaffected by chloroquine.

Since most studies of class I-restricted Tc have used cells specific for viruses, hapten-modified self antigens or allogeneic MHC molecules, it was thought that these T cells recognized surface antigens which could associate with MHC class I in the plasma membrane. However, data clearly show that this is not true in most, if not all, cases. For example, Townsend and colleagues have studied murine Tc clones specific for the nucleoprotein (NP) of influenza virus. These clones recognize and kill target cells transfected with the *NP* gene and the appropriate class I molecule. Through the use of deletion mutants and synthetic peptides, short sequences of NP were identified as representing intracellularly processed epitopes recognized by the T cells.

Many subsequent studies have confirmed that antigen recognition by class I-restricted Tc, like that of class II-restricted T cells, requires antigen processing to a peptidic form that can associate with MHC molecules. Similarly, the

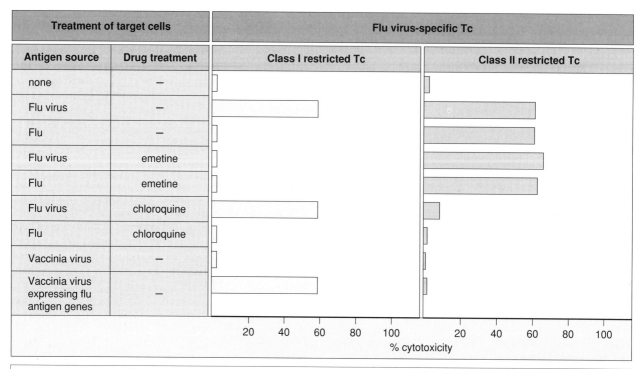

| Treatment of target cells | | Flu virus-specific Tc | |
Antigen source	Drug treatment	Class I restricted Tc	Class II restricted Tc
none	—		
Flu virus	—		
Flu	—		
Flu virus	emetine		
Flu	emetine		
Flu virus	chloroquine		
Flu	chloroquine		
Vaccinia virus	—		
Vaccinia virus expressing flu antigen genes	—		

Fig. 7.6 Recognition of influenza virus infected cells by class I and class II-restricted Tc. Target cells expressing both class I and II molecules were infected with virus (Flu virus), or incubated with inactivated antigen preparation (Flu) in the presence or absence of emetine (an irreversible inhibitor of protein synthesis) or chloroquine (to inhibit processing of exogenous antigens). Target killing by class I-restricted Tc required *de novo* protein synthesis, but was unaffected by chloroquine. Class II-restricted killing, on the other hand, was inhibited by chloroquine but did not require protein synthesis. Thus, class I-restricted Tc appeared to recognize viral antigens newly synthesized by infected target cells, whereas class II-restricted Tc seemed to recognize only a processed form of added viral antigen. This conclusion was supported by the use of target cells infected with Vaccinia virus vectors carrying Flu antigen genes; only class I-restricted Tc recognized these targets. Based on data of Morrison *et al*, 1986.

epitopes involved in target cell sensitization can be defined experimentally by synthetic peptides around nine amino acids long. That naturally processed antigen presented by class I molecules is in a peptide form has been supported by the X-ray crystallographic structures of class I molecules such as HLA-A2, Aw68 and B27, where electron density not assigned to the class I heavy chain occupied the epitope binding groove (see Chapter 4). It was clear early in these studies that peptides were anchored at the ends of the peptide groove of class I molecules. The extra electron density corresponding to a mixture of different peptides in class I molecules was not well resolved, indicating varying conformations in the middle. However, the regions corresponding to the ends of the peptides were fixed, consistent with similar interactions with the pockets of the class I molecule at the N- and C-termini.

Studies of influenza virus nucleoprotein (NP) have provided further evidence that cytoplasmic processing of newly synthesized molecules leads to their expression in association with class I MHC molecules. NP is synthesized on free ribosomes and accumulates in the nucleus because of a nuclear targetting signal present between amino acid residues 327–345; it does not traffic intact to the cell surface. Nevertheless, murine NP-specific

Tc clones can recognize epitopes from either the N or C-terminus of the molecule in association with H-2^k or H-2^b respectively. Again, virally infected cells and cells incubated with defined peptides are recognized but exogenously added intact NP is not. Expression of NP in target cells infected with recombinant vaccinia virus containing the NP gene also allows recognition by NP-specific Tc. The pathway involved in processing antigen in these experiments is unaffected by lysosomotropic agents such as chloroquine and is not accessible to exogenous antigen.

In contrast to NP, influenza haemagglutinin (HA) is expressed intact at the cell surface. However, mutant HA molecules lacking a signal sequence reside in the cytoplasm and are still recognized by HA-specific Tc. Tc recognizing epitopes from the transmembrane region of HA, which are not accessible in intact molecules expressed at the cell surface, have also been described. Other experiments have also shown that introducing intact antigen into the cytoplasm of a target cell is enough to allow presentation by class I. For example, the soluble protein ovalbumin (OVA), which is normally recognized by class II-restricted T cells, can be introduced into the cytoplasm, or expressed there by gene transfection, allowing the stimulation of class I-restricted, OVA-specific Tc.

The role of the proteasome

The recent discovery of two genes encoding proteasome subunits, *LMP2* and *LMP7*, in the class II region of the MHC, interdigitating the *TAP* loci, provided circumstantial evidence for the involvement of this organelle in antigen processing. Proteasomes are large, evolutionarily conserved, cytoplasmic structures involved in protein turnover (*Fig. 7.7*). The 20S structure is believed to consist of the products of 14 different genes in mammals giving rise to seven α and seven β subunits which form four ring, or torus, structures to make a barrel. A similar arrangement of subunits is used to make a more complex 26S structure which is constructed by adding proteins of a different nature to the ends of the barrel. The 26S particle is involved in degrading ubiquitinated substrates. Deletion of individual proteasome subunits in yeast is lethal, which is not surprising since the proteasome is responsible for most non-lysosomal protein turnover.

The weight of evidence supports the notion that the LMP subunits replace two constitutive components. Since expression of the LMP proteasome subunits is inducible with IFNγ it has been proposed that the cell recruits the two novel components in order to tailor the proteasome to the demands of antigen processing. In the scheme which enjoys most support the LMPs subtly change the output of the proteasome so that it tends to produce peptides with C-termini suited to the binding pockets of most class I molecules. It is proposed that proteasomes with LMPs cleave more often after hydrophobic or basic amino acids as opposed to the constitutive situation which favours a tendency for cleavage after acidic residues. Actual cleavage pattern changes are probably more complex and may be imagined to reflect the needs of the APC to produce peptides with suitable C-termini as well as a suitable length for transport via the TAPs. The rules governing the precise way the LMPs influence specificity remain to be determined on proteins suitable as substrates for presentation rather than short peptides studied so far. In B cell lines lacking the *LMP* genes very little effect on antigen presentation to T cell clones is detectable so far although in mice with single defects in either *LMP2* or *LMP7* differences in responses to viral antigens *in vivo* are detectable.

Intuitively, since ubiquitin is coupled to most cellular proteins to target them for degradation, it seems reasonable to imagine its involvement in targetting proteins for prospective antigens. However, there is evidence both for and against the need for ubiquitination. Against includes early experiments which showed that modification of proteins to render them refractory to ubiquitination did not affect presentation. In some recent experiments, mutant cells exhibiting a temperature-sensitive defect in ubiquitination showed a defect in class I-restricted presentation of ovalbumin introduced into the cytosol at the non-permissive temperature. In the positive control experiment, presentation of an ovalbumin peptide synthesized from a transfected minigene was uncompromised. It is tempting to speculate that the 26S proteasome particle is at work here but more definitive evidence is lacking at present.

Mechanism of antigen-class I association

Most early experiments were consistent with antigenic peptides associating with newly synthesized class I molecules before they reach the cell surface. Experiments with the fungal antibiotic brefeldin A have been instrumental in defining where peptide–MHC interactions occur. Brefeldin A blocks the egress of newly synthesized proteins from a specialized pre-Golgi compartment, causing them to recycle back to the endoplasmic reticulum (ER). Treatment of target cells with brefeldin A completely inhibits presentation of an influenza virus class I-restricted epitope represented by amino acids 55–73 of the matrix protein (M1), to HLA-A2-restricted Tc clones (*Fig. 7.8*). Presentation of influenza virus antigens to murine H-2^k-restricted Tc is similarly inhibited. This inhibitory effect of brefeldin A is thought to be due specifically to its effect on protein trafficking from the ER although the antibiotic may block other pathways.

Mutant cell lines provided evidence that binding of peptides to class I in the ER is important for the stable expression of these MHC molecules at the cell surface. Townsend and colleagues have described a mutant murine T lymphoma cell line, RMA-S, which expresses low levels of cell surface class I molecules and is unable to process and present epitopes of NP synthesized in the cytoplasm. However, addition of synthetic peptide epitopes to the culture medium leads to a marked increase in surface class I molecules, allowing recognition by specific Tc. Similar results have been obtained with the human cell line LCL721.174 and its BxT fusion derivative T2, where an HLA-A2-restricted influenza matrix protein epitope enhances the surface expression of HLA-A2 molecules.

Subsequent analyses of these systems have shown that, in the absence of peptide, class I heavy chains can interact with β$_2$-microglobulin (β$_2$m) and some are transported to the cell surface but being unstable they are rapidly lost. Binding of peptides added to the culture medium stabilizes these class I molecules, resulting in surface class I expression. In normal cells, the association of a peptide with the peptide binding site of a newly synthesized class I heavy chain in the ER allows the β$_2$m-heavy chain complex to adopt the correct conformation for stable surface expression.

In the absence of foreign antigens, class I-binding peptides are derived from normal self proteins in wild type cells. A small proportion of class I molecules may reach the surface membrane without a bound peptide but would be short lived. In fact, in the mutant murine T lymphoma cell line RMA-S, those class I molecules that reach the cell surface can be stabilized by placing the cells at reduced temperature. It is feasible that antigenic peptides produced by proteolysis *in vivo*, such as at sites of inflammation, might bind to and stabilize free class I molecules, leading to stimulation of class I-restricted T cells. The existence of such a mechanism is conjectural.

The role of peptide transporters

In the 1980s, Townsend's group predicted that, since sections of viral antigens synthesized intracellularly ended up on the cell surface in conjunction with class I molecules, at some stage they had to traverse a membrane. But what mechanism could be used to push short, often hydrophilic peptides across a lipid bilayer? At the end of the '80s, the finding of genes within the class II region of the MHC (*TAP1* and *TAP2*) with characteristics of membrane-spanning ATP-dependent pumps provided a solution to this problem (*Fig. 7.7*).

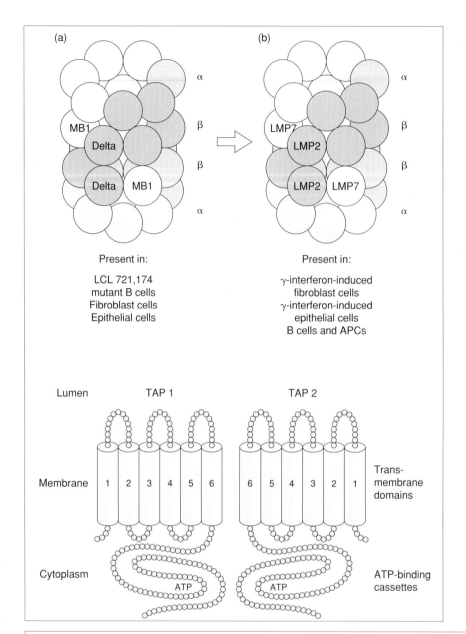

Fig. 7.7 Structure of the proteasome and the TAP molecule involved in preparing peptides for loading onto class I molecules. The 20S proteasome particle is shown to consist of a cylinder composed of four stacked rings or discs. Each ring has seven subunits in a pseudohelical arrangement. The proteasome is composed of two types of subunit, α and β. The outer rings contain α subunits and the inner rings β subunits, making the molecular organization $\alpha_7\beta_7\beta_7\alpha_7$. Each subunit may occur twice in the particle, leading to a structure comprising a complex dimer. The two β subunits designated delta and MB1 can be exchanged by the two MHC-encoded subunits LMP2 and LMP7, respectively. The locations of the subunits are still hypothetical, although the basic arrangement of α and β subunits is derived from the structure of *Thermoplasma* proteasome that is made up of 14 identical α and 14 β subunits. The presence of LMP2 and LMP7 in the proteasome particle may alter the specificity of cleavage of proteins. From Belich *et al*, 1994.

ATP-binding cassette (ABC) transporters comprise a large superfamily. The basic organization of these molecules, of two transmembrane domains and two ATP-binding cassettes, is similar although they may be encoded in a variety of different ways: on one long mRNA, or in the other extreme, each domain on a separate mRNA. A variety of different moieties may be transported by different versions. From Hyde, 1990. In the diagram, a hypothetical model of the TAP transporter shows how the transmembrane domains snake in and out of the cell membrane. Almost all of the limited polymorphism in the human TAP alleles is in the ATP-binding cassette domains. In the rat TAP2 alleles, which differ by up to 29 amino acids from each other, variable residues in the membrane domains are thought to be responsible for determining specificity for transporting different peptides across the membrane. The molecule is shown in a linear fashion as a heterodimer but in fact could be a multimer and may be arranged folded round to make a pore.

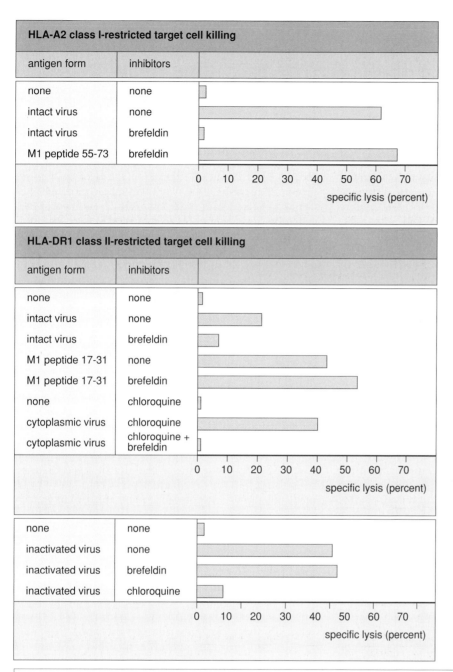

HLA-A2 class I-restricted target cell killing

antigen form	inhibitors	specific lysis (percent)
none	none	
intact virus	none	
intact virus	brefeldin	
M1 peptide 55-73	brefeldin	

HLA-DR1 class II-restricted target cell killing

antigen form	inhibitors	specific lysis (percent)
none	none	
intact virus	none	
intact virus	brefeldin	
M1 peptide 17-31	none	
M1 peptide 17-31	brefeldin	
none	chloroquine	
cytoplasmic virus	chloroquine	
cytoplasmic virus	chloroquine + brefeldin	

antigen form	inhibitors	specific lysis (percent)
none	none	
inactivated virus	none	
inactivated virus	brefeldin	
inactivated virus	chloroquine	

Fig. 7.8 Effects of brefeldin A and chloroquine on processing of influenza virus matrix protein for recognition by class I and class II-restricted T cells.
HLA-A2 or HLA-DR1 bearing B lymphoblastoid cells were incubated with different forms of influenza virus matrix protein (M1) with or without brefeldin A and chloroquine before being used as targets for specific Tc (clone Q115 specific for M1 peptide 55–73 in association with HLA-A2 [upper panel] and clone 109.2B2 specific for M1 peptide 17–31 associated with HLA-DR1 [lower panel]). The upper panel shows that class I-restricted presentation of matrix protein by cells infected with intact influenza virus is completely inhibited in the presence of brefeldin A, a reagent which traps newly synthesized class I molecules and other proteins in the ER. However, brefeldin A has no effect on the presentation of pre-processed antigen, in this case in the form of the synthetic M1 peptide 55–73. Similar experiments on class II-restricted recognition (lower panel) showed that brefeldin A has a partial inhibitory effect on processing of matrix protein in virally infected cells. When the virus was introduced directly into the cytoplasm (by absorption to the cell at 4°C and lowering the pH to below 5.0), antigen processing was still efficient in the presence of chloroquine but was completely blocked by the addition of brefeldin A but markedly reduced in the presence of chloroquine. These results indicated that both the cytoplasmic ER and endosomal processing routes can operate for this class II restricted epitope, and that the route followed depends on the form of the antigen and its mode of entry into the cell. Based on data of Nuchtern *et al*, 1989, 1990.

Mutant cell lines, in which class I molecules were retained in the ER with subsequent low surface expression, turned out to have defects in either TAP1 (.134), TAP2 (RMA-S, Bm36.1) or both (721.174, T2) and surface expression of class I as well as other associated phenotypes could be restored by transfection of the appropriate DNA clones. Other evidence for the TAPs had come from studies in the rat where a locus in the class II region called *cim*, for class I modifier, which turned out to be TAP2, was shown to influence the allogenicity of RT1A^a MHC class I molecules in recombinant inbred strains. In the *cimb* background strain, the RT1A^a class I molecule was retained in the ER. Introduction of a clone corresponding to the *TAP2a* allele restored full surface expression of RT1A^a and led to a different set of peptides associated with the class I molecule.

Biochemical characterization of the TAP1 and TAP2 proteins showed that they were associated as a heterodimer, or heteromultimer, to make a structure similar to the many other transporter family members, such as the cystic fibrosis transporter and p-glycoprotein. The more than 60 known ATP-binding cassette (ABC) transporters found from prokaryotes to mammals exhibit specificity for substrates as diverse as inorganic ions, sugars, polysaccharides, hydrophobic drugs, amino acids, peptides and proteins. Similar to other ABC transporters, TAP1 and TAP2 each consist of an N-terminal hydrophobic multimembrane-spanning domain and a C-terminal hydrophilic domain which contains the highly conserved sequence necessary for ATP binding.

Antisera coupled to gold beads, used on thin frozen sections for electron microscopy, showed that the human TAP molecules were located in the ER membrane, with the putative ATP-binding cassette facing the cytoplasm. Taken together, these data provided further indirect evidence that the TAPs constituted a transporter responsible for moving cytoplasmic proteins into the lumen of the ER.

More direct evidence for the role of the TAPs in transporting peptides into the ER has come from assays designed to measure TAP-dependent passage of peptides into the ER in cells permeabilized with streptolysin O which creates holes in the plasma membrane but leaves the ER membrane intact. First, these assays demonstrated a clear dependence on ATP for transport. Then they permitted a detailed analysis of optimum peptide composition for transport (*Fig 7.9*). The optimum length for efficient transport was around nine or more amino acids; less than seven amino acid peptides were poor competitors yet much longer peptides were effective. The most dramatic effects of amino acid composition on transport were provided by the C-terminus. Human transporters were non-selective as were rat TAPs from the a allele. In contrast, rat TAP^u alleles worked much better on peptides with hydrophobic C-termini, as did mouse transporters. In fact, peptides isolated from mouse class I molecules exclusively contain hydrophobic C-termini and, in any case, mouse MHC class I structures are probably not receptive for peptides with a charged C-terminus; no mouse alleles have an Asp residue at position 116 in the peptide binding groove, mandatory to accommodate charged C-termini.

These data were consistent with the phenotypic effects of rat *cim* alleles. It should be pointed out that rat *TAP2*

alleles can differ by as many as 29 amino acids from each other but those of humans and mice are relatively non-polymorphic. Perhaps during evolution rats have exploited TAP differences to maximize variation in handling various protein epitopes. It is interesting to note that the permissiveness of the human TAPs for peptides with charged or hydrophobic C-termini correlates with the occurrence of Lys and Arg in this position in a number of peptides isolated from HLA class I alleles. Moreover, these alleles all have an Asp residue at positions 77 and 116, forming part of the 'F' pocket in the peptide binding groove. Experiments in which various peptide epitopes were engineered with -NH$_2$ or -COOH extensions, preceded by signal sequences so that they were transported directly into the ER, showed that a precise -COOH terminus was essential for subsequent presentation by class I molecules but -NH$_2$ terminal extensions could be tolerated. These data suggest that -NH$_2$ terminal trimming may take place in the lumen of the ER to provide finished peptides of the exact size for class I binding.

In conclusion, it seems likely that the TAPs have evolved in different species to meet the requirements of the class I products that they serve. It is perhaps no coincidence that the TAP and class I genes are genetically linked, as pointed out in Chapter 4. A diagram summarizing the pathway of antigens from the cytoplasm onto the cell surface, coupled with class I molecules, is shown in *Figure 7.10*. In this working model, the MHC-encoded LMPs modify the proteasome to preferentially make peptides with appropriate -COOH termini for binding to grooves of class I molecules. The TAP transporter moves peptides of seven or more amino acids into the ER where they may be trimmed by an unidentified aminopeptidase for binding to class I molecules.

The role of calnexin and TAP binding

There is a complex series of events to coordinate loading of appropriate peptides into the class I groove which is only just being understood (*Fig. 7.10*). Initially, class I molecules are associated with a resident ER protein, calnexin. As has been shown by co-precipitation experiments in the mild detergent digitonin, they then associate directly with the TAPs. Release is presumably concomitant with peptide binding. Other factors in this scheme, which have not yet been resolved, concern whether peptides are trimmed within the ER after binding to class I molecules and whether chaperone molecules such as heat shock proteins are involved in the process.

PROCESSING FOR CLASS II-RESTRICTED RECOGNITION — EXOGENOUS ANTIGENS

Although presentation of processed antigen to T cells appears to be similar for both class I and class II MHC molecules, involving binding of peptides in the groove, the intracellular events leading to the formation of these two types of MHC–peptide complex appear to be very different in most cases. The understanding of class II peptide loading has involved cell biology and the analysis of the maturation of class II molecules in various vesicles within the cell.

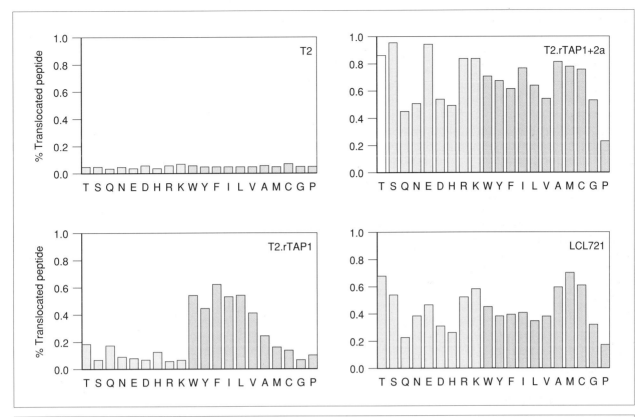

Fig. 7.9 The effect of -COOH terminal amino acids on the efficiency of peptide translocation into the ER. The TAP1/2-deficient mutant cell line T2 and T2 cells transfected with rat TAP1 plus TAP2[a] or TAP2[u] alleles, as well as wildtype LCL721 cells, were used. The peptide series RYWANATRSX was used where X is one of the 20 amino acids indicated. ^{125}I-labelled peptides were translocated into the ER of streptolysin O-permeabilized cells in the presence of ATP, recovered through an N-linked glycan and quantified by γ counting. The human and rat TAP1/2[a] transporters are fairly non-selective for the -COOH terminal amino acid. The other rat transporter (rat TAP1/2[u]) as well as mouse, which is not shown, selects for peptides with hydrophobic C-termini (green). Taken from Momburg *et al*, 1994.

Mechanism of antigen-class II association

As with the studies of class I-restricted presentation, one of the major goals of recent experiments has been the elucidation of the routes of intracellular traffic of class II molecules and the site(s) of their association with antigenic peptides. Two major possibilities have been considered:

- Recycling of class II molecules from the cell surface with peptide exchange occurring in an endosomal compartment. In some cells, particularly murine B lymphoma lines, rapid and specific endocytosis of class II molecules has been reported.
- The intersection of the class II biosynthetic pathway with a compartment containing processed antigen (*Fig. 7.11*). There is support for both pathways but the most recent evidence favours the latter as the major one. Indeed, newly synthesized class II molecules, unlike class I, do not go immediately to the surface but are delayed for 1–3 hours, presumably for peptide loading to take place. Both systems, as well as additional pathways, could function, with the relative importance varying with cell type and prevailing circumstances, such as their state of activation.

Cell biology and the role of Ii

Newly synthesized class II molecules associate with a non-polymorphic 'invariant chain' (Ii) within the cell. The Ii chain is a type II membrane protein, so unlike MHC class I and class II molecules the C-terminal portion of the molecule extends into the lumen of the ER. The Ii-class II association occurs in the ER membrane and remains during transport through the Golgi apparatus. The Ii chain is proteolytically cleaved and released before the class II molecule is expressed at the cell surface.

Electron microscopic studies using anti-Ig-coated gold particles and B cells have shown that mIg is rapidly internalized (within 2 minutes) by receptor-mediated endocytosis into endosomes, where it is found co-localized with cathepsins B and D and class II molecules. In these experiments, Ii also co-localized with the anti-Ig coated beads, indicating that the class II molecules within the endosome were primarily derived from a newly synthesized pool rather than from internalized plasma membrane.

Recent experiments on intracellular trafficking of MHC molecules have extended these observations. In the B lymphoblastoid cell line, JY, some constitutive internalization of class II did take place but no recycling back to the cell

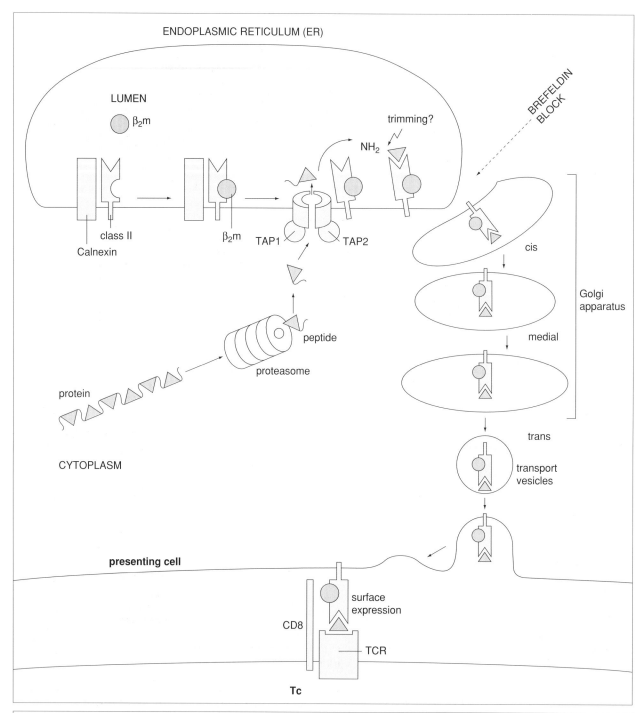

Fig. 7.10 Major proposed route of intracellular trafficking of MHC class I molecules in antigen processing and presentation. Intracellular proteins are thought to be degraded into peptides by the proteasome, two subunits of which, LMP2 and LMP7, are encoded in the MHC class II region. Proteasomes which have incorporated the MHC-encoded subunits may preferentially cleave substrates at the -COOH side of residues appropriate for binding into the pockets of class I molecules, which generally accommodate hydrophobic or basic amino acids. The peptides so produced, which may be around nine or more amino acids, are then transported into the endoplasmic reticulum via the TAP1/TAP2 heterodimer in an ATP-dependent fashion. Once in the lumen of the ER the peptides may attach to newly synthesized class I-β$_2$-microglobulin molecules which are weakly associated with the TAPs, having been released from calnexin. Trimming of the -NH$_2$ terminus of the peptide may then take place. A conformational change in the class I molecule, charged with peptide, releases it to be transported to the cell surface for antigen presentation to cytotoxic T cells carrying the CD8 surface marker. The pathway is blocked by the antifungal antibiotic brefeldin A which apparently prevents molecules leaving a pre-Golgi compartment so that they return to and are trapped in the ER.

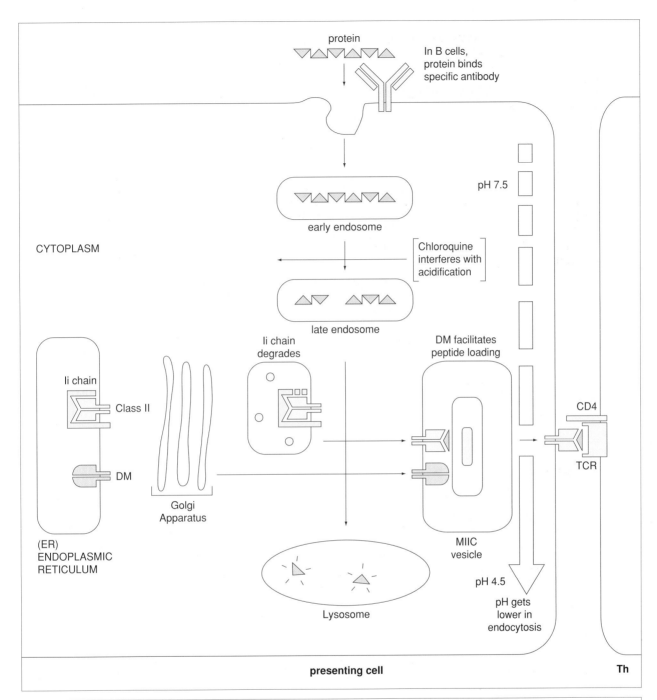

Fig. 7.11 Major proposed route of intracellular trafficking of MHC class II molecules. Most peptides in the lumen of the ER are prevented from binding to class II molecules by the invariant chain. The invariant chain appears to be necessary for chaperoning class II molecules to a post-Golgi vesicle where cleavage of the chain takes place, releasing the class II structure for peptide binding. Most class II-restricted antigenic epitopes enter the APC by endocytosis (either receptor-mediated or fluid phase) into early endosomes. In the case of B cells specific antigens to surface immunoglobulins are captured for presentation in this way. Enzymatic degradation of the endocytosed proteins occurs and at this stage the endocytic pathway is transected by the biosynthetic pathway, so that class II molecules released from invariant chain can bind peptides. The DM molecule is necessary for this process but it is not yet clear how it is involved. The newly formed class II-peptide complexes then move to the cell surface, by an unknown mechanism but most likely involving vesicular fusion with the cell surface. Blocking trafficking of early endosomes within the cell at 18°C and inhibiting endosome acidification with chloroquine both prevent class II restricted presentation via this pathway. In some cells, recycling of class II molecules to and from the cell surface by endocytosis, with exchange of peptide, may be an important pathway.

surface took place. Transport of newly synthesized class II molecules from the trans-Golgi to the cell surface was delayed for 1–3 hours. During this time the newly synthesized class II molecules traffic to an endocytic compartment. Morphological studies have shown that class II molecules pass through a post-Golgi vesicular compartment devoid of class I molecules and morphologically distinct from the Golgi, ER or lysosomes. This compartment has been suggested as a possible site of intersection with the endocytic pathway where association of antigenic peptides and class II molecules could occur. The existence of a class II-containing compartment may explain previous observations of large pools of intracellular class II molecules associated with Ii in both mouse and human B cell lines and would account for the relative insensitivity of class II-restricted presentation to inhibitors of protein synthesis.

Since Ii traffics with class II molecules to endosomes it is important to define a function for this molecule. Two main hypotheses have been invoked. In one, Ii association with class II molecules blocks premature access of peptides to the groove. This could occur either by the Ii chain binding to the groove itself or by making a conformational change in the class II molecule. Cell-free translation experiments support the notion that Ii chain and peptide binding to class II molecules are mutually exclusive. On reaching the endosome the class II-Ii complex can be cleaved by proteases to allow binding of antigenic peptides present in the compartment.

The second hypothesis suggests that Ii acts as a chaperone which binds to class II chains and steers them to the appropriate compartment for association with peptide. There is evidence that Ii chain has both of these functions.

Loading of peptides onto class II molecules takes place in a specialized vesicle within the cell, called the MIIC. These vesicles, which have some of the characteristic markers of late endosomes and some of lysosomes, have multiple membranes, looking like sectioned onions in the electron microscope.

Role of the DM molecule

DM (M in the mouse) is a molecule that has been shown recently to be involved in loading peptide onto class II molecules. DM superficially resembles other class II molecules, in that it consists of an α and a β-chain, both of which are encoded by adjacent genes — *DMA* and *DMB* in humans; *Ma* and duplicated β-chain genes *Mb1* and *Mb2* in mice — within the class II region of the MHC (Chapter 4). Unlike conventional class II genes, DM genes are not highly polymorphic. DM genes are expressed in the same tissues in which other class II molecules are found. Lack of expression of either *DMA* or *DMB* genes leads to a defective protein and B cell lines with interesting phenotypes. In these mutant cells, class II molecules are expressed at the cell surface but have an altered conformation and do not bind certain conformation-specific antibodies. Class II molecules made in these cells are unstable and dissociate into separate α and β-chains upon electrophoresis in SDS. These cells no longer process and present proteins but addition of appropriate class II-binding peptides directly to the cells is effective. Interestingly, peptides extracted

from class II molecules in DM mutant cells are mostly associated with a fragment of the invariant chain, called CLIP (for class II-associated invariant chain peptide).

These findings, plus the fact that DM molecules reside in the MIIC vesicles and do not accumulate on the cell surface, implicate the DM heterodimer in some aspect of peptide loading onto conventional class II.

Role of endocytosis

Support for an endocytic route of antigen entry into presenting cells has come from many studies using specific antibodies to a variety of APC surface molecules such as class I and II molecules themselves, transferrin receptors and B cell mIg. Antigenic epitopes bound to such targeting antibodies and those of the antibody itself, are internalized by receptor-mediated endocytosis which is much more rapid than fluid phase endocytosis and allows efficient processing and presentation to class II-restricted T cells. Since many soluble self antigens can potentially be processed for association with class II molecules it has been argued that elicitation of a strong immune response to foreign antigen *in vivo* requires antigen entry into the APC via a receptor in this manner. These receptors could be specific, as in the case of mIg and receptors for Fc, complement or mannose-containing antigens, or of lower selectivity such as macrophage uptake of non-opsonized aggregated antigenic material. The use of receptor-mediated endocytosis by mIg in APCs seems to be a particularly important mechanism, allowing the cells selectively and efficiently to present their specific antigen to class II-restricted T cells.

One piece of evidence of a role for endosome–lysosome fusion in antigen processing for class II responses is the effect of low temperatures. At 16–18°C endocytosis can occur normally, albeit at a slower rate but fusion of early endosomes with other membrane-bound compartments, such as lysosomes, is completely inhibited, along with other endosome functions. Under these conditions, presentation of antigen which has been taken up by endosomes is blocked, indicating a role for endosome–lysosome fusion in antigen processing and class II-restricted responses.

Variations

In spite of the generalized rules concerning intracellular compartments from which class I and class II molecules draw their peptides, there are situations in which class I is known to handle exogenous antigens and where class II picks up endogenously synthesized proteins that have not come from endosomes.

It is clear that although specialized machinery, namely the LMPs and TAPs, exist to ensure that peptides from cytoplasmic proteins enter the ER, proteins entering the lumen of this compartment independently, namely signal peptides which are cleaved off proteins destined for membranes or for secretion, are dealt with by class I. Certain class I molecules, HLA-A2.1 for example, are ideally suited to binding predominantly hydrophobic signal sequences that are cleaved upon entry into the ER by signal peptidase and HLA-A3 can present an epitope from HIV gp120 in T2 cells. These data suggest that class I loading is not exclusively served by the TAP system and the processing of some transmembrane or secreted proteins by cytosolic proteases renders them suitable substrates for class I binding.

There is scope for further variation in types of antigen handled by unconventional, Ib or 'non-classical', class I molecules. The H-2M3 class I structure, encoded in the *M* region, was initially followed by virtue of its capacity to deal with the mitochondrial antigen which is formylated at the N-terminal methionine. This is a feature of most bacterial proteins and the grooves of M molecules can accommodate the additional formylmethionine group because of the design of the appropriate pocket. M3 is now firmly established as a restriction element for the antigen from *Listeria monocytogenes*. There is some evidence that other class Ib molecules, such as CD1, are not dependent on TAP for surface expression in TAP-/- mice or humans and present lipoglycan antigen to T cells expressing αβ T cell receptors.

Although most class II-restricted T cells appear to recognize exogenous antigens entering the APC by endocytosis it is easy to imagine that some class II molecules could pick up peptide in the ER before the Ii chain has bound. It is also likely that some endogenously synthesized proteins find their way into endosomes. They may be imported into lysosomes directly and there is some evidence that unconventional access to lysosomes is afforded by association with heat shock proteins or by specialized intracellular engulfment mechanisms known as autophagy. Measles virus cytoplasmic antigens, for example, are predominantly recognized in association with class II.

ANTIGEN PRESENTATION TO T CELLS

Expression of peptide–MHC complexes in sufficient amounts at the cell surface may be enough to stimulate many T cell hybridomas and some long term T cell clones. This is clear from the ability of these cells to respond to antigenic peptides bound to purified MHC molecules in artificial lipid bilayers. However, most T cells, particularly resting virgin cells, require one or more additional signals before they can be activated. These co-stimulatory signals may include cytokines such as IL-1 and IL-6 as well as interactions between other cell surface molecules, either for adhesion or for signalling between the T cell and the APC. The nature of the co-stimulatory signals and the requirements of different T cell types is discussed in Chapter 8. In the absence of co-stimulatory signals, partial activation (e.g. upregulation of some surface proteins or cytokine secretion) and/or tolerance may be induced.

Since T cell activation is central to the immune response to most antigens, modulation of APC function must play an important role in immunoregulation. One mode of control is to regulate MHC expression. For example, IFNγ upregulates both class I and class II molecules on many cell types and IL-4 induces increased class II expression by B cells. The importance of MHC expression is clearly seen in some cases of virus-induced tumours (e.g. adeno- and papilloma viruses) where class I MHC expression is downregulated allowing the transformed cells to escape recognition by Tc.

Further details of MHC gene regulation can be found in Chapter 4. Regulating co-stimulatory activity also influences APC function. For example, a number of T cell-derived cytokines can regulate the expression of adhesion molecules on different APC types. Regulation of IL-1 production by APCs, such as macrophages, also plays an important role in these cells ability to stimulate T cell subpopulations requiring this cytokine as a costimulus (see Chapter 8). Direct contact with T cells appears to be necessary for the induction of co-stimulatory activity in some APCs.

ANTIGEN PRESENTING CELL TYPES

Most cells of the body express class I MHC molecules and can therefore serve, in theory, as APCs for class I restricted T cells. In practice it is likely that increased expression of class I molecules, along with the LMP/TAP machinery, under the influence of agents such as IFNγ is necessary to achieve sufficient T cell stimulation. Nevertheless, the widespread expression of class I molecules seems appropriate since it is the role of class I restricted T cells to recognize and destroy virus-infected cells as well as perhaps transformed or otherwise abnormal cells. However, the term APC is normally reserved for a more limited set of cells capable of presenting antigen in association with class II molecules. The major APC types are macrophages, dendritic cells, Langerhans cells and B cells and are sometimes referred to as 'professional' APCs. There is a paucity of information on the relative importance of different APC types *in vivo*. Most likely the role of an APC type depends on the conditions under which the body encounters antigen.

Macrophages

For many years, antigen presentation to T cells was regarded as a function exclusively restricted to cells of the monocyte/macrophage lineage and initial studies of antigen processing events used macrophages as the APC population. Because macrophages are actively phagocytic and possess an armoury of degradative enzymes they are particularly effective in processing and presenting particulate antigens such as bacteria and certain parasites. They play a major role in triggering T cell-mediated immunity to intracellular parasites and facultative anaerobic bacteria, such as various strains of *Mycobacteria*, *Listeria* and *Leishmania* and present antigens derived from the living organisms within them. Marginal zone macrophages are also thought to play a role in the processing and presentation of blood-borne antigenic material. Receptor-mediated internalization of immune complexes, via Fc and complement receptors, can markedly enhance macrophage antigen presentation.

Resting macrophages express relatively low levels of MHC class II molecules but these are markedly increased by cytokines such as IFNγ produced by T cells at sites of immune activation. Activated macrophages secrete a variety of proteases into their local environment which could degrade antigenic material for presentation.

The role of macrophages in inflammation and immunity to pathogens is discussed in Chapters 14 and 16.

B cells

Although non-phagocytic, B cells can internalize antigenic material by constitutive pinocytosis or receptor-mediated endocytosis. Using these pathways both normal and transformed B cells can process and present antigen to T cells in a non-specific manner. B cell lines have the advantage in experimental systems that they can be grown to large numbers *in vitro*.

Because B cells carry antigen-specific mIg molecules on their surface they can efficiently and specifically endocytose and process appropriate antigen. Experimentally, this allows B cells to present their specific antigen at concentrations up to 1000-fold lower than required for presentation by macrophages and dendritic cells. In effect, B cells only act as APCs for their specific antigen, idiotopes of their specific mIg or other antigens which bind to B cell surface molecules. A number of experiments have shown that the epitope specificity of mIg can influence the subsequent processing of antigen. For example, tetanus toxoid-specific EBV-transformed human B cells recognizing particular epitopes within the tetanus toxoid molecule generate epitope-dependent antigen fragments, implying a direct influence of the mIg receptor on processing. The implication here is that the specificity of the mIg in a particular B cell can influence peptides associating with class II molecules.

Processed fragments of mIg can also become associated with class II molecules in B cells. For example, the murine B lymphoma line A20 can present an idiotype of its mIg to specific T cells. Since antigen presentation by specific B cells forms the basis of cognate helper interactions between T and B cells, the specificity repertoires of the two cell types can clearly influence one another.

The outcome of antigen presentation by normal B cells appears to depend on their state of activation. Resting B cells can process and present antigen in a form that can interact with the specific T cell receptor but in most cases this does not seem sufficient to activate the T cell for cytokine secretion and proliferation. Resting B cells may not be able to supply appropriate co-stimulatory signals required by most T cells (see Chapter 8).

Langerhans cells and dendritic cells

Lymphoid dendritic cells (DCs) are non-phagocytic, bone marrow-derived cells thought to belong to a different lineage from macrophages. They are characterized by their irregular shape, constitutive expression of MHC class I and II molecules at high levels and paucity of endocytic vesicles and lysosomes. DCs are found as interdigitating cells in the T cell areas of secondary lymphoid tissues and in the thymic medulla and as veiled cells in afferent lymphatics.

A number of studies have indicated that DCs may be the major APC type involved in triggering primary T cell responses as well as secondary responses of resting memory T cells. According to this hypothesis, macrophages and B cells only act as APCs for sensitized T cells recently activated by DCs. Much of the evidence for this central role for DCs has come from *in vitro* studies of primary alloreactive and syngeneic mixed lymphocyte reactions, which involve T cell recognition of class II molecules already bearing peptide. DCs appear to be essential for these proliferative responses of resting T cells; the ability to stimulate primary responses appears to be due to their constitutive expression of a co-stimulatory factor which is not IL-1.

DCs are poorly endocytic so how can they process antigen for presentation? One suggestion is that processing is carried out by ectoproteases on the DC plasma membrane. However, DCs in peripheral lymph nodes are derived from Langerhans cells (LCs), class II-bearing bone marrow-derived cells in the epidermis of the skin. These cells, which contain cytoplasmic racket-shaped granules of unknown function known as Birbeck granules, endocytose antigenic material and process it for presentation to T cells. LCs bearing antigen also migrate from the epidermis, via the afferent lymph — where they have been called 'veiled' cells because of their distinctive appearance — to draining lymph nodes, where they form the interdigitating DCs in the paracortex and present antigen to T cells trafficking through the node (see Chapter 14). Freshly isolated LCs differ from lymphoid DCs: they process intact antigen for presentation to previously sensitized T cells or T cell hybridomas very efficiently but have a relatively low level of class II expression and little capacity to stimulate primary responses in resting T cells. However, during *in vitro* culture LCs rapidly upregulate their class II expression and co-stimulatory activity, whilst losing their ability to process antigens; these features are typical of DCs. Thus LCs in the skin may serve two functions:

- They can process antigen for local presentation to sensitized T cells at sites of immune inflammation.
- They can migrate, bearing processed antigen, to draining lymph nodes whilst differentiating into potent immuno-stimulatory DCs necessary for initiating primary responses.

Other APC types

A wide variety of cell types have some antigen-presenting ability provided they express, or can be induced to express, class II molecules. The response of T cells to the recognition of peptide–class II complexes on these cells depends on their activation requirements. For example, Kupffer cells of the liver, astrocytes in the brain, endothelial cells, articular chondrocytes and thyroid epithelial cells may be unable to present antigen to and activate resting T cells but may trigger previously activated cells.

For some cells induced to express class II molecules (with IFNγ, for example) inability to provide the appropriate co-stimulatory signals may lead to the induction of unresponsiveness rather than activation (see Chapter 8). Some investigators have speculated that this is primarily a protective measure to prevent destruction of host tissues rendered temporarily class II positive in response to the production of cytokines by T cells activated locally by 'professional' APCs. In some species including humans, guinea-pigs and rats, activated T cells express class II molecules and are able to present pre-processed antigen to other T cells; with human T cells this results in tolerance in the responding population, presumably because class II positive T cells lack the co-stimulatory signals required for full activation.

Thymic epithelial cells

Thymic epithelial cells appear to play a specialized APC role during T cell development in the thymus. Recognition of MHC-self-peptide complexes expressed by these cells is thought to be critical for the positive selection of immature thymocytes which are self-restricted. Details of the role of thymic epithelial cells in the development of T cells and T cell tolerance can be found in Chapters 6 and 12.

Follicular dendritic cells

During secondary immune responses and late in the primary response once antibody has formed, antigen-containing immune complexes localize in lymphoid follicles initiating the development of germinal centres, where acceleration and affinity maturation of the antibody responses and memory B cell development take place (see Chapter 9). Immune complexes, often transported to lymph nodes or splenic germinal centres by cells such as veiled cells, become trapped on the dendritic processes of follicular dendritic cells (FDCs), forming an antigen-retaining reticulum. FDCs have multiple dendritic processes connected to a cell body with little cytoplasm surrounding a nucleus, which is commonly bilobed with a prominent nucleolus. They posses little rough ER, Golgi or vesicles and few mitochondria. The dendritic processes which form the functional part of the cell may be short, pleomorphic structures as well as the more characteristic highly convoluted, extensive projections which interdigitate with neighbouring FDCs. They develop from a filiform appearance to more mature beaded structures, both of which bind immune complexes primarily through complement and Fc receptors, often with a spiralling periodicity of about 440–490Å. *In situ* FDCs often appear to express MHC class II antigens but recent studies indicate that these are molecules that have been released by B cells in germinal centres, perhaps from those cells dying as a result of the process of affinity maturation (see Chapter 9).

Within 1–3 days of a secondary antigenic challenge, the interaction of beaded FDC dendrites with immune complexes leads to spherical particles of 0.3–0.4µm diameter breaking off the beaded dendrite; these persist for only a few hours during the early development of the germinal centre. The production of these 'immune complex coated bodies' or iccosomes depends on the level of circulating antibody and the dose of antigen administered. Iccosomes are thought to attach to germinal centre B cells via their immune complexes to be endocytosed, allowing the B cell to process antigens trapped in the immune complexes for presentation to T cells (*Fig. 7.12*). Immune complex material accumulates in germinal centre B cells following the disappearance of iccosomes. When germinal centre B cells, isolated on the basis of binding to the lectin peanut agglutinin (PNA), were examined at different times, after secondary antigenic challenge, their ability to stimulate T cells was most prominent at approximately the same time as most B cell uptake of immune complexes was observed. Thus, FDCs appear to trap antigen in the form of an immune complex and then pass it on to B cells in a state that can be readily endocytosed for processing and presentation. *In vitro* studies have indicated that this uptake

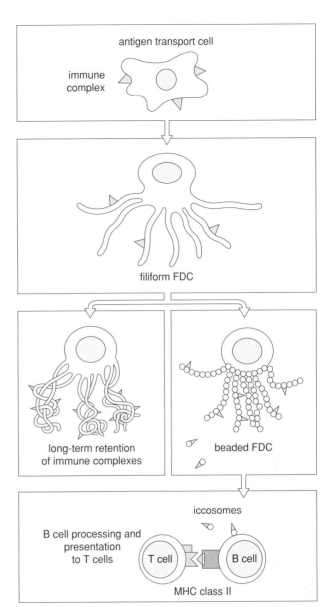

Fig. 7.12 Hypothesis for the handling of immune complexes by follicular dendritic cells. During secondary responses, antigen rapidly forms immune complexes with existing antibody. Most are rapidly cleared from the body but a small proportion are transported to follicular germinal centres, either as free complexes or on the surface of cells in the blood or lymph, where they bind to follicular dendritic cells (FDCs). Immune complexes bind to the many dendritic processes of FDCs, which can assume a beaded appearance. Within 1–3 days of immune complex formation, some immune complex-bearing bead structures (iccosomes) break off and are endocytosed by germinal centre B cells. Processing of the internalized antigenic components of the immune complexes enables these B cells to present antigen to specific T cells. Immune complexes can also be retained for long periods of time on the tightly convoluted filiform dendrites of other FDCs. Based on the observations of Szakal *et al*, 1988 and 1989.

is restricted to antigen-specific B cells, involving mIg, rather than Fc receptor- or complement receptor-mediated uptake by non-specific B cells. Tingible body macrophages containing the debris of dead lymphocytes also endocytose iccosomes but it is not known if these cells are capable of antigen processing and presentation.

Immune complexes also persist on the dendrites of FDCs for many months, if not years. This reservoir of antigenic material probably accounts for the maintenance of the secondary antibody response. It has also been suggested that antigen trapped on FDCs is critical for the maintenance of memory cells (Chapter 9).

SUMMARY

T cells recognize processed forms of antigen that can bind to the peptide binding groove of MHC class I and class II molecules. In most cases, the formation of immunogenic peptides involves intracellular degradation by proteolytic enzymes. The site of these processing events and the association of peptide with MHC molecules usually differ for class I- and class II-restricted epitopes.

Class I-restricted epitopes are derived from proteins synthesized in the cytoplasm. These proteins are then degraded, in the cytoplasm, by the proteasome and transported into the endoplasmic reticulum (ER). The binding of peptides to newly synthesized class I molecules appears to be essential for them to adopt the correct conformation for stable expression at the cell surface. Because of this, most surface class I molecules contain a peptide derived from cellular proteins.

Although some cytoplasmic viral antigens can also use this route for association with newly synthesized class II molecules, most peptides are prevented from binding to class II structures in the ER because of the association of these MHC molecules with the invariant chain (Ii). This Ii-class II association persists while the complex traffics from the ER, through the Golgi complex to a specialized vesicle, the MIIC. These Ii-class II complexes then intersect the route of traffic of antigen-containing endocytic vesicles. The Ii chain is then proteolytically removed, allowing antigenic peptides to bind before transport of the loaded class II molecule to the cell surface. Most class II restricted epitopes are derived from endocytosed antigens. In certain cell types, particularly B cells, antigens may be bound by surface receptors such as mIg and internalized to supply antigenic peptides for class II molecules.

Most T cells require signals in addition to MHC-bound peptide before they can be fully activated. Such co-stimuli include soluble molecules delivered by the APC, or signals derived from interactions with adhesion molecules. APCs differ in their ability to provide these co-stimuli as well as in their ability to process antigen. Macrophages are actively phagocytic and play an important role in processing bacterial antigens and immune complexes, while B cells can selectively process and present their specific antigen. Both of these cell types may present antigen primarily to previously sensitized T cells. However, dendritic cells appear to express co-stimulatory activity required for the activation of resting T cells. Dendritic cells are inefficient at processing antigens but seem to be derived from precursors such as Langerhans cells of the skin which can process antigen and which migrate and differentiate, with their processed antigen, to form potent immuno-stimulatory dendritic cells within secondary lymphoid tissues.

The relative importance of different APCs *in vivo* probably depends both on the nature of the antigen and its site of entry into the body. In secondary responses, highly differentiated follicular dendritic cells trap immune complexes and appear to pass them on to germinal centre B cells for processing and presentation to T cells.

FURTHER READING

Adorini L, Nagy ZA. Peptide competition for antigen presentation. *Immunol Today* 1990, **11**:21.

Androlewicz MJ, Anderson KS, Cresswell P. Evidence that transporters associated with antigen processing translocate a major histocompatibility complex class I-binding peptide into the endoplasmic reticulum in an ATP-dependent manner. *Proc Natl Acad Sci USA* 1993, **90**:9130.

Androlewicz MJ, Cresswell P. Human transporters associated with antigen processing possess a promiscuous peptide-binding site. *Immunity* 1994, **1**:7.

Austyn JM. *Antigen Presenting cells in focus.* Male D (Ed). IRL Press: Oxford; 1989.

Babbitt BP, Allen PM, Matsueda G, Haber E, Unanué ER. Binding of immunogenic peptides to Ia histocompatibility molecules. *Nature* 1985, **317**:359.

Bakke O, Dobberstein B. MHC class II-associated invariant chain contains a sorting signal for endosomal compartments. *Cell* 1990, **63**:707.

Belich M, Glynne RJ, Senger G, Sheer D, Trowsdale J. Proteasome components with reciprocal expression to that of the MHC-encoded LMP proteins. *Curr Biol* 1994, **4**:769.

Bhadwaj N, Lau LL, Friedman SM, Crow MK, Steinman RM. Interleukin 1 production during accessory cell-dependent mitogenesis of T lymphocytes. *J Exp Med* 1989, **169**:1121.

Bijlmakers MJ, Benaroch P, Ploegh HL. Assembly of HLA-DR1 molecules translated *in vitro*: binding of peptide in the endoplasmic reticulum precludes association with invariant chain. *EMBO J* 1994, **13**:2699.

Braciale TJ, Braciale VL. Antigen presentation: structural themes and functional variations. *Immunol Today* 1991, **12**:124.

Büüs S, Wederlin O. A group-specific inhibitor of lysosomal cysteine proteinases selectively inhibits both proteolytic degradation and presentation of the antigen dinitrophenol-poly-L-lysine by guinea-pig accessory cells to T cells. *J Immunol* 1986, **136**:452.

Carbone FR, Bevan MJ. Class I-restricted processing and presentation of exogenous cell-associated antigen in vivo. *J Exp Med* 1990, **171**:377.

Cresswell P. Assembly, transport and function of MHC class II moloecules. *Ann Rev Immunol* 1994, **12**:259.

Davidson HW, Watts C. Epitope-directed processing of specific antigen by B lymphocytes. *J Cell Biol* 1989, **109**:85.

Demotz S, Grey HM, Appella E, Sette A. Characterization of a naturally processed MHC class II-restricted T cell determinant of hen egg lysozyme. *Nature* 1989, **342**:682.

Elliott T. How do peptides associate with MHC class I molecules? *ImmunolToday* 1991, **12**:386.

Elliott T, Cerundolo V, Elvin J, Townsend A. Peptide-induced conformational change of the class I heavy chain. *Nature* 1991, **351**:402.

Elliott T, Smith M, Driscoll P, McMichael A. Peptide selection by class I molecules of the major histocompatibility complex. *Curr Biol* 1993, **3**:854.

Falk K, Rotzschke O, Stevanovic S, Jung G, Rammensee H. Allele-specific motifs revealed by sequencing of self-peptides eluted from MHC molecules. *Nature* 1991, **351**:290.

Gell PG, Benacerraf B. Studies on hypersensitivity. II. Delayed hypersensitivity to denatured proteins in guinea pigs. *Immunol* 1959, **2**:64.

Germain RN. MHC-dependent antigen processing and peptide presentation: providing ligands for T lymphocyte activation. *Cell* 1994, **76**:287.

Germain RN, Hendrix LR. MHC class II structure, occupancy and surface expression determined by post-endoplasmic reticulum antigen binding. *Nature* 1991, **353**:134.

Goldberg AL, Rock KL. Proteolysis, proteasomes and antigen presentation. *Nature* 1992, **357**:375.

Guagliardi LE. Koppelman B, Blum JS, Marks MS. Cresswell P, Brodsky FM. Co-localization of molecules involved in antigen processing and presentation in an early endocytic compartment. *Nature* 1990, **343**:133.

Guidos C, Wong M, Lee K-C. A comparison of the stimulatory activities of lymphoid dendritic cells and macrophages in T proliferative responses to various antigens. *J Immunol* 1984, **33**:1179.

Hammer J, Takacs B, Sinigaglia F. Identification of a motif for HLA-DR1 binding peptides using M13 display libraries. *J Exp Med* 1992, **176**:1007.

Harding C. Phagocytic processing of antigens for presentation by MHC molecules. *Trends Cell Biol* 1995, **5**:105.

Harding CV, Unanué ER. Low-temperature inhibition of antigen processing and iron uptake from transferrin: deficits in endosome functions at 18°C. *Eur J Immunol* 1990, **20**:323.

Heemels MT, Schumacher TNM, Wonigeit K, Ploegh HL. Peptide translocation by variants of the transporter associated with antigen processing. *Science* 1993, **262**:2059.

Howard JC, Seelig A. Peptides and the proteasome. *Nature* 1993, **365**:211

Hyde SC, EmsleyP, Hartshorn MJ, Mimmick MM, Gileadi U, Pearce SR, Gallagher MP, Gill DR, Hubbard RE, Higgin CF. Structural model of ATP-binding protein associated with cystic fibrosis, multidrug resistance and bacterial transport. *Nature* 1990, **346**:362.

Lanzavecchia A. Receptor-mediated antigen uptake and its effect on antigen presentation to class II-restricted T lymphocytes. *Ann Rev Immunol* 1990, **8**:773.

Long EO. Intracellular traffic and antigen processing. *Immunol Today* 1989, **10**:232

Lotteau V, Teyton L, Peleraux A, Nilsson T, Karlsson L, Schmid SL, Quranta V, Peterson PA. Intracellular transport of class II MHC molecules directed by invariant chain. *Nature* 1990, **348**:600.

Mellins E, Smith L, Arp B, Cotner T, Celis E, Pious D. Defective processing and presentation of exogenous antigens in mutants with normal HLA class II genes. *Nature* 1990, **343**:71.

Metlay JP. Pure E, Steinman RM. Control of the immun response at the level of antigen-presenting cells: a comparison of the function of dendritic cells and B lymphocytes. *Adv Immunol* 1989, **47**:45.

Michalek MT, Grant EP, Gramm C, Goldberg AL, Rock KL. A role for the ubiquitin-dependent proteolytic pathway in MHC class I-restricted antigen presentation. *Nature* 1993, **363**:552.

Momburg F, Roelse J, Howard JC. Butcher GW, Hammerling GJ, Neefjes JJ. Selectivity of MHC-encoded peptide transporters from human, mouse and rat. *Nature* 1994, **367**:648.

Monaco JJ. A molecular model of MHC class I -restricted antigen processing. *Immunol Today* 1992, **13**:173.

Morrison LA, Lukacher AE, Braciale BL, Fan DP, Braciale TJ. Differences in antigen presentation to MHC class I- and class II-restricted influenza virus-specific cytolytic T lymphocyte clones. *J Exp Med* 1986, **163**:903.

Neefjes JJ, Momberg F. Cell biology of antigen presentation. *Curr Opin Immunol* 1993, **5**:27.

Neefjes JJ, Momburg F, Hammerling GJ. Selective and ATP-dependent translocation of peptides by the MHC-encoded transporter. *Science* 1993, **261**:769.

Neefjes JJ, Stollorz V, Peters PJ, Geuze HJ, Ploegh HL. The biosynthetic pathway of MHC class II but not class I molecules intersects the endocytic route. *Cell* 1990, **61**:171.

Nuchtern JG, Biddison WE, Klausner RD. Class II MHC molecules can use the endogenous pathway of antigen presentation. *Nature* 1990, **343**:74.

Nuchtern JG, Bonifacino JS, Biddison WE, Klausner RD. Brefeldin A implicates egress from endoplasmic reticulum in class I restricted antigen presentation. *Nature* 1989, **339**:223.

Ortmann B, Androlewicz MJ, Cresswell P. MHC class I/β_2-microglobulin complexes associate before peptide binding. *Nature* 1994, **368**:864.

Parham P. Antigen processing. Transporters of delight. *Nature* 1990, **348**:674.

Peters JM. Proteasomes: protein degradation machines of the cell. *Trends Biol Sci* 1994, **19**:377.

Pierce SK, Morris JF, Grusby MJ, Kaumaya P, van Buskirk A, Srinivasan M, Crumpt B, Smolenski LA. Antigen presenting function of B lymphocytes. *Immunol Rev* 1988, **106**:149.

Ramensee HG, Monaco J. Antigen recognition. *Curr Opin Immunol* 1994, **6**:1.

Ramensee HG, Hammerling GJ, Eds. *MHC molecules and peptides. Structure and function.* Die Medizinische Verlagsgesellschaft mbH: Marburg; 1994.

Roche PA, Cresswell P. Invariant chain association with DR molecules inhibits immunogenic peptide binding. *Nature* 1990, **345**:615.

Rosenthal AS, Shevach EM. Function of macrophages in antigen recognition by guinea pig T lymphocytes. I. Requirement for histocompatible macrophages and lymphocytes. *J Exp Med* 1973, **138**:1194.

Rotzschke G. Origin, structure and motifs of naturally processed MHC class II ligands. *Curr Opin Immunol* 1994, **6**:45.

Sadegh-Nasseri S, Germain RN. How MHC class II molecules work: peptide-dependent completion of protein folding. *Immunol Today* 1992, **13**:43.

Schmid SL, Jackson MR. Making class II presentable. *Nature* 1994, **369**:103.

Schwartz AL. Cell biology of intracellular protein trafficking. *Ann Rev Immunol* 1990, **8**:195.

Schwartz RH, Fox BS, Fraga E, Chen C, Singh B. The T lymphocyte response to cytochrome c. V. Determination of the minimal peptide size required for stimulation of T cell clones and assessment of the contribution of each residue beyond this size to antigenic potency. *J Immunol* 1985, **135**:2598.

Schumacher TNM, Kantesarian DV, Heemels MT, Ashton-Rickardt PG, Shepherd JC Fruh K, Yang Y, Peterson PA, Tonegawa S, Ploegh HL. Peptide length and sequence specificity of the mouse TAP1/TAP2 translocator. *J Exp Med* 1994, **179**:533.

Shepherd JC, Schumacher TNM, Ashton-Rickardt PG, Imaeda S, Ploegh HL, Janeway CA, Tonegawa S. TAP1-dependent peptide translocation *in vitro* is ATP dependent and peptide selective. *Cell* 1993, **74**:577.

Shimonkevitz R, Kappler JW, Marrack P, Grey HM. Antigen recognition by H-2 restricted T cells. I. Cell-free antigen processing. *J Exp Med* 1983, **158**:303.

Sprent J, Schaefer M. Antigen presenting cells for unprimed T cells. *Immunol Today* 1989, **10**:17.

Streilen JW, Crammer SF. *In vitro* evidence that Langerhans cells can adopt two functionally distinct forms capable of antigen presentation to T lymphocytes. *J Immunol* 1989, **143**:3925.

Sweetser MT. Morrison LA, Braciale VL, Braciale TJ. Recognition of pre-processed endogenous antigen by class I but not class II MHC-restricted T cells. *Nature* 1989, **342**:180.

Szakal AK, Kosco MH, Tew JG. A novel *in vivo* follicular dendritic cell-dependent iccosome-mediated mechanism for delivery of antigen to antigen-processing cells. *J Immunol* 1988, **140**:341.

Szakal AK, Kosco MH, Tew JG. Microanatomy of lymphoid tissue during humoral immune responses: structure function relationships. *Ann Rev Immunol* 1989, **7**:91.

Takada Y, Strominger JL, Hemler ME. The very late antigen family of heterodimers is part of a superfamily of molecules involved in adhesion and embryogenesis. *Proc Natl Acad Sci USA* 1987, **84**:3239.

Townsend A, Bastin J, Gould K, Brownlee G, Andrew M, Coupar B, Boyle D, Chan S, Smith G. Defective presentation to class I-restricted cytotoxic T lymphocytes in vaccinia-infected cells is overcome by enhanced degradation of antigen. *J Exp Med* 1988, **168**:1211.

Townsend A, Bodmer H. Antigen recognition by class I-restricted T lymphocytes. *Ann Rev Immunol* 1989, **7**:601.

Townsend A, Ohlen C, Bastin J, Ljunggren HG, Foster L, Karre K. Association of class I major histocompatibility heavy and light chains induced by viral peptides. *Nature* 1989, **340**:443.

Townsend A, Trowsdale J. The transporters associated with antigen processing. *Sem Cell Biology* 1993, **4**:53.

Tulp A, Verwoerd D, Dobberstein B, Ploegh HL, Pieters J. Isolation and characterization of the intracellular MHC class II compartment. *Nature* 1994, **369**:120.

Yewdell JW, Bennink JR. The binary logic of antigen processing and presentation to T cells. *Cell* 1990, **62**:203.

Ziegler K, Unanué ER. Identification of a macrophage antigen-processing event required for I region-restricted antigen presentation to T lymphocytes. *J Immunol* 1981, **127**:1869.

8 T Lymphocyte Activation and Maturation

As with many cells of the body, T and B lymphocytes exist for most of their life span in a quiescent or G0 state with respect to the cell cycle (*Fig. 8.1*). In order to proliferate, such cells must re-enter the G1 phase where a variety of proteins are synthesized in preparation for DNA synthesis (S phase). The subsequent G2 and M phases proceed to produce two daughter cells. Depending on the cell type, different growth factors and other environmental triggers are required for cell cycle progression. T and B cells have similar requirements but before these cells can respond specifically to their antigen they must be triggered through their clonally restricted T cell receptor (TCR) or surface membrane immunoglobulin (mIg) molecules. These cells can also be triggered in a polyclonal, non-antigen-specific manner by a range of mitogenic agents, both experimentally and, in some cases, physiologically.

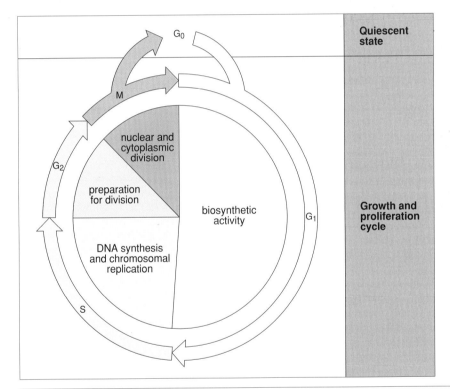

Fig. 8.1 The cell cycle. The four phases of a typical eukaryotic cell cycle are illustrated. During the G1 (gap 1) phase, a high rate of biosynthetic activity takes place allowing the cell to grow in size and prepare for DNA synthesis and the subsequent division of the cell. In the S phase, DNA synthesis and replication of each chromosome occur, producing two identical sister chromatids. A second gap (G2) allows the final cytoplasmic reorganizations required for cellular division to occur. The M (Mitotic) phase then involves chromosomal condensation, breakdown of the nuclear membrane, separation of the sister chromatids, generation of two new nuclei and finally division of the cytoplasm to form two daughter cells. In continuously dividing cell populations, the cell progeny then immediately enter G1 to begin the cycle again. However, many cells in the body enter a quiescent period, called G0, which commonly represents terminal differentiation of the cell. Deprivation of essential growth factors can also force a cell into G0. Resting T and B cells could be viewed as special examples of such growth factor deprived cells. They exist in G0 until they receive appropriate activation signals, allowing them to mediate their effector functions and to re-enter G1. In the presence of suitable growth factors such as interleukins, which the cells may produce themselves, activated cells then complete one or more rounds of cell division before returning to the G0 state to await further activation stimuli. A typical lymphocyte cell cycle may take 12–16 hours to complete, with several additional hours initially required to take the cell from G0 to G1.

The proliferation of T and B cells in response to antigen serves to expand the specifically activated clones of cells ready for a rapid and efficient response to subsequent antigen challenge. But triggering of T and B cells must also elicit various effector mechanisms to combat the antigenic threat. These include killing of virally infected cells, provision of activation, growth and differentiation signals to other cell types and production of antibodies. In some cases, the cell will also differentiate to generate memory cells. These different responses can be triggered independently of one another, although during a normal immune response they will all take place.

In this chapter, the intracellular and membrane events responsible for transmitting activation signals to post-thymic T cells and the consequences for the generation of effector cells will be considered. Although many of the biochemical and genetic events involved in mediating and regulating lymphocyte activation have been elucidated, it is often difficult to distinguish the signals involved in eliciting proliferation from those mediating effector mechanisms or differentiation; some signals are clearly critical to all these processes.

Many of the proliferative pathways are similar to those found in the growth factor-mediated responses of most mammalian cells. These include changes in the concentration of intracellular free Ca^{2+} ($[Ca^{2+}]_i$), pH, protein phosphorylation, gene transcription, mRNA processing and protein synthesis. Cell type- or subset-specific membrane proteins, cytoplasmic enzymes and genes also play a critical role in determining the outcome of the response.

T CELL ACTIVATION

Cell–cell contact

The activation of T cells during an immune response requires contact with APCs or target cells. The affinity of TCR–MHC interactions (K_d = $1-5\times10^{-5}$M) is low when compared with antibody–antigen interactions (K_d = $10^{-11}-10^{-7}$M). Therefore, the initial contact is mediated by adhesive interactions between different accessory molecules. The ability of antibodies to block adhesion has implicated both CD2 and Leukocyte Functional Antigen 1 (LFA-1) as major T cell surface molecules involved in T cell antigen recognition. The ligand for CD2 on the antigen presenting cell has been identified as CD58, also called LFA-3, in humans and CD48 in rodents. The interaction between CD2 and CD48 has been extensively studied as a paradigm for understanding the structural basis of cell adhesion. The crystal structures of the extracellular regions of rat and human CD2 have been solved and have revealed that CD2 contains two Ig domains. Both CD48 and CD58 (LFA-3) are structurally related to CD2 and have been modelled on the basis that they fold into an Ig domain. The CD2 binding site on rat CD48 has been mapped and the affinity of the soluble CD2–CD48 interaction has been measured (K_d = 60–90µm). From these studies, a picture has emerged of an interaction that is of a similar dimension to that of the TCR–MHC complex. These observations are consistent with a model in which the CD2–CD48 interaction and similar interactions with other adhesion molecules

may position the surface membranes of the T cell and antigen presenting cell at the optimal distance for the low affinity interaction between the TCR and MHC class I or class II molecule. A model of these interactions is shown in the of *Colour figures*.

Another major adhesive interaction involves LFA-1 binding to Intercellular Adhesion Molecules 1 and 2 (ICAM-1 and ICAM-2) and perhaps other, as yet unidentified, ligands. Unlike CD2–LFA-3, this interaction may be bidirectional in that both LFA-1 and ICAM-1 can be expressed by T cells as well as by some APCs. These same adhesive interactions are also important in the trafficking of lymphocytes into and through different tissues (see Chapter 14). Studies with Tc cells have shown that the initial adhesive interaction is Ca^{2+}-independent but requires Mg^{2+}. This may reflect the importance of LFA-1–ligand interactions, since this adhesion pathway has been shown to be Mg^{2+}- and temperature-dependent, whereas CD2–CD58 interactions are not.

CD4 and CD8 also promote adhesion by binding to non-polymorphic sites on MHC class II and I molecules, respectively. However, since the binding is relatively weak compared with CD2- and LFA-1-mediated associations, these interactions probably play only a minor role in intercellular adhesion. As will be discussed later, the interactions between CD4 or CD8 and MHC molecules are more important in mediating activation signals to the T cell.

In the absence of the correct Ag–MHC ligand, non-specific interactions dissociate after a short period of time, allowing the cells to part. If, however, sufficient TCRs become engaged with their specific ligand, signals are initiated which lead to activation of the T cell, with associated relocalization of some surface molecules to the region of contact between the two cells. This serves to enhance the adhesion between the cells and plays a critical role in both qualitative and quantitative aspects of signal delivery. For example, following activation, CD4 or CD8 co-localizes with the TCR at the cell-cell junction. Even in the presence of subactivating levels of specific antigen, LFA-1 molecules can redistribute into the zone of contact. This movement requires engagement of the TCR and is dependent upon Ca^{2+}. If the signal is sufficient to lead to activation of the T cell, LFA-1 associates with cytoskeletal components, such as talin, which also redistribute into the zone of contact between the cells. This association between LFA-1 and the cytoskeleton may serve to stabilize the cell-cell contacts. Recent studies have also indicated that TCR-mediated signalling leads to a rapid but transient increase in avidity of LFA-1 for its ICAM ligands. This may serve as an antigen-driven adhesion amplification pathway which stabilizes the interaction between a T cell and its APC or target, thus increasing the sensitivity of the T cell to low levels of Ag–MHC ligands.

Antigen-dependent activation pathways

Interaction of the specific receptor of a T cell with its Ag–MHC ligands results in a complex series of developmental events culminating in triggering of both the effector functions of the cell (for example, target cell killing or help for B cell responses) and the proliferation required to

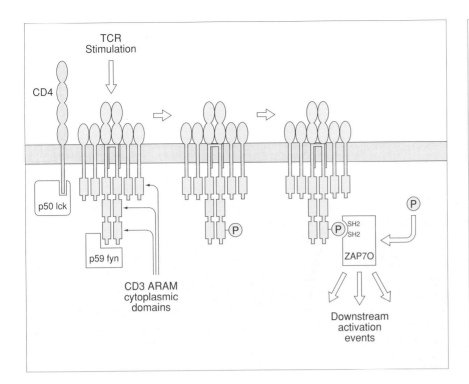

Fig. 8.2 Early signalling events in T cell activation. TCR aggregation as a result of stimulation induces phosphorylation of tyrosine residues within ARAM motifs in the CD3 cytoplasmic domains (step A). One phosphorylation event is shown, although more than one ARAM motif is likely to be phosphorylated *in vivo*. Src-family PTKs carry on this phosphorylation, either by direct interaction with the aggregated TCR complex or through co-receptor recruitment into the complex. Additional PTKs, most probably ZAP-70, bind via SH2 domains to the phosphorylated ARAM motifs (step B) and are subsequently activated by additional phosphorylation events.

expand the pool of cells capable of recognizing the antigen. A threshold number of receptors that has been estimated to be between 20–200 per cell must be occupied in order to elicit activation. This probably reflects the need for receptors to be brought into close proximity with one another. The threshold number is readily achieved at the surface of the APC and can also be mimicked experimentally by polymeric forms of anti-receptor or anti-CD3 antibodies.

Subsequent to ligand binding, signal transduction is mediated by the invariant CD3 chains of the CD3 complex. Thus, the crosslinking of chimaeric receptors in which the cytoplasmic domains of CD3ζ or ε were fused to the transmembrane and extracellular domains of other proteins initiated a series of signal transduction events that recapitulated those observed with the intact TCR complex. The CD3 cytoplasmic domains each contain a motif called an Antigen Recognition Activation Motif (ARAM) or Tyrosine-based Activation Motif (TAM). This motif, which is shared with the Igα and Igβ chains of the B cell receptor, consists of a consensus sequence (D/E)XXYXXL(X)6–8YXXL. Various studies have shown that the ARAM sequence is sufficient to couple chimaeric receptors to the T cell activation pathway. However, since one ARAM sequence is apparently sufficient to initiate the signal transduction cascade, the reason for the presence of multiple ARAMs within the TCR complex is unclear. One possibility is that they fulfil an amplification function, thus lowering the threshold of antigen to which T cells respond.

TCR-mediated phosphorylation events

TCR-mediated activation results in the induction of phosphorylation of a number of proteins, both membrane-associated and cytoplasmic. A particularly important type of

phosphorylation occurs on tyrosine residues and the ARAMs are both necessary and sufficient for the induction of tyrosine phosphorylation in T cells. Since the TCR is not a member of the class of receptors that has intrinsic protein tyrosine kinase (PTK) activity, it is likely that ARAMs associate directly with PTKs and this contention has been shown experimentally by the co-immunoprecipitation of PTK activity with antibodies to the TCR.

Two classes of cytoplasmic PTKs have been implicated in TCR function. The Src-family kinases are thought to phosphorylate the tyrosine residues within the CD3 ARAM motifs after TCR stimulation. Two members of this family, p56[lck] and p59[fyn], have been implicated in this process. p56[lck] is probably recruited into the TCR complex via its association with the cytoplasmic tails of CD4 and CD8, whereas p59[fyn] has been shown to interact directly with the antigen receptor. Thereafter, the tyrosine-phosphorylated ARAMs can recruit additional effector molecules by serving as interaction sites for the ZAP-70 kinase which contains a specialized binding domain (SH2) for phosphotyrosine residues. ZAP-70 when localized within the aggregated TCR complex would elicit subsequent biochemical responses. This model, which is depicted in *Figure 8.2*, is consistent with a number of experimental observations. For example, T cells from immunodeficient patients lacking functional ZAP-70 protein failed to proliferate following stimulation, despite both p56[lck] and p59[lck] being present in normal amounts.

Signalling role of CD4 and CD8

Antibodies to CD4 or CD8 (subsequently represented as CD4/8) can block the activation of T cells by both Ag–MHC and non-specific triggers such as mitogens or anti-receptor antibodies. This blocking effect on non-specific

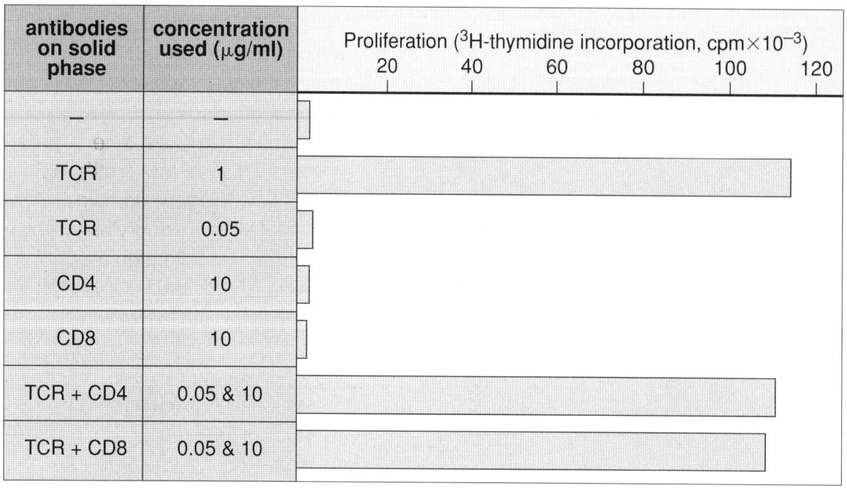

antibodies on solid phase	concentration used (μg/ml)	Proliferation (^{3}H-thymidine incorporation, cpm$\times 10^{-3}$)
—	—	
TCR	1	
TCR	0.05	
CD4	10	
CD8	10	
TCR + CD4	0.05 & 10	
TCR + CD8	0.05 & 10	

Fig. 8.3 Enhancement of TCR-mediated T cell activation through association with CD4 and CD8. Resting murine T cells were cultured with different solid phase antibodies capable of crosslinking and thus enforcing association between cell surface molecules. IL-2 was also added to enhance the proliferative response, measured by ^{3}H-thymidine incorporation after 4 days. Maximal responses could be obtained with 1μg/ml antibody to the TCR, but CD4 and CD8 antibodies at concentrations as high as 10μg/ml were non-stimulatory. However, when coupled to the same phase as a non-stimulatory dose of TCR antibody (0.05μg/ml) CD4 and CD8 antibodies could elicit maximal responses. Similar results have also been obtained through the use of heteroconjugates of such antibodies which are active in a soluble form.

signals not involving CD4/8–MHC interactions suggests that these molecules have a signalling role. Studies with antibodies coated on the same solid phase showed that bringing CD4/8 into close proximity with the TCR leads to a marked enhancement of the response (*Fig. 8.3*). Binding of CD4/8 to the same Ag–MHC complex recognized by the TCR has the same effect and leads to a co-localization of CD4/8 and TCR–CD3 to the zone of contact with the APC. Immunoprecipitation experiments have revealed that CD4/8 molecules associate with the TCR during T cell activation even in the absence of enforced interaction. When triggered by Ag–MHC on APCs or by antibody heteroconjugates, the association with the TCR is stabilized and prolonged, leading to more effective delivery of the signal. In practice, this increased effectiveness in delivering a signal means that much less ligand is required to elicit a response. In the case of CD4, interactions appear to involve two molecules associating with each TCR. Consistent with this is the recent observation that MHC class II molecules appear to exist as dimers, at least in the crystals generated for X-ray analysis (see Chapter 4).

How does this interaction between CD4/8 and the TCR affect signal transduction? The cytoplasmic tails of both CD4 and CD8 have been shown to be associated with p56^{lck}. This kinase is myristylated at its N-terminus, causing it to associate with the plasma membrane. A unique cysteine-containing N-terminal sequence of p56^{lck} binds to CD8 and CD4 via cysteine motifs in their membrane proximal 10 or 28 amino acids. Antibody-mediated crosslinking of CD4/8 has been shown to induce co-modulation and activation of p56^{lck}, with subsequent increases in CD3ζ

tyrosine phosphorylation. It is thought that the association of CD4/8 with the TCR brings p56^{lck} into close proximity with CD3ζ thus allowing more effective phosphorylation to occur. This is probably sufficient to uncouple the signalling apparatus but not to mediate activation of the cell. Indeed, the crosslinking of CD4 alone also elicits CD3ζ phosphorylation yet only serves to block a proliferative response. It seems likely that p56^{lck} also mediates phosphorylation of other proteins important in signalling, thereby modulating the response.

During activation, both CD4/8 and p56^{lck} themselves become phosphorylated. For CD4/8, phosphorylation of serine residues is thought to be mediated by protein kinase C (PKC). With CD4 and in some circumstances CD8, this leads to modulation from the surface of the cell by internalization. Phosphorylation of p56^{lck} on multiple serine residues following T cell activation appears to be mediated by a Ca^{2+}-dependent protein kinase. This multiple substitution is enough to increase the molecular weight of the protein, such that it is sometimes termed p60^{lck}. It is not clear how this affects the function of the molecule. However, tyrosine residue 505 appears to be critical in controlling its activity. Transfection of cells with the *lck* gene mutated at residue 505 leads to transformation, indicating that p56^{lck} plays an important role in regulating cell growth and differentiation. Phosphorylation by a specific tyrosine 505 kinase is thought to keep p56^{lck} inactive under resting conditions. It has been suggested that transient dephosphorylation by a specific phosphatase activates p56^{lck}, enabling it to phosphorylate its target proteins. The activity of p56^{lck} is then rapidly downregulated by a rephosphorylation of tyrosine 505.

Role of CD45 in T cell activation

CD45 is a major cell-surface glycoprotein expressed in different forms on the surface of lymphoid and myeloid cells. This molecule is able to regulate signal transduction pathways in lymphocytes. For example, antibody-mediated crosslinking of CD45 alone or, more effectively, co-crosslinking to CD3 has been shown to abolish the Ca^{2+} signal and subsequent proliferative response to some T cell activators. In contrast, CD4-mediated signals are enhanced by crosslinking to CD45 (*Fig. 8.4*). These effects are probably mediated by Ca^{2+}-independent protein tyrosine phosphatase (PTPase) activity of two domains within the 705 amino acid cytoplasmic tail of CD45. Studies with CD45-loss mutants and revertants have indicated that loss of CD45 results in increased phosphorylation of the negative regulatory carboxyl terminal tyrosine residues of Src-family PTKs, such as p56[lck] and, to a lesser extent, p59[fyn]. Induced CD45$^-$ mutants of well-defined antigen-specific T cell clones have also been shown to be unable to proliferate in response to Ag–MHC, despite having normal levels of the TCR–CD3 complex and other cell-surface molecules and despite being able to proliferate in response to IL-2. So CD45 may activate p56[lck] by dephosphorylating it, which would in turn lead to T cell activation mediated at least in part by tyrosine phosphorylation of CD3 ARAMs. In contrast, the direct interaction of CD45 with the TCR–CD3 complex could lead to dephosphorylation of CD3ζ and a downregulation of the response. Alternatively, the interaction of CD4 with CD45 may downregulate CD45 PTPase activity by p56[lck]-mediated tyrosine phosphorylation at specific sites available in the cytoplasmic tail. The different hypotheses for the role of CD45 in T cell activation are illustrated in *Figure 8.5*. PKC and calcium kinase II phosphorylation sites in the tail of CD45 may also be important in regulating PTPase activity of this molecule.

The overall effect of CD45 PTPase will probably depend on which surface proteins it is brought into contact with during the T cell activation process. These may differ from one CD45 isoform to the next, perhaps depending on differential ligand binding activities of the various isoforms. However, studies with chimaeric CD45 molecules suggest that the extracellular and transmembrane domains are not required for CD45 function. The recent generation of CD45 knockout mice and the ability to express single isoform CD45 transgenes in these mice should permit an unequivocal answer to the question of the importance of the different CD45 extracellular domains in T cell function.

Downstream effects of tyrosine phosphorylation

In addition to the TCR ARAM motifs, many other proteins are tyrosine phosphorylated upon T cell activation. The significance of these phosphorylation events is in large part unknown. However, some have been clearly implicated in the downstream signalling events that lead to IL-2 production and consequent cell division.

The enzyme phospholipase Cγ1 (PLCγ1) is tyrosine phosphorylated in response to TCR stimulation. The resulting induction of PLC activity results in the hydrolysis of

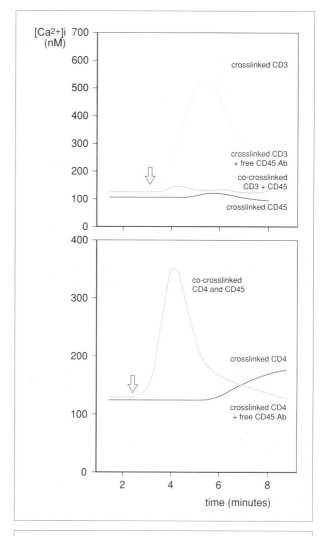

Fig. 8.4 Modulation of intracellular free calcium concentration by CD45. When peripheral blood lymphocytes are loaded with the Ca^{2+}-sensitive fluorescent dye, Indo-1, changes in $[Ca^{2+}]_i$ that occur in response to crosslinking of different suface molecules with antibodies can be followed. In the experiment shown, crosslinking of biotinylated antibodies was achieved by the addition of avidin (similar results can be obtained with unmodified antibodies crosslinked with anti-Ig). Arrows indicate the time of addition of the crosslinking agent. Top: crosslinking CD3 triggers a rapid rise in $[Ca^{2+}]_i$ which is unaffected by the addition of free antibody to CD45. However, if the CD3 and CD45 antibodies are co-crosslinked, the response is virtually ablated. Crosslinking the CD45 alone also fails to elicit a $[Ca^{2+}]_i$ response. Bottom: crosslinking CD4 results in a small, delayed rise in $[Ca^{2+}]_i$ which is also unaffected by free CD45 antibody. However, co-crosslinking of CD4 and CD45 triggers a markedly enhanced and rapid response. Based on data of Ledbetter *et al*, 1988.

phosphatidyl inositol 4,5-bisphosphate (PIP$_2$) and other phosphoinositides. The hydrolysis of PIP$_2$ yields inositol 1,4,5-triphosphate (IP$_3$) and diacylglycerol (DAG), both

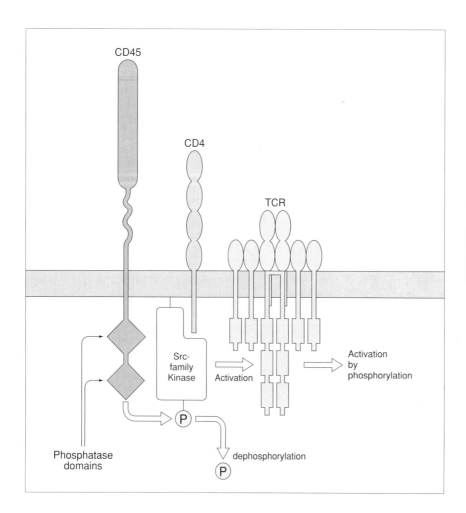

CD45

CD4

TCR

Src-
family
Kinase   Activation

Activation
by
phosphorylation

P

dephosphorylation

P

Phosphatase
domains

Fig. 8.5 Role of CD45 in T cell activation. A model for the regulation of TCR-mediated signalling by CD45 is given. Src-family kinases are inactive when phosphorylated on a tyrosine residue located at the carboxyl terminal end of the molecule, probably through interaction with their own SH2 domains. The PTPase domains within the cytoplasmic domains of CD45 may remove these phosphate residues allowing subsequent interaction with the TCR complex and activation. Adapted from Rudd *et al*, 1994.

of which play important roles as second messengers in the activation process (*Fig. 8.6*). IP_3 binds to specific receptors on the membrane of specialized Ca^{2+} storage vesicles and triggers transient release of Ca^{2+} from these stores into the cytosol. This rise in $[Ca^{2+}]_i$ is supplemented by an influx from the cell's external milieu. Recent evidence has suggested that non-voltage-gated Ca^{2+} channels in the membrane may be opened in response to IP_4 (inositol 1, 3, 4, 5-tetrakisphosphate) formed by Ca^{2+}-dependent phosphorylation of IP_3. Numerous experiments have confirmed the necessity of a rise in $[Ca^{2+}]_i$, although the relative importance of intracellular stores and Ca^{2+} influx is still not clear. However, the Ca^{2+}-mediated signal(s) can be mimicked experimentally using calcium ionophores, such as ionomycin, to raise $[Ca^{2+}]_i$.

In most circumstances, an additional signal, other than Ca^{2+}, is required to activate the T cell. This can be provided by the other product of PIP_2 hydrolysis, DAG, which activates protein kinase C (PKC), a Ca^{2+}-dependent enzyme capable of modulating the function of a variety of proteins by phosphorylating serine or threonine residues. PKC can be activated experimentally by phorbol esters such as phorbol myristate acetate (PMA); such activation triggers translocation of the enzyme from the cytosol to the membrane. Since DAG can also be generated from other phospholipids such as phosphatidylcholine, it is clear that PKC may be activated in the absence of PIP_2 hydrolysis or Ca^{2+} signals. Different PKC isoenzymes also vary in their Ca^{2+} requirements. This may be relevant to T cells, since they express particularly high levels of $PKC\beta$ which is relatively Ca^{2+}-independent.

Many experiments have shown that PKC activation effectively synergizes with calcium ionophores to elicit T cell responses, implying that Ca^{2+}- and PKC-mediated signals are fundamental to the activation process. In many different cell types, Ca^{2+}-regulated processes are mediated by activation of the multi-purpose receptor molecule, calmodulin. The Ca^{2+}–calmodulin complexes act by binding to and altering the activity of other proteins, including kinases such as the multi-functional kinase, Ca-kinase II. The phosphorylation of a series of regulatory proteins by PKC, Ca^{2+}/calmodulin-dependent and other protein kinases may ultimately control the activity of a large number of different genes required to mediate the T cell response.

The mechanism by which the TCR phosphorylates $PLC\gamma1$ is unclear. Although phosphorylation and activation requires the kinase function of $p56^{lck}$, it has been difficult to demonstrate a direct interaction of $PLC\gamma$ isoforms with either $p56^{lck}$ or the stimulated TCR complex. Such interactions may therefore be indirect.

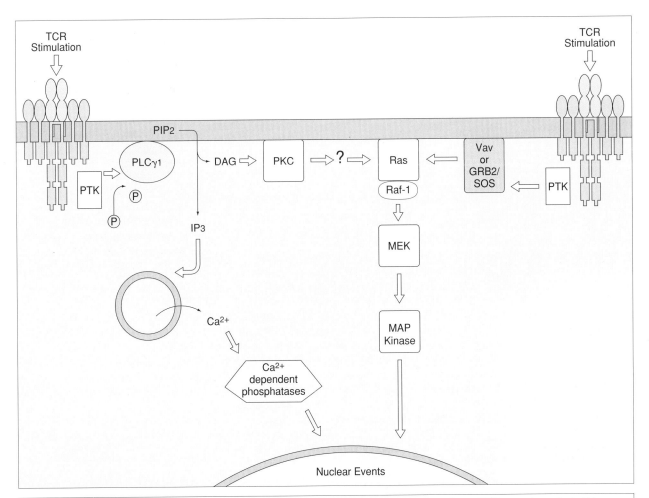

Fig. 8.6 Signalling events during T cell activation. Activated PTKs phosphorylate and activate PLCγ1 which generates the second messengers DAG and IP₃. DAG activates PKC isoenzymes which in a poorly characterized step(s) activates the Ras/MAP kinase pathway. PTKs can also activate this pathway indirectly by means of GRB2 and SOS proteins and possibly adaptor proteins such as Vav. IP₃ releases intracellular calcium stores that activate calcium-dependent phosphatases.

Stimulation of the TCR also induces a rapid activation of Ras, a 21kDa GTP binding protein with GTPase activity. Ras appears to be activated by both PKC-dependent and -independent mechanisms (*Fig. 8.6*). By analogy with Ras regulation by receptor tyrosine kinases, the PKC-independent mechanism in T cells may be via interactions with guanine nucleotide exchange proteins such as Sos and Vav and GTPase activating proteins (GAPs). The activities of these classes of proteins are modulated and GAP and Vav are tyrosine phosphorylated, by TCR stimulation.

An important downstream effector function of Ras activation is the regulation of the MAP kinase cascade. This cytosolic pathway has as its core a three-component protein kinase cascade consisting of a serine/threonine protein kinase (MAPKKK) which phosphorylates and activates a dual-specificity kinase (MAPKK) which in turn phosphorylates and activates another serine/threonine kinase (MAPK). MAPK translocates to the nucleus where it induces the expression of immediate early genes. There are multiple enzymes for each step of this cascade. The Ras/Raf/MEK/ERK pathway, where Raf corresponds to MAPKKK, MEK to MAPKK and

ERK to MAPK, has been demonstrated to link signals from receptor tyrosine kinases to the nucleus, resulting in proliferation or differentiation depending on the cell context. Ras has been shown to interact with Raf which is activated following TCR stimulation. Activated Raf in turn regulates MEK and ERK. The activation of MAP kinase has also been associated with PKC activation.

In summary, TCR stimulation results in the activation of a variety of PTKs and downstream effectors that regulate cellular responses. A summary of these pathways and the putative connections with the TCR complex is shown in *Figure 8.6*. A key cellular response that connects these surface and cytoplasmic changes to nuclear transcriptional events is the regulation of *IL-2* gene expression.

Transcriptional activation of the *IL-2* gene

Interaction of IL-2 with its receptor is necessary for progression of an activated T cell through the G1/S restriction point of the cell cycle into mitosis. The induction of *IL-2* gene expression requires integrated signals arising from the activation of PLC, Ras and a calcium/calmodulin-dependent

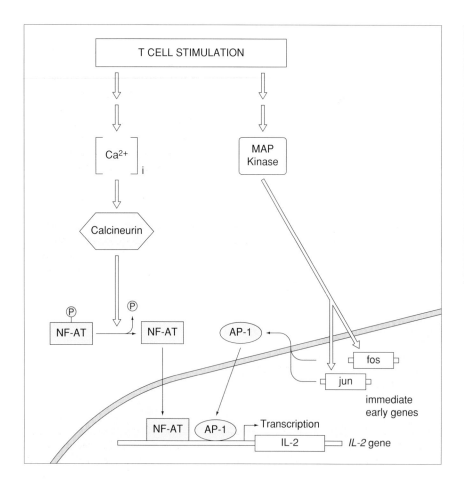

Fig. 8.7 Induction of *IL-2* gene expression. Calcineurin is a calcium-dependent phosphatase that is believed to dephosphorylate a pre-existing cytoplasmic protein, NF-AT, which then translocates to the nucleus. Activated MAP kinase induces expression of the immediate early gene products, Fos and Jun, which form the AP-1 transcription factor complex. NF-AT and AP-1 associate at the NF-AT site of the IL-2 enhancer (which also contains several other binding sites that are not shown here) to induce *IL-2* gene transcription.

serine phosphatase called calcineurin. As discussed above, PLCγ1 activation results in an increase in $[Ca^{2+}]_i$ via the second messenger IP_3. At least one critical downstream event regulated by this increase in $[Ca^{2+}]_i$ is the activation of the phosphatase activity of calcineurin.

The *IL-2* enhancer contains a binding site for a nuclear factor, NF-AT, that is induced upon T cell activation. NF-AT is a complex of at least two components. A pre-existing cytoplasmic protein, called NF-ATp (pre-existing) or NF-ATc (cytoplasmic), is translocated to the nucleus upon activation. Two candidate cDNA clones have been isolated which encode proteins related in sequence over part of their structure that also has limited similarity to the DNA-binding domain of the c-Rel gene product, a member of the NF-κB family of transcription factors. Thus, as with many other transcription factors, NF-AT$_{c/p}$ may exist as a family of proteins with subtly different functions. The nuclear component of NF-AT requires the induction of PKC, is newly synthesized and appears to be a member of the Fos and Jun families of transcription factors. These proteins are members of the 'immediate early' family of genes, so called because their transcription is induced as an early event in the activation of many cell types.

Cytoplasmic NF-ATc/p is a phosphoprotein that *in vitro* is a substrate for calcineurin. Thus, the phosphatase activity of calcineurin may activate NF-ATc/p when this translocates to the nucleus where it interacts with Fos/Jun to induce *IL-2* gene expression. The involvement of calcineurin in

T cell activation provides a mechanism for the action of two immunosuppressive drugs, cyclosporin A (CsA) and FK506, which inhibit the transcription in T cells of several lymphokine genes including IL-2. CsA and FK506 both bind to cytoplasmic proteins called, respectively, cyclophilin and FK506 binding protein (FKBP). These complexes then bind to calcineurin, inhibiting its phosphatase activity.

A scheme for the activation of the *IL-2* gene is shown in *Figure 8.7*.

CO-STIMULATORY SIGNALS IN T CELLS

In post-thymic naive T cells, signals transduced via the TCR can lead to a state of long lived immunological unresponsiveness called anergy, or to cell death. Two distinct signals are required to induce differentiation and proliferation. In addition to TCR stimulation, co-stimulatory molecules on T cells interact with ligands on antigen presenting cells. Although co-stimulatory signals are not by themselves sufficient for activation, together with TCR-mediated signals they rescue cells from anergy, inducing proliferation and differentiation to a fully functional effector cell. In this respect, they are distinct from the types of adhesion interactions discussed above. Effector T cells differ from naive T cells in that they can carry out their functions upon binding of antigen–MHC in the absence of co-stimulatory signals.

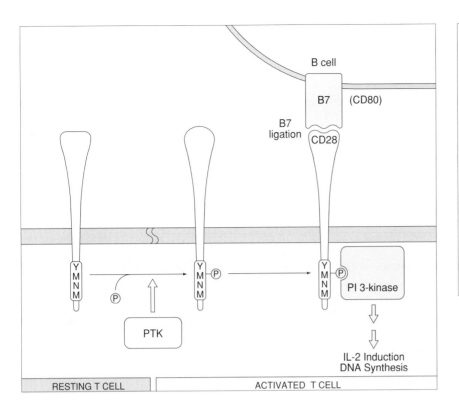

Fig. 8.8 The CD28 signalling pathway. A putative scheme for CD28 signalling is shown. A YMNM sequence within the cytoplasmic domain of the CD28 antigen is phosphorylated by PTK activity upon stimulation of the TCR. This sequence is a consensus motif (YMXM) for PI 3-kinase binding. Consequent activation of PI 3-kinase, presumably as a result of ligand binding to CD28, transmits signals to the nucleus, although the precise sequence of events and the interaction with the TCR signalling cascade has not been fully determined.

An important co-stimulatory molecule on naive T cells is the CD28 glycoprotein. A combination of antibodies to CD28 and CD3 induces naive T cells to proliferate. Furthermore, anti-CD28 will block anergy induction. Two ligands, B7-1 and B7-2, have been identified for CD28 and other as yet unidentified ligands also may exist. B7-1 is expressed on activated B cells, dendritic cells and monocytes, whereas B7-2 is also expressed on resting monocytes. A second receptor for B7, called CTLA-4, has been identified. CTLA-4 is closely related structurally to CD28 but is expressed on activated, rather than naive, T cells. CD28 is clearly a major co-stimulatory molecule as evidenced by the impairment of immune responses in CD28-deficient mice. However, these mice are not totally immunodeficient, suggesting that other co-stimulatory signals also exist. Although CTLA-4 may substitute in these mice, at least one independent co-stimulatory pathway has been defined. Thus, antibodies to the Heat Stable Antigen (HSA) glycoprotein can block the proliferative response of naive T cells to anti-CD3 and can induce anergy upon re-stimulation. The receptor for HSA on T cells is unknown.

Many other molecules, such as LFA-1/ICAM-1, can augment the immune response to antigen–MHC or anti-CD3. However, these molecules are distinguished from co-stimulatory signalling molecules in that they do not play a role in the prevention of anergy. Thus, as discussed above, they probably act to amplify the initial TCR-mediated signal but are not essential for activation.

The signalling pathway accessed by second signals would be expected to be qualitatively different from those activated by TCR stimulation in order to tip the balance between anergy and activation but must nonetheless be integrated into the TCR signalling pathway. Studies on the mechanism of CD28 signalling have revealed that the enzyme phosphatidylinositol 3-kinase (PI 3-kinase) binds to a specific motif (YMXM) in the cytoplasmic tail of CD28 (*Fig. 8.8*). PI 3-kinase is an enzyme that generates phosphoinositides in which the inositol ring is phosphorylated at the D-3 position and is becoming increasingly important as an enzyme that plays a central role in many signal transduction processes. The cytoplasmic tail of CD28 becomes tyrosine phosphorylated after CD28 crosslinking and it is likely that the essential tyrosine within the YMXM motif is phosphorylated and binds to the p85 subunit of PI 3-kinase via its SH2 domain. This recruitment of PI 3-kinase is associated with an increase in enzyme activity.

Several questions remain concerning the CD28 signalling pathway. What PTKs phosphorylate the YMXM motif within the CD28 cytoplasmic tail? PTKs such as p56[lck], p59[fyn] and ZAP-70, that are activated by TCR stimulation, are attractive candidates, although there is no direct evidence for their involvement. What are the downstream effectors of activated PI 3-kinase? CD28 ligation leads to the induction of IL-2 synthesis by a route that is distinct from the Ca^{2+}/calcineurin pathway and is insensitive to CsA and FK506. Signalling also leads to the stabilization of mRNA encoding various cytokines. A binding site, called the CD28-response element, has been identified within the *IL-2* enhancer that binds a protein that is induced after CD28 stimulation. However, the identity of this protein and the cytoplasmic second messengers that influence its activity is unknown. Finally, how does the CD28 pathway synergize with the TCR pathway to activate T cells? PI 3-kinase is also activated by TCR stimulation, probably in a tyrosine phosphorylation-independent pathway involving SH3 binding to PI 3-kinase. However, this may be suboptimal. Given these considerations, it is clear that the prospect of dissecting the interconnections between the TCR and second signal pathways is of great importance for studies on activation, anergy and autoimmunity.

DEVELOPMENT OF POST-THYMIC T CELLS

The cellular and biochemical events leading to the initial activation of virgin T cells by specific antigen have been described above. However, for the immune system to cope efficiently and effectively with the many and varied challenges received during an individual's lifetime, it must adapt so that only the most suitable effector systems are recruited. This is achieved by further differentiation of T cells. This differentiation generates effector cells with varying functions and cytokine profiles and leads to the development of memory T cells which are able to respond rapidly and more effectively to subsequent encounters with their specific antigen. The mechanisms involved in these maturation events are discussed in this chapter.

Murine T helper subsets Th1 and Th2 clones

CD4+ T cells are not homogeneous. Thus, studies of T cell clones have delineated two major subpopulations of CD4+ T cells in mice, Th1 and Th2 cells, which differ in the cytokines they secrete following activation (*Fig. 8.9*). Th1 cells synthesize IL-2, IFNγ and TNFβ, which are not made by Th2 clones. In contrast, Th2 cells (but not Th1) produce IL-4, IL-5, IL-6 and IL-10 (the characteristics of these and other cytokines are described in detail in Chapter 10). Other cytokines, such as GM-CSF, TNFα and IL-3, are made by both cell types, although the relative levels may vary. These specific patterns of cytokine gene expression can be used to categorize most murine CD4+ T cell clones. Interestingly, many CD8+ Tc and the few γδ T cell clones analysed have a cytokine production profile similar to that of Th1 cells, although only a proportion of Tc clones appear to make IL-2. Despite the fact that the cytokine profiles of most Th1 and Th2 clones are stable in culture, providing reliable populations for study, it has not yet been possible to produce antibody reagents which can specifically identify Th1 and Th2 cells on the basis of surface markers.

As might be expected from their capacity to produce different cytokines, Th1 and Th2 cells also differ in their functional activities. Thus, the production of IFNγ and TNFβ by Th1 cells enhances microbicidal activity in macrophages whereas Th2 cells synthesize cytokines that help B cells develop into antibody producing cells. Thus, in mice challenged with the protozoon parasite, *Leishmania major*, protection against infection is contingent upon macrophage activation since this parasite establishes an intracellular infection of macrophages. Microbicidal activation of macrophages is induced by IFNγ treatment and this activation is blocked by IL-4 and IL-10. These results suggest that Th1-like responses are protective against *L. major* infections, whereas Th2-like responses fail to offer protection. In this context, T cell clones, specific for *Leishmania* antigens, from mouse strains that clear infection, produce IFNγ but not IL-4. In contrast,

Cytokine	Th1	Th2	Tc
IFNγ	++	−	++
IL-2	++	−	+/−
TNFβ	++	−	+
GM-CSF	++	+	++
TNFα	++	+	+
IL-3	++	++	+
IL-4	−	++	−
IL-5	−	++	−
IL-6	−	++	−
IL-10	−	++	?
IL-7	?	+*	?

Fig. 8.9 Cytokines produced by Th1, Th2 and Tc cells. The relative ability of Th1, Th2 and Tc cells to produce different cytokines following activation is shown. The cytokines that differentiate Th1 and Th2 cells are shown boxed. *To date, one Th2 clone, D10.G4.1, has been reported to produce IL-7.

clones from strains that succumb to infection produce IL-4 as a major cytokine product.

A major difference between Th1 and Th2 subpopulations is their ability to regulate differentially the production of certain Ig isotypes. Th2 cells will trigger resting B cells presenting specific antigen to secrete IgM, IgG3 and IgA but are particularly effective in promoting IgG1 and IgE responses. Only Th2 clones appear to be capable of triggering an IgE response, probably because of the critical role of IL-4 in isotype switching to this class (see Chapter 9). In contrast, many Th1 cells can, while eliciting IgM and IgG3 responses, selectively promote the production of IgG2a, in part through the action of secreted IFNγ. Some Th1 cells are also very effective at inducing IgG1 responses, even though IL-4 has been shown to be critical for triggering production of this isotype by B cells activated with lipopolysaccharide (LPS). Optimal Th1- and Th2-triggered responses of resting B cells appear to require both cell–cell contact with the T cell and cytokine production, whereas large, pre-activated B cells respond to the appropriate cytokines alone. Overall, Th2 cells are much more efficient at providing help for antibody production by resting B cells. However, non-helper Th1 cells can clearly deliver the necessary contact-dependent signals for the production of isotypes such as IgG1 and IgE, since they will induce good antibody responses if IL-4, anti-IFNγ antibody and IL-5 are added, although IL-5 is not necessary for IgE production. Non-helper T cells can also elicit antigen-dependent proliferation of resting B cells in the absence of added cytokines. The poor intrinsic helper activity of many Th1 cells is at least partly due to the production of IFNγ, which inhibits IL-4-mediated stimulation of antibody responses, particularly of the IgE isotype. Th1 cells can also have a cytotoxic effect on antigen presenting B cells; this activity and/or the production of IFNγ may make Th1 cells appear functionally as antigen- or isotype-specific suppressor cells (see Chapter 11).

The injection of Th1 clones together with their specific antigen into the footpads of mice leads to the development of a delayed hypersensitivity (DTH) response, an inflammatory reaction resulting in swelling and a predominantly mononuclear cell infiltrate at the injection site. Th2 cells are unable to elicit this type of inflammatory response. This activity of Th1 cells can be partially ascribed to the production of IFNγ in response to the local presentation of antigen. Indeed, an important function of Th2 responses may be to play an anti-inflammatory role by combating the tissue damage resulting from Th1-like immune responses to intracellular infectious agents. Thus, a prolonged Th1 response to a widespread or prolonged infectious organism may induce tissue damage and inflammation. This pathology could be controlled by the Th2 response by both suppressing IFNγ production and suppressing its actions through IL-4 and IL-10. This regulatory effect of Th2 cells may also operate in autoimmune disease which in several experimental situations can be ameliorated by administration of IL-4. Some of the functional activities and interactions of Th1 and Th2 cells, derived largely from *in vitro* analyses, are illustrated in *Figure 8.10*. Many of these cellular interactions are also thought to play an important role in regulating both qualitative and quantitative aspects of immune responses *in vivo* (see below).

Th1 and Th2 cells appear to differ quite markedly in their requirements for activation and growth. Th1 cells use IL-2 as their autocrine growth factor and respond weakly, or not at all, to IL-4; Th2 cells produce and respond to IL-4 but will also proliferate strongly in response to IL-2. The autocrine growth of Th2 cells requires IL-1 as a co-stimulus along with TCR/CD3 signals. Activation of Th2 cells with mitogens or anti-TCR/CD3 antibodies, in the absence of APCs, results in the production of IL-4 but the ability to proliferate in response to this cytokine depends on IL-1-mediated upregulation of IL-4 responsiveness. Although IL-1 has been shown to stimulate IL-2 receptor expression on Th2 cells, a direct effect on IL-4 receptors has not yet been described but is a likely cause of the increased responsiveness. Other studies have shown that IL-4 is also required for the expression of IL-1 receptors, so these two cytokines appear to be interdependent for their effects on Th2 cells. Th1 cells do not require IL-1 as a co-stimulus for proliferation and they do not express the 80kDa IL-1 receptor.

Possible precursors of Th1 and Th2 cells

Naive T cells that have not yet responded to antigen secrete IL-2 but not IL-4 upon TCR engagement together with a co-stimulatory signal. However, these cells clearly have the capacity to develop into effector or memory T cells that can produce IFNγ or IL-4. Thus, virgin T cells can be considered to be precursor, or Th0, cells. Two alternative models have been suggested for the development of Th1 and

Th2 cells from Th0. Th0 cells may represent an uncommitted precursor cell which subsequently develops into either Th1 or Th2 depending on the signals it receives from its environment (such as different APC types, cytokines and signals from adhesion molecules). This model is depicted in *Figure 8.11*. Alternatively, separate pre-committed Th1 and Th2 precursors may secrete both sets of cytokines before switching to their pre-committed mature phenotype. This hypothesis would predict that the two types of precursor cell have different activation requirements. Currently available data cannot distinguish these two alternative models, although the former model is preferred.

Role of Th1 and Th2 cells *in vivo*

Th1- and Th2-like activities can be distinguished in *in vivo* model systems such as *Leishmania major* infection. Given the probable existence of Th1 and Th2 cells *in vivo*, the question arises as to how the relative contribution of these two subsets to an immune response is determined. In other words, how is the development of Th0 cells into Th1 or Th2 cells regulated? Several experiments have indicated that cytokines play an essential role in determining the pathway of differentiation. Thus, activation of naive T cells in the presence of both IL-2 and IL-4 in the primary culture is required to generate cells that will produce IFNγ or IL-4 upon subsequent stimulation. In the absence of IL-4, no priming for IL-4 production is observed. There appeared to be no absolute requirement for the presence of one particular type of APC for the generation of Th2 cells, although activated macrophages were particularly efficacious for Th1 cell development. This effect is mediated by the cytokine IL-12. Thus, IL-4 appears to be essential for routing Th0 cells along the Th2 pathway and IL-12 augments the Th1 pathway leading to IFNγ production.

In addition to their positive effect in inducing Th0 precursors to develop into Th1 and Th2 cells, IL-4 and IL-12 are important as inhibitors of differentiation. Thus IL-4 blocks the development of Th0 cells into IFNγ precursors both *in vitro* and *in vivo*. This effect can be abrogated by simultaneous administration of IL-12. It thus follows that the relative levels of IL-4 and IL-12 at the time of priming of naive T cells will determine the course of an immune response. For example, intracellular infection probably biases an immune response towards IFNγ production because of the induction of macrophage IL-12 production. In other immune responses, the concentration of antigen may be a determining factor. The elucidation of the mechanisms that regulate commitment to one or other functional Th subset may be of use in attempts to manipulate the immune response in diseases such as allergy where IL-4 production dominates.

Human T helper subsets

Human T cell subsets that appear to be analogous to murine Th1 and Th2 cells have been identified. Thus, human T cell clones specific for particular antigens often exhibit either a Th1- or Th2-like pattern of cytokine secretion. For example, allergen-specific T cell clones tend to secrete IL-4 and IL-5 (Th2-like profile), whereas clones specific for purified protein derivative from *Mycobacterium*

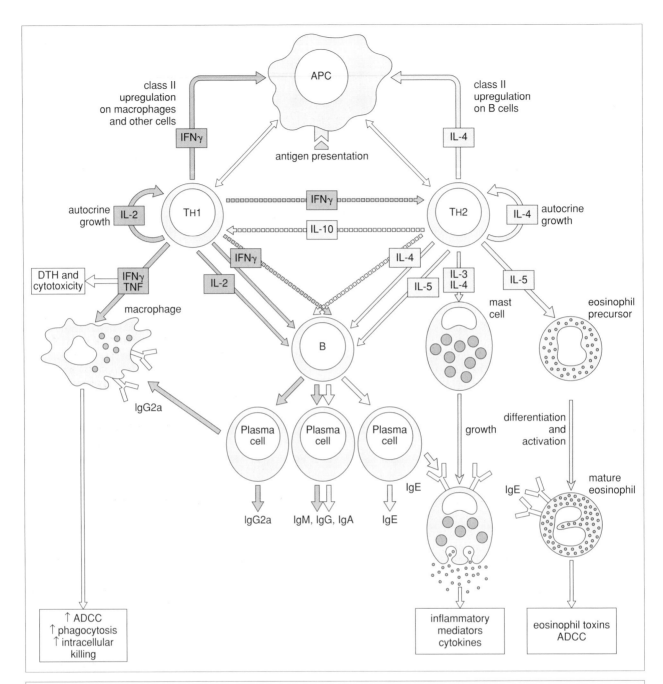

Fig. 8.10 Major effects of cytokines produced by Th1 and Th2 cells. *In vitro* defined cellular activation triggered by cytokines produced by Th1 (olive) and Th2 (green) cells are shown as 'thick arrows', and mutually inhibitory interactions as broken arrows. Thin arrows represent differentiation, other secretory events and binding of antibodies to cellular Fc receptors. The activities depicted are also thought to occur *in vivo*, allowing the immune response to adapt to combat most effectively different types of antigenic insult.

tuberculosis produce IL-2 and IFNγ (Th1-like profile). As for the murine situation, these two subsets probably arise from a bipotential Th0 progenitor cell.

The broad similarity in development and cytokine profile between human and murine Th1 and Th2 cells also extends to function. Thus, Th1 cells appear to be involved in responses leading to DTH and chronic inflammation and Th2 cells in the triggering of allergic atopic disorders. Thus,

it has become clear that there are close parallels between murine and human Th subsets, in their development, cytokine profiles and functions.

Memory T cells

When primary T cell immune responses are initiated in lymphoid tissues, naive T cells proliferate extensively and acquire effector functions. Most of these cells subsequently

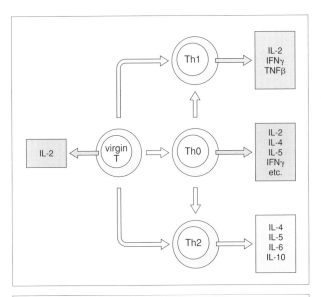

Fig. 8.11 Postulated differentiation pathways of Th1 and Th2 cells. Two alternative hypotheses of how Th1 and Th2 cells may develop from virgin T cells are illustrated. The characteristic cytokines produced by each cell population are shown. Virgin T cells, which seed the periphery following their development in the thymus, are initially capable of producing only IL-2. Following the first interaction with specific antigen, virgin T cells acquire the capacity to produce other cytokines (only characteristic cytokines are shown). One hypothesis (white arrows) suggests that this differentiation leads to the development of an uncommitted common precursor capable of producing all cytokines (shown here as Th0). Further differentiation, involving the deactivation or suppression of selected cytokine genes, leads to the development of Th1 and Th2 cells. An alternative hypothesis (green arrows) suggests that Th1 and Th2 cells are derived from virgin T cells which are pre-committed to produce their respective cytokine profiles. Intermediate states of differentiation (not shown) may occur in either pathway. For example, although Th0 cells can produce both Th1 and Th2 cytokines, individual cells may already be pre-committed to develop into one or other of the major subsets.

Phenotype	Naive T cells	Memory T cells	Activated T cells
MHC class II	–	+	+++
CD25	–	+	+++
CD2	++	+++	+++
CD11a/CD18	++	+++	+++
CD29	+	+++	+++
CD44	+	+++	+++
CD45RA	+++	–	–
CD45RO	–	+++	+++
CD54	–	+	+++
CD58	+	++	+++

Fig. 8.12 Characteristic surface markers of human CD4$^+$, naive, memory and activated T cells. Naive T cells can be distinguished from memory or activated cells by their expression of CD45RA (green) and their low or absent expression of CD29, CD44 and CD45RO (olive). Activated T cells (naive or memory) can also be identified by the expression of high levels of MHC class II, CD25 (IL-2Rα) or CD54 (ICAM-1) (grey). To distinguish a resting memory cell from an activated cell, combinations of markers are needed (e.g. CD45RO^{hi}, CD25^{lo}, MHC class II^{lo}). These markers are also thought to define similar differentiation states of CD8$^+$ and γδ T cells.

die within a week or so; however, some cells persist and form the basis of a more intense secondary response to antigen. These memory cells are long lived and, in addition to being present in greater numbers, also differ qualitatively from their naive precursors in a number of ways that allow them to respond more rapidly and effectively.

Markers

A number of different surface markers can distinguish virgin T cells from activated and memory T cells in different species. The characteristics of human memory CD4$^+$ T cells have been studied in some detail, with umbilical cord blood T cells often serving as a uniform source of virgin cells. CD45 isoforms serve as very useful markers of human virgin and activated/memory T cells, even though the functional significance of different extracellular domains is still unclear. Virgin T cells characteristically express a high molecular weight form, CD45RA, whereas activated and memory T cells predominantly express the lower molecular weight form, CD45RO. *In vitro* analyses of purified T cell populations have shown that it is the CD45RO$^+$ cells that are responsible for proliferative responses to recall antigens such as tetanus toxoid. Differential expression of CD45 isoforms may also distinguish virgin and memory subsets of CD8$^+$ T cells, as well as differentiating virgin and memory T cells in mice.

Both activated and memory cells also express higher levels of adhesion molecules, such as CD11a/CD18 (LFA-1), CD29 (VLAβ) and different VLA α-chains (see Chapter 14). Other markers can be used to distinguish activated cells from resting memory cells. Two that are most often used are MHC class II molecules (not expressed by activated mouse T cells) and the α-chain of the IL-2 receptor (CD25). ICAM-1 (CD54) has also been found at high levels on activated T cells. These three markers of activated T cells (CD25, CD54 and MHC class II) are also expressed at low levels on memory T cells. The characteristic markers of human T cells are shown in *Figure 8.12*.

Until the discovery of the differentially expressed CD45 isoforms, mouse memory T cells were distinguished by their expression of CD44 (phagocyte glycoprotein 1, Pgp1). This marker is expressed on the surface of T cells following activation and remains thereafter. In the rat, the CD45R epitope recognized by OX-22 antibody (see *Fig. 5.8*) serves to identify virgin T cells. Following activation *in vitro* or antigen exposure *in vivo*, OX-22$^+$ cells differentiate into OX-22$^-$ activated and memory T cells.

Activation requirements of memory T cells

Memory T cells are more readily activated than virgin T cells and produce cytokines more quickly, often in higher amounts. The expression of increased levels of adhesion molecules enables a memory T cell to interact effectively with an APC bearing much lower levels of Ag–MHC complexes. This is partly due to adhesion molecules increasing the interactions betwen the two cells, which allows the generation of sufficient TCR-mediated signals and partly due to activation signals delivered by the adhesion molecules themselves. Memory T cells are also less dependent on certain co-stimulatory signals provided by APCs. Biochemical differences also play an important role in enabling memory T cells to respond more rapidly and effectively although these events remain poorly characterized at present. Thus, human memory T cells respond much better to anti-CD3 and anti-CD2 antibody reagents than do virgin T cells, even though both subpopulations express similar levels of these markers. It has recently been shown that the cells which proliferate in response to anti-CD3 or anti-CD2 express the marker CD26. Both CD26$^+$ and CD26$^-$ T cells produce good Ca^{2+} responses to anti-CD3 but phosphorylation of CD3 chains is much more efficient in CD26$^+$ cells. Other activities of intracellular kinases and phosphatases, as well as their ability to associate with different surface molecules involved in T cell activation, may play an important role in the establishment and maintenance of the memory phenotype.

Trafficking

Experiments involving the cannulation of afferent and efferent lymphatic vessels of rats and sheep have demonstrated that virgin and memory T cells have different migratory patterns. Memory T cells are dispersed throughout the secondary lymphoid organs, are prominent in the thoracic duct lymph and recirculate rapidly from blood to lymph. Memory CD4$^+$ T cells are found in the afferent lymph whereas cells in the efferent lymph are mostly of the naive phenotype. This selective trafficking of memory cells to peripheral tissues may optimize the interactions of these cells with their specific antigens and help to provide a rapid effector response at the site of antigen entry into the body. In support of this hypothesis is the observation that T cells found on the epithelial surfaces of normal human lungs are primarily of the memory but not activated phenotype.

The migratory properties of memory T cells are regulated by a series of 'traffic signals' determined by the pattern of expression of families of adhesion molecules on both the lymphocyte and on the vascular endothelium of different tissues. Indeed, the pattern of adhesion molecules expressed by memory T cells migrating into the afferent lymph from different tissues is distinct, such that memory T cells are more likely to return to the tissue from which they originated. For example, gut homing memory T cells express the $\alpha_4\beta_7$ integrin which appears to be important in the interaction with the mucosal addressin cell adhesion molecule 1 (MadCAM-1) on Peyer's patch HEVs and post-capillary venules in the *lamina propria*. In contrast, T cells localized in the skin but not in the gut express a ligand (cutaneous lymphocyte associated antigen, CLA) for E-selectin, the expression of which is upregulated on skin endothelial cells upon inflammation. T cell migration to skin during inflammation is also inhibited by antibodies to LFA-1α, the integrin α_4 subunit or VCAM-1. Thus, multiple signals may be required for the efficient regulation of the accumulation of memory T cells in skin.

Life span of memory T cells

In many cases T cell memory can last for the lifetime of the host. However, estimates of the life span of a memory T cell can be complicated by the lack of markers that unambiguously identify this cell type. For example, the secondary response to antigen a month or so after priming is probably comprised, at least in part, of already activated effector T cells. This raises the issue of memory and activation state of T cells. There is evidence that the maintenance of T cell memory can depend upon the persistence of antigen. Thus, for both CD4$^+$ and CD8$^+$ T cell responses, when primed lymphocytes were deprived of contact with antigen by adoptive transfer in the absence of antigen, there was a rapid decay of memory within days or weeks of transfer.

How can antigen persist for long periods in the body? Antigen has been detected on the follicular dendritic cells in germinal centres years after administration, providing a mechanism by which CD4$^+$ cells can remain continually stimulated. However, there is no evidence that exogenous antigens on dendritic cells can enter the class I pathway of presentation. In the case of viral infections, it is possible that long term viral persistence may provide a route to maintenance of memory. However, this cannot be invariably the case and it remains probable that long term memory can persist in the complete absence of antigen.

Experiments using bromodeoxyuridine incorporation *in vivo* have revealed that most memory T cells are in interphase. Thus, if memory does indeed depend on contact with antigen, the level of antigen may not be sufficient to drive cells into the cell cycle. However, memory T cells retain activation markers such as CD44 which may indicate that they are not truly resting (G0) cells but are perhaps arrested at the restriction point late in G1.

In summary, studies on the mechanism of T cell memory have often yielded conflicting results which may reflect the complex and multifaceted nature of the phenomenon. Early memory may be a result of some persisting effector cells after the primary response has declined. Longer term memory may then depend on low level contact with antigen or with cross-reacting environmental antigen. This would explain observations that memory-phenotype T cells divide more rapidly than naive T cells. Late memory cells, persisting many years after contact with antigen, may have overcome the requirement of antigen for survival and, although semi-activated, be non-cycling. Thus, as with so much of immunology, a particular assay may measure only one aspect of a complex *in vivo* phenomenon and apparently yield conflicting results.

SUMMARY

Virgin T cells are activated by stimulation of the TCR with antigen-MHC. These surface interactions initiate a complex cascade of signal transduction events that result in cell division and acquisition of effector function.

An early biochemical event after TCR stimulation is the phosphorylation of tyrosine residues within ARAM motifs located in the CD3 cytoplasmic domains of the CD3 components. The PTKs that phosphorylate these ARAMs are unknown but the Src-family kinases, $p56^{lck}$ and $p59^{fyn}$, are good candidates. The activation of these kinases depends upon dephosphorylation of a negative regulatory site which may be regulated by the activity of PTPases such as CD45. Phosphorylated ARAM motifs are thought to recruit ZAP70 PTK to the antigen receptor complex, initiating a number of downstream events. Tyrosine phosphorylation and activation of $PLC\gamma1$, possibly by activated ZAP70, results in the generation of DAG and IP_3 which respectively activates PKC isoforms and mobilizes intracellular free calcium ion stores. PTKs also activate the MAP kinase pathway. The combined result of these activation events is the induction of *IL-2* gene expression via induction of the activity of NF-AT. This transcription factor complex comprises a pre-existing lineage specific protein that is translocated to the nucleus and members of the Fos/Jun immediate early gene family.

However, it is clear that additional surface molecules and cytokines are necessary for full lymphocyte activation. In particular, full and sustained activation of naive T cells depends upon co-stimulatory signals transduced through molecules such as CD28. These second signals activate distinct signal transduction pathways that are integrated with TCR-mediated signals to generate effector T cells.

Once activated by antigen on appropriate antigen presenting cells, T cells acquire an effector function. Helper T cells can be divided into two subsets, based on the profile of cytokine expression. Th1 cells produce IL-2, $IFN\gamma$ and $TNF\beta$ and Th2 cells produce IL-4, IL-5, IL-6, IL-10 and IL-13. This differential pattern of cytokine expression underlies functional differences between these subsets. Thus, Th1 cells are inflammatory cells that induce enhanced cellular immunity, such as microbicidal activity in macrophages, whereas Th2 cells act to help B cells produce antibodies. Cytotoxic T cells generally exhibit a Th1-like profile of cytokine secretion. The decision of a naive $CD4^+$ T cell (Th0) to differentiate into either a Th1 or Th2 effector depends in part on the cytokine environment but also on the density of ligand to which the T cell responds (affecting, for example, the degree of ligation of the TCR).

Most T cells die shortly after activation, thus providing a mechanism of limiting the immune response. However, some cells enter a memory pool such that the secondary response is much more rapid than the primary response. The maintenance of memory is complex and may have several phases depending on how long antigen persists after the initial challenge. Different mechanisms of memory may explain conflicting results of experiments addressing the requirement for persistence of antigen for the maintenance of memory.

FURTHER READING

Appleby MW, Gross JA, Cooke MP, Levin SD, Qian X, Perlmutter RM. Defective T cell receptor signaling in mice lacking the thymic isoform of $p59^{fyn}$. *Cell* 1992, **70**:751.

Baumheueter S, Singer MS, Henzel W, Hemmerich S, Renz M, Rosen SD, Lasky LA. Binding of L-selectin to the vascular sialomucin, CD34. *Science* 1993, **262**:436.

Bell EB, Sparshott SM. Interconversion of CD45R subsets of CD4 T cells *in vivo*. *Nature* 1990, **348**:163.

Berg EL, McEvoy LM, Berlin C, Bargatze RF, Butcher EC. L-selectin-mediated lymphocyte rolling on MadCAM-1. *Nature* 1993, **366**:695.

Berg EL, Robinson MK, Warnock RA, Butcher EC. The human peripheral lymph node vascular addressin is a ligand for LECAM-1, the peripheral lymph node homing receptor. *J Cell Biol* 1991, **114**:343.

Berg EL, Yoshino T, Rott LS, Robinson MK, Warnock RA, Kishimoto TK, Picker LJ, Butcher EC. The cutaneous lymphocyte antigen is a skin lymphocyte homing receptor for the vascular lectin endothelial cell-leukocyte adhesion molecule 1. *J Exp Med* 1991, **174**:1461.

Berlin C, Berg EL, Briskin MJ, Andrew DP, Kilshaw PJ, Holzmann B, Weissman IL, Hamann A, Butcher EC. $\alpha_4\beta_7$ integrin mediates lymphocyte binding to the mucosal vascular addressin MadCAM-1. *Cell* 1993, **74**:185.

Beverley PCL. Is T cell memory maintained by cross-reactive stimulation? *Immunol Today* 1990, **11**:203.

Beverley PCL. Functional analysis of human T cell subsets defined by CD45 isoform expression. *Semin Immunol* 1992, **4**:35.

Bevilacqua MP. Endothelial-leukocyte adhesion molecules. *Ann Rev Immunol* 1993, **11**:767.

Biffen M, McMichael-Phillips D, Larson T, Venkitaraman A, Alexander D. The CD45 tyrosine phosphatase regulates specific pools of antigen receptor-associated $p59^{fyn}$ and CD4-associated $p56^{lck}$ tyrosine kinases in human T cells. *EMBO J* 1994, **13**:1920.

Bradley LM, Atkins GG, Swain SL. Long-term $CD4^+$ memory T cells from the spleen lack MEL-14, the lymph node homing receptor. *J Immunol* 1992, **148**:324.

Burgess KE, Odysseos AD, Zalvan C, Drucker B, Anderson P, Schlossman SF, Rudd CE. Biochemical identification of a direct physical interaction between the CD4:$p56^{lck}$ and TiTCR-CD3 complexes. *Eur J Immunol* 1991, **21**:1663.

Butcher EC. Leukocyte-endothelial cell recognition: three or more steps to specificity and diversity. *Cell* 1991, **67**:1033.

Byrne JA, Butler JL, Cooper MD. Differential activation requirements for virgin and memory T cells. *J Immunol* 1988, **141**:3249.

Camp RL, Kraus TA, Birkeland ML, Pure E. High levels of CD44 expression distinguish virgin from antigen-primed B cells. *J Exp Med* 1991, **173**:763.

Cepek KL, Parker CM, Madara JL, Brenner MB. Integrin $\alpha_4\beta_7$ mediates adhesion of T lymphocytes to epithelial cells. *J Immunol* 1993, **150**:3459.

Chan AC, Irving BA, Fraser JD, Weiss A. The ζ-chain is associated with a tyrosine kinase and upon T cell antigen receptor stimulation associates with ZAP-70, a 70kDa tyrosine phosphoprotein. *Proc Natl Acad Sci USA* 1991, **88**:9166.

Chan AC, Iwashima M, Turck CW, Weiss A. ZAP-70: A 70kDa protein-tyrosine kinase that associates with the TCRζ-chain. *Cell* 1992, **71**:649.

Chow LML, Fournel M, Davidson D, Veillette A. Negative regulation of T cell receptor signaling by tyrosine protein kinase p50[csk]. *Nature* 1993, **365**:156.

Clipstone NA, Crabtree GR. Identification of calcineurin as a key signaling enzyme in T lymphocyte activation. *Nature* 1992, **357**:695.

Cooke MP, Abraham KM, Forbush KA, Perlmutter RM. Regulation of T cell receptor signaling by a Src-family protein tyrosine kinase p59[fyn]. *Cell* 1991, **65**:281.

Danielian S, Alcover A, Polissard L, Stefanescu M, Acuto O, Fischer S, Fagard R. Both T cell receptor TCR-CD3 complex and CD2 increase the tyrosine kinase activity of p56[lck]. CD2 can mediate TCR-independent and CD45-dependent activation of p56[lck]. *Eur J Immunol* 1992, **22**:2915.

Downward J, Graves J, Cantrell D. The regulation and function of p21[ras] in T cells. *Immunol Today* 1992, **13**:89.

Freeman GJ, Borriello F, Hodes RJ, Reiser H, Hathcock KS, Laszio G, McKnight AJ, Kim J, Du L, Lombard DB, Gray GS, Nadler LM, Sharpe AH. Uncovering of functional alternative CTLA-4 counter-receptor in B7-deficient mice. *Science* 1993, **262**:907.

Gauen LKT, Kong A-NT, Samelson LE, Shaw AS. p59[fyn] tyrosine kinase associates with multiple T cell receptor subunits through its unique amino terminal domain. *Mol Cell Biol* 1992, **12**:5438.

Glaichenhaus N, Shastri N, Littman DR, Turner JM. Requirement for association of p56[lck] with CD4 in antigen-specific signal transduction in T cells. *Cell* 1991, **64**:511.

Goodbourn S. Transcriptional regulation in activated T cells. *Curr Biol* 1994, **4**:930.

Gray D, Matzinger P. T cell memory is short-lived in the absence of antigen. *J Exp Med* 1991, **174**:969.

Gray D, Sprent J. Immunological memory. *Curr Top Microbiol Immunol* 1990, **159**:1.

Hahn WC, Menu E, Bothwell ALM, Sims PJ, Bierer BE. Overlapping but non-identical binding sites on CD2 for CD58 and a second ligand CD59. *Science* 1992, **256**:1805.

Harding F, McArthur JG, Gross JA, Raulet DH, Allison JP. CD28-mediated signaling co-stimulates murine T cells and prevents the induction of anergy in T cell clones. *Nature* 1992, **365**:607.

Hogg N, Landis RC. Adhesion molecules in cell interactions. *Curr Opin Immunol* 1993, **5**:383.

Holzmann B, McIntyre BW, Weissman IL. Identification of a murine Peyer's patch-specific lymphocyte homing receptor as an integrin molecule with an α-chain homologous to human VLA-4α. *Cell* 1989, **56**:37.

Hsieh CS, Macatonia SE, Tripp CS, Wolf SF, O'Garra A, Murphy KM. Development of T$_H$1 CD4+ T cells through IL-12 produced by *Listeria*-induced macrophages. *Science* 1993, **260**:547.

Irving BA, Chan AC, Weiss A. Functional characterization of a signal transducing motif present in the T cell receptor ζ-chain. *J Exp Med* 1993, **177**:1093.

Irving BA, Weiss A. The cytoplasmic domain of the T cell receptor ζ-chain is sufficient to couple to receptor-associated signal transduction pathways. *Cell* 1991, **64**:891.

Iwashima M, Irving BA, van Oers NSC, Chan AC, Weiss A. Sequential interactions of the TCR with two distinct cytoplasmic tyrosine kinases. *Science* 1994, **263**:1136.

Jain J, McCaffrey PG, Miner Z, Kerppola TK, Lambert JN, Verdine GL, Curran T, Rao A. The T cell transcription factor NF-ATp is a substrate for calcineurin and interacts with Fos and Jun. *Nature* 1993, **365**:352.

Jain J, McCaffrey PG, Valge-Archer VE, Rao A. Nuclear factor of activated T cells contains Fos and Jun. *Nature* 1992, **356**:801.

Janeway CA, Bottomley K. Signals and signs for lymphocyte responses. *Cell* 1994, **76**:275.

June CH, Bluestone JA, Nadler LM, Thompson CB. The B7 and CD28 receptor families. *Immunol Today* 1994, **7**:321.

Kato K, Koyanagi M, Okada H, Takanashi T, Wong YW, Williams AF, Okumura K, Yagita H. CD48 is a counter-receptor for mouse CD2 and is involved in T cell activation. *J Exp Med* 1992, **176**:1241.

Kishihar K, Penninger J, Wallace VA, Kündig TM, Kawai K, Wakeham A, Timms E, Pfeffer K, Ohashi PS, Thomas ML, Furlonger C, Paige CJ, Mak TW. Normal B lymphocyte development but impaired T cell maturation in CD45-exon 6 protein tyrosine phosphatase-deficient mice. *Cell* 1993, **74**:143.

Kopf M, Le Gros G, Bachmann M, Lamers MC, Bluethmann H, Köhler G. Disruption of the murine IL-4 gene blocks T$_H$2 cytokine responses. *Nature* 1993, **362**:245.

Koretzky G, Picus J, Schultz T, Weiss A. Tyrosine phosphatase CD45 is required for both T cell antigen receptor- and CD2-mediated activation of a protein tyrosine kinase and interleukin 2 production. *Proc Natl Acad Sci USA* 1991, **88**:2037.

Koretzky GA, Picus J, Thomas ML, Weiss A. Tyrosine phosphotase CD45 is essential for coupling T cell antigen receptor to the phosphatidyl inositol pathway. *Nature* 1990, **346**:66.

Korsmeyer SJ. Bcl-2: a repressor of lymphocyte death. *Immunol Today* 1992, **13**:285.

Koulova L, Clark EA, Shu G, Dupont D. The CD28 ligand B7/BB1 provides co-stimulatory signal for alloactivation of CD4+ T cells. *J Exp Med* 1991, **173**:759.

Lasky LA. Selectins: interpreters of cell-specific carbohydrate information during inflammation. *Science* 1992, **258**:964.

Lawrence MB, Springer TA. Leukocytes roll on a selectin at physiological flow rates: distinction from and prerequisite for adhesion through integrins. *Cell* 1991, **65**:859.

Liew FY, Millott S, Li Y, Leichuk R, Chan WL, Ziltener H. Macrophage activation by interferon gamma from host-protective T cells is inhibited by interleukin IL-3 and IL-4 produced by disease-promoting T cells in leishmaniasis. *Eur J Immunol* 1988, **19**:1227.

Linsley PS, Brady W, Grosmaire L, Aruffo A, Damie NK, Ledbetter JA. Binding of the B cell activation antigen B7 to CD28 co-stimulates T cell proliferation and interleukin 2 mRNA accumulation. *J Exp Med* 1991, **173**:721.

Liu J, Farmer JD Jr, Lane WS, Friedman J, Weissman I, Schreiber SL. Calcineurin is a common target of cyclophilin-cyclosporin A and FKBP-FK506 complexes. *Cell* 1991, **66**:807.

Mackay CR. Migration pathways and immunologic memory among T lymphocytes. *Semin Immunol* 1992, **4**:51.

Mackay CR, Marston W, Dudler L. Altered patterns of T cell migration through lymph nodes and skin following antigen challenge. *Eur J Immunol* 1992a, **22**:2205.

Mackay CR, Marston W, Dudler L. Naive and memory T cells show distinct pathways of lymphocyte recirculation. *J Exp Med* 1990 **171**:801.

Marshall CJ. Specificity of receptor tyrosine kinase signaling: transient versus sustained extracellular signal-regulated kinase activation. *Cell* 1995, **80**:179.

Mayadas TN, Johnson RC, Rayburn H, Hynes RO, Wagner DD. Leukocyte rolling and extravasation are severely compromised in P-selectin-deficient mice. *Cell* 1993, **74**:541.

Michie CA, McLean A, Alcock C, Beverley PCL. Lifespan of human lymphocyte subsets defined by CD45 isoforms. *Nature* 1992, **360**:264.

Moskophidis D, Lechner F, Pircher H, Zinkernagel RM. Virus persistence in acutely infected immunocompetent mice by exhaustion of antiviral cytotoxic effector T cells. *Nature* 1993, **362**:758.

Mossmann TR, Coffman RL. T_H1 and T_H2 cells: different patterns of lymphokine secretion lead to different functional properties. *Ann Rev Immunol* 1989, **7**:145.

Mossman TR, Cherwinski H, Bond MW, Giedlin MA, Coffman RL. Two types of murine helper T cell clone. I. Definition according to profiles of lymphokine activities and secreted proteins. *J Immunol* 1986, **136**:2348.

Mustelin T, Coggeshall KM, Altman A. Rapid activation of the T cell tyrosine protein kinase p56[lck] by the CD45 phosphotyrosine phosphatase. *Proc Natl Acad Sci USA* 1989, **86**:6302.

Ostergaard HL, Shackelford DA, Hurley TR, Johnson P, Hydman R, Sefton BM, Trowbridge IS. Expression of CD45 alters phosphorylation of the *lck*-encoded tyrosine protein kinase in murine lymphoma T cell lines. *Proc Natl Acad Sci USA* 1989, **86**:8959.

Paul WE, Seder RA. Lymphocyte responses and cytokines. *Cell* 1994, **76**:241.

Picker LJ, Butcher EC. Physiological and molecular mechanisms of lymphocyte homing. *Ann Rev Immunol* 1992, **10**:561.

Picker LJ, Kishimoto TK, Smith CW, Warnock RA, Butcher EC. ELAM-1 is an adhesion molecule for skin-homing T cells. *Nature* 1991, **349**:796.

Pingel JT, Thomas ML. Evidence that the leukocyte common antigen is required for antigen-induced T lymphocyte proliferation. *Cell* 1989, **58**:1055.

Powrie F, Mason DW. The MRC OX-22⁻ CD4⁺ T cells that help B cells in secondary immune responses derive from naive precursors with the MRC OX-22⁺ CD4⁺ phenotype. *J Exp Med* 1989, **169**:653.

Prasad KVS, Janseen O, Kapeller R, Raab M, Cantley LC, Rudd CE. Src-homology 3 domain of protein kinase p59[fyn] mediates binding to phosphatidylinositol 3-kinase in T cells. *Proc Natl Acad Sci USA* 1993, **90**:7366.

Rayter SI, Woodrow M, Lucas SC, Cantrell DA, Downward J. p21[ras] mediates control of *IL-2* gene promoter function in T cell activation. *EMBO J* 1992, **11**:4549.

Romagnani S. Human T_H1 and T_H2 subsets: doubt no more. *Immunol Today* 1991, **12**:256.

Romagnani S. Lymphokine production by human T cells in disease states. *Ann Rev Immunol* 1994, **12**:227.

Rudd CE, Janssen O, Cai Y-C, da Silva AJ, Raab M, Prasad KVS. Two-step TCRζ/CD3-CD4 and CD28 signaling in T cells: SH2/SH3 domains, protein tyrosine and lipid kinases. *Immunol Today* 1994, **15**:225.

Schreiber SL, Crabtree GR. The mechanism of action of cyclosporin A and FK506. *Immunol Today* 1992, **13**:136.

Schwartz RH. Co-stimulation of T lymphocytes: the role of CD28, CTLA-4 and B7/BB1 in interleukin 2 production and immunotherapy. *Cell* 1992, **71**:1065.

Scott P. IL-12: initiation cytokine for cell-mediated immunity. *Science* 1993, **260**:496.

Shahinian A, Pfeffer K, Lee KP, Kundig TM, Kishihara K, Wakeham A, Kawai K, Ohashi PS, Thompson CB, Mak TW. Differential T cell co-stimulatory requirements in CD28-deficient mice. *Science* 1993, **261**:609.

Shimizu Y, Newman W, Tanaka Y, Shaw S. Lymphocyte interactions with endothelial cells. *Immunol Today* 1992, **13**:106.

Shimizu Y, Shaw S, Graber N, Gopal TV, Horgan KJ, van Seventer GA, Newman W. Activation-independent binding of human memory T cell to adhesion molecule ELAM-1. *Nature* 1991, **349**:799.

Siegel JN, Klausner RD, Rapp UR, Samelson LE. T cell antigen receptor engagement stimulates c-raf phosphorylation and induces c-raf-associated kinase activity via a protein kinase C-dependent pathway. *J Biol Chem* 1990, **265**:18472.

Sieh M, Bolen JB, Weiss A. CD45 specifically modulates binding of Lck to a phosphopeptide encompassing the negative regulatory tyrosine of Lck. *EMBO J* 1993, **12**:315.

Sprent J. T and B memory cells. *Cell* 1994, **76**:315.

Springer TA. Traffic signals for lymphocyte recirculation and leukocyte emigration: the multistep paradigm. *Cell* 1994, **76**:301.

Straus DB, Weiss A. Genetic evidence for the involvement of the Lck tyrosine kinase in signal transduction through the T cell antigen receptor. *Cell* 1992, **70**:585.

Straus DB, Weiss A. The CD3 chains of the T cell antigen receptor associate with the ZAP-70 tyrosine kinase and are tyrosine phosphorylated after receptor stimulation. *J Exp Med* 1993, **178**:1523.

Tan P, Anasetti C, Hansen JA, Melrose J, Brunvard M, Bradshaw J, Ledbetter JA, Linsley PS. Induction of alloantigen-specific hyporesponsiveness in human T lymphocytes by blocking interaction of CD28 with its natural ligand B7/BB1. *J Exp Med* 1993, **177**:165.

Ucker DS. Tails of phosphorylation and T cell activation. *Curr Biol* 1994, **4**:947.

van der Merwe PA, Brow MH, Davis SJ, Barclay AN. Affinity and kinetic analysis of the interaction of the cell adhesion molecules rat CD2 and CD48. *EMBO J* 1993, **12**:4945.

van der Merwe PA, McNamee PN, Davies EA, Barclay AN, Davis SJ. Topology of the CD2-CD48 cell adhesion molecule complex: implications for antigen recognition by T cells. *Curr Biol* 1995, **5**:74.

Weiss A. T cell antigen receptor signal transduction: a tale of tails and cytoplasmic protein tyrosine kinases. *Cell* 1993, **73**:209.

Weiss A, Littman DR. Signal transduction by lymphocyte antigen receptors. *Cell* 1994, **76**:263.

Xu H, Littman DR. A kinase-independent function of Lck in potentiating antigen-specific T cell activation. *Cell* 1993, **74**:633.

9 B Cell Activation and Maturation

The human bone marrow produces 10^{10}–10^{11} B cells per day and many of these cells have a very short life span. Resting B cells undergo a complex series of events on their way to being induced to grow and then to differentiate into antibody-secreting plasma cells. This process involves an activation stage, followed by proliferation of the cell which subsequently differentiates.

CD5+ B CELLS

This chapter will focus on activation and maturation of conventional B cells but we should mention another interesting subset of B cells, marked by the CD5 antigen (Ly-1 in the mouse) which may be a ligand of CD72. CD5 is also expressed on most thymocytes and all T cells. CD5+ B cells express some classical B cell markers, such as IgM, a low level of IgD and MHC class II antigens, and do not express T cell markers. Murine Ly-1+ B cells reside primarily in the peritoneal cavity, comprising nearly half of the lymphocytes there. Human CD5+ B cells are quite rare in adults but are found in the spleens and peripheral blood of healthy individuals as well as umbilical cord blood. CD5+ B cells have been associated with the pathology of autoimmune disease and they produce many of the IgM autoantibodies.

CD5+ B cells may have a distinct precursor origin and, therefore, represent a separate lineage of B cells which appear early in ontogeny. Transplantation of murine bone marrow cells into irradiated recipients failed to regenerate the Ly-1 B cell subset. However, these cells could be transferred by grafting cells of the murine foetal omentum (connective tissue between folds of the gut), indicating that the Ly-1 B cell lineage is capable of self-regeneration in recipient mice. CD5+ B cells are the earliest cells to repopulate the host after human bone marrow transplantation, indicating that precursor cells capable of regenerating this subset reside in the bone marrow as well as the gut in humans. V gene usage of CD5+ B cells also differs markedly from other B cells in that only a limited number of germline *IGHV* gene segments is used, again indicating separate lineages. The receptors on CD5+ B cells tend to bind more than one ligand and show a preference for bacterial polysaccharides. CD5+ B cells may play a role at an early phase in infection by providing immunity to common bacterial antigens.

ACTIVATION

Early activation can proceed by two different mechanisms, one that requires contact with Th cells, T-dependent, and one that is T-independent. T-independent antigens include polyclonal B cell activators, such as bacterial cell surfaces.

For T-dependent antigens, binding of antigen allows the B cell to take up selectively and process the antigen for presentation to T cells (see Chapter 8).

Since multimeric T-independent antigens can directly activate B cells and this activation can be mimicked by antibodies to surface Ig, it is clear that the Ig receptor transmits activation signals to the cell. The initial step of activation usually involves binding of antigen to membrane forms of the B cell antibody (mIg). These surface Ig receptors are of the IgM and IgD isotype in cells which have not yet switched to other isotypes. As with T cells, other surface molecules can also transmit signals under experimental conditions, although their physiological involvement is not always clear. They include signals delivered by Th cells or by macrophages. The cell must integrate the various surface signals and translate them into an appropriate biological response, including entry into the cell cycle, proliferation and differentiation to secrete antibody. According to the strength of signals from mIg, as well as from other co-receptors, the B cell interprets its environment and responds accordingly. It has to make a value judgement on whether an antigen is noxious or not. It has also been appreciated recently that maintenance of cell survival is an important regulatory step in B cell activation.

mIg-mediated activation signals leading to gene activation

Polyclonal or monoclonal antibodies to IgM or IgD, coupled to a solid phase such as Sepharose beads, will trigger B cells into proliferative cycle (*Fig. 9.1*). Some soluble antibodies will also activate, although they need to be in the F(ab')$_2$ form to avoid negative signals mediated by Fc receptors (see below). The importance of mIg cross-linking is evident from the inability of monomeric Fab fragments to elicit activation signals. This requirement and many of the biochemical events are similar to those of T cells triggered via the TCR/CD3 complex (see Chapter 8). The receptor complexes on both B cells and T cells consist of hetero-oligomeric structures in which ligand binding and signal transduction are facilitated by sets of distinct receptor subunits. In the case of the B cells, the ligand binding portion of the receptor is surface (membrane) immunoglobulin (mIg), the tetrameric complex of heavy (H) and light (L) chains. The transducing portion consists of disulphide-linked heterodimers of Ig-α and Ig-β (now CD79a and CD79b, the products of the *mb-1* and *B29* immunoglobulin superfamily genes).

The mechanism of activation via CD79a and b is now understood in some detail. These structures interact with several cytosolic protein tyrosine kinases, triggering activation cascades that eventually reach the nucleus. Reth identified sites on CD79a and b that mediate receptor interactions with

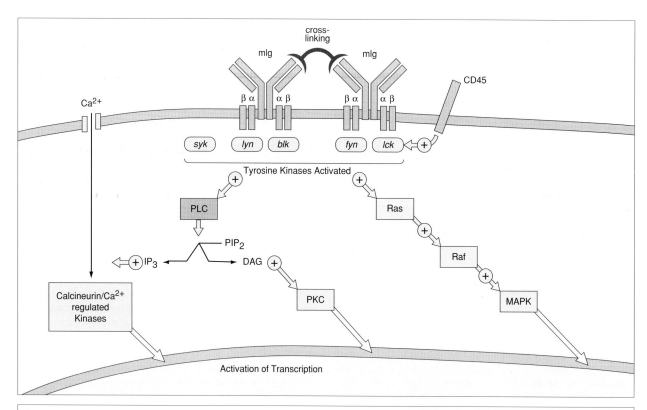

Fig. 9.1 Crosslinking of surface immunoglobulin is communicated to the nucleus. Membrane Ig (mIg) is complexed to CD79a and b (Ig-α and Ig-β) which activate signalling cascades such as the phospholipase C (PLC) cleavage of phosphatidyl inositol (4,5) bisphosphate (PIP$_2$) to inositol (1,4,5) triphosphate (IP$_3$) and diacylglycerol (DAG). Inositol trisphosphate (IP$_3$) releases Ca^{2+} ions from intracellular stores, increasing Ca^{2+} concentration and activating calcium/calcineurin-dependent protein kinases. Diacylglycerol activates α, β, and δ isoforms of protein kinase C. The small G-protein Ras GTP-binding protein is activated, resulting in activation of Raf, leading to other protein kinase signalling cascades being activated, especially mitogen-activated protein kinase (MAPK). These are driven by recruitment of signal transducers like GTPase-activating protein (GAP). A further level of control is obtained through appropriate tyrosine phosphatases, such as CD45, which plays a role in both B and T cell activation. CD45 is a receptor-like glycoprotein and is the predominant protein tyrosine phosphatase in the cell membrane. It is found on all haematopoietic cells and in the case of B cell activation it is known to augment the activation of receptor-associated kinases. It may do this by removing an inhibitory phosphate from kinases.

The primary signal may be the activation of the mIg-associated tyrosine kinase *syk*, resulting in activation of a *src*-related tyrosine kinase that phosphorylates the ARH1 motifs in the cytoplasmic domains of Ig-α and Ig-β. The other tyrosine kinases, such as *blk*, *fyn*, *lck* and *lyn*, are then recruited, resulting in association of signal transducers, including PLCγ with the receptor. Several substrates are phosphorylated but it is not known which kinase corresponds to which substrate. The second messenger pathways activated are similar to those for T cell activation.

Further along, transcription factors are activated. The signalling cascade involved is still not known but CaM-KII and PKC play a role. NF-κB transcription factor is regulated by PKCζ which has been activated by phosphatidylinositol (3,4,5) triphosphate (PIP$_3$). MAPK is a key regulatory element that targets protein kinases and signal transducers, as well as regulators of gene expression such as *c-jun*, *c-fos* and *c-myc*.

the cytoplasmic effectors. The chains have a sequence motif of around 26 amino acids in their cytoplasmic tails that is shared by cytoplasmic tails of other transducers including TCR, CD3 and FcR. This motif has been called ARH1, for antigen receptor homology motif 1, ARAM (antigen recognition activation motif) or TAM (tyrosine-based activation motif). It is characterized by a conserved amino acid sequence, part of which is Y– –L/I– – – – – – –Y– –L/I. The expression of ARH1 motifs fused to inert transmembrane proteins is enough to promote signal transduction events.

Phosphorylation of the two tyrosine residues is a critical event in signal transduction through these receptor-associated molecules. It has been suggested that the amino-terminal region of *src*-related tyrosine kinases binds to the tyrosine-phosphorylated CD79 component via the *src*-homology SH2 domains (*Fig. 9.1*).

The signals caused by activation of the kinases lead through a series of events to coordinated regulation of appropriate signal transduction events. A further level of control is obtained through appropriate tyrosine phosphatases such as CD45.

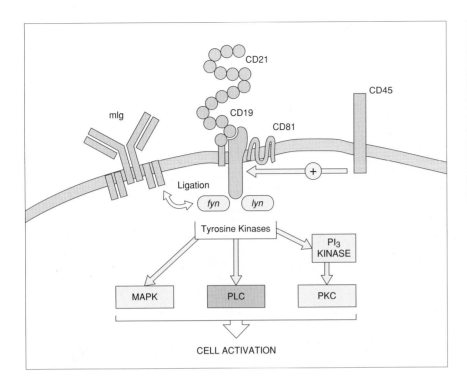

Fig. 9.2 Modulation of B cell stimulation through the CD19 complex. Binding of ligands to CD21 activates tyrosine kinases *lyn* and *fyn* which in turn amplify signalling cascades. Note that PI 3'-kinase is involved in membrane trafficking in yeast. It could have a function in activated B cells of stimulating transport of mIg plus antigen to vesicles for loading onto class II molecules.

Several substrates are phosphorylated but it is not known which kinase corresponds to which substrate. The second messenger pathways activated are similar to those for T cell activation and, ultimately, transcription factors are activated (*Fig. 9.1*).

MODULATION OF RESPONSES

In addition to mIg, stimulation of B cells is amplified by other surface interactions, including CD23 on follicular dendritic cells. The ligand for CD23, on the B cell surface, consists of at least three proteins (*Fig. 9.2*). These include a complex of CD21 (also known as CR2, complement receptor), CD81 (a serpentine protein that crosses the membrane several times) and CD19. The tyrosine kinase, *lyn*, is associated with the long cytoplasmic tail of CD19. When CD21 docks with CD23, phosphatidylinositide 3'-kinase (PI 3-kinase) is activated by CD19. Other kinases of the *src* and *syk* family are recruited as well as phospholipase C (PLC) to amplify the signal, effectively lowering the threshold of antigen stimulation required for B cell activation. Like CD79α and β, CD19 is a substrate for CD45.

The CD21 molecule may be able to change the threshold for signalling upon binding an activated complement component, C3d. This complement fragment interacts with antigen (Ag) so that the combination of C3d–Ag brings together two independent receptors, CD21 and mIg, increasing activation signalling. This strategy causes the cell to react more vigorously in the case of an infection, when a noxious antigen is present. Increased immune stimulation may be achieved by immunizing with antigen coupled to C3d.

Other participants in B cell activation include CD22 and C-type lectins CD23 and CD72. CD23 and CD72 are type II integral membrane proteins which, on ligation, can transduce a signal to the cell interior. Their predicted amino acid sequences indicate that they are both members of a large family of proteins, the Ca²⁺-dependent animal lectins. The hallmark of these lectins is a domain containing six cysteine along with certain other characteristic residues with a set spacing. CD23 and CD72 may also contain a leucine zipper motif which could promote oligomerization at the cell surface. CD72 forms a disulphide-linked homodimer. CD23 is distributed on restricted subsets of B cells. Two CD23 products, CD23a and b, formed by differential splicing, may have different signalling functions. CD72 is found on most B cells and is lost only on terminal differentiation to plasma cells.

CD23 appears to interact with IgE and CD21 as counterstructures but may be quite promiscuous with respect to ligands. Triggering can take place through either molecule with univalent antibody, suggesting that soluble ligands may exist for these lectins. This observation is consistent with other experiments which show that CD23 is necessary for IgE-dependent augmentation of immune responses. CD5 is the ligand of CD72 although others may exist. Both CD23 and CD72 can act as signalling molecules.

The physiological role of CD22 has not been established. It may act as an adhesion molecule, binding proteins with sialylated carbohydrate groups, possibly as a receptor for CD45RO. CD22 appears to modulate antigen receptor signalling by lowering the threshold of antigen stimulation required for activation. This occurs by recruiting additional *src* family and *syk* family tyrosine kinases, PLC and PI 3-kinase to amplify the signals generated by mIg. Only CD22⁺ cells can signal via the B cell receptor. CD22 may have an important role in germinal centres, where it has a high level of expression. It may have a negative role on activation unless ligated away from mIg in this environment.

T cell dependent activation

Although crosslinking of mIg provides a strong stimulatory signal, crosslinking may not be common *in vivo* except with proteins displaying repeated epitopes, such as microbial antigens. As with T cell activation (Chapter 8), B cell responses generally require two different signals to occur. Antigens that require T cell help to activate B cells are called thymus-dependent antigens and, in the absence of activating signals from appropriate Th cells, B cells that encounter such antigens may become anergic. Stimulation is helped by T cells which recognize antigen, endocytosed on the appropriate surface immunoglobulin receptor and presented on the surface of the B cell through MHC class II molecules. The T cells provide additional stimulation through co-stimulatory surface molecules and through the release of cytokines.

CD40 AND CD40L

One of the most important surface interactions between the B cell and its T cell helper is through CD40, on the B cell surface, and its ligand CD40L on the T cell. CD40 is expressed throughout the B cell lineage. Antibodies to CD40 stimulate B cells and this activation is enhanced by the presence of cofactors such as IL-4. CD40L is a membrane molecule with homology to the TNF family of cytokine receptors. It is expressed transiently after activation of almost all CD4+ T cells.

Depending on the circumstances, ligation of CD40 can result in a variety of responses including driving cells into cycle, rescuing germinal centre cells from apoptosis and promoting Ig isotype switching. Insight into the function of CD40 was provided by studying individuals defective for CD40L, suffering from the X-linked hyper-IgM syndrome (HIM). The B cells of these patients fail to switch class and are capable of producing only IgM antibodies, which are in the circulation at high levels. The phenotype can be imitated in mice by blocking the CD40 interaction with its ligand, using recombinant soluble CD40.

Activation via CD40 and subsequent class switching is intimately tied in with stimulation by cytokines. Upon Th stimulation, B cells exposed to IL-4 will switch to IgE and IgG4 production. IL-10 or IL-2 on the other hand leads to IgG1, IgG2, IgG3 or IgA production. CD40 is also necessary for the development of memory cells, as is discussed below in relation to germinal centres.

CD28 AND B7

B cells do not constitutively express the B7 molecule but it may be induced by agents such as bacterial lipopolysaccharides. This observation may explain the requirement for bacterial adjuvants in order to immunize efficiently with soluble antigen. The requirement of a second signal, in this case microbial infection, ensures appropriate T cell activation, through antigen-specific B cells. The B7 molecule interacts with CD28 on the T cell that is undergoing activation.

CYTOKINE-MEDIATED SIGNALS

Most of the biochemical events involved in T and B cell activation serve to take the cell out of its resting (G0) state into the G1 phase of the cell cycle. Signals derived from cytokine–receptor interactions then induce the cell to progress through the S phase and into proliferation. Some cytokines also induce differentiation events in the cell. As with many other receptor–ligand interactions, the complex formed between most cytokines and their receptors is rapidly internalized by the cell. This may involve receptor phosphorylation and could serve simply as a mechanism to dissociate the complex and recycle receptors to the cell surface or may also be involved in signalling mechanisms.

IL-4 has effects on a wide variety of cells and it has a potent effect on B cells, acting at a number of stages in their natural history. It mediates its biological response through a receptor, comprising the IL-4 binding receptor chain (IL-4R) and associated proteins. IL-4 is released in B–T cell interactions and is secreted in the border between the interacting cells so that it acts selectively on the antigen-specific target B cell at the point of contact. The IL-4 receptor induces a transient activation of PLC, followed by the generation of cyclic AMP (cAMP). The receptor is also involved in protein tyrosine kinase (PTK)-mediated activation of PI 3-kinase. IL-4-mediated regulation of gene expression appears to involve the Janus family of kinases JAK1 and JAK3 which mediate tyrosine phosphorylation of signal transducers and activation of transcription (STATs), such as IL-4 nuclear activated factor (IL-4 NAF) and other signal transducing factors.

Cytokines also play an essential role in regulating Ig isotype expression and IL-4 is important for switching to IgE and IgG4 (see below).

T-independent activation

Antigens which can stimulate B cells without the help of T cells are called thymic-independent. These antigens include many microbial products such as polymeric proteins and polysaccharides. One group of antigens, the B cell mitogens, can stimulate the growth and differentiation of B cells without regard to their antigen specificity, a process known as polyclonal activation. This takes place when B cells are exposed to relatively high levels of mitogens. At low concentrations, antigen-specific B cells are activated but they arise earlier than T-dependent responses and do not require priming and prior expansion of Th cells. The response to mitogens is presumably required to initiate a rapid defence against certain extracellular pathogens.

Bacterial polysaccharides, displaying repeated epitopes, are largely also thymus-independent but do not stimulate immature B cells. They probably act by crosslinking mIg, and B cell responses to this class of molecule are rapid and specific. Polysaccharides are a feature of the coats of encapsulated bacteria which are resistant to ingestion by phagocytes, unless coated by a layer of antibody. The best known of these is lipopolysaccharide, a major component of the membrane of Gram-negative bacteria. The non-polyclonal activators include highly repetitious antigens such as repeating polysaccharide structures or protein polymers which crosslink the B cell receptors. Those that do not crosslink normally require cytokines for activation to proceed as far as cell proliferation. The importance of this kind of response is illustrated by the immunodeficiency disease called the Wiskott–Aldrich syndrome. Individuals with this

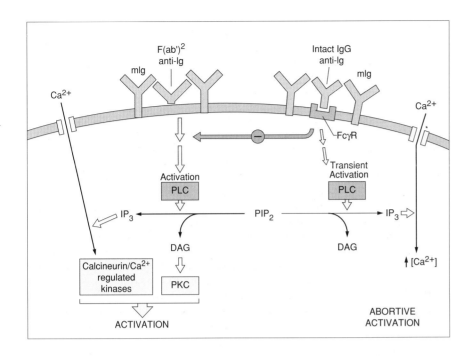

Fig. 9.3 Negative signalling via Fcγ receptor on B cells. F(ab')₂ anti-Ig antibodies can mimic antigen-mediated crosslinking of B cell mIg and activate the cell (*Fig. 9.1*). Intact anti-Ig, on the other hand, may mimic the feedback regulation induced by Ag–Ab complexes by co-crosslinking mIg to FcγR. This results in brief PLC activity, producing enough IP₃ to mediate a normal rise in [Ca²⁺]. In the absence of other signals this leads to abortive activation. The negative signal also blocks activation by F(ab')₂ anti-Ig (left).

condition fail to make antibody to polysaccharide antigens but respond normally to protein immunization. A major function of CD5⁺ B cells may be to provide anti-polysaccharide antibody.

Other modulatory interactions

ACTIVATION MARKERS

Surface expression of various markers characterizes different stages of B cell activation. These include transferrin receptors which are induced within 4 hours of activation of resting B cells with LPS or F(ab')₂ anti-Ig antibodies. This marks the transition of the cells into the G1 phase of the cell cycle. T–B collaboration results in expression of CD23 on B cells after 16–20 hours. This is probably mediated by the production of IL-2 and/or IL-4 by the T cells, since either of these cytokines can upregulate CD23 expression on B cells. IL-4 also upregulates class II expression.

NEGATIVE SIGNALS

As well as activating a cell, signals generated through antigen receptors can elicit negative signals which downregulate the response or render the cell incapable of responding to subsequent stimuli which would normally activate it. Negative signals play an important regulatory role in enabling a cell to return to its quiescent state following removal of activating signals. The induction of a state of unresponsiveness *in vivo* is important in the generation and maintenance of tolerance to self-antigens.

Evidence exists that generation of cAMP, in both T and B cells, through the activity of adenylyl cyclase, provides an off signal serving to downregulate the cell's effector and proliferative responses. Cholera toxin activates adenylyl cyclase by ADP-ribosylation of G proteins, causing prolonged cAMP production. Adenylyl cyclase is a plasma membrane bound enzyme which can be linked to receptors via stimulatory or inhibitory G proteins. There is some evidence that cAMP works by inhibiting Raf activation, although it is also likely to affect cell regulation through other mechanisms.

FCR DOWNREGULATION

The feedback regulation of murine antibody responses by specific antibodies of the IgG isotype has been demonstrated in many experiments. The effect is mediated by binding to Fcγ receptors (FcγR) on B cells (*Fig. 9.3*). These receptors can bind IgG of the G1, G2a and G2b subclasses. Co-crosslinking of FcγR to mIg on the B cell by IgG–Ag complexes or IgG anti-Ig antibodies delivers a negative signal to the B cell. Thus, while F(ab')₂ anti-Ig antibodies elicit a strong proliferative response, intact IgG antibodies, conversely, block the response to F(ab')₂ antibodies. Both forms of anti-Ig antibody elicit comparable increases in MHC class II expression and induce entry of the cell into the G1 phase.

Both intact and F(ab')₂ anti-Ig antibodies initially elicit comparable levels of inositol (1,4,5) triphosphate (IP₃) but after about 30 seconds the response to intact antibody rapidly wanes while that induced by F(ab')₂ antibodies is prolonged. Intact IgG antibody also blocks prolonged phosphatidylinositol (4,5) bisphosphate (PIP₂) hydrolysis induced by F(ab')₂ antibodies. This has been shown to be mediated by the FcγR through the use of specific antibodies to this receptor. The short-term production of IP₃ is sufficient to generate rises in Ca²⁺ comparable to those produced with F(ab')₂ and will elicit enhanced class II expression at the cell surface. More recently it has been shown that co-crosslinking FcγR to mIg uncouples the mIg receptor from its G protein, preventing transmission of activation signals. Thus, in B cells as in T cells, provision of a Ca²⁺ signal in the absence of other signals leads to abortive activation.

Thus the function of FcγR on B cells seems to be the inhibition of B cell activation and antibody production when the concentration of IgG antibodies increases and reaches a level high enough to bring together membrane Ig and FcγR. Inhibition of B cell activation can also be achieved by soluble FcγR which downregulates Ig production driven by antigen as well as lipopolysaccharide. In contrast to FcγR, the other FcR molecule CD23 (FcεRII) is involved in enhancement of activation on the B cell. It may do this by mediating the endocytosis of antigen bound to IgE and subsequently influencing release of cytokines. In addition, there is evidence that FcεR may aid activation by interacting with membrane components different to IgE.

Transcriptional control

As B cell development proceeds proteins involved in transcription of immunoglobulin are produced. E32 and Oct-2 appear early in development and are involved in transcription of Ig heavy chain. NF-κB appears at the pre-B cell stage and is required for light chain transcription. NF-κB is activated by the proteolytic cleavage of an associated molecule, IκB by the 26S proteasome, a cytoplasmic proteolytic complex (see Chapter 8). Degradation of IκB exposes nuclear localization signals on NF-κB and allows it to move to the nucleus where it is involved in the transcription of a number of genes. All B cell activators at the pre-B cell stage may work through the activation of NF-κB which has been likened to an immune system 'master switch'. Interestingly, genes homologous to NF-κB have been found in *Drosophila*. Transcription of other important B cell development genes, such as *RAG-1* and *RAG-2*, required for Ig gene rearrangement, takes place at later stages of development.

Within 15–30 minutes of B cell activation via mIg there is increased expression of the proto-oncogenes *c-fos* and *c-myc* which play a role in the proliferative response. In mice, mRNA for an early growth factor inducible gene (*Egr-1*) is rapidly upregulated by mIg crosslinking. This gene codes for a putative DNA binding protein with a zinc finger structure typical of some other transcription control proteins. Within 1–2 hours there is an increase in mRNA for class II molecules. The increased expression of class II at the cell surface serves to enhance the cell's ability to present antigen to T cells. It may also enhance the level of class II-mediated cAMP production which in turn inhibits the initial proliferative response and helps promote differentiation to antibody production.

B CELL MATURATION

Following the initial interaction between virgin B cells and antigen, usually in the presence of specific T cells, IgM antibody is produced from germline gene sequences. The ability of the immune response to adapt to combat different types of infection and other antigenic challenges is determined by the further differentiation of B cells to produce selectively antibodies of high affinity and of different isotypes. After isotype switching IgG and IgA are the predominant isotypes along with a small contribution from IgE. The mechanisms of class switching and affinity maturation lead to the production of a selected population of memory B cells which are ready to respond effectively to subsequent antigenic encounters.

Germinal centres

Antigen-activated B cells settle in lymphoid follicles where they proliferate to form germinal centres and it is in these structures that hypermutation events are triggered. Germinal centre B cells can be isolated on the basis of their avid binding to peanut agglutinin (PNA).

The formation of germinal centres is an antigen-dependent process which also requires T cell help. Three distinct phases can be identified:

- Resting follicles, initially consisting of a network of follicular dendritic cells (FDCs, see Chapter 8) with small recirculating B cells, begin to accumulate B cell blasts. These fill the spaces within the FDC network, apparently forcing the small B cells to the edge where they form the follicular mantle.
- After about 2 days, B blasts differentiate into mIg-negative centroblasts which accumulate at one pole of the follicle, adjacent to, but not in, the FDC network; this is termed the 'dark zone' in histological sections. The number of B cell blasts decreases and the FDC network fills up with non-cycling cells called centrocytes. Many of these centrocytes die *in situ* by apoptosis. These dying cells which are continually replaced by the pool of rapidly dividing centroblasts, represent B cells which have undergone somatic hypermutation but which do not produce antibody of high enough affinity to be triggered by antigen trapped within the FDC network. Isolated centrocytes can be rescued from cell death by triggering them *in vitro* with anti-Ig coated sheep erythrocytes; this is thought to mimic the *in vivo* process of antigen selection. Anti-CD40 antibodies can also rescue centrocytes from their programmed death. Expansion and escape of activated high affinity cells requires T cell help.
- The germinal centre reaction declines 2–3 weeks after antigen challenge, as plasma cells and memory B cells leave but B cell blasts can still be found in the FDC network for several months.

Thus the germinal centre appears to be the critical site for the generation of higher affinity mutants by somatic mutation and their selective activation by antigen. The many dying centrocytes are phagocytosed by macrophages within the follicle. These are called 'tingible body' macrophages since they can be seen to contain phagocytosed apoptotic bodies.

The molecular mechanisms involved in selecting centrocytes with suitable antigen binding receptors result in the interaction of CD23 with the CD21 component of the B cell-expressed CD19 complex (*Fig. 9.4*). Binding of this complex in conjunction with antigen-occupied surface immunoglobulin enhances centrocyte activation. Such cells are induced to express the *bcl-2* gene. Cells which have lost the ability to bind antigen strongly fail to express *bcl-2* and are eliminated by apoptosis. In some respects this process parallels the selection of thymocytes, although B cells are

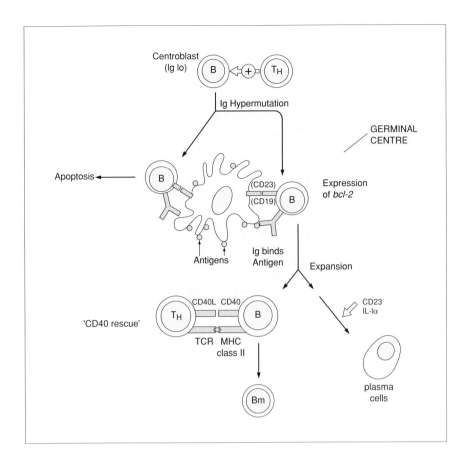

Fig. 9.4 Control of B cell activation and maturation in germinal centres. Activated B cells enter the germinal centre (top) and undergo Ig hypermutation. If they fail to encounter appropriate antigen the B cells come out of cell cycle and die by apoptosis. Engagement of antigen, by contrast, results in expression of *bcl-2*, preventing apoptosis, and permitting clonal expansion. Cells then interacting with CD40L on Th cells become long lived memory cells. Other cells, under the influence of CD23 and IL-1α become Ig-secreting plasma cells, which live for several weeks. Not all FDCs express CD23.

selected by response to foreign antigen and not during ontogeny. B cells that have bound antigen and escape apoptosis leave the germinal centre. They may then become antibody secreting plasma cells, a process which is dependent on signals received from CD23 and IL-1α. Cells activated by CD23 and cytokines secrete antibodies in large quantities. They become terminally differentiated plasma cells with a finite life span so that antibody responses eventually wane. They can no longer be influenced by Th cells since they lack surface class II and Ig.

Cells leaving germinal centres that encounter CD40L have a different fate and become memory B cells. The CD40L is expressed by T cells around the edge of the germinal centres. This CD40L is preformed and stored in cytoplasmic granules. Surface expression is elicited very rapidly by B cells presenting antigenic peptides. The CD40L/CD40 interaction also induces *bcl-2* expression, saving these cells from the default program of apoptosis. Further information on apoptosis in relation to cytotoxicity is in Chapter 15.

Class switching

During the course of a primary response, individual B cells can switch the Ig isotype they produce while retaining the same recombined *V* region and, thus, antigen specificity. Class switching is thought to occur either as a result of somatic gene recombination within the heavy chain locus or by a variety of post-transcriptional processing events.

SWITCH RECOMBINATION

Ig constant region genes (except *IGHD*) have switch regions (S) 1–4kb upstream of the first *IGHC* exon which play a role in directing the recombination of the *V* region to a *C* region downstream of that in current use (*CM* in freshly activated virgin B cells). The recombination process appears to involve 'looping out' of the intervening DNA between the *V* region and the chosen downstream *C* region, involving the alignment of similar sequences within the appropriate *S* regions (*Fig. 9.5*) The *S* region sequences are multimers (up to 150 tandem repeats) of a sequence of the form $(GAGCT)_nGGGGT$, where n = 1–7. Following alignment of the two *S* regions, endonuclease cleavage and religation processes produce a recombined heavy chain locus and a 'switch circle' of DNA containing the deleted *IGHC* genes. Switch circles have been isolated from LPS-activated murine B cells but it is not yet known how long they persist following recombination or whether they can be transcriptionally active.

Isotype switching is preceded by changes in the chromatin structure of the DNA around the switch sequences of recombining *IGHC* regions that lie 5' to each *IGHC* gene. The regions become hypomethylated and hypersensitive to DNase; they are also thought to be more accessible to the actions of enzymes and proteins involved in recombination (the switch recombinase). Analysis of a panel of B cell hybridomas revealed that of those with rearrangements on both alleles about 60% had rearranged to the same or neighbouring *IGHC* gene. This indicates

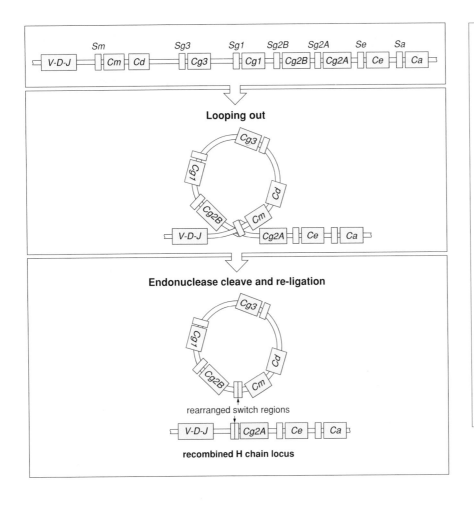

Fig. 9.5 Immunoglobulin class switch rearrangement. The germline configuration of the Ig heavy chain locus is shown at the top, with *Cm* as the nearest C-region downstream of the recombined variable (*IGHV-D-J*) gene. With the exception of *Cd*, each *C* gene is preceded by a switch region (*S*). The diagram illustrates the process for switching from IgM to IgG2a. Such class switch rearrangements involve looping out and endonuclease cleavage within recombining *S* regions. Religation then joins the DNA 5' of the breakpoint in *Sm* to that 3' of the breakpoint in *Sg2A* to produce a recombined heavy chain locus lacking *Cm*, *Cg3*, *Cg1* and *Cg2B*. The excised DNA is also religated to form a switch circle containing the deleted *C* region genes and a recombined *S* region. Modified from von Schwedler *et al*, 1990.

that switching mechanisms are not necessarily restricted to alleles bearing a functionally rearranged *V* region. As discussed below, cytokine-promoted transcriptional activity of *IGHC* genes on the non-functional allele could also play a role in class switching.

THE ROLE OF CYTOKINES IN SWITCHING

Cytokines such as IL-4, IL-5 and IFNγ can promote the production of distinct Ig isotypes. In some cases this has been shown to be due to the ability of the cytokine to direct class switching mechanisms to the appropriate *IGHC* genes. Thus, IL-4 promotes switching to IgG1 and IgE and IFNγ promotes switching to IgG2a. Although IL-5 promotes IgA synthesis it does not trigger the switch to this isotype. Transforming growth factor β (TGFβ) triggers switching to *CA* and IgA production whilst suppressing the production of other isotypes (*Fig. 9.6*). Thus the secretion of cytokines largely accounts for the known T cell dependence of Ig class switching. Signals delivered by cell-cell contact are also important, primarily in the first stages of B cell differentiation into plasma cells.

To date, cytokine-promoted switching to a number of different murine isotypes has been shown to follow a general pattern involving transcriptional activation of the appropriate *IGHC* gene regions, with the production of sterile germline transcripts, prior to the recombination events depicted in *Figure 9.7*. Similar events probably also occur in human isotype switching. One of the best analysed systems has been the IL-4 induced switching to IgG1 and IgE in LPS-activated murine B cells. For IgE, IL-4 appears to act via a specific response element upstream (*IL-4RE*) which has strong homology to a sequence in the H-2A^k MHC class II gene. Although the precise role of this site is not known, the activity of IL-4 appears to make the *SG1* and *SE* regions accessible to RNA polymerase II activity which in turn leads to the production of CH transcripts lacking IGHV-D-J coding sequences. For IgG1 but not IgE, this production of short transcripts can occur in response to IL-4 alone; LPS stimulation is required for productive switch recombination and synthesis of new isotype. The production of germline C$_\varepsilon$ transcripts by B cells in response to LPS plus IL-4 is illustrated in *Figure 9.7*. Primary germline transcription is initiated from a promoter upstream of *SE* which is thought to influenced by the 5' *IL-4RE*. The major transcript contains a small sequence coded for by a region called *Ie* which is located about 2kb 5' to *SE* in the germline configuration of the heavy chain locus. Similar sites, Iγ2b and Iα, are found in Cγ2b and Cα germline transcripts, respectively, although these do not share significant homology with one another. Because these transcripts lack *IGHV-D-J* sequences, they are detected as truncated RNA species by the relevant *IGHC* gene probes. In the case of IgE, the transcript cannot code for a protein because *Ie* has termination codons in all three reading frames.

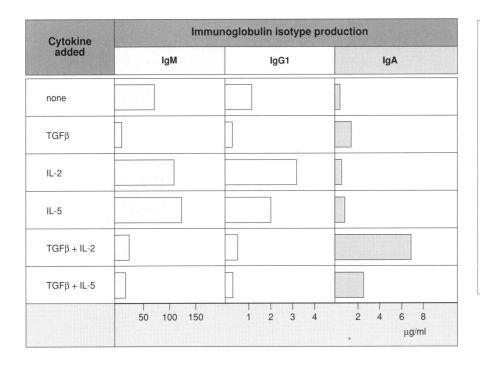

Cytokine added	Immunoglobulin isotype production		
	IgM	IgG1	IgA
none			
TGFβ			
IL-2			
IL-5			
TGFβ + IL-2			
TGFβ + IL-5			
	50 100 150	1 2 3 4	2 4 6 8 µg/ml

Fig. 9.6 Transforming growth factor-β promotes IgA responses. LPS-stimulated murine B cells produce IgM and IgG1, but no IgA. Addition of TGFβ to the culture markedly inhibits the release of IgM and IgG1, but promotes IgA synthesis. This production of IgA has been shown to involve class switching of surface IgA⁻ cells and is markedly enhanced by IL-2 and, to a lesser degree, IL-5. Neither of these cytokines alone has marked effects on LPS-stimulated B cell Ig secretion. Based on data of Coffman *et al*, 1989.

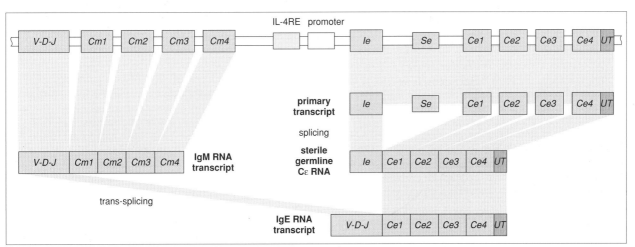

Fig. 9.7 Production of sterile germline *CE* transcripts in response to IL-4 and their possible use in IgE production. Murine B cells respond to IL-4 in the presence of LPS by producing IgE. This process involves the initial production of *Ce* transcripts lacking a variable region, but possessing an additional 5' sequence called *Ie*. Transcription initiated at *Ie* in response to IL-4 is thought to be mediated through an IL-4 response element upstream of the *Ie* sequence, and proceeds to produce a primary transcript containing *Ie*, *Se* and *Ce*, including the 3' untranslated region (UT). This is then spliced to remove the introns, including *Se*, bringing *Ie* adjacent to *Igh-c1*. Following this early transcriptional activity, DNA recombination events may follow to complete a genetic switch to IgE (not shown, but see *Fig. 9.5*). It is not yet clear whether germline *Igh-c* transcripts can be used for Ig production (as suggested here) or whether they are merely a useless byproduct of the increased accessibility of the *S* region to both recombinase and DNA polymerase enzymes. Since *Ie* has stop codons in all three reading frames, this transcript cannot yield a protein product directly, but it could theoretically be spliced to a V-region RNA sequence (such as that in an IgM RNA transcript shown here) to produce mRNA coding for IgE antibody. Such a mechanism might account for the production of IgE (and other isotypes) without the deletion of upstream *Igh-c* genes. Based in part on observations of Gerondakis, 1990 and Rothman *et al*, 1990.

It is not yet clear if the production of germline transcripts is merely an irrelevant consequence of the increased accessibility of the *S* region which is itself necessary for the initiation of switch recombination, or whether the transcripts themselves are functionally important (see below). A current working hypothesis is that cytokines, such as IL-4, regulate the transcriptional activity of recombination enhancing elements located near the *IGHC* gene (such as *Ie*, perhaps), which alters the local chromatin structure in such a way as to allow access to a recombinase enzyme system. Activation of the B cell, as with LPS, would be required for the expression of the recombinase. That activation of the recombinase system is regulated separately from the production of germline transcripts has been indicated by studies of cell lines with an introduced artificial S region recombination substrate. A cell's ability to recombine the introduced substrate did not correlate with switching of endogenous genes; however, switching did correlate with production of the appropriate germline transcripts.

SWITCHING WITHOUT *IGHC* GENE RECOMBINATION

Although genetic switch recombination may be the major mechanism for triggering the expression of mature Ig isotypes (IgG, IgA and IgE classes), the detection of 5' switch revertants *in vitro* implies that other mechanisms can be used. A number of alternative routes are possible and may even dominate in certain situations. Some B cells have been found to generate RNA transcripts which hybridize to both C_μ and $C_\gamma 1$ probes. Differential use of polyadenylation sites then leads to the production of mRNA for either IgM or IgG1 but the regulation of this process is unknown. Such cells may express both Ig isotypes. It is not clear whether a similar mechanism could be used for IgE or IgA production, since this would involve the production of very long primary transcripts which have not yet been detected. A special case of dual isotype production is the co-expression of surface IgM and IgD in mature B cells. This is also thought to occur by alternate splicing of RNA containing V_H-D-J_H, C_μ and C_δ. However, although secretion of IgD is rare, when it occurs it may involve switch recombination to the *CD* locus, even though this gene does not have a defined switch region. Homologous recombination between DNA sequences 5' to *CM* and *CD* is thought to be involved in this case.

Studies of a number of murine CD5[+] B cell lines and Epstein Barr virus (EBV)-transformed human B cell lines have shown that they are capable of producing IgG subclasses, IgA or IgE, without switch recombination; they remain surface IgM positive. For some cells, this may represent an intermediary stage of switch commitment prior to switch recombination, while for others it represents a means of transiently producing mature isotypes. Since CD5[+] B cells are long lived and are thought to recognize a limited set of microbial antigens (see below), it might be advantageous for them to be able to produce different isotypes without an irreversible commitment. It has been suggested that this route to class switching is the main one used for human IgE production.

A number of hypotheses have been put forward to explain the production of mRNA for mature isotypes without a rearrangement of heavy chain locus, although no direct evidence has yet been obtained for any of them. Trans-splicing of sterile germline C_H gene transcripts (produced in response to cytokines) to RNA containing V_H-D-J_H sequences may occur as depicted for IgE in *Figure 9.7*. Although it is more likely that the germline transcripts are usually derived from the same allele as the

V_H-D-J_H sequence, it is possible that they could also be produced by transcriptional activity of *IGHC* genes on the non-productively rearranged chromosome.

Affinity maturation

As an immune response progresses, there is an overall increase in the affinity of the antibodies produced; this is termed affinity maturation. It was originally thought that the increase in antibody affinity was due to the selective outgrowth of B cells with high affinity antigen receptors, since these would be selectively re-triggered by the diminishing antigen concentrations. Although the recruitment of B cells of high germline affinity can occur, the major mechanism for increasing antibody affinity appears to be one of somatic mutation of germline V regions followed by selective activation of cells with higher affinity.

Somatic hypermutation

Analyses of antibodies produced by B cells during the course of an immune response have shown that mutations are generated in the rearranged *V-D-J* sequences. Antibodies produced during the initial phases of a primary response use germline *V* regions but as the response progresses increasing numbers of mutations in the *V-D-J* regions are found. In secondary and hyperimmune responses almost all hybridomas have mutations. The data suggest that an ongoing process of somatic mutation and antigen selection leads to the accumulation of mutations and a stepwise increase in antibody affinity. Apparently random changes are introduced into the heavy and light chain genes and occasionally one such change leads to an increase in the affinity of the antibody. These high affinity variants are then selected to enter the pool of memory cells.

The most informative experiments so far have come from analysis of murine responses to simple haptens since a limited number of germline genes contribute. For example, in an anti-oxazolone antibody response the first 6–7 days saw usage of unmutated germline genes. In the second week somatic mutations rapidly accumulated in expressed H and L chain genes. One such sequence had 13 replacement mutations compared to the germline sequence and approximately 100-fold higher affinity for the antigen. Recent studies of splenic antibody mRNA, taken at different times after antigenic challenge, have confirmed these observations. This process of affinity maturation does not necessarily act upon the antibodies which dominate a primary response. For example, the primary response to phosphorylcholine is dominated by antibodies that express an idiotype called T15 and use a specific combination of heavy and light chains. However, the secondary response to this antigen is largely derived by somatic mutation of initially lower affinity germline sequences, producing antibodies that do not express the T15 idiotype.

Mutations which are generated at a very high rate (about 10^{-3} per base pair per generation) are found predominantly within the *V-D-J* region and the immediate 5' and 3' flanking regions. Recombinant *V-J* or *V-D* sequences seem to be the major target, since *D-J* regions in non-productively rearranged genes accumulate far fewer mutations. The chromosomal location of *V-D-J* sequences does not seem to be important for somatic mutation to operate, since randomly inserted germline Ig transgenes have also been found to mutate. The mutation mechanism was thought to be linked to class switching but this is not the case because mutations also occur in IgM antibodies and class switching can occur without somatic mutation. Hypermutation is triggered only during the proliferation of activated B cells and appears to be a transient phenomenon that is turned off as the B cell matures. This termination of somatic mutation mechanisms may be linked to class switching; it has been suggested that DNA sequences between *CM* and downstream *IGHC* genes are somehow involved in promoting mutation and that deletion of these sequences by class switching terminates the process. It is not clear if hypermutation events can be reactivated by antigen, although the accumulation of mutations during secondary and tertiary responses suggests they can.

The majority of mutations are due to single base changes although in rare cases deletion, insertion and gene conversion events have been described. Although both replacement and silent mutations are spread over the entire *V* region, replacement mutations tend to accumulate in the complementarity determining regions (CDRs). This is probably as a result of antigen selection for increased antibody affinity (see below). Mutational hot-spots have also been described in a few antibodies but vary in position from one case to the next and do not provide any clues to the mutational mechanism. Once mutations are fixed in the CDRs, non-destructive mutations may continue to accumulate in the framework regions. It has been estimated that 25–50% of mutations produce a range of structurally nonfunctional antibodies. Possible defects include an inability to associate or traffic correctly in the cell, susceptibility to proteolysis, or an inability of the membrane form to bind antigen or transmit activation signals. An example of such a destructive mutation has been described: a glycine to arginine substitution in codon 15 of the mouse λ2 chain prevents antibody secretion.

The mechanisms involved in generating somatic point mutations are thought to involve DNA repair mechanisms. Two models of mutation, based on error-prone repair and repair of mismatches in misaligned templates, are illustrated in *Figure 9.8*. Although there is circumstantial evidence in favour of both these models, it is not yet known how these processes can be selectively targeted to rearranged variable genes and do not operate on nearby *IGHC* genes. Strand selectivity of region mutations may ensure that only half of the cell's progeny carry the mutation. Further progress in unravelling the mechanisms of somatic hypermutation will require B cell lines capable of mutating in culture. An Abelson murine leukaemia virus-transformed pre-B cell line which undergoes *V* region hypermutation has been described but the rate (10^{-5} per base pair per generation) is substantially lower than that estimated to occur *in vivo*. That *V-D-J* sequences in T cells do not undergo somatic hypermutation may provide a clue to help elucidate the process. The role of somatic mutation in the generation of diversity is discussed in Chapter 4.

Clonotype selection and affinity maturation

Generation of mutations in *V-D-J* regions alone would not account for the phenomenon of affinity maturation. A process capable of selectively activating and expanding B cells producing higher affinity antibodies must also operate. In the first few days of a T-cell dependent response, activated B cells are first located in the T cell rich areas of the peri-arteriolar sheath (PALS) of the spleen. A little later, as mentioned above, antigen-activated B cells settle in lymphoid follicles where they proliferate to form germinal centres and it is in these structures that hypermutation events are triggered. At the height of the germinal centre reaction, antigen-specific hybridomas can be generated only from PNA+ B cells isolated from spleens of immunized mice. Analysis of such hybridomas produced at day 10 of the response to phenyl oxazolone revealed that the *V* region mutations differed from those seen at day 14 since about 65% were silent (i.e. did not alter the encoded amino acid). This has been interpreted to indicate that by day 10 the mutation mechanism has been activated but antigen selection of useful mutations has not yet occurred.

A potential danger of using somatic mutation to generate receptor repertoires of higher affinity is that autoreactive antibodies are likely to be generated. An example is the generation of an anti-DNA antibody from a T15 idiotype-bearing, anti-phosphorylcholine antibody by mutation of a single amino acid, Glycine, at residue 35 for an Alanine. Similar mutations almost certainly occur during a normal immune response but most autoreactive B cells probably die at the centrocyte stage due to lack of appropriate T cell help. The primary antibody response may favour localization of antigen on FDCs whereas many autoantigens will not be available in the follicle. Localization of complexes to germinal centres is important in development of the secondary response. However, autoantibodies found in autoimmune strains of mice, such as those against the nuclear antigen Sm, are thought to be derived from antibacterial antibodies by somatic mutation.

MEMORY B CELLS

A memory B cell is defined as an mIg-expressing cell which has been selected by T cell-dependent antigen-driven proliferation and somatic hypermutation and which is ready to produce a secondary immune response. The development of memory B cells is a T cell dependent process and antigens that stimulate B cells in a T-independent manner do not induce memory. T cells can influence T-independent responses (e.g. by isotype switching) but they have no effect on the generation of memory. B–T interaction is a essential for memory B cell development and the ligation of CD40 on the B cell surface is a crucial event.

Most memory B cells are thought to have undergone class switching, although this may not always involve an irreversible switch recombination of the heavy chain locus. Memory B cells are more sensitive to antigenic triggering but this is at least partly due to their higher affinity for antigen. It also seems likely that, like memory T cells,

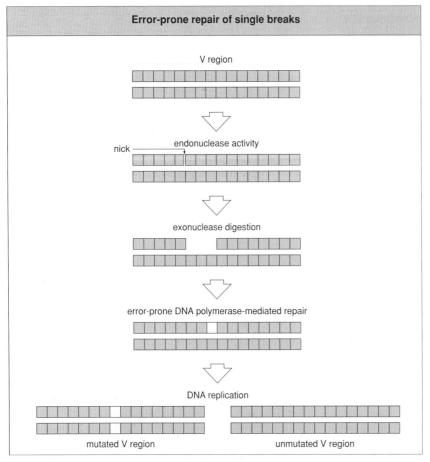

Error-prone repair of single breaks

V region

nick —— endonuclease activity

exonuclease digestion

error-prone DNA polymerase-mediated repair

DNA replication

mutated V region   unmutated V region

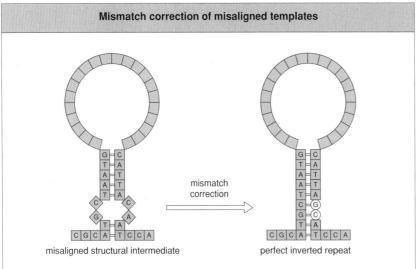

Mismatch correction of misaligned templates

mismatch correction

misaligned structural intermediate   perfect inverted repeat

Fig. 9.8 Two models of somatic mutation involving DNA repair. The process of error-prone repair of single strand DNA breaks caused by endonuclease activity is illustrated. Following nicking of the DNA, exonucleases delete several bases from the 3' end and, during repair, by a postulated error-prone DNA polymerase, base substitutions (light green) are introduced. DNA replication then copies the mutation onto both strands in one of the two daughter cells. An alternative, but not mutually exclusive, model of correction of misaligned templates is also illustrated. A conformation is adopted by imperfectly matched complementary sequences which acts as a misaligned structural intermediate used as a target for repair mechanisms. Correction of mismatched bases leads to the formation of a mutant forming a perfect inverted repeat structure.

memory B cells respond more effectively to activation signals such as antigen and T cell help. Once activated, memory B cells appear to proliferate and differentiate without somatic hypermutation mechanisms being turned on. Although successive switch recombinations have been demonstrated in B cells it is also not clear whether memory B cells are able to undergo class switching. Adoptive transfer of memory B cells into irradiated recipients

produces extensive clonal expansion and a strong antibody response to antigenic stimulation but somatic mutation and switching cannot be demonstrated.

In mice, memory B cells bear a CD45R isoform detectable by the antibody 6B2. Purification of mIgM⁻, mIgD⁻, 6B2⁺ cells enriches for IgG producing memory B cells; these are very efficient APCs and secrete antibody only following presentation to T cells or in the presence of antigen and T cell derived cytokines (a 'bystander response'). Such B cell populations are found in the recirculating B cell pool and in the static B cells of the marginal zones of the spleen.

Recent observations indicate that B cells producing antibody in the primary response are derived from precursors distinct from those of memory B cells. These are distinguishable by the level of expression of the surface marker recognized by the antibody J11D. Thus, B cells bearing high levels of J11D (J11D^{hi}) appear to represent primary virgin cells, whereas J11D^{lo} cells (only 10–15% of B cells in immunized mice) are memory cell precursors. As shown in *Figure 9.9*, J11D^{lo} B cells elicit very weak primary responses to antigen on transfer into immunodeficient mice along with specific Th cells but develop into memory cells capable of producing a strong secondary response. J11D^{hi} cells, on the other hand, elicit vigorous primary responses but little or no secondary response. Primary responses to the hapten nitrophenol (NP) are dominated by λ light chain bearing antibodies whereas the secondary response is dominated by κ-bearing antibodies. In accordance with this observation, J11D^{lo} memory precursor cells have a higher frequency of κ-chain producers. This implies that the two populations have different *V* region clonotypes. It seems likely that the J11D^{lo} population is the one that undergoes somatic hypermutation. In support of this is the observation that although J11D^{lo} B cells are not susceptible to tolerance induction, 2–5 days after activation a further interaction with their antigen in the absence of specific T cell help (e.g. with hapten coupled to the wrong carrier protein) blocks the generation of secondary B cell responses. This may reflect a model for the normal antigen-driven selection of somatically mutated B cells in germinal centres.

CD5$^+$ B cells persist for long periods of time without changing their receptor repertoire by somatic mutation. After the first few weeks of life, no more CD5$^+$ B cells are generated from mIg$^-$ precursors; the presence of CD5$^+$ B cells appears to block further differention, whereas conventional B cells are continually produced from mIg$^-$ precursors.

Maintenance of memory

Immunological memory is extremely long lived, lasting for the lifetime of the individual without further obvious antigen exposure. The mechanisms involved in the maintenance of memory B and T cells for these long peiod of time are still a matter of controversy. Two main hypotheses have been put forward:

- Memory is due to the generation of long lived resting memory T and/or B cells.
- Memory T and B cell populations are maintained by a continuous process of stimulation, recruitment and selection.

In cell transfer experiments, using syngeneic irradiated recipients, the ability to mount a memory B cell response persists for only a few weeks if the recipient is not challenged with antigen. Hapten-specific B cell blasts can be found in secondary lymphoid follicles for several months after antigen exposure. There is now strong evidence that antigens retained, in immune complexes, by the FDC network (see Chapter 7) provide a persistent stimulus for B cells, thus maintaining the memory population. The FDCs are capable of trapping and storing antigens for over a year. In addition, exposure to environmental antigens, including viruses, bacteria and other parasites, could provide intermittent immune stimulation through cross-reacting epitopes such as the highly conserved heat-shock proteins.

B cells from primed mice can respond to lower doses of antigen and the antibody they produce is generally of higher affinity. They express higher levels of class II than naive B cells to enable them to muster T cell help by antigen presentation. The antibody these B cells produce is generally of the mature IgG type. At each cycle of immunization somatic mutation of antibody sequences takes place.

SUMMARY

In many respects, B cell activation is similar to that of T cells. Engagement of surface receptor, mIg, results in a cascade of signals involving protein kinases from the membrane to the nucleus. The transducers of the signals from the membrane receptor consist of a 'sheath' of two proteins, CD79α and β. Another stimulus is obtained from CD45, a membrane-associated phosphatase. The signals are modulated by further sets of membrane molecules, including CD19, CD21 and CD81.

Activation may or may not require the help of T cells. T-dependent B cells become anergic unless they receive T cell help. An important component of such help is the engagement of the CD40 molecule on the B cell via CD40L on the T cell surface. Additional signals are provided by cytokines. T-independent antigens include bacterial polysaccharides which crosslink surface Ig. These antigens do not induce isotype switching or memory B cells. When levels of circulating Ig are high, B cell activation is downregulated by engagement of Fc receptors.

Activated T-dependent B cells proliferate and then differentiate as changes to the antibody molecules they produce take place. Germinal centres form the focus for B cell stimulation and maturation. B cells with high affinity receptors are selected in these organized foci of cells. The antibody isotype can change and somatic hypermutation results in apoptosis if antigen binding is lost. Cells expressing antibody with increased affinity for the antigen on follicular dendritic cells are selected in the germinal centre follicles. This process is controlled by Th cells which secrete cytokines that induce isotype switching.

Memory B cells express mIg which has already undergone somatic hypermutation. These cells provide a rapid, heightened response to previously encountered antigens. Memory may be maintained by the persistence of antigen in immune complexes in the follicular dendritic cell network.

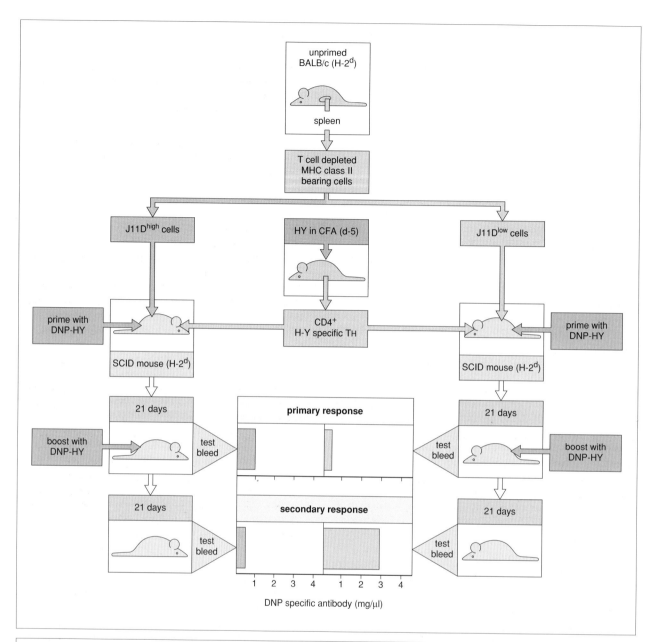

Fig. 9.9 Two separate precursor B cells generate primary and secondary responses in mice. T cell depleted, class II positive spleen cells purified from naive mice were separated into two populations on the basis of their level of expression of the J11D surface marker. These cells were transferred into mice with severe combined immunodeficiency (SCID) (a lack functional T and B cells), along with purified Th cells primed to the antigen haemocyanin (HY). The mice were challenged with the hapten dinitrophenyl (DNP) coupled to HY. The levels of anti-DNP antibodies in the blood were then monitored by radioimmunoassay as a measure of the primary response. After 21 days, the mice were boosted with the same antigen and the body levels again monitored to measure the secondary response. Only the results obtained 21 days after priming or 21 days after boosting are shown. In this experiment, J11D^{hi} cells produced a good primary response but a very poor secondary response. In marked contrast, J11D^{lo} cells elicited only a weak and somewhat transient primary response, but a strong (and prolonged) secondary response characteristic of memory B cells. Based on data of Linton *et al*, 1989.

FURTHER READING

Alt F, Marrack P (Eds). Lymphocyte activation and effector function. *Curr Opin Immunol* 1993, **5**:313.

Alt F, Marack P (Eds). Lymphocyte activation and effector function. *Curr Opin Immunol* 1994, **6**:355.

Banchereau J, Rousset F. Human B lymphocytes: phenotype, proliferation and differentiation. *Advan Immunol* 1992, **52**:125.

Berek C, Ziegner M. The maturation of the immune response. *Immunol Today* 1993, **14**:400.

Bergstedt-Lindqvist S, Moon HB, Persson U, Moller G, Heusser C, Severinson E. Interluekin-4 instructs uncommitted B lymphocytes to switch to IgG1 and IgE. *Eur J Immunol* 1988, **18**:1073.

Berton MT, Uhr TW, Vitetta ES. Synthesis of germline γ1 immunoglobulin heavy chain transcripts in resting B cells: induction by interleukin-4 and inhibition by interferon γ. *Proc Natl Acad Sci USA* 1989, **86**:2829.

Brines R. B cell special. *Immunol Today* 1994, **15**:393.

Burkhardt AL, Costa T, Misulovin Z, Stealy B, Bolen JB, Nussenzweig MC. Ig-α and Ig-β are functionally homologous to the signaling proteins of the T-cell receptor. *Mol Cell Biol* 1994, **14**:1095.

Callard RE, Armitage RJ, Fanslow WC, Spriggs MK. CD40 ligand and its role in X-linked hyper-IgM syndrome. *Immunol Today* 1993, **14**:599.

Callard RE, Turner MW. Cytokines and Ig switching: evolutionary divergence between mice and humans. *Immunol Today* 1990, **11**:200.

Cambier JC, Ransom JT. Molecular mechanisms of transmembrane signalling in B lymphocytes. *Ann Rev Immunol* 1987, **5**:175.

Charbonneau M, Tonks NK, Walsh KA, Fisher EH. The leukocyte common antigen CD45. A putative receptor-linked protein tyrosine phosphatase. *Proc Natl Acad Sci USA* 1988, **85**:7182.

Clark EA, Ledbetter JA. Leukocyte cell surface enzymology: CD45 LCA, T200 is a protein tyrosine phosphatase. *Immunol Today* 1989, **10**:225.

Coffman RL, Lebman DA, Shrader B. Transforming growth factor β specifically enhances IgA production by lipopolysaccharide-stimulated murine B lymphocytes. *J Exp Med* 1989, **170**:1039.

DeFranco AL. Structure and function of the B cell antigen receptor. *Ann Rev Cell Biol* 1993, **9**:377.

Ehlich A, Schaal S, Gu H, Kitamura D, Muller W, Rajewsky K. Immunolgobulin heavy and light chain genes rearrange independently at early stages of B cell development. *Cell* 1993, **72**:695.

Esser C, Radbruch A. Rapid induction by transcription of unrearranged sg1 switch regions in activated murine B cells by interleukin-4. *EMBO J* 1989, **8**:483.

Esser C, Radbruch, A. Immunoglobulin class switching: molecular and cellular analysis. *Ann Rev Immunol* 1990, **8**:717.

Farrington M, Grosmaire LS, Nonoyama S, Fischer SH, Hollenbaugh D, Ledbetter JA, Noelle RJ, Aruffo A, Ochs HD. CD40 ligand expression is defective in a subset of patients with common variable immunodeficiency. *Proc Natl Acad Sci USA* 1994, **91**:1099.

Finkelman FD, Holmes J, Katona IM, Urban JFJ, Beckmann P, Park L, Schooley KA, Coffman RL, Mosmann TR, Paul WE. Lymphokine control of *in vivo* immunoglobulin isotype selection. *Ann Rev Immunol* 1990, **8**:303.

Fish S, Zenowich E, Fleming M, Manser T. Molecular analysis of original antigenic sin. I. Clonal selection, somatic mutation and isotype switching during a memory B cell response. *J Exp Med* 1989, **170**:1191.

French DL, Laskov R, Scharff MD. The role of somatic hypermutation in the generation of antibody diversity. *Science* 1989, **244**:1152.

Frietas AA, Rocha BB. Lymphocyte lifespans: homeostatis, selection and competition. *Immunol Today* 1993, **14**:25.

Gerondakis S. Structure and expression of murine germ-line immunoglobulin epsilon heavy chain transcripts induced by interleukin-4. *Proc Natl Acad Sci USA* 1990, **87**:1581.

Gold MR, Defranco AL. Biochemistry of B lymphocyte activation. *Advan Immunol* 1994, **55**:221.

Gray D, Skarvall H. B cell memory is shortlived in the absence of antigen. *Nature* 1988, **336**:70.

Hardy RR, Hayakawa K. CD5 B cells, a foetal B cell lineage. *Advan Immunol* 1994, **55**:297.

Harnett MM, Klaus GGB. G-protein regulation of receptor signalling. *Immunol Today* 1988, **9**:315.

Hartley SB, Cooke MP, Fulcher DA, Harris AW, Cory S, Basten A, Goodnow CC. Elimination of self-reactive B lymphocytes proceeds in two stages: arrested development and cell death. *Cell* 1993, **72**:325.

Hoyos B, Ballard DW, Bohnlein E, Siekevitz M, Green WC. Kappa B-specific DNA binding proteins: role in the regulation of human interleukin gene expression. *Science* 1989, **244**:457.

Irsch J, Irlenbusch S, Radl J, Burrows PD, Cooper MD, Radbruch AH. Switch recominbation in normal IgA1+ B lymphocytes. *Proc Natl Acad Sci USA* 1994, **91**:1323.

Janeway CA, Golstein P. Lymphocyte activation and effector functions. *Curr Opin Immunol* 1993, **5**:313.

Kishihara K, Penninger J, Wallace VA, Kundig TM, Kawai K, Wakeham A, Timms E, Pfeffer K, Ohashi PS, Thomas ML, Furlonger C, Paige CJ, Mak TW. Normal B lymphocyte development but impaired T cell maturation in CD45-Exon 6 protein tyrosine phosphatase-deficient mice. *Cell* 1993, **74**:143.

Klaus GGB, Bijsterbosch MK, O'Garra A, Harnett M, Rigley KP. Receptor signalling and cross-talk in B lymphocytes. *Immunol Rev* 1987, **99**:19.

Kocks C, Rajewsky K. Stable expression and somatic hypermutation of antibody V regions in B cell differentiation. *Ann Rev Immunol* 1989, **7**:537.

Lassoued K, Nunez CA, Billips L, Kubagawa H, Monteiro RC, LeBien TW, Cooper MD. Expression of surrogate light chain receptors is restricted to a late stage in pre-B cell differentiation. *Cell* 1993, **73**:76.

Lenardo MJ, Baltimore D. NF-κB: A pleiotropic mediator of inducible and tissue-specific gene control. *Cell* 1989, **58**:227.

Linton PJ, Decker DJ, Klinman NR. Primary antibody forming cells and secondary B cells are generated from separate precursor cell subpopulations. *Cell* 1989, **59**:1049.

Machamer CE, Cresswell P. Biosynthesis and glycosylation of the invariant chain-associated HLA-DR antigens. *J Immunol* 1982, **129**:1564.

MacLennan ICM, Chan E. The dynamic relationship between B cell populations in adults. *Immunol Today* 1993, **29**:29.

MacLennan ICM, Liu Y-J, Joshua DE, Gray D. *The production and selection of memory B cells in follicles.* Berlin: Springer-Verlag; 1989.

Marx J. Cell communication failure leads to immune disorder. *Immunol* 1993, **259**:896.

Moller GE. Germinal centres in the immune response. *Immunol Rev* 1992, **126**:1.

Moller GE. The B cell antigen receptor complex. *Immunol Rev* 1993, **132**:5.

Parker DC. T cell-dependent B cell activation. *Ann Rev Immunol* 1993, **11**:331.

Patel KJ, Neuberger MS. Antigen presentation by the B cell antigen receptor is driven by the αβ sheath and occurs independently of its cytoplasmic tyrosines. *Cell* 1993, **74**:939.

Rajewsky K. B cell lifespans in the mouse — why to debate what? *Immunol Today* 1993, **14**:40.

Rothman P, Chen YY, Lutzker S, Li SC, Stewart V, Coffman R, Alt FW. Structure and expression of germline immunoglobulin heavy chain epsilon transcripts: interleukin-4 plus lipopolysaccharide-directed switching to Cμ. *Mol Cell Biol* 1990, **10**:1672.

Snapper CM, Mond JJ. Towards a comprehensive view of immunoglobulin class switching. *Immunol Today* 1993, **14**:15.

Swain SL, Reth M. Lymphocyte activation and effector functions. *Curr Opin Immunol* 1994, **6**:355.

Brines R (Ed). B cell signalling special. *Immunol Today* 1994, **15**:393.

van Rooijen N. Direct intrafollicular differentiation of memory B cells into plasma cells. *Immunol Today* 1990, **11**:154.

von Schwedler U, Jack HM, Wabl M. Circular DNA is a product of the immunoglobulin class switch rearrangement. *Nature* 1990, **345**:452.

10 Cytokines and Chemokines

Cytokines are mediators of short range signals between cells. They control the growth differentiation, effector function and survival of cells. They comprise families of molecules such as interleukins, lymphokines, monokines, growth factors, interferons and chemokines. The signals they transmit are transduced via specific receptors on target cells. Interleukins were defined as molecules that transmitted signals between leukocytes, monokines as products of monocytes which affected lymphocytes and lymphokines as soluble mediators generated following lymphocyte activation. As many of these molecules also influence non-lymphoid cells the term cytokine is probably more appropriate. Cytokines manifest an incredible array of biological effects which frequently overlap. A key feature of many of these molecules is their pleiotropy and redundancy. This latter feature has been exemplified by gene deletion experiments as very few cytokines appear to be essential for cellular activity. It would seem that under these conditions of genetic loss of a cytokine certain key roles can be compensated for by another cytokine. In adult animals, however, removal of a cytokine by means of a specific antagonist or antibody can have profound effects.

In vivo the activity of most cytokines is usually restricted to those cells in the immediate vicinity of release and clearly only those expressing the relevant receptors. Because of the pleiotropic effects of many of the cytokines a limitation of spread is of obvious biological value. Several cytokines bind to elements of the extracellular matrix and this together with the presence of soluble receptors ensures restriction of action to local sites.

STRUCTURE OF THE CYTOKINES AND THEIR RECEPTORS

The complete characterization of many of the cytokines has made it possible to classify them according to structure, biological activity and the structure of their receptor (*Fig. 10.1*). The structural motifs identified in cytokines are displayed in *Figure 10.2*. This grouping based on structure also relates to biological function of the cytokines in a fairly broad sense. The cytokine receptors can also be subdivided into groups as they complement the cytokine structural groups. An example of such a family group is given in *Figure 10.3*. The presence of shared subunits in some cytokine receptors may contribute to the observed pleiotropy in cytokine activity (*Figs. 10.1, 10.3* and *10.4*). With regard to signal transduction via many of these receptors the cytokine facilitates the necessary aggregation of receptor subunits. Such subunit association initiates signal transduction events.

Chemokines are small molecular weight molecules many of which act in the inflammatory response as chemoattractants. They therefore are important in innate immunity and the recruitment and activation of neutrophils, eosinophils and macrophages. On the basis of sequence usage around the conserved cysteines (C-X-C or C-C) the chemokines have been divided into two groups (see Chapter 14).

Most of the cytokines with a 4-α-helical structure bind to a receptor with a ligand binding domain called a haemopoietin domain. The interferons (IFNs) bind to an IFN receptor domain. Although the sequences of these two domains are not similar it is thought that they give rise to a similar tertiary structure. The receptors for these cytokines are heterodimers with a ligand binding unique chain with no catalytic activity and a shared common chain bearing intracellular domains necessary for signal transduction. Thus IL-2, 4, 7, 9 and IL-13 have a specific receptor component and a shared γ-chain subunit. In the case of IL-4, 7 and IL-13 the specific receptor component is a homodimer but in the case of IL-2 it is a heterodimer comprising an α (p55 or Tac antigen) and β (p70) subunit (*Fig. 10.5*). Signal transduction is mediated by the common subunits. IL-3, 5 and GMCSF bind to an α-subunit with low affinity and the generation of a high affinity receptor capable of signal transduction is accomplished by the interaction with the common β-chain.

Cytokine structure	Receptor class	Shared chain	Cytokine
4-α-helical short chain	haemopoietin domain	common γ	IL-2, IL-4, IL-7, IL-9, IL-13, IL-15
4-α-helical short chain	haemopoietin domain	common β	IL-3, IL-5, GM-CSF
4-α-helical short chain	IFN-γR		IFNγ
4-α-helical long chain	haemopoietin domain	gp130	IL-6, IL-11
β-sheet	serine/threonine kinase		TGFβ
β-sheet	Ig-like		IL-1α, IL-1β
β-sheet	TNFR p75, p55		TNFα, TNFβ, CD40L, CD27L, FASL

Fig. 10.1 Structural groups of cytokines and receptors.

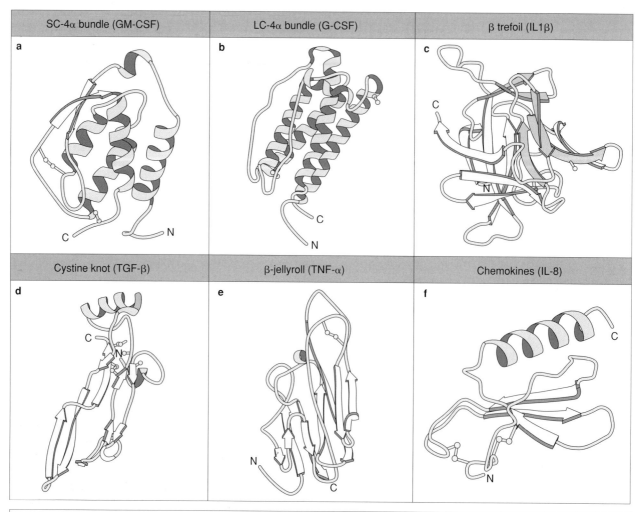

SC-4α bundle (GM-CSF)	LC-4α bundle (G-CSF)	β trefoil (IL1β)
a	b	c

Cystine knot (TGF-β)	β-jellyroll (TNF-α)	Chemokines (IL-8)
d	e	f

Fig. 10.2 The structural motifs for cytokine members of the 4-α-helical, the β-sheet and the chemokine families. (a) represents the 4-α-helical short chain structures, (b) the 4-α-helical long chain structures, (c), (d), and (e) different forms of β-sheet and (f) the chemokine structure. These structures were taken from Nicola, 1995.

IL-6 and LIF share a common receptor subunit, gp130, which mediates the signalling function of the receptor complex (*Fig. 10.6*). Following association of the IL-6/IL-6R complex to two gp130 molecules, disulphide bonded homodimerization of the two gp130 molecules takes place. Phosphorylation of gp130 occurs through tyrosine kinase activity.

The tumour necrosis factor (TNF) family of receptors is subdivided into type I and type II receptors. A key feature of this family of receptors is the presence in the extracellular region of several copies of a domain containing six cysteine residues. Some of the members of this family (p55 TNF receptor, Fas and CD40) share a cytoplasmic domain capable of transmitting cytotoxic effects (*Fig. 10.7*).

The receptors that fall into the kinase receptor family share intracellular catalytic sequences rather than extracellular domains. Some of these receptors have tyrosine kinase activity and others (e.g. TGFβ receptors) serine/threonine kinase activity. Unlike the other receptor families where the assembly of different chains is needed for receptor function many receptor kinases are single polypeptide chains which dimerize

following ligand binding. *Figure 10.6* describes the intracellular events resulting from signalling via a kinase receptor.

The chemokine receptors are G-protein coupled and differ from the other receptors by spanning the membrane seven times and displaying three extracellular and three cytoplasmic loops (*Fig. 10.8*). Following ligand–receptor interaction, G-protein associates with the cytoplasmic domain of the receptor and the G-protein α-subunit is activated, setting in train a cascade of events. In the case of IL-8/IL-8R interaction, the α-subunit of the activated G-protein in turn activates phospholipase C, generating inositol triphosphate (IP_3) and diacylglycerol (DAG). Ca^{2+} is released from intracellular stores by IP_3 and DAG activates protein kinase C.

It is not possible in this chapter to give a detailed description of the structural, functional and biological characteristics of all the cytokines and their receptors, therefore, a few selected members are described in detail which have major impact on immune function and the others have a limited description in the accompanying figures.

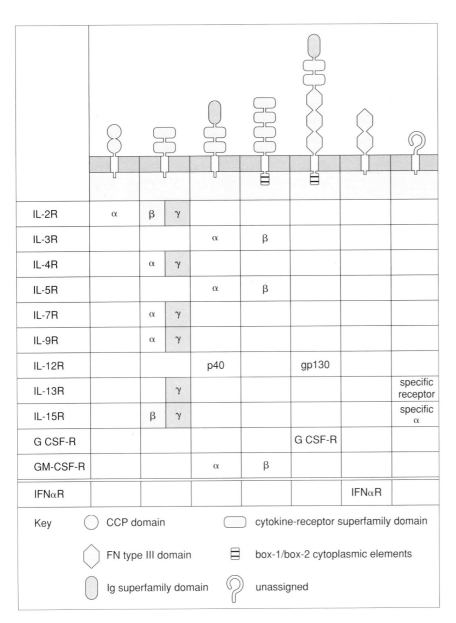

	1	2	3	4	5	6	7
IL-2R	α	β	γ				
IL-3R			α	β			
IL-4R		α	γ				
IL-5R			α	β			
IL-7R		α	γ				
IL-9R		α	γ				
IL-12R			p40		gp130		
IL-13R			γ				specific receptor
IL-15R		β	γ				specific α
G CSF-R					G CSF-R		
GM-CSF-R			α	β			
IFNαR						IFNαR	

Key:
- ◯◯ CCP domain
- ⬡ FN type III domain
- ⬭ Ig superfamily domain
- ▭ cytokine-receptor superfamily domain
- ▤ box-1/box-2 cytoplasmic elements
- ↺ unassigned

Fig. 10.3 Diagrammatic representation of members of the haemopoietin/interferon receptor family. This figure is based on that of Nicola, 1995.

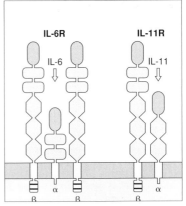

Fig. 10.4 Shared receptor subunits in the IL-6 and IL-11 receptors. Some cytokine receptors have common subunits. These may contribute to pleiotropy. Based on the study of Nicola, 1995.

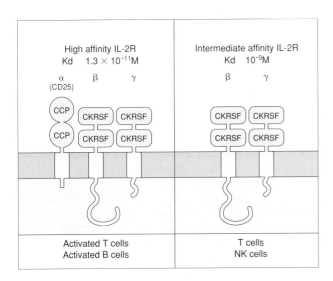

High affinity IL-2R
Kd 1.3×10^{-11}M

α (CD25)   β   γ

Activated T cells
Activated B cells

Intermediate affinity IL-2R
Kd 10^{-9}M

β   γ

T cells
NK cells

Fig. 10.5 The IL-2 receptor. The IL-2 R contains three polypeptide chains. The α-chain comprises a low affinity IL-2R. The β-chain can also bind IL-2, while the γ-chain does not. Heterodimer formation between αγ and βγ gives rise to intermediate affinity IL-2R. High affinity receptor is formed when all three chains combine to give a heterotrimer. This γ-chain is also found in IL-4R, IL-7R, IL-9R and IL-13R.

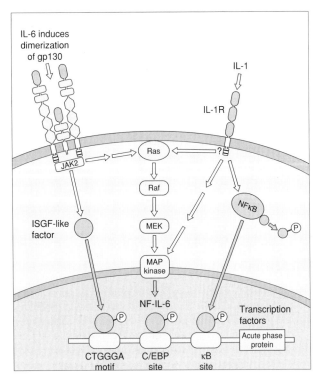

Fig. 10.6 Induction of acute phase proteins by IL-6 and IL-1. Following binding of IL-6 to IL-6R this chain associates with the signal transducing gp130 chain which itself does not bind IL-6. IL-6 binds to IL-6R with a relatively low binding affinity (K_d = 5nM) but following association with gp130 this affinity is increased (K_d = 40–70pM). Homodimerization of gp130 activates JAK2 and initiates a Ras-dependent MAP kinase cascade leading to activation of the transcription factor NF-IL6. Ligation of the IL-1R can independently activate MAP-kinase and NF-κB. NF-IL6 and NF-κB in concert with an ISGF-like factor activate the genes for acute phase proteins.

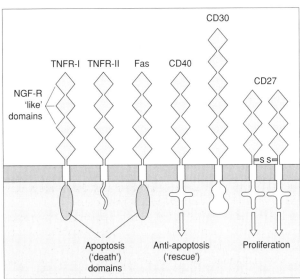

Fig. 10.7 The TNF receptor families. TNFα and β interact as homotrimers with their receptors. Other members of this receptor family include Fas, CD40 and nerve growth factor. An apoptotic domain is found in the intracellular portions of Fas, TNFRI and NGFR p75. CD40 on the other hand transmits a survival (anti-apoptotic) signal on engagement.

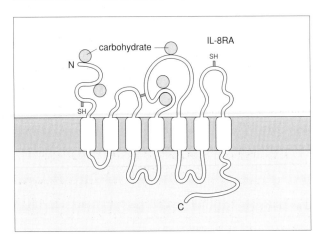

Fig. 10.8 Diagrammatic representation of the IL-8 receptor.

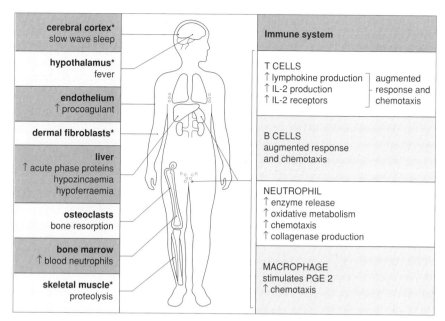

Fig. 10.9 Effects of IL-1. IL-1 acts on many different cell types and consequently may be recognized in many different bioassays. Some of the main activities are listed in the diagram. * indicates that IL-1 induces PGE2 synthesis in these cells. Some of these activities are ultimately through an effect on IL-6 release.

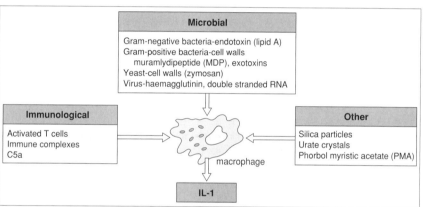

Fig. 10.10 Stimuli for IL-1 release. Cells of the mononuclear phagocyte lineage are major sources of IL-1 at sites of inflammation and immune reaction. They are induced to release IL-1 in response to the depicted stimuli.

IL-1 cytokines, receptors and receptor antagonist

Interleukin 1 has a wide range of biological activities, being produced mainly by activated macrophages and acting on many different cell types (*Fig. 10.9*). This is reflected in the great number of alternative names by which it was known before being cloned. IL-1 exists in two forms, IL-1α and IL-1β, encoded by two different genes and with limited sequence homology (20% for the human cytokine). Both forms however bind to the two IL-1 receptors and have the same biological functions. They are synthesized in precursor form which in the case of pro-IL-1β is processed by an aspartate specific protease called IL-1 converting enzyme (ICE). ICE itself has structural similarities with a nematode gene, *ced-3*, which initiates a cell death programme in *C. elegans*. It has been suggested that IL-1 may be released from macrophages during apoptosis. IL-1 production is elicited by a wide range of stimuli (*Fig. 10.10*). The IL-1 receptor antagonist (IL-1RA) has structural homology with IL-1β, is made by the same cells which make IL-1 and binds to the IL-1 receptors blocking their function. IL-1RA may play a physiological role in limiting IL-1 activity. There are two IL-1 receptors, both of which in humans bind the IL-1s and the IL-1RA and are widely distributed on a variety of cell types. However, only the type I receptor can signal and therefore the type II receptor could itself function as an IL-1 antagonist.

IL-1α and β are key inflammatory cytokines playing central roles in the immune response. These cytokines induce fever, cachexia, bone resorption, muscle proteolysis, angiogenesis and an increase in the acute phase proteins. In some cases the effects are direct, in others indirect through induction of other cytokines such as IL-6 or TNFα and in yet others through synergy with other cytokines such as GM-CSF. As IL-1 has been implicated in the pathogenesis of rheumatoid arthritis (RA) and septic shock there has been considerable interest in the development of antagonists. IL-1RA and soluble type II IL-1R are able to suppress immune responses and may be part of the normal homeostatic response to an excess of IL-1α and β.

CYTOKINES PLAYING A MAJOR ROLE IN T CELL FUNCTION

These cytokines and their characteristics are listed in *Figure 10.11*. A more detailed appraisal of their role in T cell function follows.

Cytokine	M_r(kD)	Chromosomal location		Source	Target cell	Receptor
		Murine	Human			
IL-1α	17	2	2q	macrophages	T cells, B cells macrophages and others	type I, type II both single chain
IL-1β	17	2	2q	epithelial cells	T cells, B cells macrophages and others	type I, type II both single chain
IL-2	15.5		4q	T cells	T cells, B cells NK cells	α, β, γ
IL-3	20–32	11	5q	T cells	progenitors mast cells macrophages basophils eosinophils	α, β same β as IL-5 and GM-CSF
IL-4	18–20	11	5	T cells basophils/ mast cells	T cells, B cells mast cells monocytes progenitors	single chain
IL-5	12 24 dimer	11	5	T cells mast cells	eosinophils basophils B cells	α, β same β as IL-3 and GM-CSF
IL-6	21–26	5	7p	macrophages fibroblasts, T cells mast cells	T cells, B cells hepatocytes osteoclasts	ligand binding chain + gp 130
IL-7	25	3	8q	stromal cells	T cells, pro and pre-B monocytes	single chain
IL-8	8–10	no mouse IL-8 known	17q	monocytes macrophages T cells, fibroblasts neutrophils keratinocytes endothelial cells NK cells	neutrophils T cells, B cells basophils monocytes keratinocytes endothelial cells	Type A Type B single chain
IL-9	14	13	5q	T cells	T cells, macrophages	single chain
IL-10	17–21	1	1	T cells, Ly1+B monocytes keratinocytes	B cells, T cells mast cells	single chain
IL-12	p35, 24–33? p40, 34–44	?	3p	B cells, monocytes macrophages	T cells NK cells	single chain
IL-13	9–17	11	5q	T cells	monocytes macrophages human B cells	shared receptor subunit with IL-4
IL-14	50–60	mouse IL-14 not known	?	T cells, B cell tumours, FDC	B cells	?
IL-15	14–15	?	?	monocytes epithelial cells	T cells, LAK	?
GM-CSF	20–30	11	5q	T cells macrophages endothelial cells	progenitors T cells	α, β same β as IL-3 and IL-5
IFNγ	20–25	10	12q	T cells, NK	many cell types	α, β
TNFα	17	17	6p	macrophages T cells, B cells	many cell types	Type I (p80) Type II (p60)

Fig. 10.11 Characteristics of cytokines. The major sources of cytokines with characteristics, targets and principal effects are listed. Some cytokines such as IL-1 and IL-6 have several sources and most cytokines act on more than one cell type.

IL-2

IL-2 was originally described as a T cell growth factor (TCGF) but it is now known to have activity on a variety of other cell types including NK cells, B cells, macrophages and monocytes. Additionally, it influences the growth of oligodendrocytes. The synthesis and secretion of this cytokine is triggered by activation of mature T cells. The binding of IL-2 to its high affinity receptor, either in paracrine or autocrine mode, initiates clonal expansion of activated T cells. As only activated T cells express high affinity receptors and secrete IL-2 this leads to control of T cell expansion. Expression of the *IL-2* gene is under inducible control by *cis*-acting regulatory sequences within the *IL-2* enhancer and binding sites have been identified in this region for NFAT, NF-κB, AP-1 and octamer proteins. Additionally, as with many other cytokines post-translational control is exercised over mRNA stability through an AU rich motif in the 3' untranslated region of the IL-2 message. Resting T cells express both the β and γ-chains of the IL-2R constitutively giving rise to a receptor of intermediate affinity. It is only when the α-chain combines with the other subunits that a high affinity receptor is formed with a fast rate of association ($t_{1/2}$ = 20–40s) and a slow dissociation rate ($t_{1/2}$ = 255min). Both IL-2 and IL-2Rα chain expression are tightly controlled through regulatory motifs which are absent in the β and γ-chains of the IL-2R. In the case of the α-chain the importance of NF-κB in this regulatory process is underlined by the sustained expression of α-chain in HTLV-1-induced T cell leukemias through κB transcription factor induction by the Tax transactivator protein induced by HTLV-1.

High affinity IL-2R expression is induced on B cells by IL-4 and Ig receptor binding. The activity of IL-2 on other cell types (NK, macrophages, neutrophils and LAK cells) is mainly through the intermediate affinity IL-2R.

A key role for the IL-2R γ-chain (which is also found in IL-4R, IL-7R and possibly IL-9R and IL-13R) in immune responses is highlighted by the consequences of its genetic malfunction. Mutations in the IL-2R γ-chain are responsible for X-linked severe combined immunodeficiency (SCID) in humans. In contrast mice in which the *IL-2* gene has been 'knocked out' have normal thymus and normal peripheral T cells. On certain genetic backgrounds rather than being immune deficient, genetic ablation of the *IL-2* gene resulted in the development of an autoimmune ulcerative colitis perhaps due to a failure of regulation of the immune response to a gut microorganism.

IL-4

IL-4 is produced by a subpopulation of T cells and by mast cells. Its production follows T cell activation or crosslinkage of FcεRI or FcεRII receptors on basophils or mast cells. IL-4 affects many cell types promoting the growth of T cells, B cells, mast cells, myeloid cells and erythroid progenitors. It promotes class switching in B cells to IgE and augments IgG1 production. Mice in which the *IL-4* gene has been 'knocked out' by targeted gene disruption are unable to make IgE and cannot elaborate normal levels of IgG1. IL-4 transgenic mice on the other hand express very high IgE levels. Its effect on T cell development is to drive the Th response to a Th2 type at the expense of a Th1 response. As shown in Chapter 11 (see *Fig. 11. 12*) this has a deleterious effect on the recovery of animals from *Leishmania* infection which can be corrected by administration of anti-IL-4 antibody. IL-4 blocks the differentiation of a Th0 cell to a Th1 and instead promotes differentiation of Th2 cells. Its counterbalancing cytokine is IL-12 which crossregulates IL-4. IL-4 has also been shown to initiate cytotoxic responses against tumours *in vivo* mediated by cytotoxic eosinophils and T cells. *In vitro*, it has furthermore been shown to inhibit the growth of a variety of human malignant cells.

The pleiotropic activity of IL-4 is reflected in the range of cell types which express IL-4R. This high affinity receptor is found on T cells, B cells, mast cells, myeloid cells, fibroblasts, muscle cells, neuroblasts, stromal cells, endothelial cells and monocytes.

IL-7

Interleukin 7 is produced by stromal cells and promotes the growth of T and B cell progenitors, mature T cells as well as facilitating the differentiation of both T cell progenitors and Tc cells. IL-7 also induces secretion of IL-1α, IL-1β, IL-6 and TNFα by monocytes. Its ability to enhance the generation of Tc as well as LAK cells even in the absence of IL-2 suggests that this cytokine may prove useful in tumour therapy. Removal of IL-7 *in vivo* by antibody treatment results in a profound effect on B cell precursors as well as thymocyte development underlining the influence of this cytokine on B and T cell development. On the other hand targetted expression of IL-7 to the lymphoid compartment results in elevated B and T cell numbers both centrally and in the periphery with the maintenance of a normal distribution of T cell subsets and myeloid cells.

IL-9

Interleukin 9 is produced by some activated T cells and Hodgkin's lymphoma cells. It is a T cell growth factor which acts in synergy with other cytokines. For example together with IL-2 it causes proliferation of mouse thymocytes and together with IL-4 it enhances IgE and IgG production by B cells. Its ability to stimulate directly the growth of murine T cell lymphoma cells *in vitro* suggested a link to T cell tumour development which was substantiated by the observations that IL-9 transgenic mice spontaneously develop thymomas, that IL-9 mRNA expression can be detected in lymph nodes of some lymphoma patients and the existence of an autocrine loop for the *in vitro* proliferation of a Hodgkin's lymphoma.

IL-10

Interleukin 10 has important biological effects on T cell function. It is made by Th0 and Th2 subsets of murine T cells and Ly1+B cells and its production is inhibited by IFNγ. IL-10 was called cytokine synthesis inhibitory factor because of its ability to inhibit cytokine synthesis by activated Th1 cells and NK cells. This effect on T cells is indirect, being mediated by a primary effect on macrophages.

IL-10 downregulates MHC class II expression on macrophages and inhibits LPS-induced production of IL-1, TNFα, GM-CSF and G-CSF. It also inhibits IFNγ-induced production of reactive oxygen intermediates and NO by macrophages. This suggests that IL-10 may be an anti-inflammatory cytokine which is able to downregulate Th1 responses. However, paradoxical effects of this cytokine have been seen. In transgenic non-obese diabetic (NOD) mice where IL-10 secretion is targeted to the β cell the spontaneous development of IDDM is accelerated. This may be partly because the cytokine can function as a chemoattractant and also because it can act synergistically with IL-2 and IL-7 in the proliferation of thymocytes and T cells. IL-10 also synergizes with other cytokines to stimulate proliferation of B cells and mucosal mast cells. Together with TGFβ it causes IgA production by B cells. Interestingly there is a 70% homology between IL-10 and the *BCRF1* gene of Epstein Barr virus (EBV). The implications of this for the virus are that the ability of the BCRF1 product, like IL-10, to suppress IFNγ production and macrophage activity together with its ability to increase the survival and growth of B cells may be important in the survival of this virus.

In its capacity as a modulator of macrophage activity IL-10 is able to ameliorate the effects of septic shock induced by TNFα.

IL-12

This heterodimeric cytokine manifests some effects which are almost reciprocal to those of IL-10. IL-12 is made by B cells and monocytes/macrophages and acts synergistically with IL-2 to induce IFNγ production by T cells and NK cells. It is a key factor in the development of Th1 cells stimulating both their proliferation and differentiation. It enhances the cytotoxic activity of both T cells and NK cells. This effect on NK cells may be the explanation for the ability of IL-12 to increase the survival of SCID mice infected with *Listeria monocytogenes*. The ability of IL-12 to increase NK lytic activity may have therapeutic potential as it has been shown to be able to enhance the NK activity of cells from patients immunosuppressed due to cancer or HIV infection.

IL-12 also depresses IgE production independent of its effect of increasing IFNγ production.

IL-12 is a key cytokine for directing the T cell response to that of a Th1 type. If BALB/c mice are injected with IL-12 at the time of infection with *L. major* their production of IFNγ is enhanced and concomitantly the production of IL-4 is diminished. Thus IL-12 and IL-4 are cytokines which crossregulate one another's activities. However, these effects in the case of IL-12 are seen only at early time points whereas IL-4 effects are maintained. Recent studies of Szabo *et al.* suggested that the molecular basis for these temporal differences in the influence of IL-4 and IL-12 on Th1 and Th2 responses is reflected in receptor function in the T cell subpopulations. The IL-4R and the IL-12R remain expressed and functional on Th1 cells whereas on Th2 cells functional defects in IL-12R signalling have been identified following commitment to the Th2 lineage.

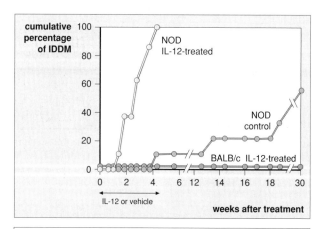

Fig. 10.12 Onset of IDDM is accelerated by IL-12. Female NOD mice aged 8–10 weeks were either injected i.p. with recombinant IL-12 or control vehicle (PBS containing 1% normal mouse serum). As a control, age-matched female BALB/c mice were injected with recombinant IL-12. Data from Trembleau *et al*, 1994.

In terms of autoimmune pathology it is clear that Th1-mediated pathologies such as IDDM will be exacerbated by this cytokine. Thus, Trembleau *et al.* have shown that administration of IL-12 to NOD mice accelerates the development of IDDM (*Fig. 10.12*).

The restricted activity of this cytokine on T cells and NK cells is reflected in the presence of the IL-12R only on those cell types.

Other cytokines are being discovered and their functional activities described. IL-15, for example, is produced by a variety of cell types, particularly epithelial cells and monocytes. Thus far it has been shown to stimulate CTL proliferation and also to facilitate their generation. This, together with its ability to enhance LAK activity, suggests a similarity to IL-2. The observation that responses to IL-15 are inhibited by IL-2Rβ chain antibody further support the functional overlap. IL-15 cannot however carry out all the functions of IL-2 as it has been shown that an IL-2 dependent cell line does not respond to IL-15. There clearly must be discrete differences between the two cytokine receptors, perhaps, the presence of a unique IL-15 binding chain associated with the IL-2Rβ subunit.

CYTOKINES ACTING ON B CELLS

The cytokines IL-1, IL-2 and IL-4 affect B cell function as well as T cell function. IL-2 stimulates the growth and differentiation of B cells. The ability of IL-4 to induce class switching in B cells has been documented above. The following section, however, deals in more detail with other cytokines having more specific effects on B cells.

IL-5

Interleukin 5 is a glycoprotein produced by activated T cells. The functional unit of activity is a disulphide

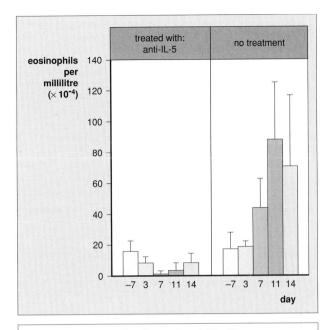

Fig. 10.13 Role of IL-5 in eosinophilia. Mice were injected with larvae of *Nippostrongylus braziliensis* at day 0, which normally induces eosinophilia (right); however, animals treated with anti-IL-5 antibody on the same day as the parasitic challenge do not develop eosinophilia (left). Control groups treated wih anti-IL-4 antibody also developed the eosinophilia.

bonded dimer. Dimerization possibly enables a higher affinity interaction with the receptor which is expressed on eosinophils, basophils and activated murine B cells. On B cells, IL-5 acts as a late acting B cell differentiation factor, playing a major role in the production of IgA. This effect on IgA synthesis may not be a primary function but the result of synergistic interactions with other cytokines such as IL-6. It has also been suggested that IL-5 induces the expression of IL-2R on B cells. However, IL-5 is perhaps better known for its effect on eosinophil differentiation (*Fig. 10.13*). It not only induces the generation of eosinophils from both human and mouse bone marrow precursors but also upregulates expression of CD11b on human eosinophils and activates IgA induced eosinophil degranulation.

T cell production of this cytokine is stimulated by parasitic infections. For example, *Trichinella spiralis* infection elicits the production of large numbers of eosinophils which is inhibitible by anti-IL-5 antibody. Transgenic mice expressing high levels of IL-5 develop an eosinophilia.

Pathologically IL-5 has a key role to play in allergic diseases. Large numbers of eosinophils accumulate in the lung following antigen challenge of asthmatic patients leading to the late manifestations of this allergic response. Eosinophils have been implicated in asthmatic lung damage through release of eosinophil major basic protein and neurotoxin from their granules. It therefore seems that the late asthmatic response is a result of a DTH response

together with eosinophilia resulting from the T cell activation and production of IL-5.

The IL-5R complex is composed of a specific ligand binding α-chain and a β-subunit which is common to IL-3R and the GM-CSFR (*Fig. 10.3*). Murine IL-5 binds with low affinity to the α-subunit but with high affinity to the heterodimeric receptor. Signalling through the receptor involves tyrosine phosphorylation of the β-subunit but the details of specific signalling events remain to be clarified.

IL-6

Interleukin 6 is a pleiotropic cytokine produced by many cell types including T cells (*Fig. 10.14*). Its effect on B cells is to promote growth and facilitate maturation of the B cells causing Ig secretion. The levels of IL-6 are elevated in a variety of diseases and this cytokine has been implicated in their pathology. As it promotes the growth of Kaposi's sarcoma cells and renal mesangial cells it has been suggested that IL-6 is involved in the development of Kaposi's sarcoma in AIDS patients and of mesangial proliferative glomerulonephritis. This is supported by the observation that IL-6 transgenic mice had a mesangial proliferative glomerulonephritis in addition to having a plasmacytosis and high circulating IgG1 levels. It is a key mediator of the acute phase response directly acting upon hepatocytes to synthesize CRP, complement components and other acute phase proteins.

Resting B cells do not express the IL-6R but are induced to express the IL-6R following activation. IL-6 interacts with the single chain IL-6R initiating interaction with gp130 and its dimerization (see *Fig. 10.6*). Activation of a tyrosine kinase occurs following homodimerization leading to phosphorylation of gp130 and signal transduction. The phosphorylation of a transcription factor which acts on the promoter region of several acute phase proteins results in its translocation to the nucleus.

IL-7 AND IL-10

Interleukin 7 has been described in the T cell section but it must be remembered that this cytokine which is secreted by stromal cells has a great effect on the development of progenitor B cells.

IL-10 also affects both T cells and B cells acting synergistically with other cytokines on the growth of haematopoietic lineages including that giving rise to B cells. Its homology with the Epstein Barr virus *BCFR1* gene and the influence this virus can have on B cell growth and survival further emphasizes its role in B cell function. Antibody mediated depletion of IL-10 *in vivo* results in a reduced IgM and IgA response with an increase in IgG2 and a depletion of Ly1⁺ B cells suggesting that this cytokine is important for the expansion of this B cell population. Recent studies of SLE patients suggest that the increased B cell responses in this population may be attributable not only to IL-6 but also to IL-10. Peripheral blood lymphocytes (PBL) from SLE patients continue to secrete IgG and anti-DNA antibodies on transfer to SCID mice which is not inhibitible by anti-IL-6 antibodies. In contrast anti-IL-10 antibodies inhibited the autoantibody production

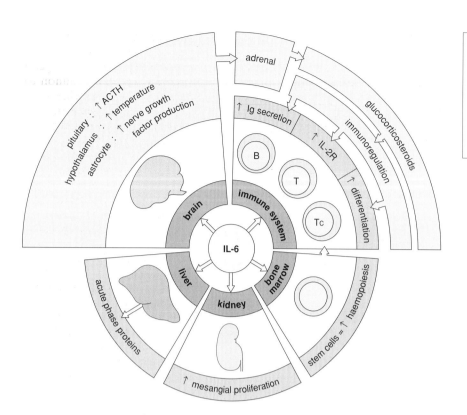

Fig. 10.14 Pleiotropic actions of IL-6. Some of the major functions of IL-6 affecting the immune system. Actions on the brain and bone marrow stem cells can modulate the numbers and activities of cells in the immune system.

without significantly affecting the total amount of IgG produced. There has also been some suggestion that IL-10 like IL-14 (see below) may induce bcl-2 expression and prevent B cell death.

IL-13

The marked structural homology between IL-4 and IL-13 and the close juxtaposition of their genes on the chromosome suggest that gene duplication occurred. IL-13 is predominantly expressed in activated Th2 cells and regulates human B cell and monocyte activity. It acts as a co-stimulant together with receptor or CD40 engagement of human B cells. Interaction between CD40 and CD40L in the presence of IL-13 induces isotype switching and IgE synthesis as does IL-4. In the mouse activity of IL-13 appears thus far to be restricted to macrophages whereas with human monocytes it has been shown to prevent the cytokine (IL-1α and β, IL-6, IL-8 and TNFα) production induced by LPS.

IL-14

Interleukin 14 is thought to play a role in the development of B cell memory. It enhances the proliferation of activated B cells and inhibits the synthesis of immunoglobulin. It has thus far been characterized only in the human, being produced by follicular dendritic cells and activated T cells. Its presence in germinal centre T cells and follicular dendritic cells suggests that during a secondary immune response sIgD$^-$ B cells migrating through the lymph node encounter antigen, become activated, express IL-14R and following binding of IL-14, increased bcl-2 expression prevents apoptosis and permits B cell memory development.

The presence of lymphoma cells or leukemia cells in a variety of malignant conditions able to proliferate to IL-14 suggests that this cytokine may be implicated in their expansion and survival. Increased production of IL-14 together with IL-6 and IL-10 has been found in SLE patients which is also interesting in view of the hypergammaglobulinaemia and monoclonal gammopathies often associated with this condition.

CYTOKINES THAT MODULATE INFLAMMATION

IFNγ

Although IFNγ was originally recognized as an anti-viral agent its immunomodulatory activities may be of more biological importance. It is a pleiotropic cytokine influencing the growth, differentiation and activity of T cells, NK cells and B cells (*Fig. 10.15*). This monomeric glycoprotein is made by activated T cells (Th0, Th1 and CD8$^+$) and NK cells but the active moiety is a dimer which interacts with two receptors causing their aggregation and subsequent activation. IFNγ is a powerful enhancer of MHC class I expression on many different cell types and induces MHC class II expression on some cells. It is a powerful activator of macrophages inducing NO synthase, TNFα and IL-1. This may, in part, explain how this cytokine increases the ability of macrophages to kill intracellular parasites and tumour cells. IFNγ also acts synergistically with many other cytokines, for example, together with TNFα it mediates cytotoxicity in a variety of cell types.

TGFβ

Transforming growth factor β (TGFβ) has achieved increasing prominence in studies of the immune system. It exists

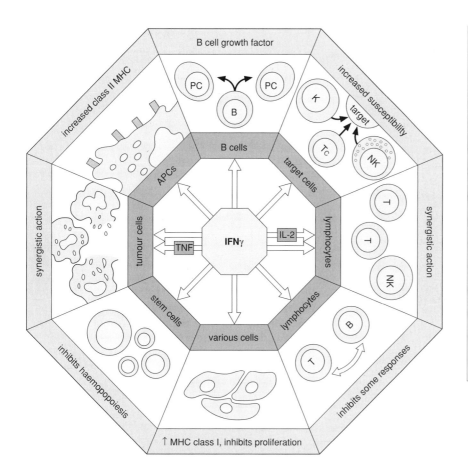

Fig. 10.15 Multiple effects of IFNγ. IFNγ is produced by Th1 cells following antigen specific activation. IFNγ enhances MHC class II expression on APCs and also can induce class II expression on many cells of the body which do not normally express IFNγ. IFNγ is thought to synergize with other B cell stimulating factors, as a lateacting differentiation factor. IFNγ can act together with TNFα to induce the production of reactive oxygen and nitrogen intermediates in macrophages. IFNγ also synergizes with TNFα to enhance the susceptibility of target cells to Tc and NK cells. Its antiviral actions are reflected in its ability to inhibit protein synthesis which also appears as a paradoxical inhibition of B cell and T cell proliferation in some systems.

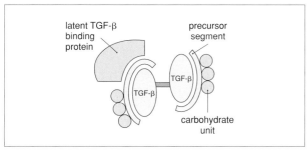

Fig. 10.16 TGFβ is secreted as an inactive homodimer. The TGFβ disulphide-bonded homodimer derived from the C-terminal regions of two precursor molecules is secreted together with two segments from the N-terminal portion of the precursor molecule. This inactive form is bound by a latent TGFβ binding protein through a disulphide bond to one of the N-terminal domains of the precursor. Activation of latent TGFβ is caused by proteases such as plasmin and cathepsins.

in three isoforms and belongs to a superfamily which includes the inhibins and activins, molecules which have been found to play an important role in embryonic development as well as wound healing and bone formation. TGFβ is not secreted in its active form but possibly is acted upon by proteases leading to the release of the bioactive homodimer (*Fig. 10.16*). The activity of the active molecule may be limited by its binding to extracellular matrix components such as decorin, fibronectin, thrombospondin and others as well as to α_2-macroglobulin in the blood. TGFβ is a powerful immunosuppressant depressing the proliferation of T cells, B cells and NK cells and the activity of macrophages. It has also been reported to act as a switch factor for B cells increasing IgA and IgG2b production. TGFβ has been implicated as a mediator of oral tolerance (Chapter 12). The anti-inflammatory properties of this molecule are emphasized by the observation that mice deprived of TGFβ by targeted gene disruption develop generalized inflammatory infiltrates.

TNFα AND TNFβ

TNFα is a 17kDa molecule which following processing is secreted as a biologically active homotrimer. In its unprocessed precursor form TNFα exists as a type II membrane protein attached by its signal sequence. It is produced by a variety of cell types including macrophages, T cells, B cells, NK cells, astrocytes and Kupffer cells. TNFα is produced in response to bacteria, viruses, cytokines (GM-CSF, IL-1, IL-2, IFNγ), immune complexes, complement component C5a and reactive oxygen intermediates. TNFβ, on the other hand, is a 25kDa protein secreted by activated T and B cells which can exist in membrane form when bound by a transmembrane protein, LT-β. Both proteins belong to a family of proteins including CD40L, CD30L and CD29L (*Fig. 10.7*). The location of TNFα, TNFβ and also LT-β within the human and mouse MHC regions of chromosomes 6 and 17 respectively have meant that these molecules may be responsible for some MHC-linked genetic effects. The sequence similarities between the three molecules together with the conservation of the TNF complex linkage groups across species suggest that these molecules arose by gene duplication. Expression of these genes is tightly controlled with many regulatory sites being present in the 5' region of the genes. A biallelic polymorphism has been identified in this region which may have pathological consequences in the homozygous form under certain environmental conditions. This is exemplified by an association of the *TNF2* allele with coeliac disease and with the increased risk of neurological complications of cerebral malaria. Postranscriptional regulation may be accomplished by controlling the rate of precursor mRNA splicing in the case of TNFβ and message stability in the case of both TNFα and TNFβ.

TNFα was previously known under a variety of other names including cachectin, necrosin and macrophage cytotoxin or cytotoxic factor. Together with IFNγ, TNFα can be shown to be cytotoxic for many tumour cells. For example, it has been shown to have a high success rate in curing patients with melanoma and other tumours following infusion alone or in combination with IFNγ. It has also been shown to cause septic shock, be involved in cerebral malaria and to play a role in inflammatory diseases such as rheumatoid arthritis.

TNFα is however also a powerful modulator of immune responses mediating the induction of adhesion molecules, other cytokines and the activation of neutrophils. Its involvement in the development of a protective immune response against *Mycobacterium tuberculosis* has been highlighted by recent experiments of Flynn, Bloom and colleagues. In these studies both neutralization of TNFα by antibody treatment and targeted disruption of the TNF p55 receptor (see below) rendered the mice more susceptible to the lethal effects of infection with mycobacteria (*Fig. 10.17*). The macrophages from TNFR p55-/- mice were unable to make large quantities of reactive nitrogen intermediates (RNI) at early time points following mycobacterial infection. This may have been a direct effect on macrophages or an indirect effect through a blockade of TNF mediated activation of NK IFNγ production. IFNγ is known to induce NO synthase activity in macrophages and hence increase levels of RNI. As RNI are known to be necessary for macrophage mycobactericidal action this may be one way in which ablation of the TNF p55 receptor affects disease susceptibility.

TNFβ also manifests a wide range of activities affecting not only lymphocytes but also bone, endothelial and neuronal cells. Its ability to enhance adhesion molecule expression on endothelium may in part explain why transgenic expression of TNFβ in pancreatic β cells initiates inflammatory infiltration of the islets.

Two different high affinity TNF receptors have been identified which bind both TNFα and TNFβ with equal affinity. Although all cell types express TNF receptors, the

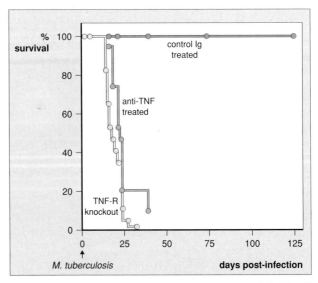

Fig. 10.17 The effect of lack of TNFα on survival of mice infected with *Mycobacterium tuberculosis*.
C57BL/6 mice were infected with *Mycobacterium tuberculosis* and treated either with a monoclonal anti-TNFα (grey) or with a control hamster monoclonal (dark green). TNFR p55-/- mice were also infected and their survival curves are shown in green. Data from Flynn *et al*, 1995.

type II (or type A) receptor, p75, is expressed predominantly on myeloid cells while the type I (type B) or p55 receptor is expressed on many different cell types. Receptor expression is modulated by vitamin D_3, IL-2, IL-1, GM-CSF and TNF itself. The X-ray crystal structure of the interaction of p60 with TNFβ shows that three receptor molecules interact with the homotrimer. Following receptor crosslinking by the TNF trimer a phosphorylcholine-specific phospholipase C is activated generating diacylglycerol (DAG) and activation of a sphingomyelinase releases ceramide from sphingomyelin and activates a Mg^{2+}-dependent protein kinase. It is probable that the two receptors have different signal transduction pathways. Gene disruption of the type I receptor generates mice resistant to TNF-induced toxic shock and increases their susceptibility to *Listeria monocytogenes* as well as mycobacteria (*Fig. 10.17*). Soluble forms of the receptor are found in patients with cancer.

Chemokines

These molecules comprise a group of related small molecular weight cytokines some of which are of fundamental importance in the innate immune response. All members of this family have similar structures and bind to seven transmembrane spanning receptors belonging to the rhodopsin superfamily. Members of the α chemokine family all have two cysteines separated by an intervening residue (C–X–C) in their structurally conserved motif and are extremely active molecules which are produced by many different cell types including monocytes, lymphocytes, granulocytes, bronchial epithelial cells, endothelial cells and keratinocytes (*Fig. 10.18*).

Chemokine	Source	Stimulant	Target	Effect
IL-8	many cell types including monocytes, macrophages, NK, T, neutrophils	IL-1α, β, TNFα, IL-3, IFNγ, PHA, viruses, bacteria	neutrophil T cell B cell monocytes basophils	chemotaxis, degranulation, respiratory burst, lysosomal enzyme release chemotaxis ↓ IL-4 induced IgE ↑ adhesion histamine release, chemotaxis
PF-4	platelets	platelet activators	T cell fibroblast endothelial cell	immunostimulant, ↓ bone resorption chemotaxis, ↑ proliferation ↑ ICAM-1
MIP-2	monocytes, macrophages	LPS	neutrophil	chemotaxis, degranulation
IP-10	monocytes, macrophages, T, keratinocytes, fibroblasts, endothelial cells	IFNγ, LPS	T cell	chemotaxis, ↑ endothelial and extracellular matrix adhesion
NAP-2/β-TG	monocytes, macrophages, platelets	platelet activation	neutrophils fibroblasts chondrocytes	chemotaxis, superoxide release ↑ proliferation ↑ glycosamino-glycan synthesis

Fig. 10.18 Characteristics of some of the chemokines.

In the human these molecules have been mapped to human chromosome 4. These molecules act as chemo-attractants causing the influx of neutrophils, monocytes, T cells and basophils. Studies of IL-8 effector function have revealed that this chemokine causes an increased expression of CD18, CD11a, CD11b and CD11c. As well as acting as a chemoattractant for neutrophils and basophils IL-8 also activates these cells causing a respiratory burst in neutrophils and histamine and leukotriene release by the basophils. Increased levels of IL-8 have been associated with several pathological conditions. In RA the elevated IL-8 probably contributes to the increased presence of neutrophils in the synovial fluid and may contribute to the synovial inflammation. IL-8 is also an angiogenic factor which may contribute to the increased vascularization of some tumours. Its presence in lung tissue and fluids almost certainly reflects an involvement in the pathology of active sarcoidosis and pulmonary fibrosis. IL-8 has been identified only in humans but MIP-2 which is found in mice has many overlapping functional characteristics and competes with IL-8 for binding to the IL-8R.

The β chemokines are distinguished by having two cysteines adjacent to one another (CC) in the conserved motif instead of a CXC. These chemokines have been localized to human chromosome 17.

MIP-1α which belongs to this family is produced by T cells, B cells, macrophages, Langerhans cells and neutrophils. It is a chemoattractant for monocytes, eosinophils, B cells and killer cells and additionally inhibits stem cell replication. RANTES is another member of this family which is produced by T cells and macrophages and is chemotactic for both memory T cells and eosinophils.

Expression of the chemokines appears to be tightly regulated. The short half life of IL-8 mRNA expression is probably due to the AU rich regions in the 3' untranslated end of this message.

All chemokines bind to receptors with characteristic seven transmembrane domains which are G-protein linked members of the rhodopsin superfamily. Two high affinity IL-8R (IL-8RA and IL-8RB) have been cloned and characterized. An additional receptor, the chemokine receptor (CK), has been found on erythrocytes and is somewhat promiscuous in that it will bind both α (IL-8 and MGSA) and β (MCP-1 and RANTES) chemokines. The CK receptor has been shown to be the Duffy blood group antigen. This antigen is known to be a receptor also for the malaria parasite, *Plasmodium vivax*. The physiological significance of this receptor may be that it is a means of clearing excess chemokine from the circulation and ensuring that chemokine gradients are maintained.

SUMMARY

The structures and biological functions of many cytokines and their receptors have been established. This has made it possible to begin to determine their role in the functioning of both a normal and pathological immune response. This understanding will permit the genesis of new therapeutic strategies (see Chapter 17) aimed at restoring normal immune function and controlling deranged activities in a more precise or directed manner.

Elucidation of the sequences and structures has enabled the evolutionary relationships between these molecules to be clarified and to provide insight into the reasons for the pleiotropic effects so frequently observed.

FURTHER READING

Banner DW, D'Arcy A, Janes W, Gentz R, Schoenfeld H-J, Broger C, Loetscher H, Lesslauer W. Crystal structure of the soluble human 55kDa TNF receptor-human TNFβ complex: implications for TNF receptor activation. *Cell* 1993, **73**:431.

Callard RE, Gearing AJH. *The Cytokine Factsbook*. Harcourt Brace & Co: London; 1995.

Coffman RL, Lebman DA, Shrader B. Transforming growth factor β specifically enhances IgA production by lipopolysaccharide-stimulated murine B lymphocytes. *J Exp Med* 1989, **170**:1039.

Coffman RL, Savelkoul HE, Lebman DA. Cytokine regulation of immunoglobulin isotype switching and expression. *Semin Immunol* 1989, **1**:55.

Flynn JL, Goldstein MM, Chan J, Triebold KJ, Pfeffer K, Lowenstein CJ, Schreiber R, Mak TW, Bloom BR. Tumour Necrosis Factor α is required in the protective immune response against *Mycobacterium tuberculosis* in mice. *Immunity* 1995 **2**:561.

Horuk R. The interleukin 8 receptor family: from chemokines to malaria. *Immunol Today* 1994, **15**:169.

Kishimoto T, Taga T, Akira S. Cytokine Signal Transduction. *Cell* 1994, **76**:253.

Nicola NA (Ed). *Guidebook to Cytokines and their Receptors*. Oxford University Press: Oxford; 1995.

Paul WE, Seder RA. Lymphocyte Responses and Cytokines. *Cell* 1994 , **76**:241.

Sanderson CJ, Campbell HD, Young IG. Molecular and cellular biology of eosinophil differentiation factor IL-5 and its effect on human and mouse B cells. *Immunol Rev* 1988, **102**:29.

Szabo SJ, Jacobsen NG, Dighe AS, Gubler U, Murphy KM. Developmental commitment to the Th2 lineage by extinction of IL-12 signalling. *Immunity* 1995, **2**:665.

Trembleau S, Penna G, Bosi E, Mortara A, Gately MK, Adorini L. Interleukin 12 administration induces T helper type I cells and accelerates autoimmune diabetes in NOD mice. *J Exp Med* 1995, **181**: 817.

Trincheri G. Interleukin-12: A proinflammatory cytokine with immunoregulatory functions that bridge innate resistance and antigen-specific adaptive immunity. *Ann Rev Immunol* 1995, **13**:251.

Wilson AG, Duff GW. Genetic traits in common diseases. *BMJ* 1995, **310**:1482.

11 Immunoregulation

The immune response, like all biological systems, is subject to a variety of control mechanisms which serve to restore the immune system to a resting state when responsiveness to a given antigen is no longer required. An effective immune response is an outcome of the interplay between antigen and a network of immunologically competent cells. The nature of the immune response both qualitatively and quantitatively is determined by many factors including the form and route of administration of the antigen, the nature of the antigen presenting cell, the genetic background of the individual and any history of previous exposure to this antigen or a cross-reacting antigen, or even antibody to the antigen. Some of these factors are dealt with in detail elsewhere and are only dealt with briefly in this chapter. Emphasis will be given to the role of various cells and their products in integrating and modulating the immune response.

REGULATION BY ANTIGEN

T cells and B cells are triggered by antigen following effective engagement of their antigen-specific receptors. In the case of the T cell, this engagement is not of antigen itself but of processed antigenic peptide bound to MHC Class I or Class II molecules (see Chapter 7). The nature of an antigen, its dose and the route of administration have all been shown to influence profoundly the outcome of an immune response.

The nature of the antigen

Different antigens elicit different kinds of immune responses. Polysaccharide capsule antigens of bacteria generally induce IgM responses whereas proteins can induce both cell mediated and humoral immune responses. Intracellular organisms such as parasites or viruses induce a cell-mediated immune response whereas soluble protein antigens induce a humoral response. An effective immune response removes antigen from the system and, since repeated antigen exposure is required to maintain T and B cells in an active expanding phase, the cell returns to a quiescent state.

Some antigens (for example those of intracellular parasites) may not be cleared so effectively and thus a sustained immune response arises resulting in pathological consequences.

The dose of the antigen

Very large doses of antigen often result in specific T and sometimes B cell unresponsiveness (high zone tolerance). T-independent polysaccharide antigens have been shown to generate tolerance in B cells following administration in high doses. In some situations clonal deletion of antigen specific cells occurs through apoptosis in high antigen concentration. Activated T cells are sensitive to apoptotic death under certain conditions, for example that of growth factor deprivation. Infection with high doses of certain strains of lymphochoriomeningitis virus (LCMV) leads to an overwhelming viral antigenic load and although antigen specific CTL are initially generated, they rapidly disappear following activation leading to viral persistence in the host. Tolerance to LCMV is maintained in such animals by deletion of newly developing LCMV-specific CTL following encounter with the persisting high titres of virus. It has been shown by transferring T cells from a transgenic mouse expressing an $\alpha\beta$ TCR from a CTL specific for a peptide of LCMV that deletion of CTL occurs (*Fig. 11.1*). As these transferred T cells can be shown to be initially activated and

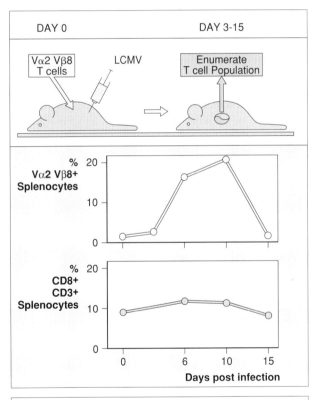

Fig. 11.1 Deletion of virus specific CTLs following high dose infection. Adult C57BL/6 mice were infected with 10^7 PFU lymphocytic choriomeningitis virus (LCMV). 10^3 TCR transgenic T cells specific for LCMV glycoprotein amino acids 32–42 and H-2D^b were transferred into these persistently infected mice. At this time point their endogenous CTL are exhausted. The *in vivo* fate of transgenic TCR (Vα2 Vβ8) expressing CD8$^+$ T cells was followed by antibody staining of splenocytes and FACS analyses at different times following cell transfer. TCR transgenic T cells are eliminated from the periphery. Data from Moskophidis *et al*, 1993.

then deleted irrespective of the time after infection this suggests that deletion of these T cells is not due to a lack of cytokines such as IL-2. Tolerance and its underlying mechanism(s) is dealt with in more detail in Chapter 12.

The route of administration

The route of administration of antigen has been shown to influence the immune response. Antigens administered subcutaneously or intradermally evoke an immune response whereas those given intravenously, orally or as an aerosol may cause tolerance or an immune deviation from one type of CD4[+] T cell response to another. Thus when ovalbumin or myelin basic protein (MBP) is fed to rodents the animals do not respond effectively to an immunogenic challenge with the corresponding antigen. Antigen, both partially degraded and intact, is absorbed from the gut and can be found in sera within 1 hour of feeding. Transfer of such serum containing antigen to naive animals prevents the induction of DTH responses to the antigen. Following feeding of MBP animals are protected from the development of the autoimmune disease, experimental allergic encephalomyelitis (EAE). This approach may have potential therapeutic value also in allergy as recent studies have shown that oral administration of a T cell epitope of the Der p1 allergen of house dust mite could tolerize to the whole antigen. With regard to mechanism(s) of such tolerance induction, both anergy and immune deviation have been implicated. Similar observations have been made when antigen is given as an aerosol. Studies in EAE have shown that aerosol administration of an encephalitogenic peptide can inhibit disease induction either with encephalitogenic peptide or with spinal cord homogenate (*Fig. 11.2*).

A clear example of the effect of route of administration on the outcome of the immune response is provided by studies of infection with LCMV. Virus can be effectively cleared by CD8[+] Tc cells following priming with a dominant LCMV peptide, GP33. Immunity to LCMV can be shown after priming with peptide s.c. in incomplete Freund's adjuvant, however, if the same peptide is repeatedly injected i.p. the animals become tolerized and cannot clear the virus (*Fig. 11.3*).

GENETIC CONTROL OF IMMUNE RESPONSES

There are many ways in which genetic factors may play some role in influencing the immune response. It has long been recognized that the ability to make an immune response to any given antigen varies between individuals. Familial patterns of susceptibility to *Corynebacterium diphtheriae* infection suggested that resistance or susceptibility might be an inherited characteristic. This proposal was supported by the finding that different strains of guinea pigs displayed different resistance patterns to diphtheria and that this characteristic was inherited. In 1943, Fjord–Scheibel showed, by selection of high-responder and low-responder guinea pig strains, that the production of diphtheria anti-toxin was controlled by a single gene, inherited as a Mendelian dominant trait. This study was also the first demonstration of the dominance of high responsiveness. Ninety percent of offspring

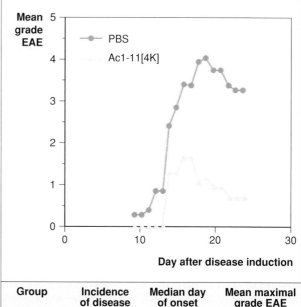

Group	Incidence of disease	Median day of onset	Mean maximal grade EAE
PBS	9/9	14	4.1±1.4
Ac1-11[4K]	6/8	16	1.7±1.7

Fig. 11.2 Aerosol administration of peptide modifies the development of EAE in PL/J mice. Mice were treated with a single dose of 100μg peptide Ac1–11[4K] of MBP — the encephalitogenic region of the antigen in this strain — by inhalation; control mice received the carrier alone. EAE was induced 7 days later with the peptide given this time in adjuvant. Data from Metzler *et al*, 1993.

of the two high-responder animals were anti-toxin producers in the first generation, whereas it took five generations of inbreeding low-responders before 90% of their offspring were low-responders.

With the development of inbred mouse strains it became possible to analyse genetic influences more rigorously and it was conclusively demonstrated that genetic factors play a role in determining immune responsiveness. It was furthermore shown that immune response (Ir) genes within the MHC (see Chapters 4 and 7) play a fundamental role in influencing the response against infectious agents.

Considerable advances have been made in recent years: the elucidation of the structures of MHC class I and MHC class II, the analyses of polymorphic residues in the MHC and their influence on peptide binding, the ability to monitor the T cell repertoire following the generation of reagents and molecular methods for TCR detection, the development of transgenic mice; all these have contributed to an explosion of information about genetic factors influencing the immune response. However, genetic influences on the immune response are not always linked to the MHC. For example, severe combined immunodeficiency is due to the lack of a recombinase activating gene and leukocyte adhesion deficiency is caused by mutations in the β_2 integrin subunit which lead to a failure of expression.

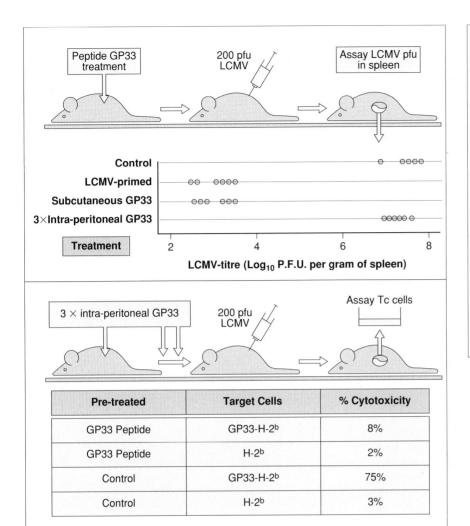

Fig. 11.3 Peptide induced inactivation of LCMV specific Tc. C57BL/6 mice were either primed with LCMV or injected with 100µg LCMV peptide, GP33. The peptide was given either s.c. or three times i.p. with adjuvant. Following infection of such primed mice with LCMV those animals given peptide i.p. failed to develop protective immunity whereas those primed with either peptide s.c. or LCMV itself developed neutralizing antibody against the virus. Analysis of Tc activity in these mice showed that mice given i.p. peptide failed to develop Tc specific for GP33 whereas those mice given adjuvant alone efficiently lysed the H-2^b targets loaded with GP33 peptide. Data from Aichele *et al*, 1994.

Pre-treated	Target Cells	% Cytotoxicity
GP33 Peptide	GP33-H-2^b	8%
GP33 Peptide	H-2^b	2%
Control	GP33-H-2^b	75%
Control	H-2^b	3%

MHC-linked immune response genes

As discussed in previous chapters, the immune response depends upon the activation of clones of lymphocytes. In the case of T cells, these recognize antigen only when it is presented to them as peptide complexed to class I or class II major histocompatibility molecules. Thus CD8$^+$ Tc cells specific for LCMV glycoprotein will lyse only virally infected target cells derived from an MHC class I matched mouse strain (*Fig. 11.4*); this recognition was learnt during ontogeny (*Fig. 11.5*). The peripheral T cell repertoire is influenced both by the range of endogenous polymorphic self antigens and by the MHC antigens of the individual. The ability of peptide to bind to MHC is affected by the amino acid sequences in the binding sites of the MHC molecules. The elucidation of the three dimensional structure of MHC molecules has permitted the positions of the polymorphic residues to be assigned. These have been shown to reside in the groove in which peptide is bound and to influence affinity between a given peptide and the MHC. Thus the extensive sequence polymorphism of MHC molecules has a profound impact on peptide binding and, as a consequence, on T cell activation. It is now established that, during development T cells are

subjected to two selection processes in the thymus: positive selection, based on an interaction of the TCR with MHC on thymic cortical epithelium and negative selection, a result of a high-affinity interaction between the TCR and MHC–peptide presented on bone marrow-derived cells in the thymus medulla (Chapter 6).

The expressed peripheral T cell repertoire can therefore be shaped by both positive and negative selection, thus affecting the immune response.

MHC-LINKED GENE CONTROL OF THE RESPONSE TO INFECTION

MHC-linked genes have been shown to play a role in the immune response to infectious agents and also to self antigens. In some cases the gene involved is an MHC gene itself but in others it is thought to be a gene that is simply linked to the MHC.

The first observation that genes (*Ts-1* and *Ts-2*) within the MHC could influence the response to parasites involved the susceptibility to *Trichinella spiralis*. It is interesting that such an effect should be noted with an antigenically complex organism, particularly as these parasites express different antigens at different stages in their life cycle, with different APCs

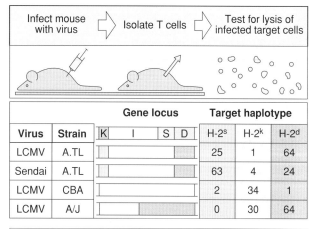

		Gene locus				Target haplotype		
Virus	**Strain**	K	I	S	D	H-2^s	H-2^k	H-2^d
LCMV	A.TL					25	1	64
Sendai	A.TL					63	4	24
LCMV	CBA					2	34	1
LCMV	A/J					0	30	64

Fig. 11.4 Class I restriction of virus-specific Tc cells.
The cytotoxic cells of virus-infected adult mice of different strains were tested for their ability to kill virus infected target cells of different H-2 haplotype (k, s and d). The strain A.TL is H-2K^s and H-2D^d and its cells kill target cells infected with lymphocytic choriomeningitis virus (LCMV) only if the targets share the H-2K^s or the H-2D^d haplotypes. Haplotype identity between the cells and targets at MHC Class II loci does not produce cytotoxicity. This shows that the antiviral cytotoxic T cells are class I restricted. Note that the cytotoxicity to LCMV is determined mostly by the *H-2D* locus. By comparison, in A.TL mice infected with Sendai virus, the cytotoxicity is principally determined by the H-2K locus. Infection of CBA mice with LCMV confirms the importance of genetic restriction in these responses, while the infection of A/J mice with LCMV confirms the finding that cytotoxicity to LCMV is strongest to the H-2D-matched infected targets. Different viruses may associate preferentially with particular H-2K or H-2D MHC molecules to present a target for cytotoxic cells.

being involved in their presentation. If different recombinant mouse strains are infected with *T. spiralis* it can be seen that resistance or susceptibility is affected by the *H-2E* locus. Mouse strains which express H-2E appear to be susceptible while those strains which do not express H-2E are resistant. An additional MHC-linked gene has been shown to influence the response to *T. spiralis* but in this case it is not an MHC-encoding gene itself but another gene in linkage disequilibrium. This gene, which has been designated *Ts-2*, maps between *S* and *D*, close to the *TNF* genes.

The *H-2E* subregion has also been shown to influence susceptibility to *Leishmania donovani*. Using H-2 congenic mice it was shown that H-2E-expressing mice were unable to combat visceral leishmaniasis. Direct involvement of the H-2E product in this susceptibility was shown by the ability of anti-H-2E antibody but not the anti-H-2A antibody to enhance parasite clearance. Furthermore comparison of the response to *L. donovani* of NOD mice which do not express H-2E and NOD-E mice which express H-2E as a result of insertion of an MHC encoding transgene demonstrated that the mice expressing H-2E were not able to clear the parasite from the liver and spleen as effectively as NOD mice.

In humans, a comparison of the HLA haplotypes associated with severe malarial anaemia revealed that the HLA haplotype (DRB1*1302, DQB1*0501) which is common in West Africans is rare in other racial groups and provides protection from the lethal consequences of infection by *P. falciparum*. DRB1*1302 has been shown to bind different peptides from DRB1*1301 due to a single amino acid difference in the β-chain. This would clearly influence the response to the malaria parasite.

MHC-LINKED GENE EFFECTS ON AUTOIMMUNE DISEASE

MHC associations have been found with several autoimmune diseases. For example, insulin dependent diabetes mellitus (IDDM), an autoimmune disease in which the beta cells of the pancreas are destroyed by cells of the immune system, is associated with HLA-DR3 and HLA-DR4. The highest risk is in fact seen in HLA-DR3/4 heterozygotes. Because of linkage disequilibrium, although the original associations were seen with DR, they are in reality with DQ. Molecular genetic analysis has permitted the association to be analysed in more detail and it seems that the primary association in Caucasians is with DQB1*0302. In rheumatoid arthritis the predominant association is with HLA-DR4 or DR1 in several ethnic groups; there is little association with HLA-DQ. The way in which these disease associations contribute to susceptibility remains unclear but possible explanations include repertoire differences through positive and negative selection on different class II genes, or preferential binding of disease-inducing epitopes on bacteria or viruses to particular MHC molecules. In this context, analysis of the amino acid sequences of peptide binding grooves of HLA-DR4 and DR1 has demonstrated the presence of differently charged residues in susceptible or resistant subtypes of HLA-DR.

BXSB male mice spontaneously develop the autoimmune disease, systemic lupus erythematosus (SLE) with MHC genes playing a critical role in disease development. The BXSB, like other H-2^b mice, does not express H-2E due to a deletion in the *Ea* promoter region. Introduction of a transgenically encoded *Ead* gene which permits H-2E expression in the BXSB increases survival, prevents the hypergammaglobulinaemia and reduces the development of autoantibodies and glomerulonephritis characteristic of SLE (*Fig. 11.6*). The mechanism by which this protection is afforded is not clear but it is suggested that an Eα peptide competes with autoantigenic peptide for presentation by H-2A^b.

Another example of linkage disequilibrium is that provided by the association of autoimmunity in the (NZB × NZW) F1 mouse with the H-2^z of the NZW parent. It has been clearly demonstrated that this association was not with an MHC gene itself but with the *TNFa* gene closely linked to the MHC genes. The NZW *TNFa* allele gives rise to the production of low amounts of TNFα. If the concentration of this cytokine is increased, the mice are protected from the development of lupus nephritis (*Fig. 11.7*).

Other MHC-linked genes have recently been identified which may influence immune responses. These are genes which are involved in the generation by proteolysis and transport of antigen peptide fragments. These genes are polymorphic and such polymorphism has functional consequences.

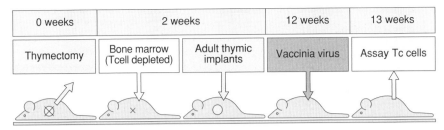

Donor bone marrow	Recipient	Thymic donor	Killing of infected targets	
			Type A	Type B
A × B	A × B	A	+	−
A × B	A × B	B	−	+

Fig. 11.5 Role of thymic MHC haplotype in T cell development. Eight week-old mice of MHC haplotype AxB were thymectomized, irradiated and reconstituted with bone marrow which had been specifically depleted of T cells by treatment with anti-Thy-1.2 and complement. Each mouse was then given a subcutaneous graft of adult thymus of either type A or type B haplotype (grafted tissue was first irradiated to destroy mature T cells). About 20% of animals survived this treatment and recovered immune function. Ten weeks after grafting, they were infected with *Vaccinia* virus and the spleen cells from these mice were tested 1 week later for their ability specifically to kill virally infected target cells of haplotype A or B. Animals reconstituted with a type A thymus were able to kill targets of haplotype A and those with a type B thymus killed haplotype B targets. Data from Zinkernagel *et al*, 1978.

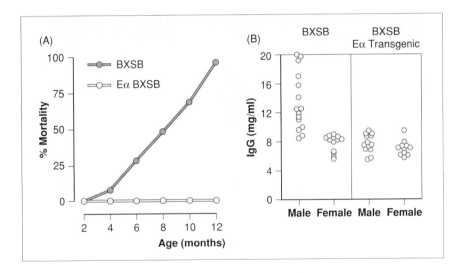

Fig. 11.6 The effect of transgenic expression of Eα in BXSB mice. (A) mortality and (B) serum IgG levels are depicted. Based on data by Merino *et al*, 1993.

For example, in the rat different allelic forms of the *cim* locus affect peptide loading into the class I MHC, which in turn affects the ability of the class I MHC molecule to be recognized as an alloantigen. It is therefore possible that some of the MHC-linked disease associations which have been identified are attributable to similar genes, involved in proteolysis and transport of antigen peptides to the MHC molecules for presentation to cells of the immune system.

Non-MHC-linked immune response genes

The immune response is also governed by some genes outside the MHC region. This has been shown very clearly both in the genetic analyses of susceptibility and resistance to autoimmune diseases, allergy and in studies of the immune responses to infectious organisms including mycobacteria, listeria, salmonella and rickettsia — diseases where the cell-mediated response is particularly important. Individuals with defects in the complement component C3 show an increased susceptibility to bacterial infections and a predisposition towards immune-complex disease. High IgE production in some allergy prone families has been shown to be associated with the presence of an 'atopy gene' on human chromosome 11q.

THE EFFECT OF NON-MHC-LINKED GENES ON THE RESPONSE TO INFECTION

Macrophages play a key role in the immune system. Genes regulating their activity may therefore determine the outcome

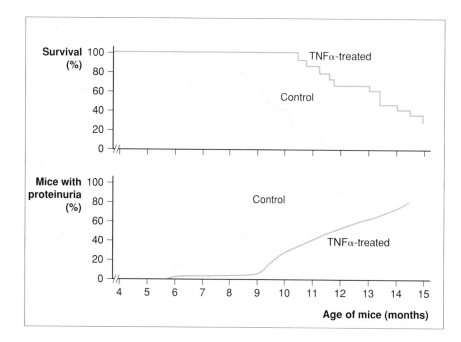

Fig. 11.7 Role of TNFα in protection against lupus nephritis. Upper: Twenty (NZB × NZW) F₁ female mice were treated with recombinant murine TNFα. Their survival is compared with age- and sex-matched F₁ controls. Lower: Cumulative frequency of significant proteinuria (≥ 300mg/dl) in (NZB × NZW) F₁ mice treated with TNFα, and in controls. Data from Jacob and McDevitt, 1989.

of many immune responses. A good example of such genetic control of macrophage function is provided by the *Lsh/Ity/Bcg* gene. This gene governs the early response to infection with *Leishmania donovani, Salmonella typhimurium, Mycobacterium bovis, M. lepraemurium* and *M. intracellulare*. Its influence is on the the early phase of macrophage priming and activation and it has wide-ranging effects. Recent studies have identified *Nramp* as a potential candidate for *Bcg* in the mouse. As *Nramp* encodes a membrane protein with homology to known transport proteins the suggestion has been made that it may be implicated in the transport of NO_2^- into the phagolysosome and thus facilitate the killing of intracellular organisms. However, until *Nramp* has indeed been formally shown to encode the Bcg product either by transfection or transgenesis this is purely hypothetical.

Biozzi generated two lines of mice by selective inbreeding based on their responsiveness to erythrocyte antigens. These high-responder and low-responder Biozzi mice make quantitatively different amounts of antibody in response to antigenic challenge. The basis for these differences has in part been attributed to genetic differences in macrophage activity. These high- and low-responder strains also differ markedly in their ability to respond to parasitic infections and this does not necessarily correlate with the amount of antibody they make.

Eosinophils play an important role in the host response to parasitic infection. It has been shown that the degree of eosinophilia after infection is genetically determined, with marked differences seen in different inbred strains of mice. Similar observations have been made in guinea pigs and sheep, where a consistent correlation has been found between resistance to nematode infection and the extent of eosinophilia.

NON-MHC–LINKED GENES AFFECT DEVELOPMENT OF AUTOIMMUNE DISEASE

Most autoimmune diseases have been shown to be influenced not only by MHC-linked genes but also by genes not linked to this complex. Recently, major advances have been made in mapping the loci which govern susceptibility to the autoimmune disease insulin dependent diabetes mellitus (IDDM). This work has been largely carried out using the NOD mouse strain which spontaneously develops an autoimmune disease similar to IDDM in man. At least 10 genetic loci have been identified in the NOD mouse (Idd-1,2,3,4 to 10) with only one locus (Idd-1) linked to the mouse MHC on chromosome 17 and thought to encode MHC class II antigens. The other genes have been mapped to other chromosomes but their identity and functional roles in determining resistance or susceptibility remain to be clarified.

One way in which non-MHC linked genes could determine resistance or susceptibility to autoimmunity would be through an effect on the Th1 or Th2 bias of the immune response to autoantigen. This is seen in the experiments of Scott and colleagues, 1994, where double transgenic mice expressing a TCR specific for influenza haemagglutinin (HA) presented in the context of H-2Aᵈ and HA in the β cells developed IDDM when these two transgenes were expressed on a B10.D2 background but not when the strain background was BALB/c. Analysis of the cytokine production by T cells following presentation of HA *in vitro* showed a Th2 bias (more IL-4 production) when the T cells were derived from the BALB/c double transgenic mice (*Fig. 11.8*).

The development of SLE in BXSB male mice described above is associated with the Y chromosome-linked autoimmune acceleration gene (*Yaa*) which accelerates disease onset in autoimmune prone mice.

When the lymphoproliferative (*lpr*) gene is introduced into mouse strains it causes the development of a characteristic clinical syndrome. The mice develop anti-DNA antibodies, rheumatoid factor, circulating immune-complexes and glomerulonephritis. There is also a lymphadenopathy in these mice involving an expansion of CD4⁻8⁻ T cells in the periphery. These T cells are not

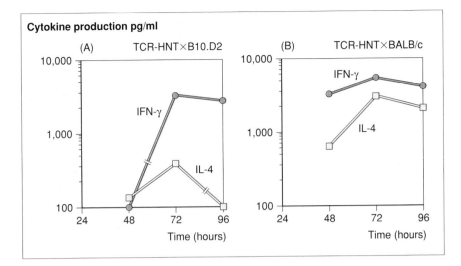

Cytokine production pg/ml

(A) TCR-HNT×B10.D2

(B) TCR-HNT×BALB/c

Fig. 11.8 Background genes influence cytokine production and affect the bias towards Th1 or Th2 responses. TCR transgenic mice expressing a TCR specific for influenza haemagglutinin (TCR-HNT) were crosssed to B10.D2 or BALB/c mice. Spleen cells from these F_1 mice were stimulated *in vitro* with the haemagglutinin peptide recognized by TCR-HNT T cells and IFNγ and IL-4 production measured at different time points thereafter. Data from Scott *et al*, 1994.

monoclonal but have differently arranged TCRs. It was suggested that the syndrome was due to a defect in negative selection but it was difficult to see how a gene such as *lpr* could mediate this effect. Recently, it has been shown that mice with the *lpr* gene have a defect in the Fas antigen which is encoded by a gene on chromosome 19 in the mouse. The Fas antigen is a cell surface protein which is a member of the tumour necrosis/nerve growth factor family and mediates apoptosis. The defect in Fas antigen arising from the *lpr* mutation results in the failure of apoptosis. However, this defect does not appear to affect negative selection and the generation of a normal repertoire of mature single positive T cells in the thymus. It is proposed that the defect results in the expansion of double negative T cells in the periphery and an acceleration of an autoimmune syndrome. The defect in apoptosis is also expressed in B cells and permits the accumulation of autoreactive B cells in the periphery. Recent studies suggest that lymphocytes may undergo programmed cell death in the liver. Defects in the Fas pathway appear to result in accumulation of cells in the liver.

Other studies further suggest that the *gld* gene, which has been shown to result in a similar autoimmune phenotype to that seen in *lpr/lpr* mice, may arise from a related defect. It is proposed that the *gld* encoded protein is the ligand for the Fas antigen and thus mice which are *gld/gld* do not express the ligand, have a defect in apoptosis of peripheral B and T cells and develop autoimmunity. The *gld* gene is located on chromosome 1 in the mouse and thus provides yet another example of a gene which affects immune function but which is not MHC linked.

THE ROLE OF THE ANTIGEN PRESENTING CELL IN IMMUNE REGULATION

The nature of the APC initially presenting the antigen may determine whether responsiveness or tolerance ensues. As stated in Chapter 8 for effective activation of T cells it is important that co-stimulatory molecules are expressed by the APC. For example, if antigen is presented to T cells by a 'non-professional' APC where no co-stimulation is provided unresponsiveness results. When naive T cells are exposed to antigen by resting B cells they fail to respond and indeed become tolerized. Presentation by dendritic cells or activated macrophages which express high levels of MHC Class II as well as co-stimulatory molecules such as those of the B7 family and ICAM-1 results in highly effective T cell activation. The involvement of B7 in CTL activation is nicely demonstrated in triple transgenic mice where the peripheral T cells express an αβ TCR specific for the LCMV glycoprotein peptide 32–42 and H-2D^b and both B7-1 and LCMV glycoprotein is selectively expressed in pancreatic beta cells. In double transgenic mice expressing only LCMV-gp in the β cells and the LCMV specific CTL in the periphery β cell destruction does not occur spontaneously. However, when B7 is expressed in the β cells through transgenesis activation of the CTL occurs and the β cells are destroyed resulting in the development of insulin dependent diabetes mellitus (*Fig. 11.9*).

Adjuvants may facilitate immune responses by inducing expression of high levels of MHC and co-stimulatory molecules on APC.

Skin Langerhans cells, dermal dendritic cells and macrophages are thought to endocytose or phagocytose cutaneously administered antigen and then migrate to the draining lymph node where T cell activation takes place. Following chronic UVB irradiation a generalized impairment of skin APC function occurs and immune responses such as contact hypersensitivity fail to occur.

The importance of APC function in determining the outcome of an immune response is shown in studies of diffuse cutaneous leishmaniasis where it has been proposed that deficiencies in local cytokine production or signalling may lead to impaired APC function and consequently an induction of parasite-specific anergy. This is supported by the absence of MHC Class II or ICAM-1 on skin keratinocytes, a deficit of CD1a and HB15$^+$ Langerhans cells and reduced expression of cytokine genes encoding IL-6, TNFα and IL-1β.

Transgene for			Incidence of diabetes	
Anti-LCMV TCR	LCMV peptide	B7	% Incidence	Age
	+	+	0	→ 11 mo
+		+	0	→ 11 mo
+	+		0	→ 11 mo
+	+	+	100%	14 weeks

Fig. 11.9 Role of costimulatory molecules in immunoregulation. Expression of B7-1 and LCMV gp on pancreatic β cells together with transgenic expression of a TCR specific for LCMV gp leads to IDDM. Double transgenic mice, expressing TCR together with beta cell LCMVgp (GP-TCR), do not spontaneously develop IDDM. Expression of B7-1 on β cells (GP-B7-TCR) therefore permits IDDM to be initiated spontaneously. GP-TCR mice develop IDDM after infection with LCMV. Data from Harlan *et al*, 1994.

REGULATION OF THE IMMUNE RESPONSE BY T CELLS

T cells can suppress immune responses

T cells clearly modulate the immune response in a positive sense by providing T cell help. Furthermore, the kind of help which is generated (Th1 *versus* Th2) affects the nature of the immune response, favouring either humoral or cell-mediated immunity. Additionally there is clear evidence that T cells are capable of downregulating immune responses (*Fig. 11.10*). The production of different cytokines by different Th cell subpopulations probably provides an explanation for certain observations regarding the regulation of the immune response by T cells. Cross-regulation of Th subsets has been demonstrated where cytokines, such as IFNγ, secreted by Th1 cells can inhibit the responsiveness of Th2 cells and IL-10 produced by Th2 cells downregulates B7 and and IL-12 expression by APC which in turn inhibits Th1 activation. Thus preferential activation of Th1 or Th2 cells may result in an immune deviation and may provide the explanation for the early studies demonstrating that T cells can modulate IgE responses. The selective biasing of responses may prove therapeutically useful as described above in the treatment of allergy.

Early studies of Leishmania infection in mice showed that whereas most mouse strains developed a localized lesion in response to cutaneous infection with *Leishmania major* BALB/c mice developed a fatal disseminated visceral disease. Furthermore T cells from infected BALB/c mice were shown to depress DTH responses on transfer to recipient mice (*Fig. 11.11*). It is now known that BALB/c mice develop a dominant Th2 response to *L. major* and that treatment of this strain with anti-IL-4 at the time of infection permits the emergence of a Th1 response and a cure of the infection (*Fig. 11.12*). Studies with the IL-4 'knockout' mouse have confirmed these findings.

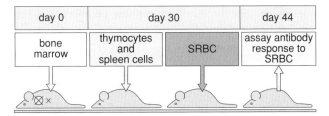

Spleen cells		Log$_2$ antibody response
1	8 × 10^7 SRBC-primed splenocytes	6
2	—	4
3	8 × 10^7 SRBC-tolerized splenocytes	0

Fig. 11.10 Suppressor cells in immunological tolerance. Thymectomized and irradiated mice were reconstituted with bone marrow cells. After 30 days they were recolonized with thymocytes and spleen cells and challenged with SRBC. At day 44, recipients given splenocytes primed with an immunogenic dose of SRBC made a strong response (1). Animals receiving no spleen cells had a moderate response (2). Animals receiving cells from mice tolerized to SRBC (with a high dose of antigen) did not respond (3), indicating that cells from tolerized animals actively suppress the response in the recipient. Data from Gershon and Kondo, 1972.

Of particular interest has been the observation, made in many experimental models of autoimmune disease, that CD4$^+$ T cells, generated following administration of high doses of autoantigen, often given in a soluble or disaggregated form, prevent further induction of autoimmunity. For example, CD4$^+$ T cells have been shown to prevent the

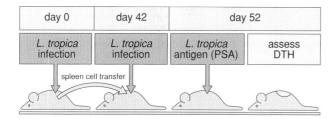

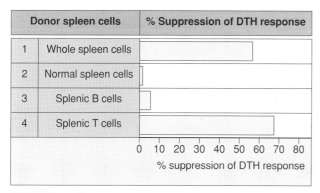

	Donor spleen cells	% Suppression of DTH response
1	Whole spleen cells	
2	Normal spleen cells	
3	Splenic B cells	
4	Splenic T cells	

0 10 20 30 40 50 60 70 80
% suppression of DTH response

Fig.11.11 Suppressor cells in Leishmaniasis. BALB/c mice were infected with *Leishmania tropica* and after 42 days the spleen cells from these animals were transferred to recipients which were then also infected. After 10 days, the ability of the recipients to mount a delayed type hypersensitivity (DTH) reaction was measured following sensitization with protein-soluble antigen (PSA) from *L. tropica*. DTH reflects the ability of these animals to resist the infection. Animals that had received whole spleen cells showed a 57% suppression of their DTH response (1), by comparison with control animals which received spleen cells from uninfected donors (2). When the splenocytes from the infected donors were fractionated before transfer, it was found that B cells could not produce the suppression (3) whereas T cells could (4). This indicated that T cells contribute to disease susceptibility. Based on data of Howard *et al*, 1982.

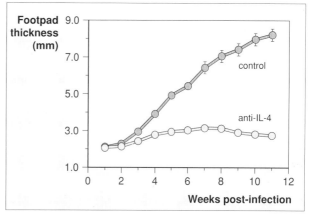

Fig.11.12 Immune deviation in *L. major* infection. Disease progression in an infection by *L. major* was measured by footpad thickness over 11 weeks following infection. Treatment of animals with anti-IL-4 blocks disease progression, indicating a deleterious effect of IL-4 in immunity to this parasite. Data from Sadick *et al*, 1990.

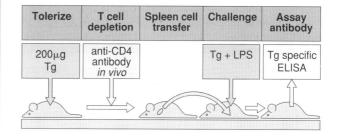

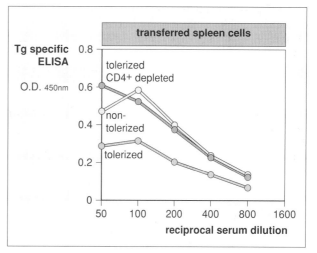

Fig. 11.13 Tolerance transfer by CD4+ T cells. Mice were injected with 200µg of mouse thyroglobulin (Tg) to induce tolerance. (A control group was not tolerized.) Part of the tolerized group was further treated *in vivo* with depleting anti-CD4 antibodies, to remove T-cells. For each mouse, spleen cells were transferred into an irradiated syngeneic recipient. The recipients were then challenged with mouse thyroglobulin and LPS and their anti-Tg antibody response was assayed using ELISA. Anti-CD4 treatment removed the ability to transfer tolerance. Data from Parish *et al*, 1988.

development of autoantibodies to thyroglobulin (*Fig. 11.13*) and additionally thyroiditis. Furthermore, administration of a non-depleting anti-CD4 antibody to mice at the same time as an immunogenic dose of thyroglobulin not only prevents the development of autoimmunity in the mouse but results in the development of a population of CD4+ T cells which can transfer specific tolerance to naive recipients. The exact mechanism by which T cells exert such a negative influence is not entirely clear. However, recent experiments suggest that the production by Th cells of cytokines such as TGFβ, IL-4 and IL-10 can either partially or totally suppress an immune response.

CD8+ T cells have also been shown to regulate immune responses. As described, oral tolerance can be established to MBP. CD8+ T cells have been found in the spleens of such tolerized animals which can adoptively transfer resistance to EAE *in vivo*. These T cells not only suppress T cell responses to MBP *in vitro* but additionally perform bystander suppression to other unrelated antigens. This effect is thought to be mediated by TGFβ (*Fig. 11.14*).

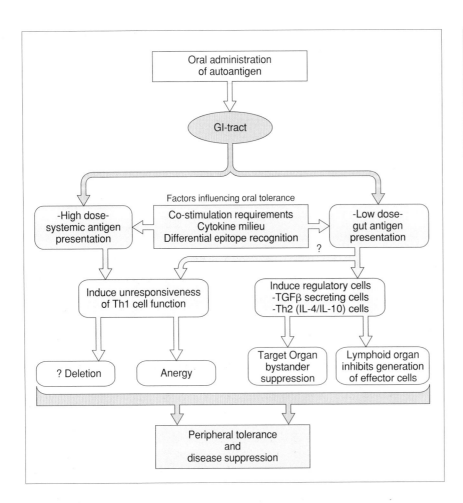

Fig. 11.14 Oral tolerance. Oral administration of antigen results in the generation of T cells, both CD4$^+$ and CD8$^+$ T cells, which are able to downregulate some immune responses by secreting IL-4 or TGFβ respectively. Based on studies of Weiner *et al*, 1994.

The role of such CD4$^+$ or CD8$^+$ T cell-mediated regulatory effects in normal physiology has been questioned. The observation that CD4$^+$ T cells can be found in unmanipulated normal animals which are able to prevent autoimmunity supports their importance in normal homeostasis. Furthermore, the observation that certain dysregulated immune responses arise in rats and mice when CD4$^+$ Th2 cells, which normally make IL-4 and IL-10, are removed strongly suggests that regulation of the immune response by CD4$^+$ Th2 cells is a normal physiological process and not an artefact.

Regulation by veto cells and CTL

It is clear that deletion of self-reactive T cells in the thymus is one way in which self tolerance is generated but it is also apparent that such mechanisms can also occur in the periphery.

Experiments have been described which demonstrate the ability of T cells to kill autoreactive cells. By labelling the donor (AxB) F$_1$ cells with fluorescein isothiocyanate (FITC) prior to injection into parental A strain it has been possible to follow their fate *in vivo*. The donor cells remain in the recipient for several days and can be removed by cell sorting prior to assay for veto function *in vitro*. By this means it has been possible to demonstrate that the donor F$_1$ cells do not need to be present in the culture for their veto function to be manifested. Limiting dilution analyses have been carried out to assess the frequency of Tc

precursors in spleen cells from recipients of F$_1$ cells and have shown that the reduced Tc activity is attributable to an inactivation *in vivo* of the recipients specific alloreactive Tc precursors. It has been suggested that the veto phenomenon rather than idiotype-specific suppression may be invoked to explain allograft tolerance (*Fig. 11.15*). It has also been shown that the presence of donor T cells is necessary for the maintenance of the tolerant state.

REGULATION OF THE IMMUNE RESPONSE BY IMMUNOGLOBULIN

Enhancement of the immune response by IgM

Antibody itself has been shown to exert feedback control. Passive administration of IgM antibody together with antigen specifically enhances the immune response to this antigen whereas IgG antibody suppresses the response. This was originally shown with polyclonal antibodies but has subsequently been confirmed using monoclonal antibodies. Mice were injected with monoclonal IgM to sheep red blood cells (SRBC) 2 hours before immunization with SRBC. The antibody response to SRBC was measured and compared with animals which received no IgM. The response was enhanced and dependent upon the antigen dose used.

The ability of passively administered antibody to enhance or suppress the immune response depending on

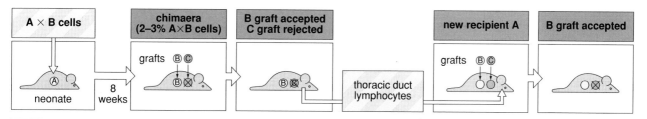

Fig. 11.15 Veto cells in allograft specific suppression. Chimaeras are formed by the injection of (A × B) F$_1$ cells into a haplotype A neonate. When fully grown these animals will accept a type B graft while not accepting a control (type c) graft. Thoracic duct lymphocytes from these mice can transfer specific tolerance to a new recipient (right). Removal of CD8$^+$ (A × B) cells from the developing chimaera prevents the development of tolerance indicating that this population maintains the tolerance. Based on the studies of Fink *et al*, 1988.

the class has several clinical consequences. Certain vaccines (e.g. mumps and measles) are not generally given to infants before 1 year of age, as the levels of maternally derived IgG remain high for at least 6 months after birth. The presence of such passively acquired IgG at the time of vaccination would result in the development of an inadequate immune response in the baby. The phenomenon of IgM enhancement has been used in model systems to demonstrate its potential to bypass the depressing effect of maternal antibody on the immune response of offspring. Studies in murine malaria have shown that succcessful vaccination of offspring of immune mothers can be achieved if monoclonal IgM to the parasite, *Plasmodium yoelii*, is administered together with the formalin-fixed parasite vaccine.

The mechanisms by which antibody modulates the immune response are not completely defined. In the case of IgM enhancement there are two possible interpretations. One of these involves the development of an anti-idiotypic response to the administered monoclonal, which amplifies the immune response (see below). The other involves an effect of passively administered antibody on the uptake, processing and presentation of antigen, due to the binding of the IgM-containing immune complexes to certain APCs through their Fc receptors.

Suppression by IgG

While IgM antibodies enhance the specific antibody response IgG monoclonal antibodies can be shown to suppress specifically the response if administered just prior to or at the time of immunization. This suppression is also observed *in vitro* following IgG and antigen administration *in vivo*. The mechanism of suppression is poorly understood. It has been claimed that IgG may act by masking antigenic determinants but this is difficult to reconcile with the complete suppression observed to a complex antigen by a monoclonal IgG with specificity for a single determinant. It is possible that the monoclonal facilitates opsonization and clearance of the antigen. Additionally, engagement of FcγRII by the IgG antibody and cross-linking it to the mIg receptor by antigen may inhibit B cell responses.

The ability of passively administered antibody to down-regulate immune responses can be turned to clinical advantage. In the case of Rhesus (Rh) incompatibility, the administration of anti-RhD antibody to Rh$^-$ mothers prevents primary sensitization by foetally derived Rh$^+$ blood cells.

Regulation by immune complexes

In the previous section one of the possible ways in which antibody (either IgM or IgG) was shown to modulate the immune response involved an Fc-dependent mechanism and immune-complex formation with antigen. Immune-complexes themselves can inhibit or augment the immune response. The immune response of patients with malignant tumours is often depressed and it has been postulated that this is the result of the presence of circulating immune-complexes composed of antibody and tumour cell antigens. Rheumatoid factors (RFs) are autoantibodies with specificity for IgG Fc. Although RFs are found in high titres in the sera of many patients with rheumatoid arthritis or animal models of this human autoimmune disease they comprise a normal component of any immune response. One way in which RFs could increase the efficiency of an immune response would be by crosslinking IgG bound to microorganisms thus facilitating complement fixation, lysis and opsonization. In a secondary immune response, antigen–antibody complexes could be taken up not only by macrophages and antigen-specific B cells but also by B cells expressing RF as their specific Ig receptor. These B cells could then present antigen to T cells and increase not only the antigen specific component of the response but also the synthesis of RF itself. Such a role for RF-secreting B cells has been proposed in rheumatoid arthritis.

REGULATION OF THE IMMUNE RESPONSE VIA THE IDIOTYPE NETWORK

Tolerance to self-antigens is established during ontogeny (see Chapter 12). Individual antigen-specific receptors on B and T cells are only present at low levels during the neonatal period and these levels are insufficient to generate tolerance to those epitopes which are formed by amino acids in or around the binding site. These epitopes are unique to any given receptor or antibody. Although antibodies are present in the serum, tolerance develops to their Fc portions only because these are present in sufficient concentration. Tolerance does not develop to the unique sequences in the heavy and light chains which determine the antigen binding specificity because each one is present in only a low amount. Individual T cell receptors and immunoglobulins are therefore immunogenic by virtue of these unique sequences, known as idiotypes (Ids). Antibodies formed against these antigen-binding sites are called anti-idiotypic antibodies and they are capable of influencing the outcome of an immune response. Niels Jerne proposed that idiotypic interactions within the immune system formed a physiological network. According to this theory, when an antibody response is induced by antigen, this antibody will in turn invoke an anti-idiotypic response to itself. This hypothesis is conceptually very appealing but the role of such an idiotype network in controlling a normal immune response has been hotly debated.

Terms describing network interactions

Idiotypes (Ids) are the specific set of epitopes (idiotopes) expressed by antigen receptor molecules of B cells and T cells. They may be encoded in the germline *V* region genes or they may be generated by the process of recombination and mutation involved in producing functional variable regions. Some require the presence of two associated domains of the right specificity (e.g. heavy and light chains of specific subgroups). The relationship of Ids to the immunoglobulin genes is discussed in Chapter 2. Since both antigen and anti-Id bind to Id, sometimes they will have structural similarities to each other. In other words, the anti-Id partly mimics the antigen and its structure and in these situations is essentially the image of the antigen. This is referred to as the 'internal image', since it is generated by the immune system itself as opposed to the antigen which is external. Anti-Ids can often mimic the functions of antigen by cross-linking the antigen receptors of lymphocytes; however, internal image anti-Ids go beyond functional mimicry of antigen and structurally resemble that part of the antigen which binds to the Id.

Physiological and non-physiological network interactions

It has been suggested that regulatory interactions may occur through recognition by T cells of shared idiotopes or 'regulatory' idiotopes expressed on a large proportion of antigen-specific B cell receptors and presented presumably as peptide fragments in the context of MHC class II by these B cells.

The physiological relevance of the idiotype network has been questioned. It is clear, however, that the immune response can be manipulated through network interactions. This is shown in *Figure 11.16* by the differential effect of administering anti-Id to the T15 idiotope in neonates and adult mice. The T15 idiotope is commonly expressed on anti-phosphoryl choline antibodies and administration of anti-T15 to mice *in utero* or *postpartum* has a long lasting effect on the T15 component of the anti-phosphoryl choline response.

Physiological network interactions

There are several situations in which it has been possible to show network interactions under physiological conditions. It has been shown during a normal immune response to phosphoryl choline, for example, that an anti-T15 response can be detected in mice following the peak response to phosphoryl choline (T15 dominated). Immunization of mice with ungulate insulins initially stimulates an anti-insulin response followed by an anti-Id response to the anti-insulin. Some of this anti-Id has anti-insulin receptor

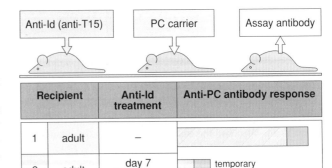

Recipient		Anti-Id treatment	Anti-PC antibody response
1	adult	–	
2	adult	day 7 high dose	temporary suppression
3	neonate	day 42 low dose	long-lasting suppression

Fig 11.16 Anti-id induced suppression in neonates and adults. Mice were pretreated with anti-T15.Id, during either the neonatal period or as adults. They were subsequently immunized with the hapten PC coupled to a carrier. The total antibody was measured along with T15 component of the response (hatched area). Normal adult mice make a good response to PC which is dominated by T15 (1). Adult mice pretreated with anti-Id are temporarily suppressed with the loss of the T15 component, accounting for the reduction in the total anti-PC response (2). Mice treated with anti-Id in the neonatal period undergo long-term suppression of their T15⁺ B cells, but generate T15⁻ PC-specific cells to compensate (3).

activity. The presence of spontaneously arising anti-insulin and anti-insulin receptor antibodies has been documented in the sera of humans and animals spontaneously developing diabetes. It is not clear whether these autoantibodies themselves exacerbate the disease by increasing the requirement for insulin.

The presence of anti-idiotypic antibodies to acetyl choline receptor antibodies in neonatal offspring of mothers with myasthenia gravis has been suggested to play a role in protecting these babies from neonatal myasthenia gravis.

Using the network

Although doubt exists regarding the relative importance of network interactions in the normal regulation of the immune response there is little doubt that network interactions can be used to develop important experimental and therapeutic reagents. The usefulness of these reagents lies in the fact that internal image antibodies can be used either to isolate receptors to act as vaccines or to target specific B cells.

ANTI-IDIOTYPES IN RECEPTOR BIOLOGY

Experimentally anti-idiotypic reagents provide powerful tools in the investigation of receptor-ligand interactions. Once an antibody to a ligand has been obtained, the generation of anti-Ids provides some internal image antibodies which can then be used either to detect or isolate the receptor thus obviating the need to have purified receptor in the first instance. This approach has been successfully used in studies of receptors for endocrine hormones, neurotransmitters and neuropeptides.

ANTI-IDIOTYPES IN VACCINE DEVELOPMENT

Once an antibody has been shown to mediate protective immunity an internal image, Ab1, can be raised and used as a surrogate antigen for vaccination. This may be important for those situations in which the relevant antigen is unknown or cannot be cloned because it is a carbohydrate or glycolipoprotein. This approach has been used successfully in the experimental induction of protective immunity to several viruses (Newcastle disease, Sendai, Reovirus, Rabies, Cytomegalovirus and Hepatitis B), bacteria (*L. monocytogenes*, *E. coli* and *Streptococcus pneumoniae*) and parasites (*S. mansoni* and *T. rhodesiense*).

In the case of the development of HIV vaccines initial interest in the use of an idiotype approach stemmed from the observation that the virus uses CD4 as its receptor for entry into T cells, macrophages and dendritic cells. Mutations in the virus would be unlikely to affect recognition of CD4 and therefore anti-Ids to anti-CD4 antibody might recognize the virus. Initial studies *in vitro* showed that such anti-Ids were able to neutralize virus and *in vivo* in monkeys this approach was able to elicit neutralizing antibodies. However, the uncertainty regarding the ability of idiotype vaccines to elicit relevant cellular immune response consistently has limited the use of this strategy.

The response to some T-independent antigens (polysaccharides) develops relatively late in ontogeny in both mice and humans. Neonatal mice cannot be vaccinated against *E. coli* K13, even when this polysaccharide capsule antigen is made into a T-dependent antigen by coupling it to a carrier. Stein and Soderstrom, 1984, performed a series of particularly interesting experiments on the response of mice to *E. coli*. These workers raised an IgG1 monoclonal anti-Id to an *E. coli* specific IgM monoclonal known to be capable of transferring passive protective immunity. Treatment of neonates with either IgM or its IgG1 anti-idiotype enabled them to resist a lethal *E. coli* infection. In this context, the anti-Id known to have paratopic specificity can act as an internal image of the antigen (surrogate antigen) under conditions in which the antigen itself is not efficacious. Furthermore, injection of mothers with the anti-Id immediately after delivery resulted in transmission of the anti-Id and hence protective immunity, via the milk to the suckling offspring. This study has also been extended to demonstrate that immunity to *E. coli* can be induced in CBA/N mice which are genetically unresponsive to polysaccharides. Such a study emphasizes the unique potential of the anti-idiotype vaccine approach.

ANTI-IDIOTYPE IN TUMOUR IMMUNOTHERAPY

Theoretically, if a tumour specific antigen can be identified, an anti-Id raised against an antibody to this antigen should invoke a specific immune response against the tumour. In practice it has proved difficult to identify such tumour specific antigens. However, in the case of T and B cell lymphomas their antigen specific receptors distinguish them from other cells and can be used as potential targets for immunotherapeutic intervention. Anti-idiotypes to B cell Ig receptors have been raised and used to remove B lymphoma cells from mouse bone marrow *in vitro*. *In vivo* this approach has been problematic. The following factors could

influence the success of such therapy: the presence of large quantities of secreted tumour Ig (Id) could prevent the anti-Id from gaining access to the target lymphoma and result in immune complex formation; Ig undergoes somatic mutation and thus cells failing to express receptor or expressing mutated receptors would escape therapeutic intervention; the development of an immune response against the anti-Id itself. By introducing a human Fc into the mouse immunoglobulins (this is called 'humanizing') it is possible to limit the response against the therapeutic immunoglobulin. Improved toxicity is achieved by coupling a toxin or its subunit, anti-neoplastic drugs or radioisotopes to the immunoglobulin. Toxins used include ricin A-chain, blocked ricin, saporin and diphtheria toxin.

MODULATION OF IMMUNE RESPONSES BY NERVOUS AND ENDOCRINE SYSTEMS

It has long been suspected that events occurring in the central nervous system (CNS) could affect an individual's immune responses. These could be modulated either directly via the innervation of the lymphoid organs or indirectly by the release of hormones such as corticosteroids or polypeptides such as the endorphins and enkephalins. Evidence has now accumulated that tri-directional communication occurs between the nervous system, endocrine organs and the immune system (*Fig. 11.17*). Likewise it is also clear that events which affect the neurological or psychological state of an individual, such as fear or stress, can also affect the development of lymphocytes, their migration properties or their responsiveness. A few examples of this type of effect will illustrate the point.

- It is noted that mice stressed daily by confinement for 1 hour in a small box are unable to recover from an inoculation of Sendai virus which would ordinarily be below the lethal dose.
- Rats which are stressed by exposure to light, noise or frequent handling have a reduced antibody response to immunogens such as sheep erythrocytes.
- Monkeys separated from their mates show reduced lymphocyte mitogenic responses. This effect is also seen in man, in recently bereaved individuals and during the stress of examinations. Interestingly the level of lymphocyte mitogenic responses in rats is directly related to their position in the social hierarchy.
- It is possible to produce conditioned immunosuppression in mice by administering cyclophosphamide in association with a conditioning stimulus. The animals subsequently show reduced responses to an immunogen when given the conditioning stimulus alone. Conversely, a conditioning stimulus can enhance antibody responses if it was initially associated with an immunogenic stimulus.

In general, it is found that conditions, broadly classified as 'stress', result in a reduced ability to mount immune responses. However, if the stressor is modifiable or controllable so that the animal can cope with the stress there is a reduced likelihood of a deficit in the immune reponses.

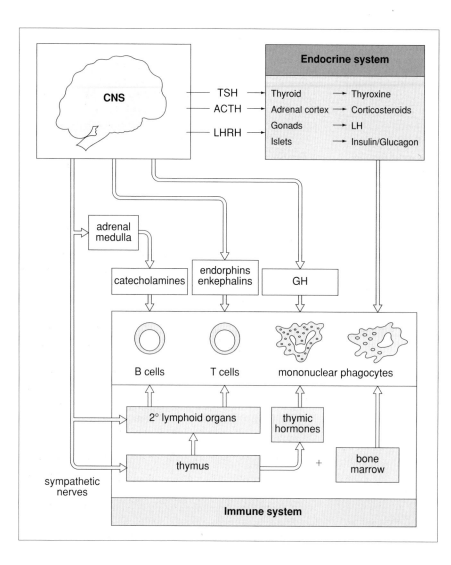

Fig. 11.17 Interconnections between the CNS, endocrine and immune systems. The CNS can modulate the immune system directly via sympathetic innervation, acting either on the blood supply to lymphoid organs or directly on lymphocytes. Alternatively, it can act by releasing pituitary hormones, some of which (e.g. growth hormone, GH) act directly on lymphocytes and mononuclear phagocytes, while others act indirectly by stimulating release of hormones from other endocrine glands, which then act on the leukocytes.

While neurological and endocrine effects on the immune response clearly occur and mechanisms of communication between the systems have been established, it is often impossible to detail the precise chain of events which occur in any particular response. In many cases the effects are mediated by corticosteroids but this is not the only means of control. For example, conditioned immunosuppression may be induced in adrenalectomized animals. Finally one must stress that on balance, neuroendocrine modulation of immune responses is secondary to the principal controls, namely, antigen, cytokines and direct interactions between cells of the immune system.

Innervation of lymphoid organs

Both primary and secondary lymphoid tissues are innervated by the sympathetic nervous system. The nerve fibres are associated with both blood vessels and cellular elements including lymphocytes and macrophages. The small unmyelinated fibres which innervate lymphoid organs come from a two step pathway with the cell bodies lying in the spinal cord and ganglia. Usually the fibres enter the lymphoid organs in association with the blood vessels before arborizing in the parenchyma. In general, it is the T cell areas of spleen and lymph nodes which receive the innervation, although this is not necessarily true during ontogeny. In the thymus, the outer cortical layer containing the least mature thymocytes has the densest innervation. In spleen 99% of sympathetic fibres run into the PALS, where they are seen in both the superficial and deep levels and other fibres arborize through the marginal zone and are associated with marginal zone macrophages. In lymph nodes the fibres are particularly dense in the subcapsular plexus but some also run down into the medulla via the medullary cords. Noradrenalin is the principal transmitter on this pathway but neuropeptide Y, VIP and substance P have also been identified.

The observed innervation of lymphoid tissues suggests that the sympathetic nervous system could modulate immune functions either by direct action on cells or by affecting the local blood supply. For example, since it appears that 25% of lymphocytes passing through the circulation of a lymph node will migrate across the HEV, merely increasing blood flow through a node will increase migration into that node. The proposal that lymphocytes receive direct signals from sympathetic nerves has been supported by the observation that tyrosine hydroxylase positive (noradrenergic) fibres running through the T cell areas of the splenic PALS or the lymph node cortex have boutons containing neurotransmitter granules in close apposition (6nm) to lymphocytes and at some distance from smooth muscle of the vascular system. This gap is as narrow as some synapses in the CNS and there appears to be some specialization of the apposed membrane on the lymphocytes. Furthermore, α-adrenergic and dopaminergic receptors have both been identified on lymphocytes.

The function of the sympathetic innervation has been studied using chemically sympathectomized animals treated with 6-OH DOPA, although this treatment also ablates adrenalin production from the adrenal medulla. In one experiment, localization of lymph node cells from sympathectomized mice into lymph nodes of normal mice was reduced, while migration of normal cells into sympathectomized organs was enhanced. In general, infusions of catecholamines, dopamine or their agonists *in vivo*, usually result in enhanced lymphocyte output from secondary lymphoid tissues. In some cases there is a differential effect on lymphocyte subpopulations, with high plasma adrenalin producing an initial fall in the CD4:CD8 ratio followed by a delayed (one hour) increase. The effects of sympathectomy on immune responses have been very variable with both enhancement and suppression of PFC responses quoted.

The role of central sympathectomy has also been studied and has been found to suppress the primary immune response to T-dependent antigens by up to 90%. The effect may be due to Ts activity since spleen cells from centrally sympathectomized mice could suppress the PFC response to sheep erythrocytes in normal animals. However, the interpretation of this type of experiment is difficult, since the suppression does not occur in hypophysectomized animals and this suggests that central sympathectomy may act via endocrine pathways, possibly the hypophyseal–adrenocortical axis. Other experiments in which selective areas of the brain have been ablated may also end in impaired immune responsiveness, paticularly in relation to the numbers of T cells and NK cells found in peripheral lymphoid tissues. Again, the interpretation of these experiments is very difficult, since a direct effect on a T cell-mediated response may be counteracted by an enhancing effect on B cell proliferation. In addition, many of the procedures are stressful for the animals and such effects may interact with the intended effects of the experimental procedures.

ACTH and corticosteroids

Lymphocyte numbers in the peripheral circulation and immune responsiveness follow a cycle of diurnal variation. For example, in mice the numbers of circulating lymphocytes and mononuclear cells peaks at midnight and is at its lowest at midday. Likewise, the response to injected tumours was also lowest at midday. These cycles follow the diurnal variation in the production of pro-opiomelanocortin (POMC) in the hypothalamus, which may be broken down into melanotropin, adreno-corticotrophic hormone (ACTH) and various endorphins and enkephalins. ACTH acts on the adrenal cortex to induce corticosteroids and these hormones have been shown to be strongly immunosuppressive. An example of the importance of these hormones in controlling immune responses

is seen in experimental allergic encephalo-myelitis (EAE) in rats. The LEW strain which is susceptible to EAE tends to produce low levels of corticosteroids, whereas the PVG strain produces high levels of these hormones and is not. However, adrenalectomized PVG animals cannot produce the corticosteroids and do develop EAE; this variation is not the only trait controlling susceptibility to EAE.

Lymphocytes can also participate in the control of corticosteroid production. Following the demonstration that blood mononuclear cells could also produce ACTH, it was found that over 50% of leukocytes would respond to low levels of corticotropin releasing factor (CRF) by the synthesis of POMC and ultimately ACTH itself. This response is suppressed by dexamethasone, a synthetic corticosteroid analogue and so lymphocytes appear to respond in a similar way to pituicytes. The functional significance of ACTH production by lymphocytes is still debated. Some B cell lines can both produce and respond to ACTH, where it appears to act in concert with IL-4 and IL-2 to enhance growth, although it has no activity by itself. In other cases plaque forming cell responses to both T-dependent and, to a lesser extent, T-independent antigens were suppressed by exogenous ACTH at nanomolar concentrations. This in turn hints at differential effects on different lymphocyte subpopulations with B cells being stimulated and T cells suppressed by ACTH. It has been suggested that the lymphocyte contribution to the total plasma ACTH pool is low but nevertheless it might be important locally in lymphoid organs.

Endocrine receptors and neuropeptide receptors

Receptors for more than 20 different peptide hormones have been identified on lymphocytes or mononuclear phagocytes. Some of the more important ones are listed in *Figure 11.18* but the relative importance of each of these hormones in modulating immune reactions is an open question. The roles of the endogenous opiates α, β and γ-endorphin are particularly interesting since, like ACTH, these are released from POMC and their levels are raised during stress. α-endorphin which constitutes the N-terminal portion of β-endorphin suppresses plaque-forming cell responses. However, β-endorphin at low doses enhances responses. This has lead to the suggestion that there are two sites on β-endorphin, one of which can suppress and one of which enhances. This allows some measure of control of immune responses by these peptides, depending on the level and balance of the opioids which are available to responding lymphocytes.

Finally, one should mention the possible role of neuroendocrine modulation of the effector stages of the immune response, particularly in type I and type IV hypersensitivity reactions. Substance P and vasoactive intestinal peptide (VIP) released from peripheral nerves both act on smooth muscle and can therefore modulate the effects of mast cell mediators such as histamine. Substance P causes contraction of smooth muscle from ileum, whereas VIP relaxes it. VIP therefore antagonizes the histamine-induced vasoconstriction occurring in asthma and both can modulate inflammatory responses by controlling the patency of resistance vessels. Several mediators, including dynorphin, β-endorphin and substance P can also act directly on mast cells to cause granule release and, in the case of substance P,

Hormone	Produced	Targets	Principal effects
Glucocorticoids	adrenal cortex	T and B cells	↓ Ab production, ↓ NK activity ↓ cytokine production
ACTH	pituitary activated lymphocytes	T and B cells	glucocorticoid induction, variable effects on antibody production, cytokine production and proliferation
Enkephalins	pituitary	T and B cells	low dose T cell activation, high dose suppression
β-endorphin	pituitary	T and B cells	variable effects — usually suppresses cellular activation and antibody synthesis
Melatonin	pituitary	T cells/ thymocytes	↑ Ab synthesis ↑ MLC proliferation
Catecholamines	adrenal medulla sympathetic nerves	B cells > T cells	↑ cell mobilization, accelerated immune responses
Thyroxine	thyroid	lymphocytes	↑ plaque forming cells, ↑ T cell activation
Prolactin	pituitary	T cells, B cells, macrophages	↑ macrophage activation, ↑ IL-2 production
Growth hormone	pituitary	mononuclear cellls	↑ macrophage activation, ↑ Ab synthesis
Vasopressin and oxytocin	pituitary	T cells	↑ proliferation

Fig. 11.18 Hormones that act on leukocytes. Some of the major hormones that have been shown to bind specifically to leukocytes are listed, togeher with their principal effects. At least 10 other hormones are known to bind to lymphocytes via specific receptors.

eicosanoid production. In contrast to these mediators, somatostatin, also released from peripheral nerves, appears to modulate responses by inhibiting basophil activation and in some cases blocking release of other neurotransmitters. Clearly, the fine control of these reactions is very complex and the detailed role of each mediator is still under investigation.

SUMMARY

The maintenance of an immune response is ultimately controlled by the availability of antigen. Following stimulation with antigen and accessory cell-derived co-stimulatory signals, T and B cells move from a resting G0 state into G1, produce a variety of cytokines, express receptors for cytokines and progress to cell division and in the case of the B cell secrete immunoglobulin. Once antigen is removed the cells gradually return to a quiescent state.

Genetic factors also influence the immune response. Differences in APC function can clearly affect the ability of different strains of animals to respond effectively to antigen. The inability of a given antigenic determinant to associate with a particular MHC antigen would render individuals with that haplotype unresponsive to that epitope. The expressed T cell repertoire is also modified by MHC and polymorphic self antigens and this may affect the immune response. T cells have been shown to play a role, not only by providing help for an effective immune response but also by possibly biasing or depressing immune responses. There is now good evidence for two distinct subpopulations of CD4+ T cells which secrete different cytokines. Differential activation of these subsets profoundly influences the subsequent immune response. Imbalance in these subsets can lead to pathological states.

Immunoglobulins themselves can both enhance or suppress B cell and cell-mediated immune responses depending on the isotype and epitope specificity. This can be accomplished in a variety of ways including antigen clearance, more efficient antigen localization and presentation or through idiotypic interactions.

The immune response is also clearly influenced by the central nervous and endocrine systems either through innervation or through release of hormones which may influence the production of or response to cytokines. The integration of all these levels of control is essential for the maintenance of health in a changing environment.

FURTHER READING

Aichele P, Kyburz D, Ohashi PS, Odermatt B, Zinkernagel RM, Hengartner H, Pircher H. Peptide-induced T cell tolerance to prevent autoimmune diabetes in a transgenic mouse model. *Proc Natl Acad Sci USA* 1994, **91**:444.

Blalock JE, Smith EM, Meyer WJ. The pituitary-adrenocortical axis and the immune system. *Clin Endocrinol Metab* 1985, **14**:1021.

Calabrase JR, Kling MA, Gold PW. Alterations in immunocompetence during stress, bereavement and depresssion: focus on neuroendocrine regulation. *Am J Psychiatry* 1987, **144**:1123.

Eisenberg RA, Sobel ES, Reap EA, Halpern MD, Cohen PL. The role of B cell abnormalities in the systemic autoimmune syndromes of *lpr* and *gld* mice. *Semin Immunol* 1994, **6**:49.

Felten DL, Felten SY, Bellinger DL, Carlson SL, Ackerman KD, Madden KS, Olschowski JA, Livnat S. Noradrenergic sympathetic neural interactions with the immune system: structure and function. *Imm Rev* 1987, **100**:225.

Fink PJ, Shimonkevitz RP, Bevan MJ. Veto cells. *Ann Rev Immunol* 1988, **6**:115.

Gaulton GN, Greene MI. Idiotypic mimicry of biological receptors. *Ann Rev Immunol* 1986, **4**:253.

Gershon RK, Kondo K. Infectious immunological tolerance. *Immunol* 1972, **21**:903.

Goodnow CC, Adelstein S, Basten A. The need for central and peripheral tolerance in the B cell repertoire. *Science* 1990, **248**:1373.

Harlan DM, Hengartner H, Huang ML, Kang Y-H, Abe R, Moreadith W, Pircher H, Gray GS, Ohashi PS, Freeman GJ, Nadler LM, June CH, Aichele P. Mice expressing both B7-1 and viral glycoprotein on pancreatic beta cells along with glycoprotein-specific transgenic T cells develop diabetes due to a breakdown of T lymphocyte unresponsiveness. *Proc Natl Acad Sci USA* 1994, **91**:3137.

Herman A, Kappler JW, Marrack P, Pullen A. Superantigens: mechanisms of T cell stimulation and role in immune responses. *Ann Rev Immunol* 1991, **9**:745.

Holt PG. Immunoprophylaxis of atopy: light at the end of the tunnel? *Immunol Today* 1994, **15**:484.

Howard JG, Hale C, Liew FY. Genetically determined response mechanisms to cutaneous Leishmaniaisis. *Trans R Soc Trop Med Hygeine* 1982, **76**:152.

Husband AJ, Ed. *Psychoimmunology.* CRC Press Inc: Boca Raton; 1993.

Hutchings PR, Cooke A, Dawe K, Waldmann H, Roitt IM. Active suppression induced by anti-CD4. *Eur J Immunol* 1993, **23**:965.

Jacob CO, McDevitt HO. Tumour necrosis factor-α in murine autoimmune lupus nephritis. *Nature* 1988, **331**:356.

Jerne NJ. Towards a network theory of the immune system. *Ann Immunol Paris* 1974, **1235**:373.

Mason D, MacPhee I, Antoni F. The role of the neuroendocrine system in determining genetic susceptibility to experimental allergic encephalomyelitis in the rat. *Immunol* 1990, **70**:1.

McCann SM, Ono N, Khoram O, Kentroti S, Aguila A. The role of brain peptides in neuroimmunomodulation. *Ann N Y Acad Sci* 1987, **496**:173.

Merino R, Iwamoto M, Fossati L, Muniesa P, Araki K, Takahashi S, Huarte J, Yamamura KI, Vassali JD, Izui S. Prevention of systemic lupus erythematosus in autoimmune BXSB mice by a transgene

encoding I-E alpha chain. *J Exp Med* 1993, **178**:1189.

Metzler B, Wraith DC. Inhibition of experimental autoimmune encephalomyelitis by inhalation but not oral administration of the encephalitogenic peptide: influence of MHC binding affinity. *Int Immunol* 1993, **5**:1159.

Moskophidis D, Lechner F, Pircher H, Zinkernagel RM. Virus persistence in acutely infected immunocompetent mice by exhaustion of antiviral cytotoxic effector T cells. *Nature* 1993, **362**:758.

Nagata S, Suda T. Fas and Fas ligand: lpr and gld mutations. *Immunol Today* 1995, **16**:39.

Nossal GJV. Negative selection of lymphocytes. *Cell* 1994, **76**:229.

Parish NM, Roitt IM, Cooke A. Phenotypic characteristics of cells involved in induced suppression to murine experimental autoimmune thyroiditis. *Eur J Immunol* 1988, **18**:1463.

Payan DG, McGillis JP, Goetzl EJ. Neuroimmunology. *Adv Immunol* 1987, **39**:299.

Powell D, Mason D. Evidence that the T cell repertoire of normal rats contains cells with the potential to cause diabetes. Characterization of the CD4+ T cell subset that inhibits this autoimmune potential. *J Exp Med* 1993, **177**:627.

Powrie F, Leach MW, Mauze S, Menon S, Caddle LB, Coffman RL. Inhibition of Th1 responses prevents inflammatory bowel disease in *scid* mice reconstituted with CD45RB^hi CD4+T cells. *Immunity* 1994, **1**:553

Rozzo SJ, Eisenberg RA, Cohen PL, Kotzin BL. Development of the T cell receptor repertoire in *lpr* mice. *Semin Immunol* 1994, **6**:19.

Sadick MD, Heinzel FP, Hokaday BJ, Pu RT, Dawkins RS, Locksby RM. Cure of Leishmaniasis with anti-interleukin-4 monoclonal antibody. Evidence for a T-cell dependent interferon-γ-independent mechanism. *J Exp Med* 1990, **171**:115.

Schwartz RH. A cell culture method for T cell clonal anergy. *Science* 1990, **248**:1349.

Scott B, Liblau R, Degermann S, Marconi LA, Ogata L, Caton AJ, McDevitt HO, Lo D. A role for non-MHC genetic polymorphism in susceptibility to spontaneous autoimmunity. *Immunity* 1994, **1**:73.

Stein KE, Soderstrom T. Neonatal administration of idiotype or antiidiotype primes for protection against Escherichia coli K13 infection in mice. *J Exp Med* 1984, **160**:101.

Tapo FJ, Caceras-Dittmar G, Sanchez MA. Inadequate epidermal homing leads to tissue damage in human cutaneous leishmaniasis. *Immunol Today* 1994, **15**:160.

Vidal SM, Malo DM, Vogan K, Skamene, Gros P. Natural resistance to infection with intracellular parasites: isolation of a candidate for Bcg. *Cell* 1993, **73**:469.

von Boehmer H. Positive selection of lymphocytes. *Cell* 1994, **76**:219.

Weiner HL, Friedman A, Miller A, Khoury SJ, Al-Sabbagh A, Santos L, Sayegh M, Nussenblatt RB, Trentham DE, Hafler DA. *Ann Rev Immunol* 1994, **12**:809.

Zinkernagel RM, Pircher HP, Ohashi P, Oehen S, Odermatt B Mak T, Arnheiter H, Burki K, Hengartner H. T and B cell tolerance and responses to viral antigens in transgenic mice: implications for the pathogenesis of autoimmune versus immunopathological disease. *Imm Rev* 1991, **122**:133.

Wicker A, Todd A, Patterson LS. Genetic control of autoimmune diabetes in the NOD mouse. *Ann Rev Imm* 1995, **13**:179.

12 Tolerance and Autoimmunity

The term tolerance defines a state of specific immunological non-responsiveness to an antigen which arises as a result of previous exposure to that antigen. This is a purely functional definition of a state which may be achieved in a variety of ways, including clonal deletion of specific T or B cells, clonal anergy, effector cell blockade and the development of T cells capable of regulating or suppressing specific immune responses. Advances in elucidating the mechanisms underlying tolerance are attributable to the use of transgenic mice coupled with the availability of antibodies recognizing specific TCR Vβ or Vα-chains. Several key questions about tolerance induction — where it happens and how it is brought about — have been addressed and in some cases answered.

Immunological non-responsiveness due to administration of exogenous antigen is called 'acquired immunological' tolerance whereas non-responsiveness to endogenous antigens is termed 'natural immunological' or 'self' tolerance. The relationship between natural and induced states of tolerance is unclear but several systems have been described in which self tolerance is broken and autoimmune responses induced. These autoimmune states can often be regulated by inducing a state of acquired immunological non-responsiveness.

Early studies of tolerance suggested that exposure to foreign or non-self antigens during embryonic life resulted in development of specific non-responsiveness to those antigens. In 1945, Owen observed that dizygotic twin cattle which share a common placenta are frequently chimaeric as a result of sharing blood cells during embryonic life. Such cattle can accept skin grafts from one another, manifesting a state of naturally induced tolerance. Similarly, studies of patients with antibodies against a wide range of HLA antigens as a result of blood transfusions, pregnancies or graft rejection, often do not make antibody against their non-inherited maternal HLA antigens. As reactivity against non-inherited paternal antigens is seen, this suggests that exposure to maternal antigens during embryonic life renders these individuals specifically tolerant.

In 1949, Burnet and Fenner emphasized the necessity of distinguishing self from non-self and suggested that this process is learnt by the immune system during ontogeny. Since, in theory, the immune sytem could respond against a whole universe of antigens, it is necessary to prevent the development of responses against self antigens and hence autoimmunity. In a classic experiment carried out by Triplett, complete removal of the pituitary from the tree frog during early life enabled the animal to reject grafted pituitary tissue, whereas if only a part of the pituitary was extirpated, these frogs tolerated the grafted tissue. This suggested that self antigens were recognized during ontogeny and that tolerance to them was established as a result. Other observations are consistent with these observations. Studies of C5 deficient animals showed that individuals incapable of making this serum protein, normally present in serum at 50–85μg/ml, are not tolerant to C5, whereas normal animals are tolerant. A similar observation has been made with the clotting component of serum, Factor VIII.

The experiments of Hanahan addressed the role of antigen expression during ontogeny and the development of self tolerance. Transgenic mice were generated in which the SV40 genes were placed under the control of an insulin promoter, such that expression of the viral transforming genes was targeted to the insulin producing pancreatic beta cells. These animals developed insulinomas and the SV40 T antigen was detected on the surface of insulinoma cells. However, one mouse line failed to develop insulinomas and further studies revealed that this line did not express the viral antigens until late in ontogeny. Therefore, these mice did not become tolerant to the viral antigens and could make an effective immune response against those cells expressing them.

In some cases, states of incomplete or partial tolerance are observed. This simply means that only some arms of the immune response against an antigen are affected. For example, delayed hypersensitivity may be blocked while antibody responses remain intact or it may be that only some classes of immunoglobulin are affected. Isotype shifts are frequently observed in states of partial tolerance. Partial tolerance almost certainly reflects immune deviation in which predominantly Th1 or Th2 responses are induced and their respective cytokines influence the immune response which predominates (Chapters 10 and 11). It has been shown that alloantigen administration to neonates induces tolerance to relevant allogeneic skin grafts in adult life, this regimen expands T cells that produce IL-4 and so provides help for antibody responses. Cytokines which are induced following antigen exposure profoundly affect the subsequent immune response (Chapter 10) and the cytokine profile is influenced by the nature of the antigen presenting cell. This in turn may be affected by the route and dose of the antigen which is administered.

MECHANISMS OF B CELL TOLERANCE INDUCTION

B cells reactive with self antigens are present in normal individuals, although they produce antibodies which are usually of low affinity — often IgM. Many of these antibodies appear to be polyspecific recognizing many different antigens as detected by ELISA. In some cases these antibodies recognize either denatured or modified self antigens, which Grabar has suggested aids the removal of effete molecules. In contrast, individuals with some autoimmune diseases make IgG antibodies which recognize self determinants with high affinity and so cause pathology; for example, anti-TSH receptor antibodies in patients with Graves' disease. The experiments of Klinman and others suggested that the bulk of autoreactive B cells might be purged from the B cell repertoire during ontogeny. The deleted cells would be those B cells with high affinity for the autoantigen; thus lower affinity B cells might escape this form of tolerance induction. As in studies of T cell tolerance the use of transgenic mice has clarified the process of the development of B cell tolerance to self antigens. Additionally, as in studies of T cell tolerance, the timing of exposure to antigen and the presence or absence of co-stimulatory signals can influence whether tolerance or reactivity prevails.

B cells are deleted in the bone marrow

Nemazee and Bürki generated transgenic mice (H-2^d) expressing a transgene encoding IgM anti-class I H-2^k alloantibody on the membrane of 20–50% of their B cells. When these mice were mated with normal H-2^k mice, B cells bearing the transgene-encoded B cell receptor (detectable by means of an anti-idiotypic reagent) were no longer present in the F$_1$ offspring and no idiotype was detectable in their sera. This suggested that the B cells expressing the transgene-encoded immunoglobulin had been deleted. However, since the possibility remained that these results could arise from the transgene-encoded antibody (anti-H-2^k) being made in cells which also contained the antigen (F$_1$ mice are H-2^k × H-2^d), Nemazee and Bürki proceeded to study the B cells of bone marrow reconstituted irradiation chimaeras (*Fig. 12.1*). In these animals the donor bone marrow cells were derived from the IgM anti-H-2^k transgenics (H-2^d) and the recipients were either H-2^d or (H-2^d × H-2^k) F$_1$ mice expressing the target antigen. In those chimaeras expressing the target antigen, B cells bearing the transgene-encoded idiotype were not detectable and such animals had markedly reduced total numbers of splenic B cells suggesting that they had been clonally deleted. The lack of B cells with high density of B220 suggested that deletion had occurred during the transition from pre-B to mature B cell, the stage where mIg is expressed.

Goodnow and colleagues have made similar observations by crossing IgM anti-hen egg lysozyme (HEL) transgenic mice (IgM anti-HEL) or anti-HEL IgM + IgD transgenic mice (IgM/IgD anti-HEL) with mice expressing a transgenically encoded membrane form of HEL (HEL^{mem}) on all cells. Transgenic Ig is detectable by an Ig allotype marker and also by its ability to bind HEL. These double transgenic mice lacked serum anti-lysozyme antibody and B cells expressing the transgenic Ig on their surface. Although immature self-reactive bone marrow B cells expressing HEL binding Ig receptor (albeit at a lower density) and low levels of B220 had a very high turnover, it was not higher than that found in non-transgenic mice and, additionally, these self-reactive B cells did not appear to die by apoptosis. When the immature bone marrow B cells (B220^{lo} IgD$^-$) from double transgenic mice were cultured in the presence of thymocytes from a non-transgenic animal surface IgM levels returned to normal (*Fig. 12.2*) and B220 levels increased. IgD was also expressed demonstrating that these B cells were not committed to die nor had there been an irreversible arrest of development. Indeed they were able to secrete antibody following LPS stimulation. Such changes were not seen when these B cells were co-cultured together with thymocytes from a HEL^{mem} transgenic mouse (*Fig. 12.2*).

BCL-2 PREVENTS ELIMINATION OF AUTOREACTIVE B CELLS IN THE BONE MARROW

When anti-HEL IgM/Bcl-2 double transgenics were used as donors of bone marrow transferred into non transgenic or HEL^{mem} recipients it was found that the presence of the *bcl-2* transgene prevented the elimination of immature autoreactive B cells and permitted them to accumulate in the periphery. However, their developmental arrest was still manifest (B220^{lo}, L-selectin^{lo}, CR2$^-$, CD23$^-$) and maturation occurred only in the absence of membrane HEL (*Fig. 12.3*).

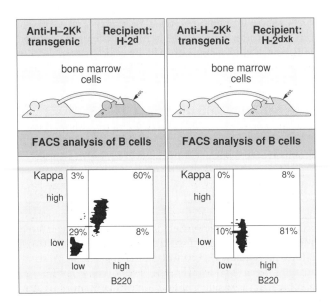

Fig. 12.1 B cells are tolerized by clonal deletion. Irradiation chimaeras were generated by transferring bone marrow from a transgenic mouse expressing an immunoglobulin receptor specific for H-2^k into mice bearing H-2K^d or F$_1$ animals also expressing H-2K^k. Mature B cells expressing surface Ig (anti-kappa) and B220 were detected in the bone marrow by double label FACS analysis. B cells expressing the transgenic Ig receptor were deleted in F$_1$ recipients expressing the H-2K^k antigen (right) but were not deleted in H-2K^d mice (left). Furthermore, cells expressing high levels of B220 were reduced in the bone marrow of chimaeras expressing H-2K^k. This data supports a deletion mechanism for B cell tolerance. Data from Nemazee and Bürki, 1989.

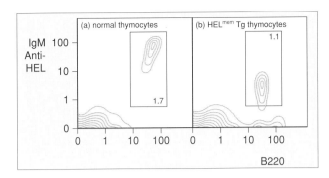

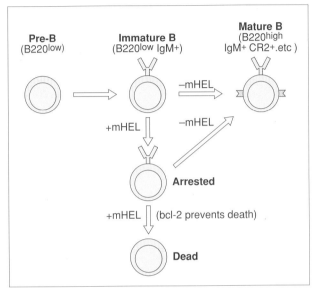

Fig. 12.2 Culture of self reactive immature B cells in the absence of self antigen restores normal phenotype. FACS-isolated immature B220^{low} IgD$^-$ bone marrow cells from double transgenic anti-HEL/HEL^{mem} mice were stained with antibodies recognizing the IgM allotype of the immunoglobulin transgene and B220 following (a) culture with non transgenic or (b) HEL^{mem} transgenic thymocytes for 32hr at 37°C. Culture with thymocytes lacking HEL leads to increased expression of surface IgM anti-HEL. Boxes indicate percent of total B cells. Data from Hartley *et al*, 1993.

Fig. 12.3 Elimination of self reactive B cells at the immature stage. Goodnow and colleagues have summarized their observations as depicted in this figure. The presence of the antigen HEL arrests the development of immature B cells. Their death is prevented by expression of *bcl-2*, although this does not prevent the developmental block. From Hartley *et al*, 1993.

B cells can be deleted in the periphery

An example involving peripheral deletion has been provided by studies of mice expressing transgenically a naturally occurring NZB IgM autoantibody to mouse erythrocytes. When these transgenic mice (IgM anti-RBC) were compared to normal mice it was found that the numbers of mature bone marrow and splenic B cells were greatly reduced. This reduction in the numbers of mature conventional B cells was not affected by transgenic co-expression of *bcl-2*. The remaining B cells had low surface expression of transgenically encoded mIg, suggesting that these B cells were anergized. By comparison, the numbers of Ly1$^+$ peritoneal B cells were not so markedly affected. Approximately 50% of the IgM anti-RBC transgenic mice developed an autoimmune haemolytic anaemia. It was established that the autoantibodies were produced by those peritoneal B-1 or Ly1$^+$ B cells (IgM^{hi} B220^{lo}) which, unlike conventional B cells (IgM^{lo} B220^{hi}), were not reduced. As i.p. injection of mouse erythrocytes eliminated the Ly1$^+$ B cells in the peritoneal cavity through apoptosis and resolved the anaemia it was suggested that the B-1 subset was not tolerized in the bone marrow but may be tolerized by antigen in the peritoneum (*Fig. 12.4*).

BCL-2 PREVENTS DELETION OF B CELLS IN THE PERIPHERY

This deletion of peritoneal autoreactive B cells was inhibited by *bcl-2* transgene expression indicating that peripheral deletion mechanism(s) differ from those in the bone marrow in this model. These findings contrast in some ways from those of Goodnow and colleagues described above as there was no increase in the numbers of immature B cells in the *bcl-2* transgenic mice expressing Ig recognizing RBC. The differences could be attributable to differences in amount, cellular location and timing of expression of the self antigens in the bone marrow as well as differences in the affinity of the transgenic Ig for its antigen. Furthermore the assay systems differ in that the HEL/anti-HEL^{mem} *bcl-2* experiments utilized irradiation chimaeras whereas the RBC/anti-RBC experiments were all carried out *in situ*.

The ability of Bcl-2 protein to prevent apoptosis of B cells is not restricted to the Ly1$^+$ B cell pool. Cross-linkage of mIg in the absence of a co-stimulation signal from a T cell leads to apoptosis. If normal mice are injected i.p. with anti-Ig antibodies — the peritoneal cavity contains little free Ig which would neutralize the injected antibody — there is an elimination of B cells. FACS analyses of the B cells before and after treatment showed that both B-1 and B-2 B cells were deleted and the use of F(ab')$_2$ fragments showed that it was not necessary for the Fc receptor to be bound for apoptosis to be initiated. This deletion does not occur in *bcl-2* transgenic mice.

The B cells of autoimmune prone mice (NZB or [NZB × NZW] F$_1$) are refractory to this form of death

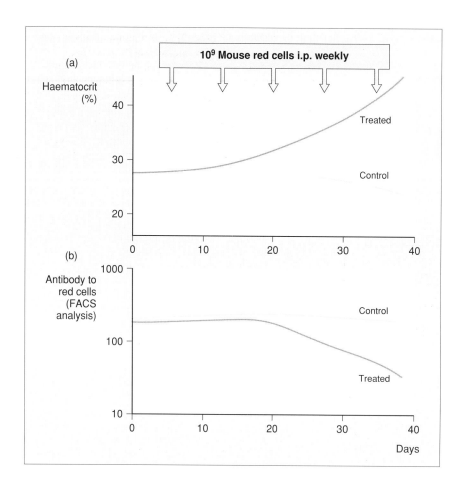

(a)

Haematocrit (%)

10^9 **Mouse red cells i.p. weekly**

Treated

Control

(b)

Antibody to red cells (FACS analysis)

Control

Treated

Days

Fig. 12.4 Intraperitoneal injection of self antigen prevents autoimmunity. Mice suffering from haemolytic anaemia as a result of expression of transgenically encoded IgM anti-RBC autoantibody were injected i.p. with RBC. This treatment resulted in an elevation of the haematocrit (a) and a reduction (b) in the levels of bound autoantibody. Data from Murakami *et al*, 1992.

signal through their Ig receptor (*Fig. 12.5*). However, this reduced susceptibility to B cell apoptosis via receptor cross linkage in these mouse strains does not appear to be due to increased levels of *bcl-2* expression in their B cells. This has led to the suggestion that some fundamental defect in the elimination of self reactive B cells may lead to the pathogenesis that develops in these animals.

Tolerance through B cell anergy

Single transgenic mice have been constructed where HEL is expressed and secreted under the inducible control of the metallothionein promoter or constitutively with the albumin promoter. Different transgenic lines expressed different levels of HEL in the blood ranging from high (10^{-8}M or 120ng/ml) to low (10^{-10}M or less). Following immunization with HEL it was possible to show that peripheral tolerance to HEL was established through different routes in the different transgenic lines. Those transgenic mice expressing low levels of HEL were tolerant only at the T cell level and could be induced to make high affinity anti-HEL antibody if immunized with HEL coupled to a carrier. Transgenic mice expressing high levels of HEL were tolerant in both the B cell and T cell compartments and following immunization with HEL coupled to a carrier such as SRBC could make only a low affinity anti-HEL antibody response (*Fig. 12.6*). To analyse this system further, double transgenic mice were generated expressing HEL in soluble form and also a high affinity anti-HEL antibody (see above). The double transgenic mice did not

contain the serum anti-HEL antibody present at high levels in the single Ig transgenic mice. However, the double transgenic mice did contain normal numbers of HEL binding allotype expressing B cells. Detailed FACS analysis showed that these B cells had up to 100-fold reduction in the level of mIgM expression but no reduction in the level of IgD expression. All other markers such as B220, L-selectin, MHC class II, CD22, CD23 and CD21 were normal. Furthermore these B cells were normally distributed throughout the B cell areas in the spleen and lymph node. Thus although apparently maturationally normal and residing in the follicular mantle zone, the B cells from double transgenic mice were functionally inactive or anergic. Anergy was found in double transgenic mice where the levels of soluble HEL were sufficient to cause 45% occupancy of the available B cell receptors but not in those where only a 4.5% occupancy was achieved. Downregulation of mIgM results from retention of mIgM within the endoplasmic reticulum and this together with a desensitization of the remaining receptors (both IgM and IgD) which results in a diminished tyrosine kinase activity and Ca^{2+} flux contributes to the anergic state. Further insight into the mechanism of negative signalling was achieved by the demonstration that HEL/anti-HEL transgenic mice which also carried the motheaten viable (*me*[v]) gene have a reduced threshold for the development of B cell anergy. The motheaten allele encodes a disrupted cytosolic protein tyrosine phosphatase, PTP1C, which in the *me*[v] mutation results in an aberrantly sized product with 10–20% the wild type activity. Introduction

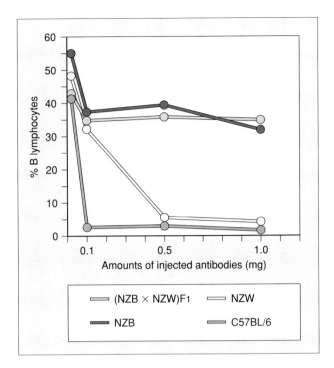

Fig. 12.5 Peritoneal B cells from autoimmunity-prone mice are not deleted by cross-linkage of their Ig receptor. NZB and (NZB × NZW) F$_1$ mice spontaneously develop autoimmunity whereas NZW and C57BL/6 mice do not. Surface Ig receptors of peritoneal B cells were cross-linked by i.p. injection of different doses of anti-IgM antibody followed by an anti-mouse Ig antibody. The numbers of peritoneal B cells were estimated 12 hours later. Data from Tsubata *et al*, 1994.

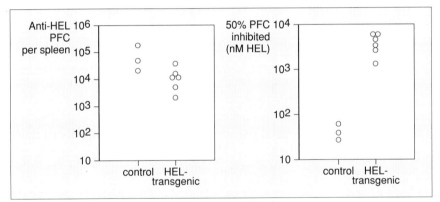

Fig. 12.6 Low affinity B cells are not tolerized.
Transgenic mice which expressed HEL showed both B and T cell tolerance to HEL. However, a B cell response was elicited via a T cell bypass when transgenic mice were immunized with HEL coupled to sheep red blood cells (SRBC). In this situation T cells specific for SRBC provide help for HEL-reactive B cells and transgenic mice can be induced to secrete anti-HEL antibody (left). The antibody secreted by the transgenic mouse was of lower affinity than that secreted by a comparably immunized non-transgenic mouse (control). The concentration of HEL required to inhibit the antibody response (plaque forming cells [PFC]) of the transgenic is 100 times greater than that required in the control mice. High affinity B cells are either absent or unable to respond. Data from Goodnow *et al*, 1990.

of the *me^v* gene into the double transgenic mice results in a reduced threshold for HEL induced B cell inactivation indicating that PTP1C is involved in B cell negative signalling.

B cells can escape deletion in the bone marrow through receptor editing.

Several lines of transgenic mice have been made which recognize endogenous self antigens. In many lines of mice such as those described above, B cells bearing receptors capable of recognizing self antigens are negatively selected in the bone marrow.

However, it has been shown that the B cells themselves may not necessarily be deleted or irrevocably arrested in their development. If the expressed receptor is revised such that it no longer binds self antigen the B cell may mature and be found in the periphery. For example, the studies of Weigert and colleagues showed that in a transgenic mouse expressing the heavy and light chain genes encoding autoantibodies to double stranded DNA (dsDNA) normal peripheral B cell numbers were found in the mice. These transgenic mice did not develop autoimmunity and none of the hybridomas generated from their spleens reacted against dsDNA although some reacted against single stranded DNA (ssDNA). Examination of heavy and light chain usage by the hybridomas revealed that light chains found in spontaneous anti-dsDNA autoantibodies were not represented. This has led to the suggestion that B cells may escape deletion if they can utilize different light chain rearrangements in their Ig receptor. It has been shown that immature sIg B cells express RAG mRNA when they encounter the autoantigen and undergo secondary light chain rearrangements thus generating a different receptor specificity. If the new receptor does not recognize self antigen the immature B cell does not die but continues normal B cell development. This process has been termed 'receptor editing'. Although these studies have been carried out in transgenic mice the findings are consistent with the finding of a high frequency of secondary *IGK* gene rearrangements in normal B cells. As most *Vk-Jk* gene rearrangements are inversional this ensures retention of the entire *Vk* gene repertoire should further revision be required.

T CELL TOLERANCE

Many T cells capable of recognizing self antigen are deleted in the thymus through central tolerance. As the avidity threshold for tolerance induction in the thymus is less than that required for activation in the periphery this provides an efficient means of generating tolerance to many self antigens. In addition to deletion it has been shown that thymocytes may be rendered functionally inactive or anergic following presentation of self antigen by thymic epithelial cells. This tolerance would apply only to those self antigens expressed in the thymus or able to reach it. Additionally, as some tissue specific peptides would be presented to CD8+ T cells in the context of MHC class I molecules, some form of peripheral tolerance mechanisms must apply. Tolerance within the CD4+ T cell pool may provide one mechanism but other mechanisms also operate.

Peripheral T cell tolerance

Transgenic mice have provided valuable insights into the mechanisms by which T cell tolerance may be obtained to self antigens expressed in the periphery. Transgenic mice have been constructed in which a foreign antigen, an MHC or a viral antigen, is expressed under the control of a tissue specific promoter. In most cases the animals were found to be tolerant to the transgene product even though no thymic expression of the transgene was evident, thus excluding central tolerance. In those situations where antigen is present in the thymus it is likely that not all antigen reactive cells are actually deleted. This has been shown both for CD4+ T cells as well as CD8+ T cells.

After central tolerance peripheral CD4+ T cells remain which are capable of low avidity T cell interactions

The β-chain of mouse haemoglobin occurs in two allelic forms, Hbbs and Hbbd. It has been shown that a single epitope, Hbd (64–76), which binds to H-2Ek, is a self antigen in CBA/J (Hbbd) mice but a foreign antigen in CE/J

mice (Hbbs). Variants of Hbd (64–76), for example with a serine at position 69, have been shown to modify T cell function *in vitro* and have thus been called altered peptide ligands (APL). The influence of such events on *in vivo* T cell function has been explored in a transgenic mouse model in which a transgenic TCR β-chain derived from a hybridoma specific for Hbd (64–76) has been introduced. When the transgene-encoded β-chain paired with an endogenous α-chain a primary reactivity to an APL was found and it was shown that some T cell responses were directed primarily against the Ser 69 variant. For some T cell responses Hbd (64–76) was itself found to behave as antagonist (*Fig. 12.7*). To explore the *in vivo* consequences of such a reactivity pattern the transgenic mice were crossed to CBA/J mice whose haemoglobin contains the Hbd (64–76) epitope. As Hbd (64–76) is known to be expressed together with H-2Ek on cortical epithelial cells of this strain it is perhaps not surprising that T cells capable of a high avidity interaction with Hbd (64–76) were deleted in the thymus. This is reflected in the demonstrable shift in the Ser 69 dose curve required to elicit a response in these peripheral transgenic T cells and the increased CD4 dependency of this response. If this was used as a model of self tolerance the implication would be that these autoreactive T cells would only become activated in conditions of high

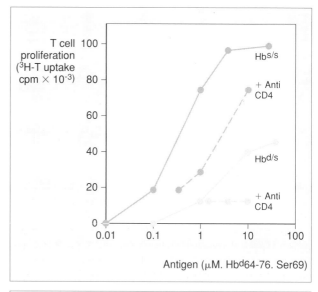

Fig. 12.7 Low avidity self reactive T cells are present in the periphery. Transgenic mice expressing a TCR in which the endogenous α-chain pairing with the transgenic β-chain produces T cells capable of recognizing a Ser 69 variant of Hbd (64–76). The non mutated, naturally expressed Hbd (64–76) acts as an antagonist. Comparison of T cell responsiveness to increasing doses of the Ser 69 variant in transgenic mice on a Hbs/s or Hbd/s background showed responsiveness only at higher doses in Hbd/s mice. Analysis of the effect of anti-CD4 on T cell responses to the Ser 69 variant showed a greater requirement for CD4 in T cell activation in the Hbd/s mice. Data from Hsu *et al*, 1995.

antigen concentrations and presentation on cells providing adequate co-stimulation.

Tolerance through ignorance

It is arguable that tolerance through ignorance is not true tolerance as tolerance may be defined as a functional state which arises as a result of previous encounter with antigen. Self tolerance has long been known to be broken when self antigen is released from a sequestered or privileged site. However, Zinkernagel and colleagues provided a model system which permits a detailed study of this phenomenon. Transgenic mice were constructed which expressed a D^b-restricted TCR specific for the LCMV glycoprotein (gp) peptide 32–42. This epitope is a dominant CTL epitope in LCMV infection of C57BL mice. This transgenic line has been used extensively to demonstrate that central tolerance can occur at various stages of T cell ontogeny, that the avidity of the interaction for negative selection is less than that required for T cell activation in the periphery and that thymic epithelium can mediate deletion.

Other transgenic mice were constructed in which LCMV gp was expressed under the control of an insulin promoter (RIP-gp) thus directing expression of the viral protein to the β cells of the pancreas. Single transgenic RIP-gp mice were able to develop effective CTL responses against LCMV gp and moreover developed insulin dependent diabetes mellitus (IDDM) following infection with LCMV. These single transgenic mice also developed antibody responses against LCMV gp equivalent to that found in non-transgenic mice. Expression of LCMV gp in the pancreatic β cells therefore did not functionally affect the activity of LCMV CTL or the B cell response to virus. Study of the double transgenic mice generated by breeding RIP-gp mice with the TCR transgenics revealed that the T cells were not deleted, there was no reduction in T cell CD8 expression levels and IDDM did not develop spontaneously although T cells from the double transgenic mice were shown to recognize LCMV gp *in vitro*. Infection of these double transgenic mice with LCMV resulted in IDDM. It is clear from this study that potentially autoreactive CTL are present yet do not manifest their cytolytic activity until they are activated following infection. Although the pancreatic β cell expressed LCMV gp it was unable to activate the CTL itself. The inability to activate the CD8+ T cell appeared to be due to a lack of co-stimulation as transgenic introduction of B7 into the β cells elicited spontaneous IDDM in TCR/RIP-gp/RIP-B7 triple transgenic mice (see Chapter 11).

T cell tolerance through anergy

Several different lines of transgenic mice have been generated by expressing an alloreactive TCR specific for K^b and additionally K^b on different peripheral sites due to the use of tissue specific promoters (*Fig. 12.8*). The TCR was detected by means of an anti-clonotype. All the lines of mice were tolerant of K^b skin grafts and failed to reject EL4 cells, a K^b expressing tumour cell line. In all cases, K^b expression was restricted to the peripheral tissue and none was expressed in the thymus as evidenced by the following:

- Lack of detection of K^b in the thymus by PCR.
- The failure of thymus grafts from K^b transgenic mice to confer the tolerant phenotype.
- Normal positive selection of CD8+ clonotype positive T cells.

In all cases, the mice were specifically tolerant of the alloantigen K^b and as T cells were present in the periphery this suggests that the T cells were functionally inactive or anergic *in vivo*.

Anergy through downregulation of TCR and co-receptors

The level of expression of CD8, Thy-1 and TCR was downregulated in both Alb-K^b and GFAP-K^b transgenic mice. This downregulation could be reversed *in vitro* in the TCR x GFAP-K^b transgenic mice by *in vitro* culture of spleen T cells with antigen (*Fig. 12.9*).

Another interesting example of T cell anergy through TCR downregulation occurs during pregnancy (Tafun *et al*, 1995). The female TCR transgenic mice above were mated with mice with a different MHC haplotype. Females mated with H-2^b males but not other haplotypes downregulated their anti-H-$2K^b$ TCR+ cells and were unable to destroy H-2^b tumours. After parturition TCR levels returned to normal as did the ability to reject EL4 cells.

Double transgenic TCR x 2.4 Ker-K^b (keratin promoter with H-$2K^b$) mice were tolerant of K^b bearing skin grafts but showed no reduction in TCR or co-receptor expression on peripheral T cells. As the peripheral T cells expressed enhanced levels of activation markers CD44 and CD2 it was assumed that they had encountered antigen. The expression of antigen on epithelial cells was able to maintain the tolerant state which was shown to be reversible as transfer of spleen cells from TCR x 2.4 Ker IV transgenic mice to nude H-2^d recipients conferred the ability to reject K^b expressing skin grafts.

Promoter	TCR construct specificity	Expression	K^b Skin graft acceptance	EL4 growth inhibition	*In vitro* K^b CTL
Albumin	K^b	liver	+	+	+
C reactive protein	K^b	inducible in liver	+	+	+
Keratin IV	K^b	epithelium	+	+	+
Glial fibrillary acidic protein	K^b	cells of neuroectoderm origin	+	+	+

Fig.12.8 T cell receptor transgenics used to examine tolerance mechanisms in which K^b is only expressed in the periphery.
The different double transgenic lines were called TCR × ALB-K^b, TCR × CRP-K^b, TCR × 2.4 Ker-K^b and TCR × GFAP-K^b respectively.

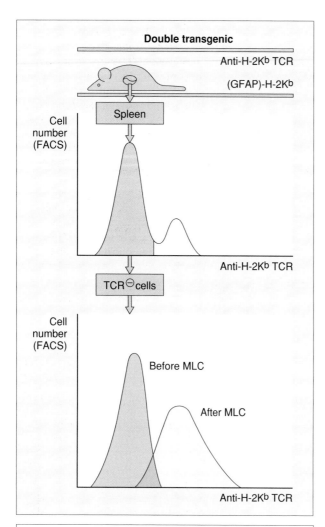

Fig.12.9 Upregulation of clonotype expression following *in vitro* culture with antigen. Spleen cells from TCR anti-H-2K^b/H-2K^b double transgenic mice of haplotype H-2$^{d/k}$ were separated by FACS into TCR$^+$ and TCR$^-$ populations (upper panel). Clonotype negative splenic T cells were cultured in mixed lymphocyte culture in the presence of alloantigen (H-2^b). FACS analysis for TCR anti-H-2K^b clonotype expression showed that upregulation of the clonotype could be seen following culture of clonotype negative cells with K^b expressing cells (lower panel). Data from Arnold *et al*, 1994.

Peripheral antigen concentration affects downregulation of TCR

The influence of antigen concentration on the levels of expression of TCR and co-receptors has been shown in TCR x CRP-K^b double transgenic mice. C reactive protein (CRP) synthesis is induced in the hepatocytes by a variety of agents including LPS. In TCR x CRP-K^b transgenic mice 30% of the CD8$^+$ T cells expressed normal levels of TCR and the remainder had much reduced levels of expression. After induction of CRP with LPS a further reduction in the number of cells with normal TCR expression was seen and even a reduction in the total number of CD2$^+$ CD4$^-$ T cells (*Fig. 12.10*). This

suggests that an increase in the peripheral concentration of the antigen caused a further downregulation of TCR and co-receptor in some T cells and a deletion in others.

These and other transgenic studies suggest that CD8$^+$ T cells which recognize self antigen expressed only in the periphery may not be deleted but become functionally inactive. As with CD4$^+$ T cells there is also data to suggest that CD8$^+$ T cells that escape central tolerance do so because they have a lower avidity for the antigen–MHC class I complex.

Oldstone, von Herrath and colleagues have constructed transgenic mice expressing LCMV nucleoprotein (NP) under the control of the *Thy-1.2* promoter (Thy-1.2-NP) and thus express LCMV NP in all T cells. In H-2^d mice all high affinity CTL specific for NP were deleted in the thymus through central tolerance but low affinity CTL were spared. If parallels were to be drawn between this and true autoantigens which may be expressed both in the thymus and in the periphery, incomplete deletion of autoreactive T cells might occur and only T cells capable of low affinity interactions with peptide–MHC complexes are released into the periphery.

Peripheral tolerance through deletion

The superantigen staphylococcal enterotoxin B (SEB) stimulates CD4$^+$ and CD8$^+$ T cells expressing Vβ8. If SEB is injected into adult mice a large number of CD4$^+$ and CD8$^+$ Vβ8$^+$ T cells are deleted. If SEB is given to thymectomized mice it has been shown that an initial proliferative response is followed by an 80% loss of those cells bearing Vβ-chains reactive with the superantigen. Similar results have been found with SEA and deletion of Vβ3$^+$ T cells. A possible explanation for these observations is that superantigens induce deletion because they are being presented on non-professional APC with an absence of co-stimulatory molecules. Recent experiments by Vella and colleagues have shown that this deletion was minimized by concomitant injection of LPS (*Fig. 12.11*) and that this rescue is not due to an involvement of B7-1 or B7-2 but perhaps partly through the elaboration of TNFα by activated macrophages.

Peripheral tolerance through deletion may also be achieved through the action of veto cells (Chapter 11); T cells reactive against graft alloantigens may be deleted in this way.

EXPERIMENTAL INDUCTION AND MAINTENANCE OF TOLERANCE

There are many situations where it would be appropriate to try to generate immunological tolerance. Many factors influence the outcome of an immune response and additionally the ease of tolerance induction. An understanding of the basis of these variables will lead to better protocols for inducing and maintaining tolerance.

Age of the animal

Following Owen and Traub's demonstration that exposure to antigen *in utero* results in tolerance to the antigen, Billingham *et al.* induced tolerance to allografts by injecting

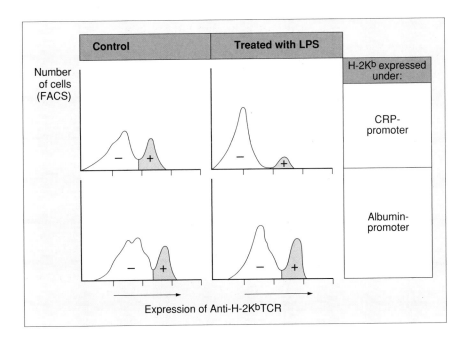

Fig. 12.10 Peripheral antigen concentration affects the downregulation of clonotype expression. Production by the liver of C reactive protein (CRP) but not albumin is increased by LPS injection. Clonotype analysis of TCR single transgenic and TCR x CRP-K^b and TCR x Alb-K^b double transgenic mice. CD8$^+$ splenic T cell-enriched populations were analysed. Upregulation of H-2K^b by LPS leads to the loss of the cells expresssing anti-H-2K^b TCR. Data from Arnold *et al*, 1994.

allogeneic spleen and bone marrow cells into embryonic or neonatal mice. Similar observations were made by Hasek and colleagues in the chicken, in which chimaerism was obtained by embryonic parabiosis. The observation that tolerance is more readily induced and is of longer duration in immature animals has been amply confirmed.

These ontogenic differences reflect the differential sensitivity of immature and mature B and T cells to signals transduced by their antigen-specific membrane receptors. This is seen in the experiments of Nossal *et al.* in which the ability of anti-IgHμ antibody to tolerize adult and newborn splenic B cells was investigated. Thirty times more antibody was required to inhibit B cell mitogenesis or antibody formation by mature B cells than was necessary for newborn B cells. This greater sensitivity of immature B cells to tolerance induction has also been shown using a range of antigens. The *in vitro* studies of Matzinger and Guerder show that immature T cells die when presented with antigen on dendritic cells which are the most potent antigen presenting cell for mature T cells, suggesting that the outcome of signalling through the TCR is much dependent on the maturational status of the T cell.

Genetic background

Strain differences have been observed in the ease and maintenance of tolerance induction in mice; for example, the autoimmune mouse strain (NZB × NZW) F₁ was found to be difficult to tolerize and the tolerance induced was of short duration (see above). All murine strains that develop symptoms similar to human systemic lupus erythematosus (SLE) have been shown to be resistant to tolerance induction with hapten-substituted or disaggregated immunoglobulin. However, this may not be universally true for all antigens as one of the autoimmune mouse strains (MRL/lpr) can be tolerized to haptenated syngeneic spleen cells. Cinader and Hutchings and colleagues have shown that SJL mice manifest some abnormalities in tolerance induction; this is particularly interesting as this strain is highly susceptible to the

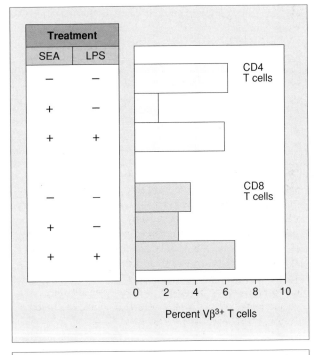

Fig. 12.11 SEA causes deletion of Vβ3$^+$ T cells which is prevented by LPS. Mice were injected with 0.04μg SEA and then 24 hours later with 50μg LPS. The percentage of splenic CD4$^+$ and CD8$^+$ Vβ3$^+$ T cells was determined by flow cytometry 9 days after SEA injection. Data from Vella *et al*, 1995.

experimental induction of many autoimmune conditions. Unlike most mouse strains, SJL mice cannot develop T cells that can specifically regulate the experimental induction of thyroid autoimmunity or haemolytic anaemia.

Composition of the antigen

The physical properties of the antigen are critical in determining its efficacy as a tolerogen. In general, agents that are poorly degraded are good tolerogens; for example, supra-immunogenic doses of polysaccharides or polymers composed of D-amino acids are slowly catabolized, thus they persist and maintain the state of tolerance. The experiments of Dresser highlighted the fact that disaggregated soluble antigen is a powerful inducer of tolerance in adult animals. The reason for this may be that when soluble antigen is internalized by APC they fail to be activated such that the necessary co-stimulatory molecules such as B7 are expressed. Antigen presentation to a T cell in the absence of co-stimulation may lead to anergy.

A particularly effective way of inducing tolerance is to inject the antigen coupled to splenocytes. This leads to an immune deviation or split tolerance as Th1 or DTH responses to the antigen are depressed while Th2 or antibody responses remain intact. This means of specifically depressing the DTH response approach has been used to prevent chronic inflammatory demyelinating disease induced by Theiler's murine encephalomyelitis virus (*Fig. 12.12*). This bias of the immune response towards a Th2 type at the expense of a Th1 response may have arisen through presentation of antigen by B cells. This is clearly suggested by the observations of Day and colleagues who prevented rat EAE by ensuring that B cells presented a myelin basic protein (MBP) derived encephalitogenic peptide — the peptide was coupled to anti-IgD to direct it to the B cell.

Dose of antigen

The studies of Mitchison showed that the dose of antigen could influence the degree and duration of tolerance. In general it was found that supra-immunogenic doses of antigen could sometimes cause immunological unresponsiveness; detailed dose curves were carried out by Mitchison, clearly demonstrating that for some T-dependent antigens tolerance could be induced at two dose ranges, one lower and one higher than that used for optimal immunization (*Fig. 12.13*). In the case of T-independent antigens such a biphasic dose curve was not observed. Cell transfer studies showed that at low antigen doses the T cells were tolerized whereas at higher doses B cells as well as T cells could be tolerized. This was called low and high zone tolerance, respectively. The dose of antigen required to tolerize mature T cells is many times lower (sometimes a thousandfold) than that required to tolerize mature B cells. The amount of antigen required to cause B cell tolerance depends on the affinity of the B cell Ig receptor for the antigen. High affinity B cells can be tolerized at lower concentrations of antigen than low affinity B cells. This may explain why in some cases of incomplete tolerance only low affinity antibody is found; similar considerations may be found for T cells.

High doses of LCMV have been found to lead to clonal exhaustion of CTL (see Chapter 11). When mice are infected with high doses of virus not only does CTL exhaustion occur but also the virus persists. This inability to clear the virus completely may arise because LCMV having exhausted mature CTL then causes central tolerance in any newly arising LCMV-specific CD8+ T cells.

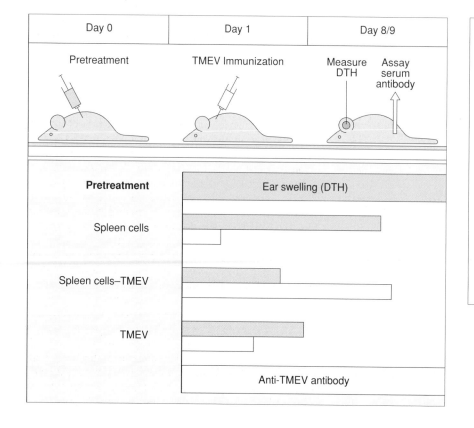

Fig. 12.12 Immune deviation results in a depressed cell-mediated response to Theiler's virus. SJL mice were injected i.v. with either 5x10⁷ spleen cells coupled to Theiler's virus (TMEV-SP) or 50μg inactivated Theiler's virus (TMEV). Mice were immunized with 25μg UV-irradiated TMEV in adjuvant s.c. 24 hours later. Seven days later mice were challenged in the ear with UV-inactivated TMEV and the ear swelling measured to indicate the extent of the DTH response. Sera were taken from the mice and assessed for TMEV specific antibody. Data from Peterson *et al*, (1993).

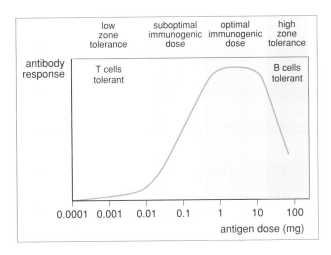

Fig. 12.13. High and low zone tolerance. Immunization of animals (e.g. the rabbit) with a T-dependent antigen produces a characteristic dose response curve of antibody levels. In the supra-immunogenic region (high zone) B cells are tolerant, while T cells may be tolerized in the sub-immunogenic (low zone) region.

Route of antigen administration

The outcome of an immune response often depends upon the route of antigen administration. Subcutaneous or intramuscular injection is usually immunogenic, whereas oral or aerosol administration is often very good at inducing tolerance. Injecting antigen intravenously or intrathymically has also been a good way of providing a tolerogenic signal. It is possible that antigen introduced intravenously or orally undergoes a process of biological filtration such that immunogenic complexes are removed, leaving the tolerogenic monomeric antigen as the first form to interact with the immunocompetent cells. It is also possible that different antigen presenting cells (e.g. 'non professional' APC) gain access to antigen following immunization through different routes and/or that immune deviation occurs following immunization through different routes. Intrathymic injection of antigen may conceivably cause clonal deletion or anergy of antigen reactive T cells. However, it has also been shown that with some antigens such injections can result in an immune deviation or split tolerance where tolerance induction inhibits a Th1 response but spares the Th2 response to antigen.

Intravenous administration of HEL has been shown to prevent subsequent immune responses to this antigen. As it was found that non-responsiveness *in vitro* could be reversed by addition of IL-2 it was suggested that soluble HEL had anergized the responsive T cells. Intravenous and oral routes of immunization have also been shown to generate T cells which are capable of adoptively transferring antigen specific tolerance. CD4$^+$ T cells (i.v. tolerance) or CD8$^+$ T cells (oral tolerance) have been shown to mediate this function (see Chapter 11). In the latter case, IFNγ and TGFβ have been implicated as mediators of tolerance. It is known that oral or inhaled soluble protein antigen stimulates primarily IFNγ production in draining lymph nodes and high concentrations of this cytokine are known to bias the T cell response towards a Th1 type of response. This would therefore lead to an immune deviation with suppression of IgE production. TGFβ suppresses many immunological activities including the proliferation and effector function of B cells, T cells and NK cells. The basis, both cellular and molecular, for tolerance induction is currently being investigated. The availability of transgenic mice expressing defined T and/or B cell antigen receptors provides systems more amenable to detailed analysis.

Manipulations facilitating tolerance induction

A variety of approaches is being used to develop regimens which would faciltate tolerance induction through either specific ablation of the whole of an immune response to a given antigen or deviation of the response from a damaging to an innocuous one. Some of these approaches have been discussed in Chapter 11 but a few additional examples are given below.

In order to prevent graft rejection it clearly would be advantageous to develop a regimen which specifically enabled the recipient to develop tolerance to the alloantigens and thus perceive the graft as self. An ability to prevent primary responses and to tolerize primed or memory responses has great therapeutic potential, since it is applicable to damaging responses against both foreign antigens such as allergens and against self antigens as occur in autoimmune disease.

It has been suggested that many of the protocols employed in transplantation to ward off rejection episodes are successful because they either minimize available T cell help (e.g. treatment with anti-CD4, Cyclosporin A or FK506) or they deplete mature cells (e.g. total lymphoid irradiation or cyclophosphamide) leaving immature cells that are more readily tolerized. Monoclonal anti-CD4 either alone or in combination with anti-CD8 antibodies has proved successful in inducing and maintaining tolerance to a variety of antigens. In terms of generating tolerance to skin graft alloantigens it is clear that combined antibody therapy is more efficient (*Fig. 12.14*). In the case of generating long term tolerance to self antigens the use of a non depleting anti-CD4 antibody alone has proved sufficient even when the T cells have already been primed. As the anti-CD4 antibody does not delete CD4$^+$ T cells but downregulates CD4 expression it is possible to examine the functional state of the tolerized cells. Waldmann and colleagues carried out an interesting series of experiments in which they examined the basis for tolerance development to AKR/J bone marrow in CBA/Ca mice which have many minor histocompatibility mismatches. These animals also differ at their Mls-1 locus, AKR being Mls-1^a and CBA/Ca being Mls-1^b. Since CD4$^+$ Vβ6$^+$ T cells are deleted by the retroviral superantigen encoded by Mls-1^a

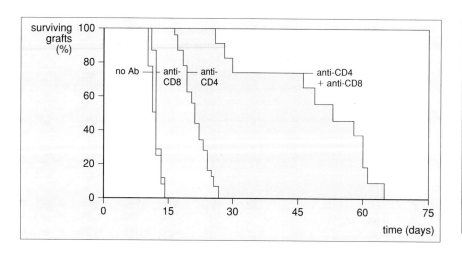

Fig. 12.14 Role of CD4⁺ and CD8⁺ T cells in graft rejection. CBA mice were grafted with BALB/c skin differing at the MHC and minor loci. Graft survival in animals treated for 30 days with anti-CD4 and anti-CD8 or a combination of both antibodies is shown. Anti-CD8 alone had no effect on graft survival, while anti-CD4 enhanced it but treatment with both antibodies was most effective. Based on data of Waldmann, 1989.

during their ontogeny in AKR/J mice, analysis of the CD4⁺ Vβ6⁺ T cells in the periphery of these bone marrow chimaeras provides an indication of whether the CBA/Ca recipient has developed tolerance to this minor antigen. The results were very clear: the mice were specifically tolerant to AKR antigens and Vβ6⁺ T cells in the periphery of these bone marrow chimaeras were unable to respond to stimulation with a mitogenic anti-Vβ6 antibody (*Fig. 12.15*). This clearly indicates that the peripheral Vβ6⁺ T cells of the CBA/Ca recipient had been rendered anergic by treatment with anti-CD4 antibody in the presence of alloantigen.

There is good data suggesting that antigen-specific tolerance induced by anti-CD4 results in the generation of cells which are able to transfer tolerance adoptively and indeed prevent the functioning of already primed cells. The actual mechanism by which this occurs is still unclear but is thought to be due to a cytokine-mediated effect of the tolerant T cells. The studies of Waldmann and colleagues suggest that tolerant T cells may be able to generate a tolerant milieu which is no longer dependent on their presence. In this sense the tolerance is said to be infectious.

Manipulations preventing tolerance induction

Certain situations favour tolerance induction whereas other situations mitigate against it; for example, several studies have

shown that treatment of neonatal or irradiated bone marrow chimaeras with Cyclosporin A (CsA) results in the development of some autoimmune conditions or what appears to be graft versus host disease. This suggests that the drug may interfere with the normal tolerogenic processes which occur during ontogeny. Sprent, Jenkins and their co-workers established that the normal clonal deletion of T cells in response to self-superantigens does not occur in CsA treated mice; it is tempting therefore to speculate that by interfering with thymocyte activation this drug spares the maturing T cells from deletion and permits their entry into the periphery. CsA must also prevent these cells from being anergized either centrally or in the periphery, since once drug treament is withdrawn these autoreactive T cells become active. An alternative explanantion is that following removal of CsA there is an imbalance in the CD4⁺ T cell subpopulations such that Th1 cells predominate. Such an imbalance has been shown to predispose to autoimmunity and graft versus host disease. Some infections may prevent anergy induction perhaps through modification of the cytokine milieu; for example, T cells can be rescued from anergy induced by superantigen following infection with *Nippostrongylus brasiliensis*.

IL-2 has also been shown to modulate tolerance induction. Neonatal spleen cells do not make IL-2 following concanavalin A stimulation; this age related ability to

Treatment	Proliferation response to:		Vβ6⁺,CD4⁺ spleen cells
	BALB/c	AKR	
Control	+	+	2.9–3.8%
Tolerized	+	−	2.8–3.7%

Fig. 12.15 Tolerance and anergy to Mls-1ᵃ. Adult thymectomized CBA/Ca (H-2ᵏ, Mls-1ᵇ) mice were injected with a non-depleting anti-CD4 antibody and an anti-CD8 antibody for 2 weeks. Two days after the beginning of antibody treatment, 2x10⁷ AKR (H-2ᵏ, Mls-1ᵃ) bone marrow cells were infused and 8 weeks later the ability of the spleen cells to respond to AKR, BALB/c (H-2ᵈ) or anti-Vβ6 was assessed. The numbers of Vβ6⁺ CD4⁺ T cells were also determined by flow cytometry and shown to be unaffected by the tolerance regimen. Control mice received the antibody treatment but not the AKR bone marrow cells. Data from Qin *et al*, 1990.

secrete IL-2 may play a role in tolerance induction. A number of experiments have shown that administration of a tolerogenic signal in the presence of IL-2 abrogates the induction of tolerance (*Fig. 12.16*). Administration of IL-2 *in vivo* not only blocks tolerization to alloantigen but also tolerance induced by antigen-coupled spleen cells. This hypothesis is supported by the observation that regimens which downregulate IL-2 production favour tolerance induction whereas those which cause IL-2 release (e.g. graft versus host disease) prevent tolerance induction.

Termination of self tolerance and methods of inducing autoimmunity

Tolerance does not normally develop to antigens which are sequestered from the immune system, such as sperm antigen and lens crystallin. Thus autoantibodies can often be detected following tissue trauma which allows contact between these antigens and the immune system.

In those individuals genetically unable to make a normal self antigen such as C5 or factor VIII tolerance is never developed to these antigens. Thus antibodies may be generated to these components when they are administered.

If we assume that during ontogeny T or B cells which bear receptors capable of engaging self-peptide–MHC complexes or self antigen respectively with a high affinity are deleted or rendered functionally inactive then autoreactive lymphocytes in the periphery are either those which have never seen the autoantigen or are those bearing only low affinity receptors. Autoreactivity could therefore be induced if new T cell help were to be provided. The studies of Weigle and colleagues clearly demonstrated that tolerance to human gamma globulin (HGG) could be broken if the tolerized animals were immunized with bovine gamma globulin (BGG), an antigen which shares some determinants with HGG but also has some antigenic differences. These differences can give rise to a Th cell response, sometimes referred to as a T cell bypass which provides the necessary help for B cells to respond to antigens on BGG. Since some of these B cell epitopes are shared between HGG and BGG, the subsequent antibody response contains antibodies to some epitopes which are shared between HGG and BGG. Tolerance to self antigens can be broken in a similar way. Thus immunization of mice with rat RBC results in the initiation of an autoantibody response against mouse RBC. These autoantibodies are wholly cross-reactive between rat RBC and mouse RBC (*Fig. 12.17*). The same principle applies to autoreactive DTH responses or to autoreactive CTL; provision of T cell help may be all that is required to generate an autoreactive response. This T cell help could arise not just from an exogenous cross-reacting antigen but from a modified self antigen. The development of autoimmune disorders in response to treatment with some drugs can arise in this way; for example, some patients treated with α-methyl DOPA develop an autoimmune haemolytic anaemia, possibly as a result of the drug combining with self RBC and thus generating a modified antigen. As the B cell receptor is able to mutate somatically it can be seen that there is the potential to generate high affinity B cell responses to self following adequate provision of T cell help and the genesis of cytokines necessary for the development and maturation of the B cell response (see Chapter 10). Therefore it can be readily seen how infection with a microorganism bearing an epitope shared with a self antigen may precipitate an autoimmune attack through the genesis of a T cell bypass comprised of T cells specific for non-self antigens.

Another way in which a microorganism sharing antigenic determinants with a self antigen may initiate autoimmune pathology is by being present in high concentration and being taken up, processed and presented by a professional APC bearing an array of co-stimulatory molecules. Thus low

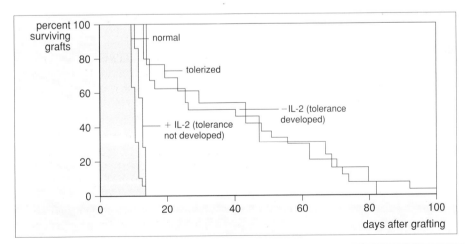

Fig. 12.16 Neonatal tolerance is not developed in the presence of IL-2. Tolerance to allogeneic stimuli can be developed if neonates are given large numbers of semi-allogeneic cells. For example, CBA mice are tolerized to C57BL/10 ScSn alloantigen, by neonatal administration of semi-allogeneic (CBAxC57BL/10 ScSn) F₁ bone marrow. Such tolerized mice accept skin grafts from C57BL/10 mice better than normal mice. This is shown by the skin graft survival time in normal compared to tolerized animals. Control mice which received medium without IL-2 developed tolerance and did not show accelerated graft rejection. However, if IL-2 is administered immediately after tolerization, tolerance is not developed. Data from Malkovsky and Medawar, 1984.

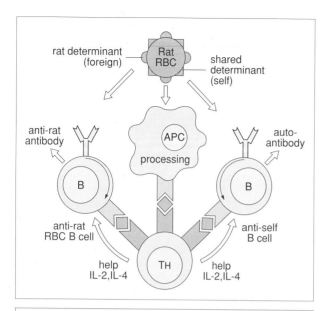

Fig. 12.17 Termination of self tolerance by cross-reacting antigens. Rat RBCs and mouse RBCs share some antigenic determinants but differ in others. Th cells are generated which recognize those foreign determinants and provide help for B cells specific for both cross-reacting antigens and foreign antigens. This produces autoantibodies to mouse RBCs.

avidity self reactive T cells which have escaped central and peripheral tolerance mechanisms can be activated.

It is also theoretically possible that an infection with an intracellular organism — bacteria, virus or parasite — may influence processing and presentation of normal self antigens such that different peptidic self epitopes are generated. Such neo-self antigens would be capable of initiating an autoimmune response against the infected cell.

When certain mouse strains are immunized with thyroglobulin extracted from the thyroid gland it is found that they develop an autoimmune thyroiditis as well as thyroid autoantibodies. It is not only important that the antigen is given together with adjuvant (LPS or complete Freund's adjuvant) but also that the thyroglobulin is iodinated. Thyroglobulin, a 300kDa protein with four potential iodination sites, is normally stored in the thyroid follicles and it is converted by a peroxidation reaction in the thyroid epithelial cells to the hormones T_3 and T_4. The small amounts of thyroglobulin in the circulation are normally poorly iodinated and therefore tolerance to these iodinated epitopes is unlikely to develop. T cells specific for iodinated peptide have been isolated from thyroglobulin primed mice and been shown to transfer thyroiditis to naive syngeneic mice. In this case, T cells which have not been deleted from the repertoire but which normally never see high enough concentrations of antigen to activate them are induced to respond. The presence of adjuvant in the immunization regimen ensures that thyroglobulin epitopes are presented by professional APC together with the appropriate co-stimulation.

As in any normal immune response the susceptibility to induced autoimmune pathology is under genetic control.

Thus thyroiditis is readily induced in $H\text{-}2^k$ and $H\text{-}2^s$ but not in $H\text{-}2^b$ or $H\text{-}2^d$ haplotype mice. Tolerance to self antigens may be broken in mice and rats following thymectomy and graded low doses of irradiation. If this procedure is carried out in PVG rats with MHC $RT1^c$ the rats predominantly develop autoimmune thyroid disease but in PVG $RT1^u$ rats insulin dependent diabetes mellitus (IDDM) mainly develops. It is known that thymectomy and low dose irradiation leads to a perturbation in T cell subsets in the rat with the dominant emergence of $CD45RC^{hi}$ $CD4^+$ T cells. The relative deficit of a Th2 population has been shown to predispose towards the genesis of autoreactivity (see Chapter 11). The disease bias manifest in the two different congenic rat lines may reflect the relative ability of the MHC class II molecules to present autoantigenic peptides.

Once an immune response against a self target organ has been initiated this can lead to further release of self antigen and responses against a wider array of self determinants. Some of these may be towards sequestered antigens to which self tolerance has never been established but additionally, increased concentrations of self antigens may facilitate responses against cryptic determinants on self antigens at the inflammatory site. This determinant spreading of an autoimmune response has been validated in several systems. Thus although an initiating trigger may elicit a restricted response once tissue pathology has occurred the response widens. This is clearly demonstrated in studies of experimental allergic encephalomyelitis (EAE) where, following injection of myelin basic protein (MBP) or spinal chord homogenate together with adjuvant, disease is attributable to $CD4^+$ T cells utilizing a $V\beta8$ chain in their TCR and recognizing an immunodominant epitope on MBP. With time the response spreads to other determinants on MBP and other antigens and correspondingly the T cell response widens. In most spontaneous autoimmune conditions there is no evidence of the dominant usage of a particular TCR possibly because such an analysis is usually performed when the disease is well established.

AUTOIMMUNE DISEASE

It should be emphasized that although most individuals can be induced to manifest autoreactive responses, few develop autoimmune disease. This may be because the original agent, for example mycoplasma in the case of autoimmune haemolytic anaemia following mycoplasma infection, is removed by a productive immune response against it. In the case of drug-induced diseases, once the drug treatment is stopped the patient usually recovers from the autoimmune disorder. There are several possible, not mutually exclusive, explanations for the continuation of disease in susceptible individuals:

- The agent involved in the initiation of the autoimmune disease may still be present and therefore constantly stimulating T cells.
- Following tissue damage, a cascade of autoreactivity may be set in motion through the release and exposure of the immune system to normally sequestered antigens for example, this may be the case in the presence of anti-insulin antibodies in patients with IDDM, since such

antibodies may arise following release of pro-insulin from dead or dying beta cells and its subsequent presentation by macrophages or dendritic cells in the inflammatory lesion.

The self reactive cells that are clearly present in normal individuals are held in check by some regulatory process. The demonstration that autoimmune pathology can result from an imbalance in T cell subpopulations provides support for this view.

Most spontaneous autoimmune conditions are under polygenic control with the MHC playing a key role in determining susceptibility or resistance. The concordance for disease in monozygotic twins for autoimmune diseases like IDDM and rheumatoid arthritis (RA) is less than 50%, indicating the involvement of environment in disease development. The NOD mouse, an excellent spontaneous animal model of human IDDM, has provided an invaluable tool for the analysis of the genetic elements predisposing to IDDM as well as providing insight into the pathological processes that may lead to specific beta cell destruction. Backcross and congenic studies have permitted the identification of at least 13 loci as playing a role in IDDM. Analogous studies have been carried out in studies of renal disease in the (NZB × NZW) F$_1$ mouse, an animal model of SLE, by Drake and colleagues. It has been possible to evaluate the role that the MHC might play in NOD IDDM through the construction of NOD transgenic mice. The MHC of the NOD mouse contains an unusual H-2A molecule which is Aα^d Aβ^{g7}. This beta chain has several amino acids in common with Aβ^d but has several distinctly different amino acids. In particular, at positions 56 and 57 Aβ^{g7} has a histidine and a serine respectively whereas most other Aβ chains have a proline and an aspartate at these positions. The location of these amino acids at one end of the antigen binding groove suggests that they may influence binding of diabetogenic peptides and hence tolerance induction. The H-2A molecule is equivalent to HLA-DQ and the observation that in some ethnic groups the presence of a charged residue at position 57 of the DQ beta chain afforded protection from the development of IDDM suggested an equivalent scenario for murine IDDM. Transgenic NOD mice have been constructed in which the introduced genes encode Aβ-chains expressing proline at position 56 or aspartate at position 57. In both situations, the development of IDDM was markedly reduced supporting the role for this locus in determining resistance or susceptibility to this autoimmune condition. In this case, resistance is dominant. Complementary observations have been made in RA and in an animal model of this chronic inflammatory condition, collagen induced arthritis. In RA, susceptibility has been shown to be linked to particular HLA-DRB1 alleles sharing sequence homology in the region encoding amino acids 67–74. In the animal model disease development requires expression of H-2A^q. Transgenic introduction of the Aβ^q gene into a resistant H-2^p expressing mouse strain renders it susceptible. As there are only four amino acid differences between Ab^q and Ab^p this suggests that the arthritogenic peptide may be unable to bind into the I-A^p binding groove. In this situation responsiveness is dominant.

The *H-2E* locus has been implicated in playing a protective role in animal models of IDDM and RA. NOD mice do not express H-2E despite the presence of a functional Eβ^{g7} as a result of a deletion in the promoter region of the *Ea* gene. Transgenic introduction of an Eα^d into NOD mice permits expression of a functional H-2E molecule and prevents IDDM. Mice which are susceptible to collagen induced arthritis are H-2^q and do not express H-2E due to a non functional *Eb^q* gene. If susceptible mice express H-2E through crossing with an H-2E^d-expressing strain the mice are completely protected from the experimental induction of arthritis.

Activated T cells have emerged as key mediators in pathology either possibly directly as CTL or through their ability to produce cytokines capable of recruiting other T cells, macrophages and polymorphs. The products of T cells (e.g. IFN-γ, TNFα and TNFβ), macrophages (free radicals such as NO, IL-1, TNFα) and polymorphs (free radicals, eosinophil granule proteins) can cause tissue damage if not regulated. The ability of local cytokine production to influence an organ specific autoimmune disease such as IDDM is clearly shown by the studies of Sarvetnick and colleagues in which transgenic expression of IFNγ in the pancreatic beta cells elicited a chronic inflammatory state and tissue destruction.

B cells play a direct role in the development of some autoimmune pathologies such as Graves' disease and myasthenia gravis where autoantibodies to the TSH receptor and the acetylcholine receptor respectively influence cellular function. More generalized effects of autoantibody are seen in pemphigus vulgaris and SLE. In the former case the auto-antibodies are directed against a desmosome protein found in keratinocytes and mucous membrane epithelia and in the latter case through formation of antigen–antibody complexes which become deposited at many sites including the kidney. The ability of the B cell Ig receptor to undergo somatic mutation in the presence of T cell help means that there is always the possibility for the emergence of high affinity autoreactive B cell responses provided there is T cell activation. The possibility exists that the chronicity of some autoimmune conditions might be indirectly attributable to B cells either through the genesis of immune complexes which maintain T cell activation or through presentation of self antigens.

Current therapeutic approaches include those which target T cells and inflammatory cytokines. These will be discussed further in Chapter 17.

SUMMARY

Tolerance can be generated and maintained in a variety of ways. Great advances have been made in recent years in formally demonstrating that some of the theories proposed many years ago are fundamentally correct. Evidence has been found for both clonal deletion and clonal anergy of B and T cells. Using transgenic technology it has been possible to show that clonal deletion of T and B cells occurs at early stages in their development. It has also been possible to show that antigen-specific T or B cells may be present but functionally inactive in the periphery.

Some forms of tolerance can be experimentally induced by administering antigen such that the T cell response is biased either to a Th1 or to a Th2 response or that the T cells secrete TGFβ.

Tolerance to self antigens can be broken in several ways. Since most normal individuals can be induced to develop autoreactivity but few develop autoimmune disease, it is clear that clonal deletion of all autoreactive cells does not occur. In some cases autoreactive T cells do not cause pathology because they do not see self antigen: tolerance through ignorance. In other cases the T cells bear low affinity receptors and require high antigen concentrations and co-stimulation to become activated. Provision of T cell help or co-stimulation can initiate T or B cell autoreactive responses.

There is also some evidence for maintenance of self tolerance through regulation of autoreactive T cells, as imbalance in CD4+ T cell subpopulations can lead to autoimmunity. Therapeutic regimens which restore that balance can prevent autoimmune pathology.

FURTHER READING

Adams TE, Alpert S, Hanahan D. Non-tolerance and autoantibodies to a transgenic self antigen expressed in pancreatic β cells. *Nature* 1987, **325**:223.

Alferink J, Schittek B, Schonrich G, Hammerling GJ, Arnold B. Long life span of tolerant T cells and the role of antigen in the maintenance of peripheral tolerance. *Int Immunol* 1995, **7**:331.

Arnold B, Schonrich G, Ferber I, Alferink J, Hammerling GJ. Peripheral T cell tolerance: distinct levels and multistep mechanisms. In *Transgenics and targeted mutagenesis in immunology*. Bluethmann H, Cohashi PS (Eds). Academic Press: San Diego; 1994.

Bluethmann H, Ohashi PS. *Transgenesis and targeted mutagenesis in immunology*. San Diego: Academic Press; 1994.

Cyster JG, Goodnow CG. Protein tyrosine phosphatase 1C negatively regulates antigen receptor signaling in B lymphocytes and determines thresholds for negative selection. *Immunity* 1995, **2**:13.

Day MJ, Tse AGD, Puklavec M, Simmonds SJ, Mason DW. Targeting autoantigen to B cells prevents induction of a cell-mediated autoimmune disease in rats. *J Exp Med* 1992, **175**: 655.

Decker DJ, Klinman NR. Inter-relating B cell subpopulations and environmental regulation with the expression of three tiers or repetoire diversity. *Int Rev Immunol* 1992, **8**:159.

Drake CG, Rozzo SJ, Vyse TJ, Palmer E, Kotzin BL. Genetic contributions to lupus-like disease in NZB x NZW F₁ mice. *Imm Rev* 1995, **144**:51.

Foster I, Hirose R, Arbeit JM, Clausen BE, Hanahan D. Limited capacity for tolerization of CD4+ T cells specific for a pancreatic beta cell neoantigen. *Immunity* 1995, **2**:573.

Fowell D, Mason D. Evidence that the T cell repertoire of normal rats contains cells with the potential to cause diabetes. Characterization of the CD4+ T cell subset that inhibits this autoimmune potential. *J Exp Med* 1993, **177**:627.

Goodnow CC, Cyster JG, Hartley SB, Bell SE, Cooke P, Healy JI, Akkarajn S, Rathmell JC, Pogue SL, Shokat KP. Self tolerance checkpoints in B lymphocyte development. *Adv Imm* 1995, **59**:279.

Hartley SB, Cooke MP, Fulcher DA, Harris AW, Cory S, Basten A, Goodnow CC. Elimination of self reactive B lymphocytes proceeds in two stages: arrested development and cell death. *Cell* 1993, **72**:325.

Holmdahl R, Vingsbo C, Mo JA, Michaelsson E, Malmstrom V, Jansson L, Brunsberg U. Chronicity of tissue specific experimental autoimmune disease: A role for B cells. *Imm Rev* 1995, **144**:139.

Hsu BL, Evavold BD, Allen PM. Modulation of T cell development by an endogenous altered peptide ligand. *J Exp Med* 1995, **181**:805.

Lee M-S, Sarvetnick N. Immunological studies utilizing cytokine transgenic mice. In *Transgenesis and targeted mutagenesis in immunology*. Bluethmann H, Ohashi PS (Eds). San Diego: Academic Press; 1994.

Malkovsky M, Medawar PB. Is immunological tolerance (non-responsiveness) a consequence of interleukin-2 deficit during recognition of antigen. *Immunol Today* 1984, **5**:340.

Miller SD, McRae BL, Vanderlugt CL, Nickevich KM, Pope JG, Pope L, Karpus WJ. Evolution of the T cell repertoire during the course of experimental immune-mediated demyelinating diseases. *Imm Rev* 1995, **144**:225.

Murakami M, Tsubata M, Okamoto A, Shimuzu S, Kumagai H, Imura H, Honjo T. Antigen-induced apoptotic death of Ly-1 B cells responsible for autoimmune disease in transgenic mice. *Nature* 1992, **357**:77.

Nemazee D. Promotion and prevention of autoimmunity by B lymphocytes. *Curr Biol* 1993, **5**:866.

Nemazee DA, Bürki K. Clonal deletion of B lymphocytes in a transgenic mouse bearing anti-MHC class I antibody genes. *Nature* 1989, **337**:562.

Nisitani S, Tsubata T, Murakami M, Okamoto M, Honjo T. The bcl-2 gene product inhibits clonal deletion of self reactive B lymphocytes in the periphery but not in the bone marrow. *J Exp Med* 1993, **178**:1247.

Ohashi PS, Hengartner H, Battegay M, Zinkernagel RM, Pircher H. Thymocyte selection and peripheral tolerance using the lymphocytic choriomeningitis virus as a model antigen. In *Transgenesis and targeted mutagenesis in immunology*. Bluethmann H, Ohashi PS (Eds). San Diego: Academic Press; 1994.

Parish NM, Hutchings PR, O'Reilly L, Quartey-Papafio R, Healey D, Ozegbe P, Cooke A. Tolerance induction as a therapeutic strategy for the control of autoimmune endocrine disease in mouse models. *Imm Rev* 1995, **144**:269.

Peterson JD, Karpus W, Clatch RJ, Miller SD. Split tolerance of Th1 and Th2 cells in tolerance to Theiler's murine encephalomyelitis virus. *Eur J Immunol* 1993, **23**:46.

Qin S, Cobbold Sp, Pope H, Elliot J, Kioussis D, Davis J, Wladman H. Infectious transplantation tolerance. *Science* 1993, **259**:974.

Radic MZ, Erikson J, Litwin S, Weigert M. B lymphocytes may escape tolerance by revising their antigen receptors. *J Exp Med* 1993, **177**:1165.

Schönrich G, Momburg F, Malissen M, Schmitt-Verhulst A-M, Malissen B, Hammerling GJ, Arnold B. Distinct mechanisms of extrathymic T cell tolerance due to differential expression of self antigen. *Int Immunol* 1992, **4**:581.

Tsubata T, Murakami M, Honjo T. Antigen-receptor cross-linking induces peritoneal B cell apoptosis in normal but not autoimmunity-prone mice. *Curr Biol* 1994, **4**:8.

Vella AT, McCormack JE, Linsley PS, Kappler JW, Marrack P. Lipopolysaccharide interferes with the induction of peripheral T cell death. *Immunity* 1995, **2**:261.

Von Herrath MG, Dockter J, Nerenberg M, Gairin JE, Oldstone MBA. Thymic selection and adaptibility of cytotoxic T lymphocyte responses in transgenic mice expressing a viral protein in the thymus. *J Exp Med* 1994, **180**:1901.

Waldmann H. Manipulation of T cell response with monoclonal antibodies. *Ann Rev Immunol* 1989, **7**:407.

Zanelli E, Gonzalez-Gay MA, David CS. Could *HLA-DRB1* be the protective locus in rheumatoid arthritis? *Immunol Today* 1995, **16**:274.

13 Complement

The complement system is a large group of molecules constituting nearly 10% of the total serum protein and forming one of the major defence systems of the body. Complement regulatory molecules are present in serum and on cell surfaces, while the seven distinct receptors for activated complement fragments are distributed on different leukocyte populations. Functions of the system include the control of inflammatory reactions, clearance of immune complexes, cellular activation and anti-microbial defence. The system also plays a role in development of immune responses and is a major effector system in autoimmunity and hypersensitivity.

Molecules of the complement system interact with each other in an enzyme cascade, generating fragments which act as opsonins, chemoattractants and adhesion molecules which bind to specific receptors on different populations of lymphocytes and phagocytes. In many ways the complement system, together with auxiliary cells (e.g. mast cells and platelets), acts as a functional link between the adaptive immune system and evolutionarily older defence mechanisms. There are three distinct pathways which can activate the system and there are striking structural and functional similarities between the components of the classical and alternative pathways. There are also homologies between C1 of the classical pathway and components of the recently described lectin pathway. Hence it is very likely that the molecules involved in each pathway have arisen by gene duplication and diversification, with the classical pathway evolving as an adjunct to the development of antibody-producing B cells. *Figure 13.1* lays

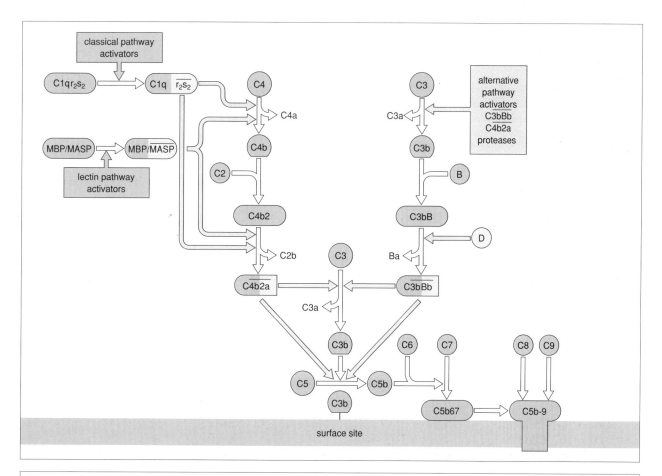

Fig. 13.1 Summary of complement activation pathways. The activation steps of the classical, alternative and lectin pathways are set out in parallel. Enzymatically active components and enzymatic cleavage is shown in green. In the presence of a suitable surface site and bound C3b, the C3 convertases cleave C5 to initiate the lytic pathway resulting in insertion of membrane attack complexes (MAC) of C5b-9 into cell membranes.

out the three main activation pathways of the complement system in a way which emphasizes their functional and structural homologies.

ACTIVATION PATHWAYS

There are two major sets of complement system molecules: those involved in the classical and lytic pathways are designated C1–C9, while alternative pathway molecules are referred to as factors (e.g. factor B and factor D). The components of the lectin pathway are mannan-binding protein (MBP — not to be confused with myelin basic protein) and MBP-associated serine protease (MASP). The activities of these pathways are regulated by a series of control proteins, some of which are designated by abbreviations of their common names such as C1 inhibitor (C1inh). Seven of the components are serine proteases which can split other components. Fragments generated in these reactions or by further breakdown are indicated by small letters — C3a, C3b, C3c etc. — and the enzymatically active components or complexes are shown by a superscripted bar, such as C3bBb. Components which have become inactivated, either by enzymatic cleavage or by internal rearrangement, are prefixed 'i', for example iC3.

The central role of C3

The activation of C3 is the central reaction of the complement cascade. C3 consists of disulphide linked α and β-chains and activation of the molecule occurs by cleavage of the α-chain via either the classical or alternative pathway. C3b covalently deposited on a surface may become a focus for the assembly of membrane attack complexes (MACs) generated from components C5–C9 of the lytic pathway. The importance of this step may be assessed from the observation that homozygous C3 deficiency is an exceptionally rare disorder usually associated with life threatening infections.

C3 has a most unusual feature, an internal thiolester bond formed between Cys and Gln residues in the α-chain, producing a ring structure which is normally inaccessibly buried inside the molecule (*Fig. 13.2*). Cleavage of C3 via the classical or alternative pathway causes the release of C3a (a 77 amino acid residue polypeptide) from the N-terminus, allowing a conformational change to occur in C3b which results in exposure of the thiolester bond. The exposed bond is very reactive and can interact with amine (–NH$_2$) and hydroxyl (–OH) groups on proteins and carbohydrates, allowing C3b to link covalently to other biomolecules. However, it is also rapidly hydrolysed by water, which means that C3b only has the opportunity to interact with molecules in the immediate vicinity of its activation site before it is hydrolyzed. It has been estimated that the halflife of the thiolester bond in metastable C3b is just 60 μsec while that in native C3 is more than 200 hours. Very rarely, C3 may undergo spontaneous rearrangement, exposing the thiolester bond producing C3i* which can also bind covalently to adjacent molecules.

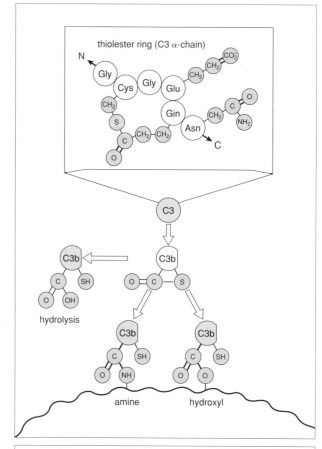

Fig. 13.2 The thiolester ring of C3 and C4. Cleavage of C3 to C3b causes the exposure of an internal thiolester ring in the α-chain formed between a cysteine and a glutamine residue with the elimination of NH$_3$. The exposed bond is extremely labile and may be hydrolysed by water, or may interact with -NH$_2$ and -OH groups on biological molecules allowing covalent attachment of C3b. A similar thiolester bond is present in C4.

This mechanism ensures that there is always a very low level turnover of C3 which can act as the primer for alternative pathway activation (see below).

It is essential that covalent binding of C3b and iC3 to host cells does not occur appreciably, since this could form a site for assembly of MACs. The actions of C3 convertases and deposition of activated C3 are therefore limited by the control proteins CR1, membrane cofactor protein (MCP, CD46) and decay accelerating factor (DAF, CD55), the latter two being widely distributed on different cell types. In the fluid phase, factor H also controls the rate of breakdown of C3b. *Figure 13.3* lists the functions of the proteins which control the activity of C3b and C4b, as well as the classical and alternative pathway C3 and C5 convertases.

The classical pathway

The classical pathway is activated by immune complexes containing IgG or IgM which bind to the C1q subunit of C1, initiating a series of steps leading to the production of

	number of CCP domains	dissociation of C3 and C5 convertases		cofactor for factor I on		localization
		classical pathway	alternative pathway	C4b	C3b	
C4bp	52 or 56	+	−	+	−	serum
H	20	−	+	−	+	serum
DAF (CD55)	4	+	+	−	−	erythrocytes leucocytes platelets
MCP (CD46)	4	−	−	+	+	B cells neutrophils T cells macrophages
CR1 (CD35)	28 or 35	+	+	+	+	erythrocytes B cells follicular dendritic cells granulocytes macrophages

Fig. 13.3 C3b and C4b control proteins. The five proteins listed are widely distributed and control aspects of C3b and C4b dissociation or breakdown. Each of these proteins contains complement control protein (CCP) domains. They act either by enhancing the dissociation rate of C3 and C5 convertases, or by acting as cofactors for the enzymatic cleavage of C3b or C4b by factor I.

a C3 convertase, $\overline{C4b2b}$. Antibody isotypes vary in their ability to bind to C1q and activate the pathway; in the human IgM, IgG1 and IgG3 are most effective and IgG2 less so; in mouse IgM and IgG2a are most effective.

C1q is linked in a Ca^{2+}-dependent complex to C1r and C1s in a molar ratio of 1:2:2 to form C1. C1q itself consists of 18 polypeptides of three different types — A, B and C. These form six disulphide linked A-B heterodimers and three C-C homodimers which are formed into six ABC subunits (*Fig. 13.4*). Each subunit has a triple helical collagen-like portion, a stalk and a globular head region which contains a site which recognizes and binds to a region in the CH2 domain of IgG (*Fig. 13.5*). Site-directed mutagenesis of mouse IgG2b indicated that a group of three residues — Asp 318, Lys 320 and Lys 322 — were essential for C1q binding. However, since they are conserved in all IgG subclasses of human and mouse, these residues alone do not determine whether or not C1q will bind; further residues in the C-terminal end of CH2 must also be involved. C1q may also bind to a site in the CH3 domain of IgM. IgM in solution adopts a star configuration but attachment to multiple antigenic sites may induce a chair or staple configuration. The conformational change associated with this is thought to allow the binding of the necessary two or three C1q heads which are required for activation of C1. The binding affinity of a single C1q head for IgG is relatively weak but when several Fc regions are clustered together, as occurs in an immune complex, the overall avidity of C1q is greatly enhanced. For this reason the complement fixing ability of immune complexes is critically dependent on size as well as their composition, with large complexes being much more efficient.

The purified C1r2-C1s2 subunit appears as a rod-like structure under EM, with the individual molecules having two linked globular domains. Models of intact C1

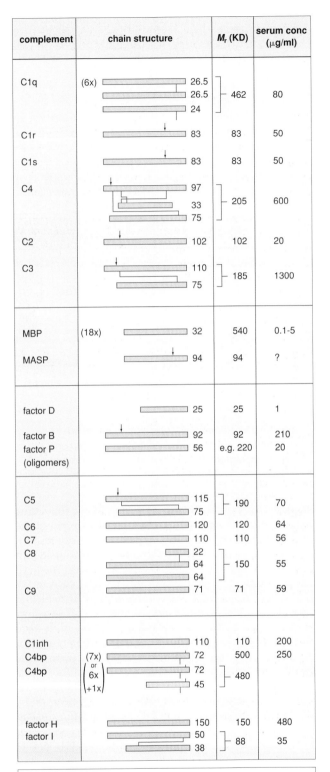

Fig. 13.4 Polypeptide chain structures of complement molecules. The polypeptides and their molecular weights in kilodaltons are shown together with their interchain disulphide bonds (black). Note that C1q is a hexamer of the basic unit and MBP is often hexameric. C4bp is a heptamer and factor P occurs as oligomers of the basic unit with trimers, tetramers and pentamers being most abundant. Arrows represent cleavage sites.

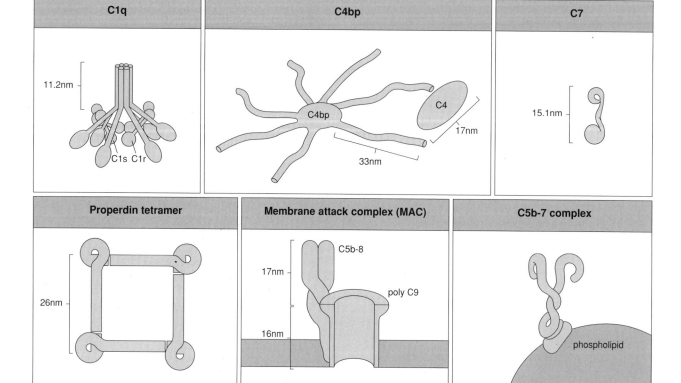

Fig. 13.5 Diagrammatic structures of selected complement components. The diagram, based on electron micrographs, illustrates some of the unusual structures of individual components and complexes, drawn to scale. See Law and Reid, 1995; DiScipio et al, 1988; and Schumaker et al, 1987.

suggest that the larger domains, containing the serine esterase catalytic sites of C1r and C1s, lie together in the centre of the C1q head and the smaller domains, responsible for interaction between C1r and C1s, lie outside. In effect, the C1r2–C1s2 subunit is wound around the head of C1q. Activation of C1 is by autocatalytic cleavage of one C1r, which can then act on the other C1r, which in turn cleaves the C1s molecules. Activation of C1r is normally limited by C1inh, which interacts reversibly with native C1. When C1q binds to at least two Fc regions it appears to alter the environment within the centre of the head, favouring activation of C1r and C1s. C1s cleaves both C4 and C2, in the ensuing steps. C1inh plays an important role in limiting the effects of C1 activation by binding to activated C1r and C1s in a 1:1 ratio, causing their release from the C1 complex. Like other serine proteinase inhibitors, C1inh presents a 'bait site'. C1r or C1s cleaves this site on C1inh and then bind to its N-terminus, becoming irreversibly inhibited. Hereditary deficiency of C1inh permits spontaneous activation of C1, leading to the generation of vasoactive kinins from high molecular weight kininogen and C2 (C2 kinin). This produces the symptoms of angioneurotic oedema.

C1s clips a 9kDa fragment with anaphylatoxic activity from C4, C4a. This exposes an internal thiolester bond in the α-chain of the large C4b fragment, analogous to that in C3b, and allows C4b to bind to –NH$_2$ and –OH

groups in nearby biomolecules. There is considerable polymorphism in C4 (see below) and the ability to link to either –NH$_2$ or –OH groups varies with different C4 isoallotypes. Those encoded at the *C4A* locus are highly reactive for –NH$_2$ and bind very poorly to –OH, while those from the *C4B* locus bind equally well to both groups. Only a small proportion of the activated C4b (<1%) binds covalently at the activation site, the remainder reacts with water to form iC4b which is rapidly catabolized. There is evidence that much of the deposited C4b binds to sites in the N-terminal portion of IgG, particularly CH1, where it may play a part in controlling catabolism of immune complexes.

In the next step, the N-terminal domain of C2 associates with C4b in a Mg^{2+}-dependent complex and is in turn split by C1s, releasing the non-catalytic fragment C2b (30kDa) and leaving the C-terminal catalytic domain (70kDa) bound in a complex with C4b to form the classical pathway C3 convertase, $\overline{C4b2a}$, which splits C3. $\overline{C4b2a}$ decays naturally with the release of C2a but this process and the initial assembly of C4b2 is controlled by C4-binding protein, C4bp.

C4bp is heptameric with an unusual spider-like shape (*Fig. 13.5*) and occurs in two alternate forms, either with seven identical α-chains or with six α-chains and a β-chain. The functional difference between the two forms is not known. The α and β-chains are folded into a series of domains referred to as complement control protein (CCP) domains. The three N-terminal domains of each α-chain contain binding sites for C4b. By binding to C4b2a, C4bp promotes dissociation of C2a and it also acts as a cofactor for factor I, another serine protease which splits C4b at two points, degrading it into C4c and C4d.

The lectin pathway

The lectin pathway is an alternative way of activating C4 and C2. It is initiated by mannan binding protein (MBP), a molecule present in serum at very variable levels (0.1–5 µg/ml). This large molecule, previously known as Ra-reactive factor (RaRF), has structural similarities to C1q. It occurs as hexamers with 18 identical polypeptide chains, arranged in units of three (cf. the ABC unit of C1q). MBP hexamers can bind to C1r2s2 but MBP may also form dimers, trimers, tetramers and pentamers, which do not. Another serine protease MBP-associated serine protease (MASP), which has 37% homology with C1r or C1s, is probably its more relevant associated protease.

MBP preferentially binds to non-reduced terminal mannose, fucose and glucosamine groups, which allows it to attach to surface carbohydrates on a variety of bacteria (*Fig. 13.6*). Conformational changes associated with this binding lead to the internal cleavage and activation of MASP, which in turn acts on C4 and C2 to generate a classical pathway C3 convertase.

The alternative pathway

The alternative pathway is activated in the presence of a variety of molecules and surfaces which provide a protected environment for the reactions involved. This pathway should really be viewed as being in a state of dynamic equilibrium, since there is always a low level of turnover of the components involved, which is rapidly upregulated in the presence of activator surfaces. Under normal circumstances the reactions are tightly controlled and limited by molecules present on mammalian cells, including DAF (decay accelerating factor), MCP (membrane cofactor protein), CR1 and by factor H which is present in serum at high concentrations. Activation of the alternative pathway is effectively due to a release from these controlling influences.

The initial seed for alternative pathway reactions is a molecule of activated surface bound C3; this may be C3b generated by the classical pathway, otherwise the low level of spontaneous iC3 produced and deposited can act as a focus. On activator surfaces, C3b will tend to bind factor B via its N-terminal Ba domain, in a way analogous to the binding of C2 by C4b. The C3bB complex is acted on by factor D, a serine protease which circulates at low levels (1µg/ml) but in an active form. Factor D releases the Ba domain from factor B, leaving the catalytically active Bb fragment associated with C3b to form the alternative pathway C3 convertase C3bBb (*Fig. 13.1*). Factor D is unique within the complement system in that it is apparently secreted in an active form, consisting of a single serine protease domain without extension. It has been separately identified as adipsin, an enzyme involved in fat metabolism.

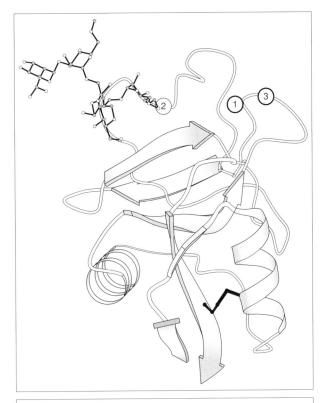

Fig. 13.6 Mannan binding protein (MBP). The ribbon diagram shows the carbohydrate-recognition domain of MBP located in loops on a segment of the molecule. The sugar group is shown in black and Ca²⁺-binding sites are numbered one to three. Based on data of Weis *et al*, 1992.

Since C3bBb generates C3b which can then form further C3bBb, the alternative pathway acts as a positive feedback loop in the presence of activator surfaces and for this reason is sometimes called the amplification loop.

It is essential that this cycle is tightly controlled in normal circumstances, so a variety of factors hold these reactions in check (*Fig. 13.7*). The binding of factor B to C3b is inhibited by factor H, which leads to an inactivation pathway in which C3b is cleaved in two places by factor I releasing C3f and leaving iC3b which is further degraded to C3c and C3dg by factor I and other serum proteases. C3dg which originally contained the thiolester ring may remain covalently bound to the particle on which it was deposited (*Fig. 13.8*). Factor H has a binding site for sialic acid residues and other polyanions in addition to its C3b binding site. This may contribute to the protection of host cells, since mammalian cells carry sialic acid residues while prokaryotic cells usually do not. Factor H also promotes the decay of C3bBb by release of Bb.

Complement C3b deposition on mammalian cells may induce death via the lytic pathway and is damaging even when the cell is not killed. Consequently there are several membrane proteins which inhibit the assembly of C3bB and promote the dissociation of C3bBb. Decay accelerating factor (DAF) present on erythrocytes, leukocytes and platelets accelerates the decay of both

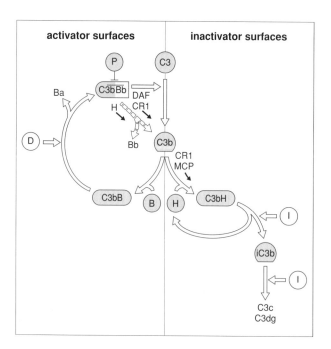

Fig. 13.7 The alternative pathway, amplification loop. The alternative pathway may act as a positive feedback loop for the generation of more C3b. This loop is controlled by a number of components: Properdin (P) can bind to the C3 convertase ($\overline{C3bBb}$) to stabilize it, whereas DAF and CR1 on cell surfaces and factor H in solution promote its decay by release of Bb. In the presence of activator surfaces factor B binds to C3b to cause further alternative pathway activation, but in the presence of inactivator surfaces factor H is bound and C3b is inactivated by factor I. CR1 and MCP on host cells also favour breakdown by this route.

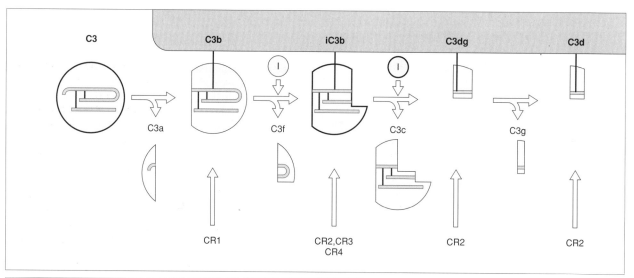

Fig. 13.8 Activation and degradation of C3. Activation of C3 occurs by release of C3a from the α-chain to produce C3b which is degraded by factor I with the release of C3f and C3c. Serum proteases cause further degradation of C3dg to C3d. The receptors which recognize each of these fragments are indicated below.

classical and alternative pathway C3 convertases. Activation of neutrophils leads to a rapid increase in the levels of surface DAF, suggesting that it is retained in intracellular stores until needed. This molecule is anchored to the membrane by a glycolipid tail, allowing it high lateral mobility. Deficiency of DAF results in abnormal C3b deposition on cells, leading to erythrocyte lysis and sometimes the symptoms of paroxysmal nocturnal haemoglobinuria. Aged erythrocytes lose DAF, which may facilitate complement-mediated clearance.

MCP is also widely distributed on leukocytes and acts as a cofactor for factor I in the degradation of C3b and C4b. The complement receptors CR1 and CR2 are less widely distributed and their primary function is thought to be in the handling of immune complexes, although they also promote $\overline{C3bBb}$ decay and degradation of C3b by factor I. Interestingly several of the proteins which control C3b and C4b, namely CR1, CR2, DAF, factor H and C4bp, are encoded in a single gene region present on chromosome 1 in humans. This is called the 'regulators for complement activation' or RCA locus.

Properdin, or factor P, was the first component of the alternative pathway to be discovered. It was once thought to be the 'activator' of this pathway but subsequent research showed that its role is in binding to and stabilizing the alternative pathway C3 convertase,

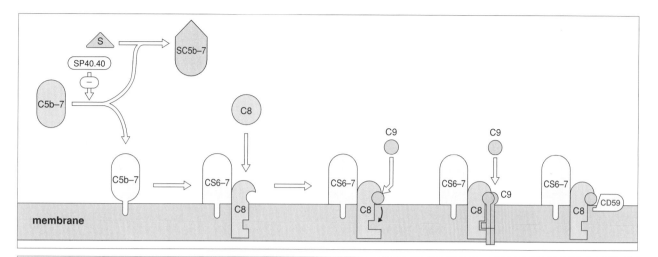

Fig. 13.9 Assembly of the MAC. C5b generated near an activator surface binds C6 and C7. C7 undergoes a transition, to expose a membrane attachment site. The transition is inhibited by SP40.40. If the C5b-7 complex fails to attach to a membrane it binds the S protein (vitronectin) and is inactive. Deposited C5b-7 binds to the β-chain of C8, probably via a site in C5b. The α-chain of C8 appears to penetrate the membrane exposing a C9 acceptor site. C9 unfolds to bind a second site on C8, while undergoing a conversion to an amphiphilic state. Further C9 molecules can now attach to the assembling MAC. In the presence of CD59 (right hand segment) the unfolding of C9 is blocked and assembly of the MAC inhibited.

producing $C\overline{3bBbP}$. It is therefore not so much an activator as an upregulator of the pathway. The structure of factor P is unusual, consisting of cyclic oligomers of a 56kDa unit (*Fig. 13.5*). Trimers and tetramers are most common. Factor P is the only component which upregulates the amplification loop. It is also a moderate acute phase protein. Hence, it provides a means of generally upregulating the activity of the complement pathways during infections.

The lytic pathway

The lytic pathway involves the assembly of MACs by the components C5–C9. Only the first step of this pathway, the cleavage of C5, is enzymatic. The subsequent steps involve a biophysical assembly in which the complex becomes amphiphilic, so that it can insert into lipid bilayers. C5 is structurally related to C3 and C4 and it too is activated by cleavage of its α-chain, releasing the N-terminal fragment C5a and leaving C5b. C5 convertases are formed by the combination of C3b with either a classical pathway or an alternative pathway C3 convertase (i.e. $C\overline{3b\,4b2a}$ or $C\overline{3b3bBb}$), in which the actual cleavage of C5 is performed by the serine esterases C2a or Bb. It appears that C3b becomes covalently bound to the C3 convertase and this in turn anchors the trimolecular complex to the surface. The fixed C3b provides a suitable attachment site for C5 where it can be acted upon enzymatically.

The first step in MAC assembly is the binding of C6 and C7 to form C5b-7, with detachment from the C5 convertase. On binding C7, the complex undergoes a transition, becoming amphiphilic and acquiring a metastable membrane-binding site. If C5b–7 fails to attach to a membrane, it may link to S-protein (also called vitronectin) in fluid phase and a functionally inactive complex SC5b–9 is formed. Apolipoprotein SP40.40 also inhibits the binding of C5b–7 to membranes. Electron micrography of C7 shows it to be an elongated molecule and the C5b–7 complex has a leaflet with a flexible stalk (*Fig. 13.5*). The stalk is formed mainly by the C6 and C7 and it is this section which is responsible for membrane binding. C6 and C7 are structurally related and the N-terminal segment of C7 also has slight homologies with C9 and the α and β-chains of C8. This has lead to the suggestion that the lytic pathway components developed by retrograde evolution in which the first member of the series was a pore forming molecule like C9. The development of C6–C8, by gene duplication and diversification, served to refine the MAC and link pore formation to the central part of the complement system.

C8 is unusual in that it consists of three polypeptide chains; the larger α and β-chains (both 64kDa) are non-covalently associated while the small γ-chain (25kDa) is linked to α by a disulphide bond and lies on the periphery of the molecule. The β-chain has an affinity for C5b–7 and there is some evidence that it binds to a site on C5b, whereas the α/γ subunit has no affinity for C5b–7. Another region on the β-chain interacts with the α/γ unit and a third domain interacts with the membrane. The α-chain of C8 has a high affinity for C9 and appears to be involved in the final assembly of the MAC (*Fig. 13.9*).

The final structure of the MAC depends on the availability of C9, since the complex may contain 1–18 molecules of C9 associated with C5b–8. When the number of C9 molecules exceeds six then typical cylindrical pore shaped complexes appear (*Fig. 13.5*), traversing the membrane. With lower levels of C9 in the complex, small aggregates are seen, which nevertheless have considerable lytic potential. C9 deficiency is common and is not associated with any severe clinical deficits. Possibly, C5b–8 alone can generate sufficient lytic activity.

C9 consists of 538 amino acids and has a beaded appearance in electron micrographs. The first C9 molecule initially attaches to a site in C8b and then undergoes a conformational change, unfolding down into the membrane where it interacts with a second site on C8b. This change is associated with loss of sensitivity to tryptic digestion, the disappearance of some epitopes, the appearance of others and an apparent doubling in length. The unwinding probably also exposes residues which can interact with acyl side-chains of the lipid bilayer. Further C9 molecules join the complex to form the sides of the tube and studies *in vitro* indicate that polymerization via cysteine residues is possible.

Two control proteins inhibit the formation of MACs on host cells. The molecule CD59 is present on the membrane of most cell types and associates with C5b–8 in such a way that it prevents the unfolding of C9 into the membrane but not its initial binding to C8b. The one case reported of CD59 deficiency is associated with PNH. Homologous restriction factor is found on erythrocytes and platelets, where it limits MAC formation by interaction with C8 and C9. The presence of this protein underlies the observation that erythrocytes are not readily lysed by homologous complement. The number of C9 molecules required to lyse a cell is variable with four to eight quoted for erythrocytes and three or more for Gram-negative bacteria. Nucleated cells can tolerate more damage before being killed, nevertheless, sublethal damage can seriously impair their function.

STRUCTURE–FUNCTION RELATIONSHIPS OF COMPLEMENT MOLECULES

The primary site of production of most serum complement components is the liver. Exceptions are C1q and factors D and P. The inflammatory cytokines TNF, IL-1 and IL-6 enhance liver synthesis of all components, except C2 and C4, by two to three-fold. Interferon-γ enhances synthesis of all components. The component molecules of C1 are produced by epithelial cells and factor D by adipocytes. In addition, activated macrophages can produce C2, C3 and C4 and factors D, P, H, I and B. While this is a minor contribution in terms of total production, it may be particularly important at sites of inflammation where local depletion is occurring. For example IL-1, IFNγ and lipopolysaccharide (LPS) have all been shown to induce factor B synthesis by macrophages. Additionally, skin fibroblasts activated with TNF produce C3 and factor B.

Several of the components are produced by the enzymatic processing of large polypeptides. For example, C4 is produced by internal cleavage of a single precursor polypeptide to leave the α, β and γ-chains of serum C4. C3 and C5 also undergo similar internal cleavages to produce their mature two chain forms, while factor I also requires enzymic processing of its precursor chains.

Complement components fall into a number of families based on common elements in their structure and similar

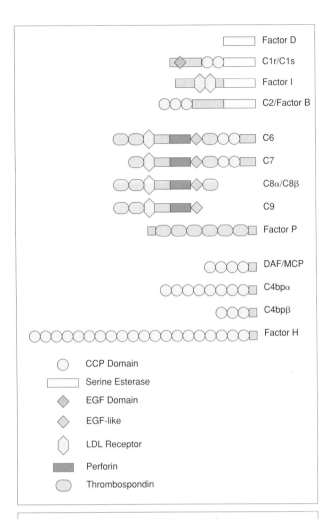

Fig. 13.10 Structural motifs in complement components. Some of the more common structures found are illustrated diagrammatically.

functions. For example, the enzymatically active components C1r, C1s, C2, FB, FI and FD are all serine proteases and they share a highly conserved catalytic site domain of approximately 25kDa. The primary structures of most of the complement components are now available from cDNA sequences but crystallographic data on their three dimensional structures are incomplete. However, sequence analysis has shown that many of the complement components are molecular mosaics, containing a variety of structural motifs which occur not only in other complement components but also in quite unrelated molecules. For example, C1r contains not just the serine protease domain but also a domain (EGF) seen in epidermal growth factor and the adhesion protein L-selectin. It also has two complement control protein (CCP) domains — structures which occur in a wide variety of molecules. Many of these structural relationships are distant; the most important are between the pairs of molecules which perform analagous functions in the classical and alternative pathways, namely C2 and FB, C1r/C1s, FD and MASP, C4 and C3. The structural subunits of the complement components are illustrated in *Figure 13.10*.

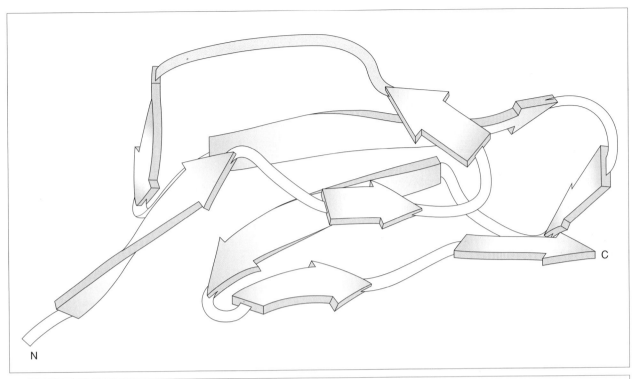

Fig. 13.11 A CCP domain. The ribbon diagram shows the tertiary structure of a CCP domain, H-16 from factor H. The structure is stabilized by two intrachain disulphide bonds near the N- and C-termini. The outer loop (coloured) is the segment which shows greatest variability between different molecules. Redrawn from Day *et al*, 1993; see also Barlow *et al*, 1993.

Molecular subunits and their functions

SERINE PROTEASE DOMAINS

The serine proteases of the complement system each have a catalytic domain of approximately 25kDa containing a triad of critical residues at the active site: His 57, Asp 102 and Ser 95, the numbering system being related to their position in chymotrypsin. With the exception of factor D, each of the proenzymes has large additional segments of polypeptide which are thought to control the binding characteristics of the proenzymes and their subsequent substrate specificity. Although factor D lacks any such extension, it is nevertheless specific for factor B, indicating that the catalytic domain alone may be sufficient to determine specificity.

COMPLEMENT CONTROL PROTEIN DOMAINS

Complement control protein domains (previously called short consensus repeats) are subunits found in many complement proteins (C1r, C1s, C2, FB), control proteins (FH, C4bp) and integral membrane proteins (CR1, CR2, DAF, MCP). These are all characterized by their ability to bind to C3 and C4, in either their native or fragmented forms. For example, FB binds via its N-terminal CCP-containing Ba portion to C3b to form C3bB and CR2 binds to the fragments C3b and C3dg. The control proteins listed in *Figure 13.3* consist almost entirely of CCP domains. These molecules, along with the C3 receptors CR1 and CR2, are all encoded in a segment of chromosome 1 in humans (1q32), referred to as the Regulators of Complement Action (RCA) locus. The tertiary structures of individual CCP domains from factor H have been determined (*Fig. 13.11*). It is notable that the overall structure is well conserved even when the primary structure homologies are quite modest. While interactions with C3 and C4 are evidently important functions of CCP domains in complement components, these sequences are also found in numerous other receptors, enzymes and structural proteins; one example is the IL-2 receptor. This implies that CCP domains are basic building blocks used in many proteins, with diverse modifications for different functions.

CCP domains consist of approximately 60 amino acid residues. They usually have four Cys residues which are linked within the unit in a 1–3, 2–4 fashion. In addition, about 12 other positions are conserved or semi-conserved. Electron microscopy and physical studies of factor H and C4bp, which contain several contiguous CCP domains, show them to be very extended, indicating that these domains are arranged like a string of beads conferring great flexibility on the molecules. The functional integrity of the domains is further emphasized by the observation that each CCP domain of factor B, for example, is encoded by a single exon. In CR1 the CCP domains are arranged in four or five groups of seven contiguous domains with up to 99% homology, termed long homologous repeats (LHRs).

Other structural units

The terminal components C6 to C9 contain three other types of structural motif first identified in other proteins. One of these is the ~60 amino acid residue domain first identified in the adhesion protein thrombospondin, termed a thrombospondin repeat (TSR). TSRs have no clearly defined single function, although most of the molecules in which they are found are involved in protein–protein or protein–phospholipid interactions. Other domains present in C6–C9 were first identified in low density lipoprotein (LDL) receptors and the epidermal growth factor (EGF) receptor. The central section of C9 also has considerable structural homology with perforin of Tc and NK cell granules (see Chapter 15), with which it shares the function of forming pores in target cell membranes. Even the peculiar structure of C1q is related to other components; the triple helical structures which form the centre of the ring are related to collagen and to similar structures found in MBP and conglutinin (a soluble receptor for iC3b found in some ruminants).

THIOLESTER RING STRUCTURE

Finally, mention should be made of the C3/C4/C5 family. C3 and C4 have the internal thiolester bond which is also found in α2-macroglobulin (see above). C5 is homologous to C3 and C4 but lacks the thiolester bond, due (in mouse) to the substitution of the critical Cys and Gln residues. The differences in reactivity of the thiolester bonds in the C4A and C4B isotypes have been outlined previously, with C4A reacting preferentially with $-NH_2$ and C4B with $-OH$ groups. Human C3 also reacts relatively poorly with $-NH_2$ groups. Interestingly, the sequence of residues in and immediately surrounding the thiolester ring is identical in both C4 isotypes but they differ at four amino acids lying at about 100 residues C-terminal to the thiolester bond and it is presumed that this region controls the specificity of the exposed thiolester bond. It is notable that deficiency of the *C4A* locus but not of *C4B*, is associated with the immune complex disease systemic lupus erythematosus. This suggests that attachment of this C4 allotype to the protein components of the complex (containing $-NH_2$ groups) facilitates their clearance.

Allotypic variants

Allelic variants of most of the complement components and receptors have been described. For example, there are more than 20 variants of C3 which vary in their electrophoretic mobility, being either fast or slow (C3F and C3S). However, many of the differences between variants do not alter the functional activity of the protein, obvious exceptions being null alleles, the alleles of MBP and the variants of C4 mentioned above.

The general principle with null alleles is that deficiencies of classical pathway components associate with immune complex diseases, primary and secondary C3 deficiencies result in pyogenic infections and lytic pathway deficiencies, with the exception of C9, permit increased susceptibility to *Neisseria* infections. Deficiency of CR3, due to the lack of CD18, produces a leukocyte adhesion deficiency, Lad type 1. However, LFA-1 and CR4 are also absent, as they share the common β-chain (CD18) with CR3 (see below).

C4 is encoded by at least two separate loci in the MHC class III region (*C4A* and *C4B*) with more than 35 known allotypes and in a few instances one of the loci is duplicated.

The allotypes vary antigenically, with most of the variants present at the *C4A* locus expressing the Rogers blood group antigen and most of those from the *C4B* locus expressing Chido. The incidence of null alleles in the C4 system is high (10–15%) but total C4 deficiency is rare and almost invariably associated with systemic or discoid lupus and severe immune complex disease of the kidney. More common is partial deficiency due to the absence of a functional protein at one of the loci. *C4B* locus alleles which bind $-OH$ groups more efficiently than *C4A* variants are also haemolytically more efficient, possibly due to the high level of carbohydrate on erythrocytes. A null allele at this locus would therefore make a shift in the overall reactivity pattern of serum C4.

The other MHC class III complement components, factor B and C2, are also polymorphic. Different types can be distinguished electrophoretically and, in some cases, by RFLP polymorphism. Three haplotypes of human C2 have been distinguished — C2C, 97%; C2A, <1% and C2B, 2% — with the C2C variant being further subdivisible by RFLP analysis. There are also three main variants of factor B (BS, 70%; BFa, 11%; BFb, 17%) with up to 16 rare alleles. The difference between the fast (F) and slow (S) forms appears to be the presence of a Gly or Arg at position 7.

There are two common allelic variants of MBP, each differing by a single amino acid and being associated with low levels of circulating MBP, presumably due to a failure to assemble normal molecules. The effect of low MBP is a reduced opsonizing capacity of the serum.

The polymorphism seen in CR1 is also instructive. It has four structural allotypes of 160, 190, 220 and 250kDa which vary by integral numbers of LHR units. The C4b binding site in CR1 is formed by the N-terminal CCP domains, meaning that polymorphism affects the distance from the membrane at which the site is available. There is also has a heritable variation in the level of CR1 expression on erythrocytes, which correlates with the presence or absence of a Hind III RFLP site but the functional consequences of this variation are not known.

COMPLEMENT EFFECTOR FUNCTIONS

The complement system has many functions in the effector phase of the immune response and this is mediated by receptors for complement fragments on different effector cell types. Receptors for C1q and fixed C3 (C3b, iC3b, C3dg, C3d) allow cells to bind to antigens, immune complexes and particles on which complement deposition has occurred (*Fig. 13.8*). There are also receptors for some of the small fragments released during activation, including the anaphylatoxins C5a, C3a and C4a, which act as short range signalling molecules.

Complement receptors

There are four receptors which bind the larger fragments of C3, called CR1 to CR4 (*Fig. 13.12*). CR1 (CD35) and CR2 (CD21) are both integral membrane proteins consisting of strings of CCP domains — 33 or more in CR1

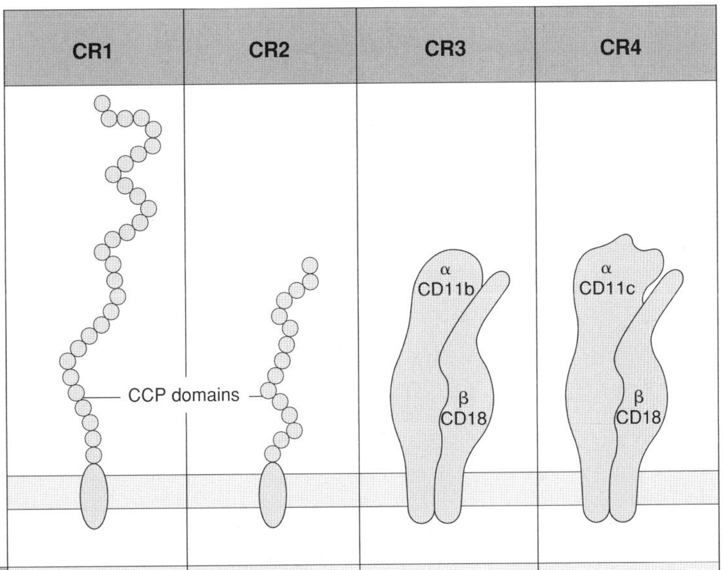

	CR1	CR2	CR3	CR4
M_r (kD)	160, 220 190,250	145	260 ⎡ α150 ⎣ β95	260 ⎡ α150 ⎣ β95
cells	erythrocytes lymphocytes granulocytes monocytes macrophages	B cells follicular dendritic cells	granulocytes monocytes NK cells macrophages	granulocytes monocytes NK cells macrophages
specificity	C4b C3b	iC3b C3dg C3d	iC3b	iC3b

Fig. 13.12 C3 receptors. Structures of the four complement C3 receptors, CR1–CR4 are shown diagrammatically, with their characteristics and the cells on which they are expressed outlined below. CR4 is often referred to as p150,95.

and 15 or 16 in CR2. They are both encoded on human chromosome 1q32 and have considerable structural homology, CR1 cDNA hybridizing to CR2 cDNA.

CR1 is present on most leukocytes, erythrocytes in primates, platelets in rodents and on some other cells where it acts as the classical 'immune adherence' receptor. The N-terminal LHR contains a C4b binding site and subsequent repeats contain C3b binding sites, the precise number varying with allotype. CR1 has at least three clearly defined functions:

• Uptake of immune complexes via neutrophils and cells of the monocyte/macrophage lineage, with the capacity to trigger macrophage activation.
• As a cofactor for factor I in C3b cleavage and dissociation of C3bBb (see above).
• As a receptor which mediates uptake of complexes onto erythrocytes or platelets for transport to phagocytes in spleen and liver.

The two N-terminal CCP domains of CR2 have a binding site for iC3b, C3dg and C3d, allowing binding to immune complexes. CR2 is present on B cells and follicular dendritic cells. On B cells it is present only on mature resting cells, disappearing as the cells start to proliferate and differentiate into plasma cells. B cells in germinal centres and mantle zones of secondary lymphoid follicles express CR2 particularly strongly. The physiological function of CR2 is

still under investigation but one suggestion is a role in localization of complexes to lymphoid follicles and the generation of B memory cells. At a cellular level, CR2 is associated with CD19 and TAPA-1 (Target for Antibody Proliferation) in a multimolecular complex. B cell activation appears to link surface IgM to the complex. In some experimental protocols ligation of CR2 with monoclonal antibodies or C3d can induce B cell proliferation, although this may require costimulation with cytokines. All these observations indicate a role in modulating B cell activation.

CR3 and CR4 are members of the β2-integrin family which also includes LFA-1. CR3 is the macrophage/NK cell marker Mac-1 and CR4 is also called gp150,95. The molecules of this family are formed of two polypeptide chains, with each member having a unique α-chain and a shared β-chain (CD18). The α-chain of CR3 is CD11b and that of CR4 is CD11c. CR3 is expressed on monocytes, neutrophils and NK cells, while CR4 has a similar distribution but is also strongly expressed on tissue macrophages. Expression of CR3 depends on the state of cellular activation, with cytokines, phorbol esters and bacterial surfaces all acting on neutrophils and monocytes to induce translocation of CR3, held as a pool in granule membranes, to the surface. This family of molecules binds in a Ca^{2+}-dependent manner to proteins containing the sequence Arg–Gly–Asp (RGD) which is found in both C3 and C4. In addition to binding iC3b, CR3 also has a distinct binding site for LPS. Other ligands for CR3 include the extracellular matrix protein fibronectin, which contains an RGD sequence, and the adhesion molecule ICAM-1, which does not. In this role CR3 appears to act as a leukocyte adhesion molecule controlling migration into tissues. For example, antibodies to CR3 have been shown to block the development of both insulin-dependent diabetes mellitus and experimental allergic encephalomyelitis (EAE) and to limit accumulation of phagocytes to the peritoneum, in response to inflammatory stimuli. In addition, ligation of CR3 by some monoclonal antibodies and some carbohydrates can trigger an oxidative burst. In summary, CR3 is involved in several aspects of phagocyte action, including cell migration, opsonic adherence and cell activation.

The collectin receptor binds to C1q, MBP and conglutinin; it was initially identified as a C1q receptor (C1qR) present on several cell types, including B cells, monocytes macrophages, neutrophils, platelets endothelial cells and fibroblasts. Binding to these cells is saturable and reversible and the affinity constant appears similar for each cell type. The receptor is related to the molecule calreticulin and it binds the collagen-like tail of C1q and MBP, although it has been found that intact C1 does not bind to the receptor on mononuclear cells. The receptor may promote uptake of antigenic particles which have fixed antibody and C1 but have lost C1r2s2 by the action of C1inh. Experimental ligation of the receptor on B cells inhibits their secretion of IL-1, indicating a possible regulatory role. In addition, the receptor can directly facilitate phagocytosis of microorganisms which have bound MBP via their surface carbohydrates.

The anaphylatoxins C3a and C5a mediate their inflammatory effects by binding to specific receptors on smooth muscle, endothelium, mast cells, basophils and platelets and are chemotactic for neutrophils and mononuclear phagocytes. There a two distinct receptors, one of which binds C3a and C4a, while the other is specific for C5a. These receptors act independently, as demonstrated by an absence of cross-tachyphylaxis on smooth muscle. The C5a receptor is a 45kDa member of the rhodopsin family of receptors, with seven transmembrane domains. On binding C5a, the receptor couples to a 40kDa G-protein which transduces the signal to the cell. The receptor binds to C5a and less effectively to C5a desArg (lacking the C-terminal Arg residue) and has 35% homology with the f–Met–Leu–Phe (fMLP) receptor which also mediates chemotaxis of phagocytic cells. The C3a/4a receptor is less well characterized, although it does not bind the desArg forms of C3a or C4a. These receptors are critical in the control of inflammation and in attracting cells to acute inflammatory sites.

Complement in inflammation

The essential features of an inflammatory response, namely an increase in blood flow, increased vascular permeability and migration of cells into the tissues, are considered in detail in the following chapter but the specific role of complement molecules is outlined here.

The anaphylatoxins C5a and C3a are most important as short range signalling molecules which diffuse from the site of an immune response to the local vasculature and can attract passing leukocytes. C3a is a 77 amino acid fragment and C5a has 74 amino acid residues; both are released from the N-terminus of the α-chain of their parent molecules and both have C-terminal Arg. C5a is the most active anaphylatoxin, 100- and 1000-fold more active than C3a and C4a respectively. It acts as a chemotactic agent for macrophages and neutrophils at concentrations as low as 1nM. C3a, C4a and C5a are inactivated by removal of their C-terminal arginine residues by a serum carboxypeptidase, termed anaphylatoxin inactivator. This enzyme contains polypeptides of 83, 55 and 49kDa, although their stoichiometry is still unclear.

In vivo C5a may synergize with other chemotactic molecules such as leukotriene B4 (LTB4) and fMet-containing peptides. Human neutrophils express about 100 000 C5a receptors but the number on macrophages varies greatly, with four to five-fold fewer receptors on inflammatory macrophages. This means that the sensitivity of an activated macrophage for the chemotactic stimulus of C5a is reduced. Binding of C5a to neutrophils induces a respiratory burst and mobilization of arachidonic acid, the precursor of the eicosanoids. In addition, it induces macrophages to release IL-1 and upregulate expression of CR1 and CR3.

Both C5a and C3a induce mast cell degranulation: this activity is essentially abrogated by removal of the C-terminal Arg residue. Histamine and 5HT released from the mast cells have powerful vasodilatory effects and cause endothelial cell retraction which together increase vascular permeability. One of the first observations of anaphylatoxin activity was on the contraction of smooth muscle and it was proposed that the anaphylatoxins could directly modulate blood vessel diameter by action on smooth muscle in the vessel wall. However, since this action can be largely blocked by anti-histamines, much of the effect of C5a and C3a in controlling vasodilation must be secondary to granule release by mast cells and basophils. Similarly, the increased permeability caused by application of C5a to vessels *in vivo* was originally thought to be due to a direct effect on the endothelium. Again, opinion is moving towards the idea that this may be a secondary effect which follows activation/migration of macrophages and neutrophils. The role of complement in the control of inflammation is summarized in *Figure 13.13*.

Opsonization and immune complex clearance

An important function of complement is in maintaining immune complexes in a soluble state and facilitating their uptake and clearance by phagocytes. Immune complexes formed near equivalence with multivalent antigens *in vitro* tend to form large lattices and interactions between the Fc portions of the antibody render them insoluble. However, in the presence of complement, C3b and C4b can attach covalently to the N-terminal domains of IgG (up to one molecule of C3b per IgG), thereby inhibiting interactions between the Fc regions and preventing insolubilization: *in vitro* the addition of serum to precipitated complexes can partially resolubilize them. This may explain why deficiencies of the classical pathway components C2 and C4 are particularly associated with immune complex deposition in tissues in diseases such as SLE and rheumatoid arthritis.

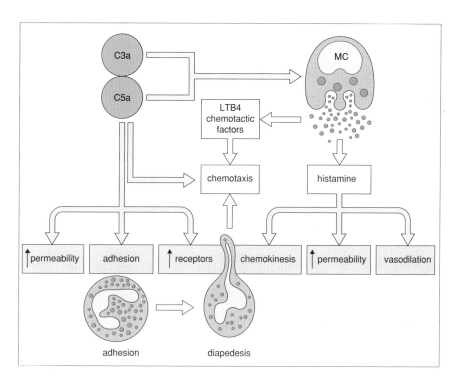

Fig. 13.13 Role of anaphylatoxins in the inflammatory response. C5a induces cellular adhesion, increased receptors on phagocytes and their chemotaxis; it also has a role (possibly indirect) in increasing vascular permeability. Both C3a and C5a induce mast cell degranulation and activation, with release of inflammatory mediators, including leukotriene B4 (LTB4) and other chemotactic factors. They may also potentiate vasodilation by a direct action on smooth muscle of the arterioles.

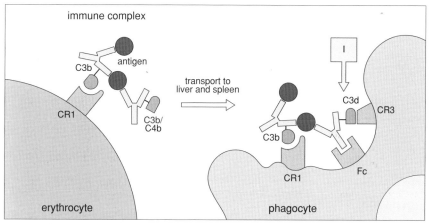

Fig. 13.14 Immune complex clearance. In primates, complexes are taken up by CR1 on erythrocytes. Platelets carry out a similar function in rodents. These are transported primarily to the liver where they may be released by factor I to be taken up by mononuclear phagocytes expressing receptors for C3d, C3dg and Fc, as well as CR1.

In primates, CR1 on erythrocytes acts as an important transport mechanism for immune complexes. In experiments where radiolabelled complexes were infused into arterial blood supplying different organs, it was shown that the majority of erythrocyte-bound complexes are stripped off by the action of factor I in the liver and transferred to tissue macrophages (Kupffer cells). In complement deficient animals, infused complexes are still removed from the circulation but they do not localize to the liver. The size of the complexes critically affects their clearance rate — large complexes fix C1q more efficiently and consequently bind more C3b and C4b and so are taken up efficiently by erythrocytes. Consequently, removal of complexes from the circulation depends on a number of variables, including the affinity and isotype of the antibody, the number of epitopes on the antigen and the efficiency of the complement system, which in turn may vary with complement allotypes.

The receptors CR1, CR3 and CR4 present on neutrophils and mononuclear phagocytes are important in allowing the attachment and internalization of immune complexes. There is a certain logic in the way that erythrocytes use CR1 to transport complexes, while phagocytes use CR1, CR3 and CR4 to take them up. CR1 recognizes C3b which is initially deposited on circulating complexes and allows their immediate uptake by erythrocytes. However, complexes which have reached the liver and have been acted on by factor I still retain their covalently bound iC3b, allowing them to attach to phagocytes via CR3 and CR4 (*Fig. 13.14*).

Binding of complexes to complement receptors on phagocytes synergizes with Fc receptor mediated attachment. The nature of the signal for internalization is unclear, although phosphorylation of the complement receptors can occur and the cytoskeleton is involved, since endocytosis is blockable by cytochalasin B. For example, binding of

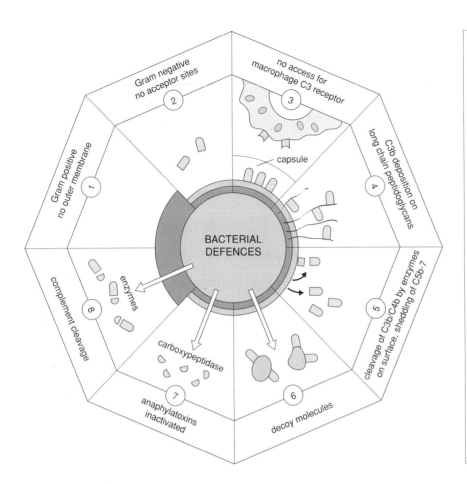

Fig. 13.15 Anti-complement defences of bacteria. 1) Gram-positive bacteria have a thick outer coat which resists complement-mediated attack. 2) Some Gram-negative bacteria lack suitable acceptor sites for C3b. 3) The anti-phagocytic capsule of some bacteria prevents complement receptors on phagocytes accessing bound C3b. 4) Some strains of Gram-negative *salmonellae* have long chain peptidoglycans which bind C3b at a safe distance from the outer membrane. 5) Surface enzymes may cleave bound C3b and C4b, while other bacteria rapidly shed the assembling MACs. 6) Several species release complement-fixing soluble molecules to decoy the complement system and consume its components.
7) Carboxypeptidases of group A *streptococci* inactivate the anaphylatoxins, while (8) other species can release enzymes which cleave the intact components before they can react.

complexes to neutrophils via C3 receptors or Fc receptors alone produces modest phagocytosis and a slight increase in cellular activity, while attachment by both receptor types induces rapid phagocytosis, an oxidative burst and lysosomal enzyme release.

Complement in the immune response

The role of complement in the development of the immune response is variable. For example, C2 and C4-deficient guinea pigs have impaired antibody responses to low doses of Tind antigens and fail to switch from IgM to IgG, whereas C4-deficient humans do not seem to be impaired in this way. The majority of antigen presenting cells express one or more types of C3 receptor; B cells have CR1 and CR2, macrophages have CR1, CR3 and CR4 and follicular dendritic cells have CR1, CR2 and CR3. Langerhans cells have also recently been shown to have a C3 receptor although it appears to be absent from the interdigitating cells of the T cell areas of lymph node. Furthermore, complement-fixing immune complexes localize to lymphoid follicles more efficiently than non-fixing complexes. These and other observations suggest that complement plays an auxiliary role in potentiating antigen uptake by APCs, although it is not mandatory for subsequent processing and presentation. It seems likely that this is most relevant for immune complexes originating in the tissues, where antibody levels may be low and which move via lymphatics to reach the lymph nodes to localize on APCs there.

There have also been reports of immunoregulation by C3a and C5a. In contrast to their similar actions in inflammation their effects on immune reponses appeared divergent. C3a appeared to be suppressive, possibly by inducing PGE2 release from macrophages, while C5a enhanced both cell-mediated and antibody responses.

Defence against pathogens

The importance of the complement system in defence against a variety of microbial pathogens is clearly seen in individuals with deficiencies of certain components. For example, individuals lacking C3, B or D are subject to a variety of recurrent bacterial infections which may be life threatening. Lack of lytic pathway components, particularly C5 to C8 is associated with recurrent neisserial infections. Activation of C3 may induce migration of leukocytes to the site of infection and its deposition on microorganisms may opsonize them for phagocytosis. Some organisms are also susceptible to MAC-mediated damage. Whether these effector mechanisms are active depends on the structure of the organism and many pathogens deploy anti-complement defences (*Fig. 13.15*)

In general, the surfaces of Gram-positive and of encapsulated Gram-negative bacteria are poor complement activators. In particular, the sialic acid containing capsules of type B *N. meningitidis* and *E. coli* group K1 are very poor activators of the alternative pathway in the absence of antibody. It is possible that sialic acid favours the binding of factor H and therefore makes these encapsulated bacteria appear to have a non-activator surface. Additionally, although complement molecules may reach the surface of these bacteria and become activated, complement receptors on phagocytes are unable to access the bound C3b and C4b. Other strategies of anti-complement defence include rapid cleavage of bound C3b (e.g. *S. pneumoniae*) and having surface structures which act as poor acceptors for C3b deposition (e.g. *H. influenzae*).

Some organisms release anti-complement molecules. These include enzymes, such as the elastase from *P. aeruginosa* which cleaves a number of complement components and a carboxypeptidase released by group A streptococci which acts as a specific C5a inactivator. An alternative strategy is to release decoy molecules which activate and thus consume complement. Examples of this group are teichoic acid released by *S. aureus* and the mucoexopolysaccharide released by *P. aeruginosa*, which is an effective alternative pathway activator.

Susceptibility of bacteria to MACs depends to a large extent on the composition of the bacterial cell wall, with Gram-positive organisms generally being resistant, while some that are Gram-negative (which have outer membranes) are sensitive. Considerable numbers of MACs are required to damage a Gram-negative bacterium and the complement system must also work in concert with lysozyme, punching holes in the outer membrane and thereby allowing the enzyme access to the peptidoglycan cell wall. MACs may also become deposited on enveloped viruses, leading to disassembly of the envelope, which is derived from the host cell membrane and loss of infectivity.

Some strains of *Salmonella* can evade the action of C5b–9 by restricting deposition to non-critical sites away from the outer membrane. Serum-resistant non-encapsulated *Salmonella* strains have a long chain form of lipopolysaccharide (LPS) in their outer membranes, constituting 2–3% of the total LPS but which preferentially binds the assembling lytic pathway components. Both the serum-resistant and serum-sensitive variants bind similar quantities of C3b and consume lytic pathway components with equal efficiency. The serum-sensitivity, due to damage caused by MACs, is critically dependent on the length of the LPS chains, with units containing more than 13 O-antigen repeats conferring resistance.

Serum-resistant and serum-sensitive strains of *N. gonhorroeae* also occur but in this case the difference cannot be accounted for by differences in the LPS side chains. C5b–9 complexes from the resistant form have different sizes from those on the sensitive form, indicating that the actual manner of deposition on the outer membrane differs.

If appropriate levels of specific antibody bind to the bacterial surface, this can circumvent many of these anti-complementary strategies.

In extreme cases, pathogens may subvert elements of the complement system for their own devices. Examples of this type include microorganisms such as *Leishmania* which can not only resist complement mediated attack but also use surface bound C3b to gain access to host macrophages via their C3b receptors, CR1 and CR3. This is conceptually different to the direct binding of Epstein Barr virus to CR2 on B cells, although the end result, infection of a particular set of host cells, is similar.

COMPLEMENT IN HYPERSENSITIVITY AND AUTOIMMUNITY

Since activation of the complement classical pathway is directed by the immune system, whenever there is a failure of immune recognition, inappropriate complement activation may occur. Consequently, in many immune complex diseases, antibody in tissues detected by immunofluorescence is often co-localized with C3 and other complement components. Deposition may occur *in situ*, such as in Goodpasture's syndrome where autoantibody to basement membranes of lung and kidney directs complement deposition to those sites. Alternatively, preformed complexes containing complement may deposit from the circulation, particularly into sites of filtration or haemodynamic stress. In some sense, the finding of complexes deposited in tissues is an indication of the failure of the correct methods of clearance by phagocytes carrying Fc and C3 receptors. This may result from overloading of the system, as occurs in some severe infections (e.g. malaria, leprosy and hepatitis) or may be due to failure of the clearance system. For example, low levels of CR1, C4, C2 or C3 might be expected to lead to slower removal of complexes and hence predispose to deposition in tissues. C3b deposited on membranes, or associated with insoluble complexes, allows binding of phagocytes which are unable to internalize the complexes. Instead they release granule contents and reactive oxygen intermediates to the exterior, causing tissue damage. Other components, although less often looked for histologically, may be equally damaging. For example, C9 is found deposited on motor endplates in myasthenia gravis, indicating MAC-mediated damage at these sites, and the peculiar sensitivity of oligodendrocytes to C9 has suggested a way in which they may become damaged in demyelinating conditions.

SUMMARY

Complement is an important effector system linking the immune system to several mechanisms which control inflammatory reactions. In addition, the lytic action of complement plays a role in defence against some pathogens and in hypersensitivity and autoimmunity. Complement may be activated by immune complexes via the classical pathway or by surfaces which favour alternative pathway activation, or by some carbohydrates. Each may lead to the covalent deposition of C3b on the activator, via a labile thiolester bond generated by C3 activation. Both classical and alternative pathways can generate C3 and C5 convertases which activate C5 as the first step of the lytic pathway, the non-enzymatic assembly of a complex of C5b–C9 which can attach to target cell membranes and cause channels to be produced which can lead to membrane disassembly and/or osmotic lysis. The activation of the system is closely controlled by soluble components, membrane receptors for activated C3 and the intrinsically limited half lives of the active components. The anaphylatoxins, C3a and C5a, play a role in the development of inflammation by inducing mast cell degranulation, activating phagocytes and acting as chemotaxins for macrophages and neutrophils. Meanwhile, C3b, C1q and MBP act as opsonins which bind immune complexes or microbial carbohydrates to receptors on erythrocytes, phagocytes, antigen presenting cells and B cells. Many of the complement components are molecular mosaics, consisting of several different types of subunit. These subunits include serine protease domains, CCP domains and segments found in other receptors; they are present in different assortments in different components, although gene diversification has produced varied but precise specificities of action for each component.

FURTHER READING

Barlow PN, Steinkasserer A, Norman DG, Kieffer B, Wiles AP, Sim RB, Campbell ID. Solution structure of a pair of complement modules by NMR. *J Mol Biol* 1993, **232**:268.

Campbell RD, Law SKA, Reid KBM, Sim RB. Structure, organization and regulation of the complement genes. *Ann Rev Immunol* 1988, **6**:161.

Colten HR. Complement deficiencies. *Ann Rev Immunol* 1992, **10**:809.

Cooper NR, Moore MD, Nemerow GR. Immunobiology of CR2, the B lymphocyte receptor for the Epstein Barr virus and the C3d complement fragment. *Ann Rev Immunol* 1988, **6**:85.

Day AJ, Barlow PN., Steinkasserer A, Campbell ID, Sim RB. Progress in determining module structures in C1r and C1s. *Behring Inst Mitt* 1993, **93**:31.

Dierich MP, Schulz TF, Eigentler A, Huemer H, Schwable W. Structural and functional relationships among receptors and regulators of the complement system. *Mol Immunol* 1988, **25**:1043.

Discipio RG, Chakravarti DB, Muller-Eberhard HJ, Fey GH. The structure of C7 and the C5b-7 complex. *J Biol Chem* 1988, **263**:549.

Holmskov U, Malhotra R, Sim RB, Jensenius JC. Collectins: collagenous C-type lectins of the innate immune defence system. *Immunol Today* 1994, **15**:67.

Law SKA, Reid KBM. *Complement in Focus,* edn 2. Male DK (Ed). Oxford University Press: Oxford; 1995.

Law SKA. The covalent binding reaction of C3 and C4. *Ann N Y Acad Sci* 1983, **421**:246.

Liszewski MK, Post TW, Atkinson JP. Membrane cofactor protein MCP or CD46: newest member of the regulators of complement activation gene cluster. *Ann Rev Immunol* 1991, **9**:431.

Lublin DM, Atkinson JP. Decay accelerating factor: biochemistry molecular biology and function. *Ann Rev Immunol* 1989, **9**:35.

Moffit MC, Frank MM. Complement resistance in microbes. *Springer Semin Immunopathol* 1994, **15**:327.

Morgan BP, Meri S. Membrane proteins that protect against complement lysis. *Springer Semin Immunopathol* 1994, **15**:369.

Painter RH. The binding of C1q to immunoglobulins. *Behring Inst Mitt* 1993, **93**:131.

Perkins SJ. Three-dimensional structure and molecular modelling of C1 inhibitor. *Behring Inst Mitt* 1993, **93**:63.

Reid KBM. Structure function relationships of the complement components. *Immunol Today* 1989, **10**:177.

Schumaker VN, Zavodsky P, Poon PH. Activation of the first component of complement. *Ann Rev Immunol* 1987, **5**:21.

Sodetz JM. Structure and function of C8 in the membrane attack sequence of complement. *Curr Topics Microbiol Immunol* 1988, **140**:19.

Stanley KK. The molecular mechanism of complement C9 insertion and polymerization in biological membranes. *Curr Topics Microbiol Immunol* 1988, **140**:49.

Weis WI, Drickamer K, Hendrickson WA. Structure of a C-type mannose binding protein complexed with an oligosaccharide. *Nature* 1992, **360**:127.

Whaley K, Loos M, Weiler JM (Eds). *Complement in Health and Disease,* edn 2. Kluwer Academic Publishers: Lancaster; 1993

14 Cell Traffic and Inflammation

The development of immune responses *in vivo* is far more complex than the interactions which are seen *in vitro*. Lymphoid tissues have distinctive compartments which allow lymphocytes, antigen presenting cells and phagocytes to develop and interact in defined microenvironments. The convergence of these cells on different tissues is a result of leukocyte migration between tissues. Indeed, the leukocytes present in blood are but the small proportion which are in transit.

There are four principal patterns of lymphocyte traffic:

- Migration of precursors into primary lymphoid tissues.
- Migration of differentiated, virgin lymphocytes into secondary lymphoid tissues.
- Migration of activated lymphocytes from lymphoid tissues into inflammatory sites.
- Migration of cells between different secondary lymphoid tissues.

Phagocytes and antigen presenting cells (APCs) also migrate between tissues. For example, neutrophils make a one way journey from bone marrow to tissues; monocytes migrate from blood into tissues, where they differentiate into macrophages and may then return to secondary lymphoid tissues; Langerhans cells move from bone marrow to colonize the epidermis but may be induced to differentiate into dendritic cells which transport antigen to lymph nodes.

There has recently been a revolution in our understanding of how cells migrate into secondary lymphoid tissues and inflammatory sites — a process controlled by the expression of adhesion molecules on endothelium in different tissues, interacting with corresponding ligands present on particular populations of leukocytes. The localization of any particular cell is not pre-determined but it will be more likely to migrate across endothelium in some tissues than others, based on the local expression of adhesion molecules. Because of this, when a population of cells is considered, the probabilistic effects of the interactions between leukocytes and endothelium produce the distinctive patterns of leukocyte traffic seen *in vivo*. It is worth remembering that a lymphocyte will usually pass through the venular circulation hundreds of times *in vivo*, before it migrates again into a tissue.

LYMPHOCYTE RECIRCULATION

Since the number of cells specific for any antigen is relatively small, traffic between lymphoid tissues is essential to enable lymphocytes to encounter their own antigen. The first definitive evidence of lymphocyte recirculation came from the pioneering work of Gowans who showed that the majority of lymphocytes in the efferent lymph from a rat lymph node came from the blood and were not merely the result of proliferation within the node. Subsequent studies showed that lymphocytes recirculate many times even in the absence of antigen (*Fig. 14.1*). For example, it occurs

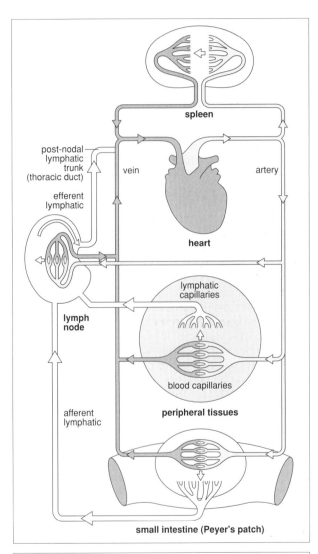

Fig. 14.1 The major routes of lymphocyte recirculation. Naive and memory lymphocytes migrate primarily to secondary lymphoid tissues, here exemplified by the spleen, lymph nodes and Peyer's patches. Different populations of T and B cells selectively localize to these sites. Following activation in the lymphoid tissues, activated and naive cells may return to the blood stream via efferent lymphatics. Memory cells re-seed distant lymphoid tissues while activated T cells migrate to non-lymphoid tissues, where they may act as effector cells in inflammatory responses.

vigorously in foetal sheep. Secondary lymphoid tissues are the major sites of recirculating lymphocyte traffic. It has been estimated that, in the rat, over 50% of lymphocytes leaving the blood enter the splenic white pulp; in sheep, a lymph node may extract 25% of all lymphocytes which pass through the high endothelial venules. In general, naive lymphocytes do not recirculate to such a degree as memory cells, nevertheless, thoracic duct cannulation for a few days produces a generalized depletion of lymphocytes from all the drained nodes, implying that most lymphocytes have the capacity to recirculate. Antigen, mobile APCs and naive lymphocytes all converge on secondary lymphoid tissues where immune responses can develop. The response of a lymph node to antigen is reflected in the output of cells into its efferent lymph. Within a few hours of antigen stimulation a local inflammatory response develops, producing an increase in blood flow to the node of up to 25 times normal. This gives rise to an increase in lymphocyte traffic into the node. The second phase takes place 1–2 days after antigen stimulation and is seen as a marked increase in the output of small lymphocytes into the efferent lymph. This output is devoid of antigen-specific cells which are selectively retained within the node. These cells are thought to be retained following recognition of antigen on appropriate APCs. After about 2 days, cell proliferation has increased markedly within the nodes and blast cells begin to appear in the efferent lymph; this emigration peaks at about 4 days (earlier in the secondary response). The blast cells again show specific homing properties. For example, gut IgA-producing B cells tend to move to mucosal areas. However, lymphoblasts also have a higher affinity for peripheral tissue endothelium. This migration disseminates activated antigen-specific cells and marks the beginning of the effector stage of the immune response.

The rate of movement of lymphocytes into peripheral tissues is normally much lower than through secondary lymphoid organs and the cells usually migrate through in a few hours — much faster than the rate of movement through lymph nodes. Nevertheless, this traffic is very important in maintaining immunological surveillance throughout the body. When tissue damage occurs or patrolling lymphocytes encounter antigen, mechanisms are activated which upregulate leukocyte traffic to that site. This is one of the three key features of inflammation — the others being increased blood flow and enhanced vascular permeability. Studies *in vivo* using Indium-labelled cells have shown that lymphoblasts selectively migrate into areas of inflammation, or to sites of delayed hypersensitivity reactions.

Movement between lymphoid tissues

Long-lived recirculating lymphocytes consist primarily of memory T and B cells and virgin T cells. Normally, virgin B cells have a relatively short lifespan and do not enter the recirculating population, except during the early stages of a primary response or following experimental suppression of normal B cell development. Lymphocytes may enter lymph nodes either via the afferent lymphatics or by crossing the vascular endothelium. In humans and most other animals this occurs across specialized high endothelial

venules (HEV). These structures are absent from some animals (e.g. sheep), although the lymph node vascular endothelium still supports lymphocyte traffic. In peripheral nodes, the majority of cells enter from the blood, while a higher proportion of cells entering central lymph nodes do so via afferent lymphatics.

High endothelial venules

High endothelial venules (HEV) consist of one or two layers of columnar endothelial cells which are present in most secondary lymphoid tissues but not in spleen, bone marrow or thymus. The origin of these HEV is related to the differentiation of secondary lymphoid tissues and they are present in athymic mice and rats. HEV may be induced in other tissues but only at sites of chronic inflammation which is thought to be a function of persistent cytokine secretion. Within lymph nodes, HEV are confined to the paracortical T cell areas. They are also present in mucosa-associated lymphoid tissues including Peyer's patches (see *Fig. 1.6*).

High endothelial cells are linked by macular (spot) tight junctions, express non-specific esterase and selectively take up sulphate ions to be incorporated into sulphated glycolipids, some of which act as HEV-specific adhesion molecules (see below). Indeed, the sets of adhesion molecules expressed by HEV constitute in part their distinctive phenotypes: the precise set of adhesion molecules expressed on a high endothelial cell depends on its location.

Selective migration across HEV

Migration of lymphocytes into lymphoid tissues is controlled by adhesion molecules on the lymphocytes interacting with receptors on the HEV. There is considerable selectivity in this movement, ensuring that cells preferentially localize to appropriate tissues. For example, lymphocytes isolated from gut-associated lymphoid tissue tend to localize to Peyer's patches when reinfused, while splenocytes preferentially return to the spleen. Other experiments, in which cells were sorted and labelled before reinfusion into the host animal, showed that small lymphocytes (including the memory population) tended to localize to lymph nodes. Different lymphocyte populations also migrate selectively into different lymphoid tissues. B cells are over-represented in Peyer's patches by comparison with their percentage in blood. Conversely, they migrate less well to peripheral lymph nodes where T cells are prevalent. There is also evidence for selective recruitment of different T cell subsets to particular lymph nodes. For example, the proportion of CD8+ T cells in lymph nodes can be ranked as follows: cervical nodes > other peripheral nodes > mesenteric lymph nodes. Such differences can be accounted for by selective expression or action of particular adhesion molecules on different lymphocyte subsets interacting with locally expressed ligands on HEV in the different lymphoid tissues.

Movement into non-lymphoid tissues

Immune responses in non-lymphoid tissues induce the migration of neutrophils, monocytes and lymphocytes into the area. The acute inflammatory response is characterized by an early influx of neutrophils, with lymphocytes and

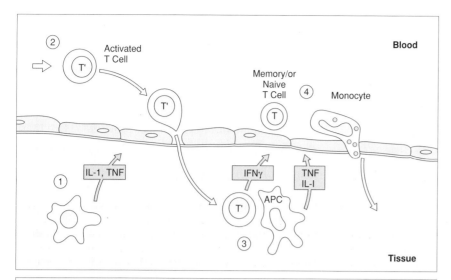

Fig. 14.2 Initiation of inflammatory reactions *in vivo*. Tissue damage or activation of mononuclear phagocytes in the tissue leads to release of IL-1, TNFα and other cytokines which can signal to the local endothelium, inducing adhesion molecules and favouring leukocyte migration (1). Alternatively, activated T cells, which have recently entered the circulation show high migratory capacities and patrol the tissues (2). Should these active T cells encounter their specific antigen on local antigen presenting cells (APC), they will be induced to release IFNγ and interact with tissue cells to release further inflammatory cytokines (3). Newly induced adhesion and signalling molecules on the endothelium will now recruit effector cells and other T cell populations (4).

mononuclear phagocytes starting to enter the lesion from one day later; they may then become the predominant cell type in chronic inflammatory sites, such as the rheumatoid joint or the CNS plaques of multiple sclerosis. The phased arrival of cells at an inflammatory site depends on a number of factors including sequential expression of adhesion molecules on the endothelium and the availability and numbers of different leukocyte populations in the blood. The population balance of cells in inflammatory sites at any moment (seen histologically) also depends on the longevity of the cells and on whether they are retained at the site.

The scheme outlined in *Figure 14.2* attempts to explain the development of an inflammatory reaction *in vivo*. Initially cytokines (e.g. IL-1, TNFα) from local non-lymphoid cells can signal to endothelium to upregulate leukocyte immigration. Alternatively, if patrolling lymphocytes encounter their antigen on local APCs, they too can induce endothelial adhesion molecules. After the initial neutrophil influx, activated CD4+ lymphocytes are usually the first to enter the inflammatory site. If they encounter their antigen, they release IFNγ and induce effector cell immigration, inluding macrophages and CD8+ T cells. Should the antigen persist, a chronic reaction develops, with induction of new adhesion molecules on the endothelium, permitting migration of non-activated lymphocytes. In contrast, clearance of the antigen leads to a waning of cytokine secretion, downregulation of the endothelial adhesion molecules and a fall in leukocyte immigration. This is accompanied by a reassertion of negative controls on the T cells and other effector cells at the site.

It has been debated whether lymphocytes selectively leave the blood in response to their own specific antigen, or whether extravasation occurs at random and antigen-specific cells are retained at the site of the immune reaction. Although MHC class II molecules can be induced readily on endothelial cells *in vitro* by IFNγ, it is usually present only *in vivo* at sites of strong immune reactions (although different species do vary in this respect). Consequently, there is little scope for an antigen-specific element in the interactions between endothelium and CD4+ T cells. However, if an immune reaction is in progress in the body, there will be a higher proportion of newly activated, antigen-specific cells in the circulation. Since these cells preferentially migrate across endothelium at inflammatory sites, this could produce a *de facto* selective migration of relevant antigen-specific cells to that site.

MOVEMENT OF ANTIGENS AND ANTIGEN PRESENTING CELLS

If an antigen gains direct access to the blood, it will initially localize primarily on marginal zone macrophages in the spleen. Antigens present in the gut may be directly sampled by Peyer's patch M cells and intra-epithelial lymphocytes which can transport them to the T and B cell areas of the patch. Similar events occur in mucosa-associated lymphoid tissues of the bronchus. Antigens entering most other peripheral tissues will be transported to local lymph nodes, either free in the lymph or on cells. Free antigens tend to localize first on phagocytes in the subcapsular sinus before reaching other areas of the node. Antigens can then bind to dendritic cells in the cortex before reaching follicular dendritic cells (FDCs) which preferentially take up antigen complexed with antibody and complement. Both mature and virgin lymphocytes gain access to APCs in the T cell areas but only mature recirculating cells contact the FDCs, where, if activated by T_{dep} antigens, they participate in the formation of germinal centres. Antigen may also be transported to lymph nodes, bound to macrophages or as complexes on B lymphocytes which are then passed to FDCs.

In the skin, a specialized group of cells expressing MHC class II, the Langerhans cells, migrate from the epidermis to transport antigen to the local lymph nodes. Ultraviolet light or application of antigen to skin potentiates this movement. These cells appear as veiled cells in afferent lymph and become the interdigitating APCs in the paracortex. Veiled cells have also been found in intestinal lymph destined for the mesenteric nodes and cells of this lineage are thought to be present in most tissues of the body.

Afferent lymph normally contains very few macrophages or other APCs (except B cells), although class II-negative, antigen-laden macrophages have been found in thoracic duct lymph. The functional relevance of these cells is not known but they may transport antigen to the spleen in order to disseminate the immune response further.

ADHESION MOLECULES

Migration is controlled by the expression of adhesion molecules on leukocytes which interact with corresponding ligands on endothelium. Expression of individual adhesion molecules on leukocytes depends both on their cell lineage and on their state of differentiation and activation. Endothelial cells also express a wide variety of different adhesion molecules. Expression patterns vary between different tissues within the body, as well as between different sections of the vascular bed. They can be modulated by endothelial activation in response to cytokines and other inflammatory mediators. Different cytokines induce different sets of endothelial adhesion molecules which are expressed in sequence to control the various phases of leukocyte migration.

Clearly it requires corresponding pairs of adhesion molecules on leukocytes and endothelium for attachment and migration to take place. However, expression of the correct molecules is necessary but not sufficient. Only a proportion of the expressed adhesion molecules on leukocytes may be functionally capable of interacting with receptors on the endothelium and short term signals from cytokines or from the endothelium modulate the functional avidity of the adhesion molecules.

There has been considerable progress in identifying and characterizing adhesion molecules on leukocytes and endothelium and in determining which pairs of molecules interact. However, since both endothelium and leukocytes express variable sets of adhesion molecules which vary with time and location, it has taken longer to determine which molecules contribute to each of the types and phases of cell migration. This has also been complicated by the realization that many adhesion molecules have binding sites for more than one ligand.

Most adhesion molecules can be grouped into families, with related structures but different ligand-binding specificities. These include the integrins, the selectins, immunoglobulin supergene family adhesion molecules and carbohydrate-containing molecules. Unfortunately, most adhesion molecules still have several different names. For simplicity, this chapter uses the most prevalent current nomenclature, with synonyms given in *Figures 14.3–14.5*.

Integrins

The integrins are a large family of molecules involved in intercellular and cell-substratum adhesion (*Fig. 14.3*). Each member is a heterodimer of non-covalently linked α and β-chains, both of which traverse the cell membrane. In some cases the α-chain undergoes post-translational cleavage, producing separate disulphide-linked polypeptides. Originally, three families of integrins were described, in which the members of a particular family share a common β-chain but each has a unique α-chain. More recently, additional chains have been identified and the α and β-chains may link in new combinations so that the family divisions are less well delineated. Therefore, the most accurate nomenclature for an integrin is given by its pair of chains, for example $α_3β_1$.

The $β_1$ family includes the 'very late antigens' VLA-1 and VLA-2 which are expressed at 2–4 weeks after T cell activation *in vitro* and are involved in binding to extracellular matrix proteins; they share the CD29 $β_1$-chain. Other molecules in this family are found on a wide variety of cells but are still referred to as VLA molecules. Molecules of this group anchor cells to elements of the extracellular matrix such as collagen (VLA-2), laminin (VLA-6) and fibronectin (VLA-5), with a high degree of specificity, while VLA-3 binds to all three of these matrix proteins. VLA-4 has two distinct binding sites, one for VCAM-1 and one for fibronectin. The attachment site on fibronectin for VLA-4 is different to that recognized by VLA-5. The $α_4$-chain can also combine with $β_7$, producing a molecule, $α_4β_7$, which binds to both VCAM-1 and MadCAM-1. VLA-4 ($α_4β_1$) and $α_4β_7$ are expressed on many circulating lymphocytes and monocytes, with levels and proportions dependent on the state of cell activation. Hence these two integrins are thought to be important in the control of transendothelial migration, whereas the other $β_1$-integrins are probably more involved in matrix interactions. The $β_2$ family consists of the molecules LFA-1 ($α_Lβ_2$), CR3 ($α_Mβ_2$) and CR4 ($α_Xβ_2$) which share the CD18 $β_2$-chain. These are expressed exclusively on leukocytes and hence are referred to as the leukocyte integrins. LFA-1 is expressed by all leukocytes (except some macrophages), albeit at different levels, and is involved in numerous immunological functions including cell migration into tissues. CR3 and CR4 mediate phagocytosis by binding to immune complexes coated with iC3b and iC4b (Chapter 13). CR3 also has binding sites for lipopolysaccharide (LPS) and ICAM-1, this latter being important in the control of neutrophil and monocyte migration. Congenital deficiency of CD18

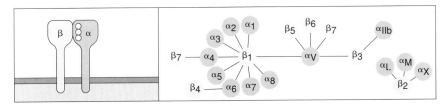

RECEPTOR	CHAINS	CD	LIGANDS	SPECIFICITY	EXPRESSION
VLA-1	$\alpha_1 \beta_1$	49a/29	Collagens Laminin	?	T Cells Fibroblasts Mesangial Cells
VLA-2	$\alpha_2 \beta_1$	49b/29	Collagens Laminin	DGEA	Activated T Cells Platelets
VLA-3	$\alpha_3 \beta_1$	49c/29	Collagen Laminin Fibronectin	RGD?	Kidney Thyroid
VLA-4	$\alpha_4 \beta_1$	49d/29	VCAM-1 Fibronectin	Composite. EILDV	Haemopoietic Cells
VLA-5	$\alpha_5 \beta_1$	49e/29	Fibronectin	RGD	Leukocytes Platelets
VLA-6	$\alpha_6 \beta_1$	49f/29	Laminin	?	Widely Distributed
LPAM-1	$\alpha_4 \beta_7$	49d/104	Mad CAM-1	Composite	Lymphocyte Subpopulations
LFA-1	$\alpha_L \beta_2$	11a/18	ICAM-1 ICAM-2 ICAM-3	Composite	Most Leukocytes
CR3	$\alpha_M \beta_2$	11b/18	iC3b, iC4b ICAM-1, ICAM-2	Composite	Mononuclear Phagocytes Neutrophils
CR4	$\alpha_X \beta_2$	11c/18	iC3b iC4b ICAM-1	Composite	Macrophages

Fig. 14.3 Integrins. A general structure of an integrin is shown top left, consisting of an α and β-chain each of which is non-covalently associated and traverses the cell membrane. The cation-binding sites on the α-chain are indicated (circles). The spider-diagram top right indicates the ways in which pairs of α and β-chains may be associated. The table gives detailed information on the integrins which are thought to be involved in the binding of leukocytes to endothelium or extracellular matrix. Binding specificity refers to sequences shown to be involved in the binding site on extracellular matrix proteins. The binding sites on the cell adhesion molecules are composite structures.

results in failure to express all three members of the family and results in the leukocyte adhesion deficiency (LAD) syndrome type-1, characterized by the failure of neutrophils to move into sites of inflammation and hence repeated bacterial infections.

The β_3 integrin family consists of the vitronectin receptor (VNR, $\alpha v \beta_3$) and Gp IIb/IIIa found on platelets. Gp IIb/IIIa has a broad binding specificity which allows platelets to bind to molecules present in damaged tissues, such as collagen, fibrinogen, fibronectin and von Willebrand factor. Its deficiency produces a chronic bleeding condition called Glanzmann's thrombasthenia.

The integrin superfamily of molecules is evolutionarily ancient and there is a high degree of sequence conservation between the different α-chains; this is also true of the β-chains. Binding of integrins to their ligands is dependent on Mg^{2+} or Ca^{2+} ions with a preference for Mg^{2+}. The α-chains of the superfamily have divalent cation binding sites which can be occupied by Ca^{2+} or Mg^{2+} (sometimes even Mn^{2+}). In LFA-1, displacement of Ca^{2+} by Mg^{2+} results in a higher binding affinity for ICAM-1 and this mechanism allows for a rapid modulation of the strength of interaction between two cells. Many of the integrins bind to molecules which contain the peptide sequence Arg–Gly–Asp (RGD). This sequence occurs in C3, C4, thrombin, fibronectin, vitronectin, laminin, fibrinogen and most types of collagen. The specific receptors have been isolated on RGD affinity columns and RGD-containing peptides can interfere with the binding of the β_1 and β_3 family integrins to their ligands. However, the binding of LFA-1 to the ICAMs (see below) is not RGD dependent, nor is the binding of VLA-4 to fibronectin or VCAM-1. Although the RGD sequence is obviously important in the binding of many integrins, it is not the only sequence recognized, nor does it determine the specificity of the adhesive interactions by itself, since most of the integrins are quite specific for their own substrate. Furthermore, the affinity of binding for the RGD tripeptide is generally 10–100-fold lower than to the correct matrix protein. This suggests that the integrin ligands have core binding regions, with flanking areas contributing to the affinity of the bond and determining binding specificity.

The transmembrane segments and short cytoplasmic segments of the β-chains are highly conserved. An exception is β_4 which has a very long (1000 residue) intracytoplasmic segment. Crosslinking these molecules at the cell surface leads to a reorganization of the cytoskeleton. Other evidence indicates that the β_1-chain is linked to actin via vinculin, talin and α-actinin. This implies that integrins can crosslink extracellular proteins to the intracellular cytoskeleton, an essential requirement for cell traction and migration through tissues. The presence of potential phosphorylation sites in the cytoplasmic segments suggests that the molecules may become activated before linking to the cytoskeleton.

RECEPTOR	CD/ SYNONYMS	Cytokine Inducible	STRUCTURE	LEUKOCYTE LIGANDS
ICAM-1	CD54	+	Ig SF Domain	CR-3 / LFA-1
ICAM-2	CD102	−		LFA-1
VCAM-1	CD106 INCAM-110	+		VLA-4
PECAM	CD31	−		CD31
MadCAM-1	Mucosal Addresssin	?+		VLA-4 / L-selectin

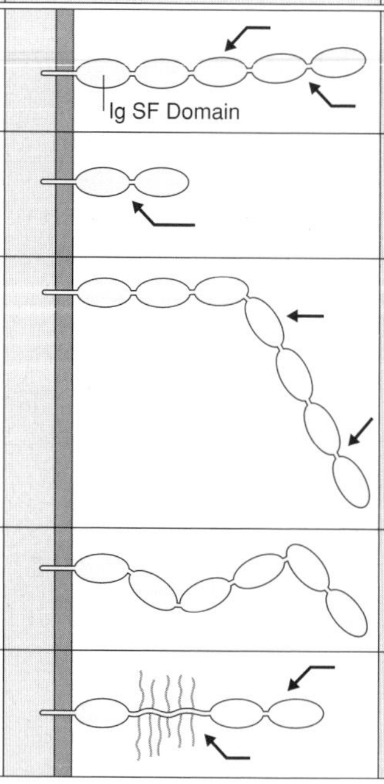

Fig. 14.4 Ig superfamily cellular adhesion molecules. The structures of five adhesion molecules which contain immunoglobulin-like domains are illustrated. Known binding sites on these molecules for the ligands listed are shown by arrows. MAdCAM-1 contains O-linked oligosacharides (dark green) which may bind L-selectin.

ICAM-1, ICAM-2, VCAM-1, MadCAM and PECAM

Several members of the immunoglobulin supergene family are expressed or induced on endothelium and act as adhesion molecules (*Fig. 14.4*). ICAM-1 (CD54) and ICAM-2 (CD102) are both receptors for LFA-1. ICAM-1 is also expressed on activated T cells, B cells and NK cells, where it contributes to the adhesion between interacting lymphocytes and between lymphocytes and APCs or target cells. ICAM-1 may be also induced on a variety of tissue cells, particularly at sites of immune reactions. ICAM-2 is present only on endothelial cells. Both of these molecules are members of the immunoglobulin supergene family, consisting of a single polypeptide chain which traverses the cell membrane. ICAM-1 has five immunoglobulin-like domains whereas ICAM-2 has only two; these are most homologous to the two N-terminal domains of ICAM-1. The binding site on ICAM-1 involves residues in both of the N-terminal domains, suggesting that LFA-1 binds at the cleft between the two domains. The ICAM-1 molecule consists of a 55kDa core polypeptide which is glycosylated to different degrees on different cell types, producing a glycoprotein of 76–114kDa. The homology between the ICAMs is about 34% and they are also related to the neural adhesion molecule, NCAM, and to myelin-associated glycoprotein (MAG), which mediates interactions involving oligodendrocytes. Unlike NCAM, ICAM-1 does not appear to undergo homophilic binding since anti-LFA-1 antibodies are capable of completely blocking ICAM-1-mediated interactions between B lymphoblasts. A third member of the ICAM family, ICAM-3, is expressed on lymphocytes but does not appear to have a role in cell migration.

The role of ICAM-1 in transendothelial migration depends on its induction by TNF, IL-1 and, to a lesser extent, IFNγ. In contrast, the role of ICAM-2 is less certain since mRNA for ICAM-2 is normally present at high levels in endothelial cells but, unlike ICAM-1, it is not induced by cytokines. For these reasons it has been proposed that ICAM-2 is normally present on endothelium and accounts for the basal levels of LFA-1-dependent, ICAM-1-independent, lymphocyte-endothelial adhesion, whereas ICAM-1 controls the enhanced movement of lymphocytes into sites of inflammation. In accord with this theory, brain endothelium, which supports very low levels of lymphocyte traffic under normal conditions, expresses only low levels of ICAM-2.

Vascular cell adhesion molecule-1, VCAM-1 (CD106), is usually a seven domain member of the Ig superfamily, although alternately spliced forms can have six or three domains. It is normally absent from endothelium but may be induced by IFNγ or TNFα *in vitro* and is seen in acute inflammatory responses *in vivo*, particularly in skin. It is confined to endothelium, although a variant form has been reported in developing skeletal muscle. The first and fourth domains of VCAM-1 contain binding sites for $\alpha_4\beta_1$ integrin, hence VCAM-1 is thought to contribute to the binding of activated lymphocytes to endothelium in acute inflammatory tissues. It has also been identified on dendritic cells, indicating a possible auxiliary role in antigen presentation.

Mucosal addressin cell adhesion molecule (MadCAM) was first identified as an adhesion molecule on HEV in lymph nodes within mucosal tissue. However, it has since also been identified at sites of inflammation, including CNS endothelium *in vivo*. The N-terminal domain has a double disulphide bond and is related to the N-terminal domains of ICAM-1 and VCAM-1. The second domain is related to the fifth domain of VCAM-1 and this is followed by a

RECEPTOR	CD/ SYNONYMS	Expressed on	STRUCTURE	LIGANDS
L-Selectin	CD62L LAM-1 MEL-14	Some Lymphocyte Monocyte Neutrophil Eosinophil	CCP Domain / EGF Domain / Lectin Domain	MadCAM-1 GlyCAM-1 CD34
E-Selectin	CD62E ELAM-1	Endothelium		Sialyl Lewis X
P-Selectin	CD62P GMP-140 PADGEM	Endothelium Platelets		Sialyl Lewis X
GlyCAM-1	SGP-50	HEV		L-selectin
CD34	CD34	Endothelium		L-selectin
PSGL-1		Neutrophil		P-selectin

Fig. 14.5 Selectins and mucin-like adhesion molecules. The table shows structures for some of the selectins and their ligands, which contain O-linked carbohydrate (dark green).

mucin-like segment containing numerous O-glycosylation sites. Interestingly, the membrane-proximal domain is related to the Cα2 domain of IgA1. This composite adhesion molecule has at least two binding regions, which allows it to interact with L-selectin, presumably via the O-linked carbohydrate (see below) and it also binds to $\alpha_4\beta_7$ integrin via the N-terminal domain(s). Differential glycosylation allows the molecule to have different relative activities on different tissues. For example, on HEV of Peyer's patches a poorly glycosylated form would bind lymphocytes expressing $\alpha_4\beta_7$, while on mucosal HEV a heavily glycosylated form would also bind lymphocytes via L-selectin. It has been proposed that a lymphocyte which expresses $\alpha_4\beta_1$ on activation has the opportunity to migrate to inflammatory tissues by attaching to endothelial VCAM-1. However, if it failed to move to an inflammatory site, switching to $\alpha_4\beta_7$ expression would allow the cell to return to a lymph node. The presence of the IgA-like domain is also intriguing. It has been hypothesized that this domain might allow interaction with Fcα receptors which are more highly expressed on gut-homing lymphocytes.

Platelet endothelial cell adhesion molecule, PECAM (CD31), is a six domain molecule found on endothelium, preferentially distributed at the lateral borders of the cells. It is also present on CD8[+] T cells and a subset of CD4[+] cells. Transfection studies suggest that it can undergo homotypic binding (cf. NCAM) and may also bind heterotypically to an unknown receptor. Crosslinking lymphocyte CD31 with specific antibody induces a transient cell activation which leads to upregulation of adhesion mediated by integrins. It is thought that homotypic interactions between lymphocyte and endothelial CD31 could activate the lymphocyte integrins, allowing them to latch onto ICAM-1, ICAM-2

and VCAM-1, if present. It is therefore debated as to whether its primary role is as an adhesion molecule or a signalling molecule.

Similar arguments apply to other surface molecules, such as LFA-3 (CD58) which is present as either a transmembrane protein or a glycosylphosphatidyl inositol (GPI)-anchored protein on endothelium and most leukocyte populations. This interacts with CD2 on T cells. Lymphocyte activation via CD2 or CD7 can enhance adhesion but this does not necessarily mean that these molecules actually contribute significantly to the binding.

The selectins

The selectins are a group of three adhesion molecules characterized by a lectin-like N-terminal domain, an epidermal growth factor (EGF) domain and a variable number of CCP domains such as those found in the complement control proteins (*Fig. 14.5*). The lectin domain recognizes terminal mannose and fucose residues present in carbohydrates or sulphated carbohydrates, in a Ca^{2+}-dependent interaction.

L-selectin(CD62L) first appears on lymphocytes late during thymocyte differentiation. It is involved in the migration of virgin T cells across HEV into peripheral lymph nodes, by interacting with heavily sialylated receptors, glyCAMs, expressed on the HEV. After transitting across HEV, L-selectin is shed from lymphocytes. A higher molecular weight form produced by differential glycosylation is present on neutrophils and contributes to their initial slowing and rolling on endothelium (see below).

P-selectin (CD62P) is a granule membrane protein present in platelets and neutrophils and in the Weibel–Palade bodies of endothelium. It rapidly redistributes as a result of granule fusion with the plasma membrane, following cell activation and is cleared quickly from the surface of endothelium. Its rapid appearance and its distribution suggest that it is involved in the haemostatic events accompanying platelet activation. But it could also contribute towards the initial slowing and rolling of neutrophils in the earliest phases of an acute inflammatory reaction.

E-selectin (CD62E) is also inducible on endothelium following TNF or IL-1 activation but, unlike P-selectin, it is synthesized *de novo* over 1–4 hours following activation. Expression of E-selectin causes a rapid increase in neutrophil binding to the endothelium. The principal ligand is the sialyl Lewis X blood group carbohydrate which is associated with the CD15 molecule, present on monocytes, macrophages and granulocytes. Since a large proportion of E-selectin is GPI-anchored, the function of the molecule appears primarily to be in slowing phagocytes, prior to the interactions of integrins and CAMs which are linked to the cytoskeleton on either cell. The early appearance of E-selectin partly explains why neutrophils are one of the first cell types to appear at inflammatory sites.

In addition to CD18 deficiency which causes the LAD syndrome and reduced phagocyte migration, a second LAD syndrome has been identified (LAD-2) in which glycosylation of molecules including CD15 is deficient. Clinically, this produces a similar pathology.

Carbohydrate-containing adhesion molecules

One principal ligand for the selectins are the carbohydrate Lewis X or Lewis A blood group determinants, present on CD15 and other cell surface molecules. Sialyl Lewis X (sLe^X) is also expressed on the leukocyte integrins and on CD66. In addition, two heavily glycosylated ligands for L-selectin of 50 and 90kDa have been identified on HEV. The 50kDa molecule is better characterized and has been designated glyCAM-1 (*Fig. 14.5*). This occurs as a dimer containing numerous sulphated O-linked carbohydrate groups and which is weakly linked to the cell membrane, probably via another molecule. GlyCAM-1 is thought to act as a scaffold for different carbohydrates in different tissues. For example, on HEV it acts as a receptor for L-selectin but it is also expressed in a non-sulphated form in mammary gland. Removal of the afferent lymphatic flow to a lymph node leads to loss of glyCAM-1. The 90kDa glycoprotein is also a receptor for L-selectin, since it was isolated by affinity chromatography, using the lectin domain of L-selectin but it is only partially characterized at present.

The molecule CD34, originally identified as a stem cell marker, is also heavily O-glycosylated and could act as an alternative ligand for L-selectin. The distribution of CD34 on endothelium is unusual. For example, it is normally present on endothelium in the CNS but is lost when immune reactions develop. Loss of an adhesion molecule might reflect a change in the signals presented to passing leukocytes, resulting in migration of a different phenotype of cell. Alternatively, loss of an adhesion molecule on the endothelium might free the leukocyte receptors to interact with a new set of adhesion molecules on the endothelium.

The molecule CD44 is present on most lymphocytes and it reacts with several cell surface and matrix components including fibronectin collagen and hyaluronate. At one time, it was thought to act as a homing receptor for HEV in lymph nodes. More recent data on glyCAM-1, MadCAM, sLe^X and their ligands have made this hypothesis untenable. Nevertheless, CD44 may still contribute to the interactions of leukocytes with matrix components in lymphoid and other tissues.

Soluble adhesion molecules

Naturally occurring soluble forms of all the selectins have been identified. It is uncertain, whether this is a physiological mechanism of controlling leukocyte adhesion (blocking *bona fide* adhesion molecules), or whether it is a side effect of rapid shedding of surface adhesion molecules — a way of quickly downregulating potential adhesion. These are not mutually exclusive.

L-selectin is shed following lymphocyte activation, or following transit across HEV. It is also released rapidly from neutrophils following stimulation with *N*-formyl-methionyl-leucyl-phenylalanine (fMLP), IL-8 or LPS. The normal physiological concentrations are just below that which could interfere significantly with lymphocyte migration. However, in HIV infection, levels may increase five-fold — sufficient to block completely L-selectin-mediated binding of lymphocytes to HEV. Soluble E-selectin is also found in blood and is taken to be a marker of inflammatory disease. The levels, however, are generally too low to interfere with binding of E-selectin to its ligands. In contrast to the other soluble selectins, soluble P-selectin is an alternately spliced variant of P-selectin, lacking the transmembrane and intracytoplasmic segment. The mechanism argues that soluble P-selectin has a genuine regulatory role. Soluble ICAM-1 and VCAM-1 have also been reported, although their significance, if any, is not known.

Control of expression and function

The interaction between leukocytes and endothelium depends on both cell types, each of which is subject to various controls. The primary control, noted above, is the expression of different sets of adhesion molecules on endothelium in different tissues and on different leukocyte populations. In addition, the activity of the adhesion molecules at any particular site can be modulated in at least three different ways.

- The level of expression of molecules at the cell surface depends on the state of activation of the endothelium or the leukocytes.
- The functional avidity of the surface molecules *in toto* can vary. For example, only a small proportion of the available molecules may be functionally active.
- The affinity of an individual adhesion molecule for its receptor can be modulated over short time-scales.

Rapid modulation of surface expression of adhesion molecules can occur when the molecules are stored in granules. This is true of P-selectin which is stored in the a-granules of platelets and the Weibel–Palade bodies of endothelium. Likewise, CR3, L-selectin and LFA-1 are

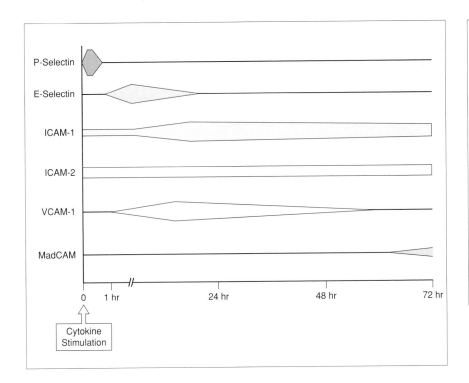

Fig. 14.6 Induction of adhesion molecules on endothelium. The time of expression of adhesion molecules on endothelium is shown diagrammatically. This is based primarily on studies *in vitro*. Note that P-selectin and E-selectin are rapidly upregulated by TNF. VCAM-1 and ICAM-1 are induced by TNF and IFNγ (rat). ICAM-1 is present at low levels and is upregulated while VCAM-1 is absent, induces faster and decays faster (CNS endothelium). ICAM-2 is not inducible. The possibility that MadCAM can be induced late in inflammatory reactions is inferred from studies *in vivo*.

held in neutrophil granules which may be quickly mobilized to the cell surface following activation. More often, however, new adhesion molecules including ICAM-1, VCAM-1 and E-selectin are synthesized over a period of hours or days, frequently in response to cytokine activation of endothelium, or specific stimulation of leukocytes. However, these two ways of upregulating expression are not mutually exclusive. For example, histamine and leukotriene C4 trigger a rapid, transient expression of P-selectin on endothelium, while IL-1, TNF and LPS produce a slower, but more sustained, increase.

The role of cytokines

Inflammatory cytokines, including TNF and IL-1, can induce adhesion molecules on endothelium in many tissues. This is important, since many cell types in the body can produce these cytokines. Therefore local cells are able to initiate leukocyte infiltration at sites of damage or pathogen invasion. These cytokines induce synthesis of ICAM-1, VCAM-1 and E-selectin on endothelium *in vitro*. ICAM-1 and VCAM-1 are induced over a time-span of hours to days, whereas E-selectin appears within hours and is lost by 24 hours after stimulation (*Fig. 14.6*). The 5′ controlling regions of the genes for these molecules contain NF-κB binding sites which become occupied following cytokine stimulation. With E-selectin, it has been shown that NF-κB is necessary but not sufficient for transcription; there are clearly other transcription factors involved including those binding to tissue-specific sites within the promoters.

Once an immune response has been initiated in the tissues, other cytokines come into play. IFNγ and IL-4 can both induce VCAM-1 and IFNγ induces ICAM-1 with an identical time course to TNF. As expected, the genes have associated interferon response elements (IREs).

T cell populations and activation

The state of lymphocyte differentiation and activation plays a critical role in determining the different patterns of cell traffic *in vivo*, noted above. Many studies have examined which adhesion molecules are expressed on different lymphocyte populations. For example, CD8+ T cells express higher levels of LFA-1 than CD4+ T cells. CD31 is expressed on all CD8+ T cells in man but only on a proportion of CD4+ T cells. In accordance with the observation that activated T cells tend to localize more effectively at sites of inflammation *in vivo*, it has been found that antigen or mitogen activation of CD4+ T cells causes them to bind more strongly to endothelium *in vitro*. If this is followed by IL-2 stimulation, then the ability to migrate is also enhanced and is accompanied by increased expression of LFA-1 and VLA-4 for several days post stimulation. Activated mouse lymphocytes also show a decreased ability to bind to lymph node HEVs associated with loss of L-selectin.

By examining cells which cross endothelium *in vitro*, it is possible to identify the phenotypes of migratory cells. In general, these cells are CD45R0+, CD45RA−, CD29+, (i.e. memory phenotype), with VLA-2, VLA-4 and LFA-1 more strongly expressed while L-selectin is lost. In these studies, activation of the endothelium with cytokines increased the numbers of migrating cells but did not select for lymphocytes of a different phenotype. However, this conclusion may apply only to the endothelial cells used (umbilical vein) in the particular set of experiments, since adhesion molecules on cells from other vascular beds vary greatly. The presence of any particular adhesion molecules on the migrating cells does not imply that these molecules are all necessarily required for crossing a particular endothelium. The phenotype of

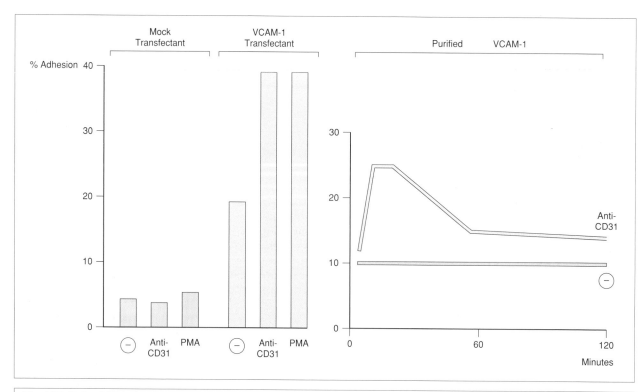

Fig. 14.7 Role of CD31 in triggering lymphocyte adhesion.
Left graph: CD8[+] T cells were bound to mock transfected L cells, or L cells transfected with VCAM-1, in the presence of anti-CD31, phorbol ester (PMA, positive control) or a negative control (-). Binding to the VCAM-1 transfectant is higher than to normal L cells, but triggering with anti-CD31 or PMA (which activates PKC) enhances adhesion considerably. Right graph: Time course of anti-CD31 triggering of the CD8[+] lymphocytes shows that the effect of crosslinking surface CD31 peaks at 10 minutes, suggesting that triggering of lymphocytes by anti-CD31 activates PKC to enhance VLA-4-mediated binding to VCAM-1. Based on data of Tanaka *et al*, 1992.

the lymphocyte may be permissive for migration into several different tissues, depending on the signals it receives from the local endothelium.

Modulation of receptor affinity

The individual affinity of many adhesion molecules can also be rapidly modulated during the process of migration, in contrast to the long term changes described above. Integrins provide the best studied example and will be discussed here.

It has been known for a long time that activation of monocytes and neutrophils with phorbol esters enhances the affinity of CR3. It is now clear that several stimuli which activate lymphocytes or phagocytes can upregulate the affinity of leukocyte integrins, as shown in anti-CD31 upregulation of VCAM-1-mediated adhesion (*Fig. 14.7*). T cells can be stimulated by antibodies to CD31, CD7 or crosslinking of CD2 and CD3. Neutrophils may be stimulated by adherence to fibronectin, as well as by fMLP, C5a and other chemotactic cytokines. All these events induce activation of protein kinase C and the kinetics of upregulation of adhesion by these mediators imply that PKC activation is involved in the short term control of adhesion. The effective affinity of LFA-1 may increase 100-fold following activation.

It has been debated how such cellular activation alters integrin affinity. One explanation is that cellular activation causes the receptors to associate with cytoskeleton and reorganize into high avidity patches on the cell membrane. Electron micrographs of leukocytes interacting with endothelium during migration does indeed show spot contacts between the cells (*Fig. 14.8*). However, surface reorganization of adhesion molecules offers only a partial explanation for affinity changes. Evidence now implies that the majority of integrins on circulating cells are in a non-functional, low affinity form which may be switched to high affinity forms following activation. The high affinity forms of some integrins can be distinguished by specific antibodies, implying that conformational changes occur in the extracellular domains. With the integrins this may relate to Ca^{2+} or Mg^{2+} binding, which alters affinity as noted above. However, it is difficult to see how changes within a cell could affect the conformation of an extracellular molecule, unless it is by causing the adhesion molecule to associate with, or dissociate from, other cell surface molecules which modulate its affinity.

In practice, activation signals may affect both receptor density and avidity. For example, fMLP stimulation of neutrophils causes mobilization of specific granules to the cell surface. These contain a number of integrins, including CR3, but the stimulus also causes an upregulation of receptor affinity. In the next step of the process, where integrins interact with CAMs on the endothelium, engagement of the receptors may lock them into a high affinity conformation, allowing an extended period of cellular interaction.

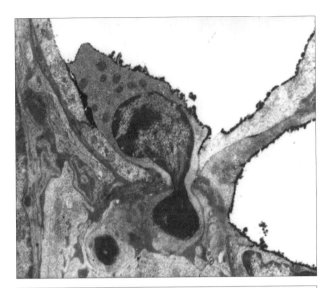

Fig. 14.8 Lymphocyte migration across CNS endothelium. The electron micrograph shows lymphocytes migrating across retinal endothelium *in vivo*. Note the localized point attachments between the endothelial cells and the lymphocytes, which persist until migration is complete. Courtesy of Dr John Greenwood and Dr Peter Munro.

MODELS OF LEUKOCYTE MIGRATION

At the cellular level, leukocyte migration is now seen as a multi-step process which requires several sets of adhesion molecules on the leukocyte to interact in sequence with corresponding receptors on the endothelium (*Fig. 14.9*).

The first step in the process is slowing and rolling of leukocytes on venular endothelium. In the venules, the haemodynamic shear force acting on the leukocytes is lowest, the negative charge on the endothelium is reduced and adhesion molecules are selectively expressed. The initial slowing is primarily mediated by the carbohydrate–lectin interactions. L-selectin on lymphocytes interacts with O-linked carbohydrates on MadCAM-1 or glyCAM-1 as cells pass through lymph node or Peyer's patch HEV. Elsewhere, interactions between L-selectin and other glycosylated molecules (e.g. CD34) contribute to the slowing. Alternatively or additionally, E-selectin induced locally on the endothelium can interact with CD15 expressed constitutively on leukocytes. Since a leukocyte normally spends only seconds passing through a venule, this initial tethering must be rapid — selectins have high association and dissociation constants and can bind their ligands within milliseconds. The tethering and rolling is essential to allow the next step to occur.

The second step involves a rapid activation of integrins on the leukocyte, induced by interaction with the endothelium. This step will occur only if suitable stimulators are present. It is debatable whether these signals are delivered by chemotactic molecules, held on the endothelial surface (see below), or whether it is direct signalling by integral surface molecules of the endothelium. Both chemotactic agents (e.g. MCP-1) and surface molecules (e.g. CD31) can induce the activation. The mechanisms may both contribute, or could be used in different circumstances to signal activation of cell types with different receptors.

The third step involves the engagement of the integrins on leukocytes with their receptors on endothelium or on the extracellular matrix. At this stage, the interacting cells are linked via molecules attached to the cytoskeleton on either side and this allows traction associated with migration. Migration itself is an active process, dependent on both cell types. Interference with G-proteins or metabolic activity of either cell blocks migration. It is not certain whether there is an additional signal which induces migration or whether the signals in step two, coupled with latching of the adhesion molecules, are sufficient. At this stage, additional adhesion molecules may also be used. For example, one study using confocal microscopy suggests that CD44 is expressed at the leading edge of the neutrophil pseudopod as it probes the basement membrane.

Once cells have migrated across the endothelium, they release enzymes which digest components of the basement membrane and allow them to move into the tissues. Endoglycosidases are synthesized by lymphocytes after antigen-specific activation and are stored in granules. Other matrix-degrading enzymes are membrane-associated. Once cells have entered the tissues, they continue to use β_1 integrins for interaction with and movement along extracellular matrix components. It is thought that collagen and laminin receptors are particularly important at this stage, although this process is less well understood than events occurring during the initial migration. At this stage the cells also move directionally in response to chemotactic agents.

Chemotactic molecules and their receptors

Chemotactic molecules are generated at sites of inflammation and diffuse towards the local capillaries; in general they are short-range signalling molecules which are relatively labile (*Fig. 14.10*). The actions of chemotactic molecules are readily measured *in vitro* and directional movement of cells occurs *in vivo* but it has been debated to what extent concentration gradients of chemotactic molecules could become established physiologically. Currently, it is thought that chemotactic molecules may act in two ways: either as an activator held on the endothelium (step two above) or in a gradient around an inflammatory site. Chemotactic molecules such as C5a also have many other functions in the inflammatory response.

A large number of molecules are chemotactic for leukocytes. Some, such as fibronectin or peptides of fibrin and thrombin, can act independently of any immunological processes. Of primary interest to immunologists are those generated by lymphocytes and macrophages, by the pathogens themselves or by the interactions of antibody and complement. These include the classical chemotactic agents, C5a, fMLP and leukotriene B4 (LTB4), as well as the recently described large family of chemokines (also called intercrines) which are related to IL-8. All of these molecules (except for LTB4) act via receptors linked to G-proteins. They are a subset of the rhodopsin superfamily of receptors, characterized by their seven transmembrane segments.

C5a, generated by the action of the complement pathways or by tissue hydrolases and bacterial enzymes, is

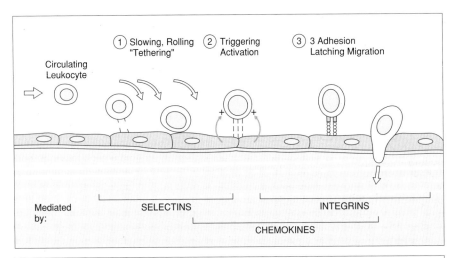

Fig. 14.9 Three step model of transendothelial migration. Circulating leukocytes are slowed in the venules by binding to endothelium, mediated primarily by selectins. They roll along the endothelium and may be brought to a halt (pavementing). They may now respond to triggering signals on the endothelium (chemokines, CD31, etc.). This upregulates integrin affinity, allowing the cells to latch onto cellular adhesion molecules (VCAM-1, ICAM-1, etc.) expressed on the endothelium and start their migratory programme. The precise combination of integrins, selectins, etc. will depend on the cell type and the vascular bed. See Springer (1994) for an elaboration of this model.

chemotactic for neutrophils and macrophages at concentrations of 1nM. Normally, C5a is rapidly inactivated by serum carboxypeptidases, producing C5a-des-Arg which is much less active. Human neutrophils have 100 000–200 000 C5a receptors (51kDa) per cell, while the numbers on macrophages vary greatly, with four to five-fold fewer receptors on inflammatory macrophages. This means that the sensitivity of an activated macrophage for the C5a chemotactic stimulus is reduced. Eosinophils apparently have two subtypes of the receptor, a high and a low affinity form, although only one gene has been identified. A model for C5a receptor binding proposes that a basic domain on C5a docks to an acidic domain at the N-terminus of the C5a receptor. This causes rearrangement of a different domain of C5a which interacts with a newly exposed site on the receptor. This causes dissociation of the $\beta_1\gamma_2$ subunit of the G-protein which then activates phospholipase C, generating IP_3 and diacylglycerol (DAG) which mobilize intracellular calcium and activate protein kinase C (PKC), respectively.

Macrophages, monocytes and neutrophils also recognize and are attracted by low concentrations (1nM) of formyl-methionyl peptides, of which the most active is fMet–Leu–Phe (fMLP). Since prokaryotes initiate translation with an fMet residue while eukaryotes do not, these peptides provide a specific signal marking the presence of invading bacteria. For different cell preparations the number of receptors ranges from 10 000–100 000 per cell. The fMLP receptor (FPR1) is 34% homologous to the C5a receptor. There is also at least one variant lower affinity form of the receptor (FPRLR). The receptor is coupled to the G-protein pathways as for C5aR and these two chemotactic agents cause cross-desensitization. This may permit

a cell to retain its appreciation of the polarity of chemotactic stimuli as it moves up a chemotactic gradient.

Monocytes, neutrophils and eosinophils have receptors for the chemotactic eicosanoids, LTB4 and 5-HETE. LTB4 is chemotactic and chemokinetic and its activities are enhanced in the presence of prostaglandin E2 (PGE2) and TNF, although these mediators do not have chemotactic activity themselves. The activity of LTB4 was first noted in eosinophil chemotactic factor of anaphylaxis (ECF-A) but the major source of LTB4 in most inflammatory reactions is probably macrophages. Thus, the first cells to enter an inflammatory site can release molecules which induce further immigration. The receptor for LTB4 has not yet been characterized.

A large number of other polypeptides have chemotactic activity and for many this is their only known action. For example, fibrin degradation products are chemotactic for neutrophils but unlike C5a, fMLP and LTB4 they do not cause cellular activation. Also in this category are substance P and TGFβ. These mediators activate G-proteins and can be chemotactic but they do not mobilize Ca^{2+} nor induce cell activation.

In the late 1980s molecular biological techniques led to the identification of a family of molecules related to platelet activating factor-4 and IL-8. This family consists of at least 18 different small proteins (8–10kDa), referred to as chemokines. They belong to two families. In the human, the 'CxC' group (α family) are located on chromosome 4 and the 'CC' group (β family) on chromosome 17. These designations refer to characteristic arrangements of the first two cysteine residues. Like C5aR, the receptors for these proteins belong to the rhodopsin family. The chemokines are basic heparin-binding cytokines with a range of functions. Only those clearly involved in immunity and inflammation

Fig. 14.10 Chemokines and chemotactic factors. The table lists those chemokines with clear relevance to immune function. The listing of target cells is based on functional or binding assays. For further details see Murphy, 1994.

FACTOR	CHARACTERISTICS	RECEPTOR	Action On NEUTROPHIL	EOSINOPHIL	BASOPHIL	MONOCYTE/MØ	T CELL
C5a	77 Amino Acid Peptide of C5 α chain	C5aR	■	■		■	
fMLP	Tripeptide with blocked N-terminus	FPR1 (Hi Aff) FPRL1 (Lo Aff)	■	■		■	
LTB4	Eicosanoid	?	■	■		■	
IP-10	α Chemokine	?				■	■
Platelet factor 4	α Chemokine	?				■	
GROα, GROβ, GROγ	α Chemokines	IL-8RB	■				
IL-8	α Chemokine	IL-8RA IL-8RB	■		■		■
MCP-1	β Chemokine	MCP-IR			■	■	■
MIP-1α	β Chemokine	MIP-Iα / RANTES. R	■				◪
MIP-1β	β Chemokine	?					◪
RANTES	β Chemokine	MIP-1α/ RANTES. R			■		◪

will be described here. Their principle actions are in chemotaxis and activation of myeloid and lymphoid cells.

The prototype for this group is IL-8 which is rapidly induced by IL-1 or TNF in a wide variety of cells, including monocytes, macrophages, T cells and endothelium. The IL-8 gene is preceded by typical cytokine-inducible elements, including an NF-κB-site, AP-1 and an interferon-response segment. IL-8 is chemotactic for neutrophils which express up to 20 000 receptors but it also acts on a population of T cells — about 10% (both CD4 and CD8) which have a much lower receptor density. Although IL-8 is chemotactic for both neutrophils and lymphocytes, it only activates other functions in the myeloid cells. Structurally, IL-8 is strikingly similar to the peptide-binding N-terminal domains of MHC molecules and it is presumed that the other chemokines have similar structures. Receptor binding leads to rises in intracellular Ca^{2+}, PKC activation and mobilization of cytoskeletal components. It also induces rapid receptor downregulation. Other members of the α family are GRO (3 proteins) and IP-10 (Interferon-inducible protein-10). These chemokines and several others all act via the two receptors for IL-8, namely IL-8RA and IL-8RB.

The β family includes macrophage inflammatory protein-1α (MIP-1α), MIP-1β and RANTES which act on the MIP-1α/RANTES receptor and Membrane cofactor-1 (MCP-1) which acts on another receptor. The details of these chemokines are given in *Figure 14.10*. What is less clear is the advantage conferred by having numerous different but closely related cytokines. A clue has emerged from studies of the subpopulations of lymphocytes which are selectively attracted by different members of the group. For example, MIP-1α promotes accumulation of CD4+ T cells, while MIP-1β favours CD8+ cells. In addition, some chemokines are chemotactic, while others activate. For example, RANTES and MCP-1 both target basophils but RANTES induces chemotaxis, while MCP-1 induces primarily histamine release. Binding studies have localized some of the chemokines to endothelium *in vivo* and the fact that the chemokines bind heparin argues that they act as flags attached to heparin groups on the endothelium and basement membranes. These observations have been assimilated into the three step model for leukocyte migration across endothelium. In this scheme, a tethered leukocyte has the opportunity to 'taste' the chemotactic molecules expressed on the endothelium and will be induced to migrate only if these are of the right type. In the later stages, the chemokines may act as directional guidance molecules for chemotactic movement and can activate cells prior to their arrival at an inflammatory site.

Chemotaxis and cellular migration

The processes by which chemotactic molecules induce directional migration are poorly understood. Leukocytes are extremely sensitive to variations in the concentrations of chemotactic factors along their length which may vary by as little as 0.1% and still induce directional migration.

In the microenvironment of the cell, the effective gradient may be steeper, as chemotactic receptors at the leading edge take up the chemotactic agent, thus preventing it from diffusing further. Following exposure to low levels of chemotactic agents, the cells polarize and send out pseudopodia. Optimal but uniform concentrations of chemotactic agents cause monocytes to polarize and induce directional movement in a randomly chosen direction but cells treated with high uniform concentrations of chemotactic agents lose their directional migration and move at random.

One mechanistic model for leukocyte migration proposes that G-actin polymerizes to filamentous F-actin at the leading pseudopod which is then swept backwards towards the telopod. This accords with observations that F-actin moves towards the back of the cell, as do CR3 and other receptors. Neutrophil chemotaxis is blockable with anti-CR3, suggesting an essential role for this adhesion molecule in migration. Most of the neutrophil CR3 is located in granules which are directed forwards to the front of the cell to fuse with the leading edge of the cell and allowing CR3 and other receptors to attach to extracellular matrix components. These receptors are then passed backwards, to be endocytosed again at the trailing edge (*Fig. 14.11*). Remodelling of plasma membrane phospholipids accompanies chemotaxis. There is some evidence that the granule-associated CR3 and that expressed on the plasma membrane are conformationally different, since they can be distinguished by antibodies. During chemotactic migration, the concentration of the chemotactic molecule must increase progressively, every few minutes, otherwise the cell detaches from the substratum. This may be related to the progressive loss of receptors for chemotactic stimuli following phagocyte activation.

The next question is how cellular activation by chemotactic agents is coupled to the molecular machinery for locomotion. Exposure of neutrophils to chemotactic stimuli results in rapid membrane depolarization, associated with an increase in intracellular Ca^{2+} and cAMP. However, rises in Ca^{2+} alone cannot account for the engagement of the cytoskeleton. Recently, a new protein (MARCKS) was described which appears to play a central role in this process. This protein is a filamentous actin-crosslinking molecule which is a substrate for PKC and binds to calmodulin. Phosphorylation causes it to be redistributed from the plasma membrane to the cytoplasm. It has been suggested that this molecule acts as a regulated cross-bridge between actin and the plasma membrane.

Another component of the process is the enzymes released by migrating cells. Chemotactic agents stimulate secretion of elastase, collagenase and cathepsins which are released soon after triggering by chemotactic stimuli. These are thought to be needed for crossing the basement membrane and for movement within tissues.

CONTROL OF BLOOD FLOW AND VASCULAR PERMEABILITY

Inflammatory reactions are a response to infection or tissue damage and often occur quite independently of the immune system, following physical injuries. The plasma enzyme

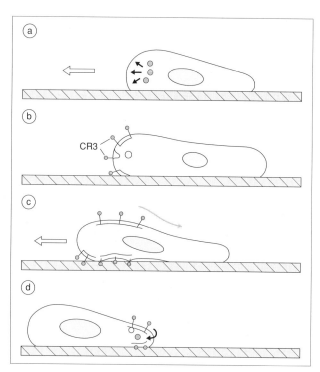

Fig. 14.11 Steps in chemotactic migration. a) A macrophage stimulated by a chemotactic agent such as fMLP, becomes polarized and moves granules towards the leading pseudopod. **b)** Granule contents are expressed and released to the plasma membrane. CR3 and LFA-1 are particularly important in this function. **c)** The adhesion molecules engage the cytoskeleton and are swept towards the trailing uropod, moving the cell forward. **d)** Adhesion molecules are endocytosed again at the trailing pseudopod to be recycled. In practice this process occurs as a continuous conveyor belt — only one set of molecules is shown here.

kinin, clotting and plasmin systems, as well as mast cells, may all be activated in inflammation, and in association with the autonomic nervous system, produce the characteristic inflammatory response. When antigenic stimuli are present, the immune system also recruits these effector systems, either directly or via the action of the complement system.

There are three principal components of an inflammatory reaction:

- Increased blood flow to the affected area.
- A concomitant increase in capillary permeability in the local vasculature.
- Increased migration of cells from the blood vessels into the affected area.

The processes controlling migration of inflammatory cells have been discussed above but the other two elements are equally important. The increase in blood flow delivers more leukocytes and serum molecules to the inflamed tissue and the increase in vascular permeability leads to exudation of the larger serum molecules — antibodies, complement, etc. — which are needed to target the effector cells. Blood flow

Mediator	Sources	Activators	Principal effects
Bradykinin	high molecular weight kininogen	factor XIIa/ kallikrein other proteases	vasodilation ↑ vascular permeability pain
Histamine	mast cell and basophil granules	IgE and antigen anaphylatoxins	vasodilation ↑ vascular permeability spasmogen chemokinesis
C3a and C5a	complement system	C3 and C5 convertases other proteases	spasmogens mast cell degranulation C5a-chemotaxis ↑ vascular permeability
PAF	basophils neutrophils macrophages	depends on cell type	platelet factor release spasmogen neutrophil activation ↑ vascular permeability
Eicosanoids (see below)	macrophages monocytes endothelial cells mast cells basophils etc.	many inducers	modulate effects of other mediators vasoactive
PGE2	cyclooxygenase pathway	many inducers	vasodilation potentiates effects of histamine, bradykinin, C5a and LTB4
PGI2	cyclooxygenase pathway	many inducers	vasodilation blocks platelet aggregation and bronchoconstriction
TxA2	cyclooxygenase pathway	many inducers	vasoconstriction platelet aggregation bronchoconstriction
LTB4	lipoxygenase pathway	many inducers	neutrophil and macrophage chemotaxis modulates increase in vascular permeability
LTD4	lipoxygenase pathway	many inducers	spasmogen ↑ vascular permeability LTB4 and LTD4 produce bronchospasm
IL-1, IL-6	macrophages endothelium some or other cells	macrophage activators (e.g. C5a)	pyrogen, PG production induces acute phase proteins activation of T cells
IFNγ, (MAF)	T cells	antigen	macrophage and K cell activation modulates inflammatory reactions
TNFα	macrophages some tissue cells	LPS IFNα Tissue damage	endothelial adhesion molecules induced cytotoxic effects fibrosis
Lymphotoxin	T cells	antigen	

Fig. 14.12 Mediators of inflammation. A list of the major inflammatory mediators excluding interleukins discussed in Chapter 10 with their principal sources and effects.

into an inflammatory site and leakage of molecules from the blood into the tissues and controlled by mediators derived from the plasma enzyme systems and from auxiliary cells, including mast cells, platelets and basophils (*Fig. 14.12*). In addition, mediators from macrophages and lymphocytes, particularly the leukotrienes and prostaglandins, can modulate capillary permeability. Some of the mediators act directly on smooth muscle or endothelium in the vessel wall, while those cytokines which act on leukocyte migration may enhance permeability indirectly; leukocyte migration across endothelium *per se* causes modest increases in vascular permeability.

The roles of different mediators can now be assessed directly by measuring the electrical resistance (current leakage) across endothelial monolayers *in vitro*, or blood vessels *in vivo*. CNS and retinal blood vessels which maintain the blood–brain barrier have very high resistances *in vivo* (up to 3000ohm/cm^2), dropping to less than 500ohm/cm^2 on stimulation (e.g. with histamine). Other vessels have much lower baseline resistance but are similarly sensitive to mediators.

Plasma enzyme systems

The kinin system is important in controlling both immunological and non-immunological inflammation. The principal mediators of the system are bradykinin, generated from high molecular weight kininogen (HMW kininogen), and lysyl-bradykinin (kallidin), generated from low molecular weight kininogen (LMW kininogen). Bradykinin is generated following the activation of Hageman factor (factor XII of the blood clotting system). Activated Hageman factor (factor XIIa) acts on prekallikrein which circulates in a complex with HMW kininogen, to generate the enzyme kallikrein. This enzyme produces internal cleavages in the complexed HMW kininogen to release the nonapeptide bradykinin and it also acts back on Hageman factor to generate more factor XIIa. These enzymes and proenzymes are all normally present in plasma.

In contrast, the pathway which generates lysyl-bradykinin is initiated by tissue damage causing the release of prokallikrein. This proenzyme is different from prekallikrein and it can be activated by plasmin, intracellular enzymes and plasma kallikrein to produce tissue kallikrein. This enzyme acts on LMW kininogen and to a lesser extent HMW kininogen to release lysyl-bradykinin and bradykinin. The actions of kallikrein are limited by C1-inh and α_2-macroglobulin but tissue kallikrein is much less susceptible to inhibition; it is inhibited only by $\alpha 1$-antiprotease. This and the fact that 70% of the available kininogen is the low molecular weight variety suggests that production of lysyl-bradykinin is of particular importance whenever tissue damage occurs.

Bradykinin is an exceptionally powerful vasoactive mediator, causing venular dilatation, increased vascular permeability, hypotension, smooth muscle contraction and activation of phospholipase A2 which leads to the generation of eicosanoids. Both bradykinin and lysyl-bradykinin are inactivated by plasma carboxypeptidases and hence are usually very transient mediators.

The role of the complement fragments C3a and C5a in the control of vascular permeability was summarized in Chapter 13. The significance of these mediators lies in the way in which the complement system links immunological events to the control of inflammation. The vasoactions of the anaphylatoxins is primarily due to their ability to cause mast cell degranulation with accompanying histamine release. Most of the direct effects of C5a on capillary permeability can be blocked by histamine receptor inhibitors (H1 and H2) but leukotrienes are also implicated. C5a may also have some indirect action on capillary permeability following its activating effect and chemotactic action on neutrophils and macrophages. As with the kinins, these polypeptides are deactivated by carboxypeptidases which localizes and limits their actions.

Cell-derived mediators

Mast cells are an important source of mediators, and being located close to blood vessels, they produce localized effects. They can be activated by immune reactions, both directly via sensitization with IgE and indirectly via C3a and C5a. Mast cells are also activated by tissue damage independently of immune reactions. Triggering of mast cells produces an influx of Ca^{2+} followed by a rise in intracellular cAMP. This induces granule release and activates phopholipase A2 to release arachidonic acid from membrane phospholipids. Arachidonic acid is converted into the eicosanoids — prostaglandins, leukotrienes and thromboxanes — via the cyclooxygenase and lipoxygenase pathways. Mast cell granules contain histamine, proteolytic enzymes, heparin, heparan sulphate proteoglycans and a high molecular weight neutrophil chemotactic factor (NCF). Basophils, which in many respects are similar to mast cells, also contain vasoactive amines. Platelet activating factor (PAF), which is newly synthesized after triggering, is also produced by basophils, neutrophils and monocytes. Enzymes released from the mast cell granules include tryptic enzymes, which can directly cleave C3 to produce C3a, and plasmin, which can cause the activation of prekallikrein, thereby activating the kinin system. These enzymes also contribute to the clearance of the inflammatory site to allow access for incoming cells.

Histamine and 5-hydroxytryptamine (5-HT) have a powerful effect on the local vasculature due to their action on H1 receptors. This includes smooth muscle contraction, increased blood flow and enhanced capillary permeability. However, histamine also acts on H2 receptors to produce a number of negative feedback effects. These include the suppression of lysosomal enzyme release from neutrophils, decreased histamine release from basophils and other mast cells and reduced neutrophil chemotaxis.

Platelets which are also sources of vasoactive amines, especially 5-HT, are activated following vascular damage and can be triggered by immune complexes by binding to their Fc receptors. There are two major types of platelet granule: the α granule contains proteolytic enzymes and cationic proteins as well as P-selectin; the so-called dense bodies contain 5-HT and adenosine diphosphate (ADP). Alterations in vascular permeability caused by 5-HT can promote the deposition of immune complexes on the endothelium; this may occur in immune complex disease. It is notable that treatment of animals with methysergide which blocks 5-HT formation, ameliorates the immune complex disease which develops spontaneously in NZB/W mice. ADP, on the other hand, contributes to inflammatory responses by promoting platelet aggregation.

Eicosanoids

Prostaglandins (PGs) and leukotrienes (LTs) are produced by many of the effector cells involved in an immune response, with endothelium, mast cells, basophils and macrophages being the most important sources. Arachidonic acid is the initial substrate for all these products and is released from membrane phopholipids by the action of phospholipase A, or indirectly by the sequential activation of phospholipase C. Arachidonic acid may be converted by cyclooxygenase into the unstable endoperoxides PGG2 and PGH2 which are the precursors of the prostaglandins and thromboxanes. Alternatively, the enzyme 5-lipoxygenase generates LTA4 which is the precursor of the leukotrienes (*Fig. 14.13*).

PGE2 is detectable in inflammatory exudates, with a maximum accumulation time at 6–24 hours after the early mediators, histamine and bradykinin. PGE2 enhances the chemotactic activities and vasoactive properties of other mediators including LTB4, C5a, histamine and kinins, although it has little such effect by itself. PGE2 alone causes pyrexia and increased blood flow. Understanding the role of prostaglandins in immune reactions is complicated by the fact that PGE1 suppresses lymphocyte activation and reduces the sensitivity of neutrophils for C5a. This suggests that prostaglandins are co-mediators which modulate the developing reactions, where the precise effect depends on the blend of prostaglandins produced.

Leukotrienes C4 and D4 also affect the vasculature. Generally speaking, they directly cause an increase in vascular permeability, while the effect on blood flow varies for different species and mediator levels. LTC4 and LTD4 are important mediators of the late response in allergic asthma, producing smooth muscle contraction and bronchospasm. Leukotrienes have been shown to inhibit lymphocyte activation and proliferation *in vitro*; they may contribute to the loss of proliferative activity at inflammatory sites *in vivo*, as lymphocytes develop their effector functions. The numerous local effects of the eicosanoids indicate that they play an important role in modulating and directing inflammatory responses.

PHAGOCYTES

Phagocytic cells, including neutrophils and macrophages, are important effector cells in acute inflammatory sites; in chronic inflammation the proportion of lymphocytes and macrophages is greater. Macrophage and polymorph effector functions depend on a number of different cellular activities which may be viewed under three headings:

- The expression of cell surface proteins.
- The intracellular activity, including that of the cytoskeleton and mitochondria and the levels of intracellular enzymes.
- The secretory capacity of the cell. More than 30 different macrophage surface receptors and over 75 different secretory proteins have been identified. These are not coordinately regulated and individual effector functions are a composite of numerous activities (*Fig. 14.14*).

Cellular activation

Macrophages develop by a series of stages during which they acquire additional receptors, metabolic functions and enhanced microbicidal and cytotoxic capacities. This process is called macrophage activation. However, it is clearly a multi-step process, in which the phagocyte responds to different activation stimuli as it progresses from the blood vessel to the inflammatory site and after it has endocytosed material. A developmental scheme, based on surface markers and functions, has been proposed in which blood monocytes can enter tissues to become either

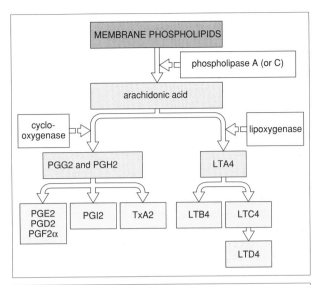

Fig. 14.13 The eicosanoids. The eicosanoids are generated from arachidonic acid which is released from membrane phospholipids, either directly by phospholipase A or indirectly by phospholipase C. Arachidonic acid may then be metabolized, either by the cyclooxygenase pathway to yield the prostaglandins and thromboxanes or via the lipoxygenase pathway to yield the leukotrienes. The most active mediators are shaded green. Some of the molecules induce inflammatory reactions, while others inhibit them. On balance the eicosanoids modulate inflammation by potentiating the effects of other mediators. Steroids exert part of their anti-inflammatory effect by inhibiting the generation of arachidonic acid, while salicylate and indomethacin inhibit the cyclooxygenase pathway.

resident tissue macrophages or immature macrophages responsive to chemotactic stimuli. The responsive cells react to inflammatory mediators and are attracted to sites of tissue damage. Inflammatory macrophages are larger than tissue macrophages and express CR3. They have increased responses to chemotactic agents, increased phagocytic abilities and higher levels of some granule enzymes and greater secretory capacities.

As mentioned above, C5a and some chemokines held on the endothelium activate migrating neutrophils and macrophages. Cytokines, particularly TNFα, released in the tissues are also an important signal to incoming cells. In particular these signals modulate expression of surface receptors and prime a cell for phagocytosis. Binding of immune complexes to Fc and C3 receptors or stimulation by bacterial products such as LPS and by cytokines, particularly IFNγ, enhance the ability of the macrophage to destroy the material it has endocytosed and may also enhance its ability to present antigen to CD4[+] T cells.

Phagocytosis

Phagocytic cells include the eosinophil and neutrophil polymorphs, in addition to the fixed and mobile cells of the mononuclear phagocyte lineage. The mechanisms of phagocytosis appear to be similar for neutrophils and mononuclear

Characteristics	Particular* regulatory stimulus	Activation stage			Effects
		immature macrophage	primed macropage	activated macrophage	
Fc receptors	interferons	+	+ +	+ +	increased phagocytosis and ADCC
C3 receptors CR1, CR3	chemotactic factors & T cell lymphokines	+	+	+ ↑	increased phagocytosis and ADCC
Mannose–Fucose receptor	MAF	+ +	+	+	decreased phagocytosis of carbohydrate-containing particles
C5a receptors	C5a	+ +	+	+	decreased sensitivity to chemotactic stimuli
f-Met-receptor		+	+	+	
LTB4	(receptor not sufficiently well-characterized for analysis)				
MHC class II	IFNγ	±	+ +	+ + +	antigen presentation to T cells
Lysosomal hydrolases	phagocytosis & lymphokines	+	+ + +	+ + +	increased microbicidal and cytotoxic ability
Secretory neutral proteases		+	+ +	+ + +	breakdown of inflammatory debris
Lysozyme	constitutive	+ +	+ +	+ +	enzymolysis of bacterial cell walls
Tumour Necrosis Factor	IFNγ & LPS	−	−	+ +	cytotoxic for tumour cells leukocyte endothelial adhesion etc.
Eicosanoids		+	+ +	+	regulate inflammatory reactions
Reactive Oxygen Intermediates (ROIs)	IFNγ, some protein antigens	−	+	+	cytotoxic and antimicrobial activities
Complement		+	+	+ +	local supplement to complement levels
IL-1, IL-6	many antigens	+ or −	+ or −	+ or −	activates T cells pyrogen induces acute phase proteins

* many inflammatory stimuli increase the various characteristics — only particularly active stimuli are noted
↑ increased activity

Fig. 14.14 Characteristic activities of macrophages.
Macrophages have a very large number of functions which summate to produce their overall activity. Many inflammatory mediators increase the activity of the various functions, but only particularly active stimuli are noted. An increase in the activity of surface receptors may be due to an increase in overall number, as occurs with the Fc receptors or be due to modulation of affinity (e.g. CR3).

phagocytes which degrade the material they have endocytosed. Neutrophils are normally viewed as terminally differentiated cells, whose function is to destroy the material which they have phagocytosed. Nevertheless, even neutrophils have some small capacity for cytokine production. By contrast, the transport and processing of antigen and its presentation is an important consequential action of phagocytosis by the longer lived macrophages. Uptake of material for all these cell types is facilitated by opsonization.

All opsonins apparently act by immobilizing the particle on the surface of the phagocyte. Macrophages can recognize particles non-specifically via surface carbohydrate receptors and specifically by their Fc receptors. There are three Fcγ receptors on human macrophages designated FcγRI–FcγRIII (CD64, CD32 and CD16). The low affinity FcγRIII receptor may be expressed as a transmembrane receptor, with a signalling capacity, or as a GPI-anchored adhesion molecule. The way in which this is controlled is not yet known. After classical pathway complement activation, antigens may also be opsonized by fragments of C3 deposited on the immune complex.

The carbohydrate receptors are thought to be important in recognition of bacteria (e.g. *Staphylococcus aureus* and *Micrococcus luteus*) and possibly also in recognition of tumour cells. This group includes the mannosyl/fucosyl receptor and sialoadhesin. Particles with surface carbohydrates can bind to phagocytes either directly to these lectin-like receptors or by the action of extracellular lectins, cross-bridging oligosaccharides on the bacteria and phagocyte. Interestingly, the mannosyl/fucosyl receptor is downregulated on activated macrophages in the presence of IFNγ, while the number of Fc receptors and the activity of the complement receptors (especially CR3) increases under similar circumstances. In essence this allows T cells to signal to incoming macrophages to make them less non-specifically adherent and to increase their capacity for immune adherence. The different classes of Fc receptor are under different regulatory controls and may be coupled to different signal transduction systems. For example, BCG (bacille Calmette– Guérin)-stimulation causes mouse macrophages to express more FcγRI and less FcγRII, while both are increased on inflammatory macrophages.

Human macrophages express two different receptors for C3 products, CR1 and CR3 (Chapter 13). CR1 is normally present at about 5000 receptors per monocyte but chemotactic agents (C5a, LTB4 etc.) can increase expression tenfold. Co-capping experiments show that Fc receptors and CR1 are interlinked via the cytoskeleton, such that they normally act synergistically. However, C3 alone can act as an opsonin, especially on activated cells where the receptors have increased lateral mobility in the membrane. In this case, the receptors act coordinately so that the particle is 'zippered' onto the membrane. CR1 becomes associated with the cytoskeleton only after it has become crosslinked during phagocytosis. CR3, with specificity for inactivated C3b (iC3b) and C3d, is confined to mononuclear phagocytes, neutrophils, NK cells and a minority of B cells. It is thought that the primary function of these two C3 receptors is to bind opsonized particles prior to phagocytosis.

The process of endocytosis of opsonized particles within macrophages involves internalization via Fc receptors centred on clathrin-coated pits in the plasma membrane. Unoccupied Fc receptors are recycled to the surface again, while immune complexes are vectored towards phagolysosomal destruction. However, this is not the end of the matter since partially degraded antigens may become subsequently associated with MHC class II molecules in antigen-presenting macrophages. This implies that they can be directed to another intracellular compartment which intercepts the class II pathway (see Chapter 7).

Microbicidal activity of macrophages and polymorphs

Bacteria and parasites taken into the phagosomes of macrophages and polymorphs are usually killed by a combination of enzymes and other anti-bacterial proteins from the lysosomes and granules, in association with reactive oxygen intermediates (ROIs). Which of these systems will be most important depends on the type of organism and the state of activation of the cell. Researchers have used macrophages from patients with chronic granulomatous diseases to resolve whether O_2-dependent or O_2-independent mechanisms are more important. These macrophages generate very few reactive oxygen products, due to an enzyme deficiency (usually an NADPH-linked oxidase or its cofactor). For example, IFNγ enhances the microbicidal activity of macrophages from these patients to *Leishmania* parasites but does not affect the metabolic deficiency. This implies that the O_2-independent systems are toxic in this case. In spite of debate on the relative importance of the various mechanisms, it is notable that organisms which can inhibit phagosome–lysosome fusion

(e.g. *M. tuberculosis*) as well as organisms which fail to trigger the cell's respiratory burst often also escape destruction. In other words, the relative importance of the different systems depends on the organism. The potential microbicidal effector mechanisms include:

- Reactive oxygen intermediates ($\cdot OH$, $O^\bullet$, O_2^- and H_2O_2).
- Toxic oxidants produced by the interaction of H_2O_2 on halides in the presence of peroxidase or catalase.
- Nitric oxide (NO).
- Cationic proteins and defensins, active at neutral pH.
- Phagosome acidification.
- Lysosomal enzymes, mostly active at acid pH.
- Growth inhibitors, including lactoferrin and arginase.

Reactive oxygen intermediates

The phagosomal membrane is originally derived from the plasma membrane and binding of particles to receptors on the plasma membrane initiates a burst of respiratory activity along with an increase in the activity of the hexose monophosphate shunt providing NADPH. Oxygen is activated by an NADPH oxidase sited in the phagosomal membrane which produces the various ROIs, O_2^-, $\cdot OH$ and singlet oxygen $O^\bullet$. The superoxide ion (O_2^-) is converted into H_2O_2 by the action of superoxide dismutase. Each of these products is highly reactive and potentially lethal for cells (e.g. singlet oxygen oxidizes double bonds). For this reason the polymorphs and macrophages protect themselves from ROIs, escaping from the phagosome by a chain of redox reactions involving glutathione. It seems likely that microorganisms may also attempt to use this kind of system to escape destruction by ROIs, as has been noted with experimental *T. brucei* infections of mice. In this case using inhibitors of glutathione synthesis leads to a rapid clearance of parasites from the blood.

Toxic oxidants

H_2O_2 is the starting material for the next step of the reactions. In the presence of myeloperoxidase and halides, such as Cl^- or I^-, hypohalites and other toxic halide compounds are generated. In the presence of myeloperoxidase, H_2O_2 can also act on amino acids to generate aldehydes, thus damaging the bacterial surface and aldehydes are themselves toxic. The myeloperoxidase for these reactions may be released into the phagosome from neutrophil azurophilic granules or may be taken up into the cell by endocytosis. Macrophages may also be able to carry out these reactions using catalase from peroxisomes, although it is not certain that catalase-catalysed reactions would be as effective as those catalysed by myeloperoxidase, particularly since many of the more pathogenic bacteria secrete catalase themselves, presumably as a protective measure. Eosinophils also generate H_2O_2 and contain very high levels of eosinophil peroxidase. This enzyme differs from myeloperoxidase in its substrate preferences but performs a related function. Eosinophils are especially effective at damaging multicellular parasites and trypanosomes, the toxic activity being greatly enhanced in the presence of halide ions. This leads to the conclusion that the pathways mentioned above are also active in eosinophils. In addition, it has been observed that secreted eosinophil peroxidase can sensitize tumour cells to the toxic effects of H_2O_2 secreted by macrophages.

Nitric oxide

Nitric oxide is generated from arginine by NO synthase. Low amounts are constitutively produced by macrophages by a calcium-dependent pathway but production is greatly increased following stimulation with inflammatory cytokines, including IL-1, TNFα and, particularly, IFNγ. These induce a separate calcium-independent synthetic pathway. Nitric oxide is particularly important in protection against parasites, pathogenic fungi and mycobacteria but not against extracellular bacteria. High levels of NO inhibit mitochondrial functions and interfere with enzymes which contain FeS cores and this is thought to contribute to its anti-microbial actions.

Defensins and other cationic proteins

Defensins are a group of small anti-microbial or cytotoxic peptides (29–35 residues) which are present in neutrophil granules and may constitute up to 5% of the total neutrophil protein. They are not generally found in macrophages, although cytokine-inducible defensins have been demonstrated in rabbit alveolar macrophages. These proteins are most effective at alkaline pH, that is, before acidification of the phagolysosome. They have a wide spectrum of activity against organisms, including *Candida*, Gram-positive and Gram-negative bacteria and spirochaetes. Some defensins apparently insert into the plasma membrane of their targets, forming voltage-regulated channels. Others interfere with receptors and signalling mechanisms.

Eosinophils also contain at least seven cationic proteins as well as major basic protein (MBP) which forms the major component of the crystalloid core of eosinophil specific granules. These proteins promote eosinophil adherence to schistosomules and MBP is directly toxic for these parasites. Charcot–Leyden crystal protein, also present in eosinophil granules, is a lectin with lysophospholipase activity. From the observed differences, it seems likely that neutrophil and eosinophil cationic proteins have distinct functions, presumably due to the fact that neutrophils destroy material internally whereas eosinophils primarily exocytose their granule contents.

Phagosome acidification

Phagosome acidification occurs at the time of lysosome fusion and is caused by the activation of proton pumps which secrete H^+ ions into the phagosome. Acid conditions enhance the activity of myeloperoxidase and favour the peroxidatic action of catalase. Acidification of the phagolysosome may by itself damage some micro-organisms. Typically, the pH falls to 3.5–4.0 and parasites such as *T. gondii* are sensitive to these conditions. In addition, the optimum pH for the majority of the lysosomal enzymes is acid.

Lysosomal enzymes

The importance of macrophage lysosomal and secreted enzymes in bacterial killing is uncertain and it is quite possible that the lysosomal hydrolases and cathepsins are primarily involved in the ultimate breakdown of the phagocytosed material, rather than as a killing mechanism. Lysozyme constitutes up to 2.5% of the macrophage protein and can act both within the phagolysosome and as a secreted protein. It breaks the bond between N-acetyl glucosamine and N-acetyl muramic acid in the bacterial cell wall peptidoglycan. This may damage Gram-positive bacteria directly but to gain access to the cell wall of Gram-negative bacteria, which have an outer lipid bilayer, it synergizes with other systems such as the complement lytic components and lysosomal defensins. Lysozyme is secreted constitutively by macrophages regardless of the activation state of the cell.

Growth inhibitors

In some circumstances a cell's ability to prevent bacterial growth by the secretion of molecules which breakdown or sequester trophic substances is important. For example, arginase limits the availability of arginine; while this presents little problem to most bacteria, it has been shown that schistosomucidal activity of macrophages correlates with their arginase secretion and tumour cells are also susceptible. Lactoferrin which sequesters iron, binds to macrophages by a specific receptor and is endocytosed and may enter phagolysosomes, where it is active at acid pH. Neutrophils can synthesize lactoferrin themselves and it is found in their granules. Overloading neutrophils with iron reduces their ability to kill some bacteria. The anti-microbial activities of macrophages are set out in *Figure 14.15*.

Secretory products

Lysozyme, mentioned above, is the major secretory product of macrophages but other lysosomal hydrolases may be released following phagocytosis of particles and in response to IFNγ. However, the secreted neutral proteases are more likely to be important in the extracellular milieu and, unlike the lysosomal hydrolases, their level of secretion varies markedly, depending on the activation state of the macrophage. Neutral proteases include collagenase, elastase, plasminogen activator and a cytotoxic proteinase. Secretion occurs in two stages, mirroring the steps required to produce activation. IFNγ primes the cells and enzyme release is triggered by phagocytosis, high levels of lymphokines and endotoxin. Activated macrophages can also secrete complement components, as well as eicosanoids, interleukin-1 and 6 and IFNβ.

In conclusion, the activation of macrophages is a complex event and not all receptors and functions are upregulated. However, in general the cell shifts from being a nonspecific effector to a cell responsive to lymphokines and capable of interaction with lymphocytes, as an antigen presenting cell. Neutrophils and eosinophils are potent but relatively short lived, effector cells responsive primarily to chemotactic and opsonic stimuli. Which of these cells will be most effective in anti-microbial activity depends largely on the invading organism and its ability to withstand the battery of enzymes, active proteins and cytotoxic metabolites produced by these cells. A summary of how the immune system can mediate inflammation is presented in *Figure 14.16*.

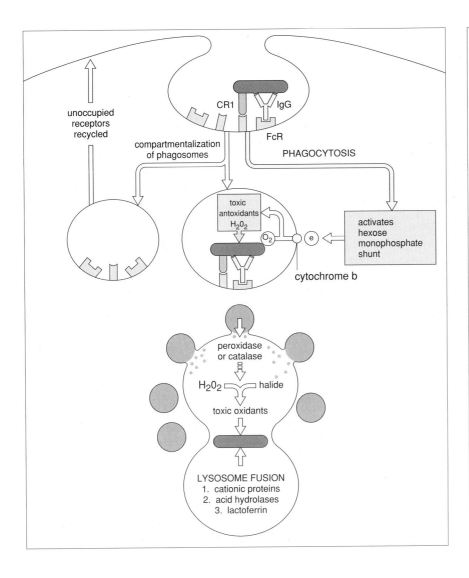

Fig. 14.15 Anti-microbial systems of macrophages. Bacteria and other particles may be opsonized by antibody or complement and become attached to macrophages via their Fc and C3 receptors. Attachment initiates phagocytosis, and the particle is endocytosed. Unoccupied receptors are recycled back to the cell surface, while the phagocytosed material proceeds through a different pathway. Phagocytosis initiates activity of the hexose monophosphate shunt which supplies electrons (e) to an enzyme in the phagosomal membrane and this generates toxic oxygen metabolites (see text) which can damage microorganisms. In the second stage, the pH of the phagosome transiently increases, at which time defensins and other cationic proteins are active. Subsequently the pH of the phagolysosome vacuole falls. and acid hydrolases and lactoferrin start to exert their cytotoxic activities. Peroxidase or catalase under these conditions causes H_2O_2 and halide ions to generate toxic oxidants such as hypohalites, which may further damage the phagocytosed particle or microorganism.

SUMMARY

Leukocyte traffic is an essential element in the immune system, since it allows the small numbers of antigen-specific cells to contact their antigen and develop in lymphoid tissues, before disseminating to other lymphoid tissues and inflammatory sites. There are two principal patterns of lymphocyte traffic:

- The migration of naïve and memory cells to, or between, secondary lymphoid tissues.
- The migration of activated cells into inflammatory sites. Different subsets of cells preferentially localize to particular tissues. This depends on adhesion molecules on endothelium reacting with counter-receptors on the leukocytes. Expression of the adhesion molecules on endothelium depends on the vascular bed, the type of endothelium and whether it has been activated by cytokines. Expression of receptors on lymphocytes, depends on the subpopulation and their state of activation.

The molecules controlling adhesion belong to several different families (selectins, Ig superfamily, etc.). Migration involves at least three steps, including tethering of the circulating leukocytes, interaction with activators expressed or held on the endothelium and then engagement of integrins on the leukocytes with cellular adhesion molecules on the endothelium. This precedes the initiation of a programme of migration. Leukocytes in inflammatory sites migrate up chemotactic gradients and may be further primed by cytokines (TNF, IFNγ etc.) and chemokines (IL-8 etc.) diffusing away from the site.

Areas of inflammation are also characterized by increased blood flow and capillary permeability, controlled by a series of mediators from the plasma kinin and complement systems and by cell-derived mediators. Mast cells, basophils, platelets, endothelium, activated macrophages and lymphocytes all release mediators which affect vascular permeability — the most important being the vasoactive amines and eicosanoids. Once at the site of inflammation, cells become activated and the microbicidal properties of macrophages and neutrophils are enhanced. Finally, antigen carried away from the site to lymphoid organs is essential in the initiation or development of the immune response to that antigen.

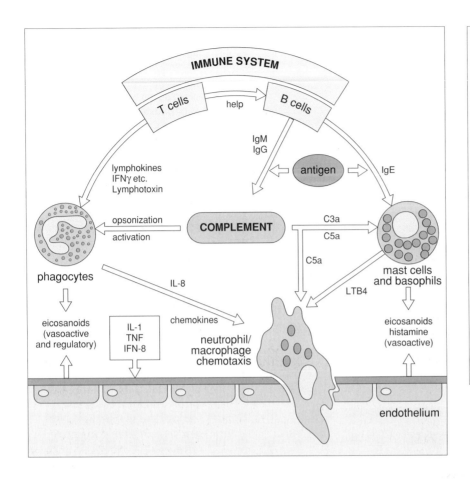

Fig. 14.16 Inflammation mediated by the immune system. The immune system can initiate inflammatory reactions either via the complement classical pathway activated by IgG or IgM and antigen, or by recruiting mast cells, sensitizing them with IgE so that they are triggered following contact with antigen. C3a and C5a also trigger mast cells and basophils, while C5a activates and is chemotactic for phagocytes. Eicosanoids released from mast cells affect the local vasculature and LTB4 is chemotactic. Additional eicosanoids are produced by macrophages and endothelium. Once present at an inflammatory site, the incoming cells are controlled by locally produced cytokines, particularly TNFα, IL-1 and IFNγ.

FURTHER READING

Bargatze RF, Butcher EC. Rapid G-protein regulated event involved in lymphocyte binding to high endothelial cell venules. *J Exp Med* 1993, **178**:367.

Bevilacqua MP. Endothelial-leukocyte adhesion molecules. *Ann Rev Immunol* 1993, **11**:767.

Bevilacqua MP, Stengelin S, Gimbrone MA, Seed B. Endothelial leukocyte adhesion molecule 1: an inducible receptor for neutrophils related to complement regulatory proteins and lectins. *Science* 1989, **243**:1160.

Briskin MJ, McEvoy LM, Butcher EC. MadCAM-1 has homology to immunoglobulin and mucin-like adhesion receptors and to IgA1. *Nature* 1993, **363**:461.

Davies P, Bailey PJ, Goldenberg MM, Ford-Hutchinson AW. The role of arachidonic acid products in pain and inflammation. *Ann Rev Immunol* 1984, **2**:335.

Diamond MS, Springer TA. The dynamic regulation of integrin adhesiveness. *Curr Biol* 1994, **4**:566.

Dransfield I, Cabonas C, Craig A, Hogg N. Divalent cation regulation of the function of the leukocyte integrin LFA-1. *J Cell Biol* 1992, **116**:219.

Foxall C, Watson SR, Dowbenko D, Fennie C, Lasky LA, Kiso M, Hasegawa A, Asa D, Brandley BK. The three members of the selectin family recognize a common carbohydrate epitope, the sialyl Lewis X oligosaccharide. *J Cell Biol* 1992, **117**:893.

Gamble JR, Khew-Goodall Y, Vadas M. TGFβ inhibits E-selectin expression on human endothelial cells. *J Immunol* 1993, **150**:4494.

Gearing AJH, Newman W. Circulating adhesion molecules in disease. *Immunol Today* 1993, **14**:506.

Gleich GJ, Adolphson CR, Leiferman KM, Schafer AI, Kroll MH, Spivak JL. The biology of the eosinophilic leukocyte. *Ann Rev Medicine* 1992, **44**:85.

Gowans JL, Knight EJ. The route of recirculation of lymphocytes in the rat. *Proc R Soc Lond Biol* 1964, **159**:257.

Hartwig JH, Thelen M, Rosen A, Janmey PA, Nairn AC, Anderem A. MARCKS is an actin filament cross-linking protein regulated by protein kinase C and calcium-calmodulin. *Nature* 1992, **356**:618.

Holzmann B, McIntyre BW, Weissmann IL. Identification of a murine Peyer's patch-specific lymphocyte homing receptor as an integrin molecule with an α-chain homologous to human VLA-4 α chain. *Cell* 1989, **56**:37.

Hynes RO. Integrins: versatility modulation and signaling in cell adhesion. *Cell* 1992, **69**:11.

Islam LN, Wilkinson PC. Chemotactic factor-induced polarization, receptor redistribution and locomotion of human blood monocytes. *Immunol* 1988, **64**:501.

Issekutz TB. Effects of six different cytokines on lymphocyte adherence to microvascular endothelium and in vivo lymphocyte migration in the rat. *J Immunol* 1990, **144**, 2140.

Issekutz TB. Lymphocyte homing to sites of inflammation. *Curr Opin Immunol* 1992, **4**:287.

Jalkanen S, Nash GS, de los Toyos J, MacDermott RP, Butcher EC. Human lamina propria lymphocytes bear homing receptors and bind selectively to mucosal lymphoid high endothelium. *Eur J Immunol* 1989 **19**:63.

Johnston GI, Cook RG, McEver RP. Cloning of GMP-140 a granule membrane protein of platelets and endothelium: sequence similarity to proteins involved in cell adhesion and inflammation. *Cell* 1989, **56**:1033.

Jung TM, Gallatin WM, Weissmann IL, Dailey MO. Downregulation of homing receptors after T cell activation. *J Immunol* 1988, **141**:4110.

Larsen GL, Henson PM. Mediators of inflammation. *Ann Rev Immunol* 1983, **1**:335.

Lasky LA, Singer MS, Dowbenko D, Imai Y, Henzel WJ, Grimley C, Fennie C, Gillett N, Watson SR, Rosen SD. An endothelial ligand for L-selectin is a novel mucin-like molecule. *Cell* 1992, **69**:927.

Mackay CR, Morton WL, Dudler L. Naive and memory T cells show distinct pathways of lymphocyte recirculation. *J Exp Med* 1990, **171**:801.

Mollison KW, Mandecki W, Zuiderweg ER, Fayer L, Fey TA, Krause RA, Conway RG, Miller L, Edalji RP, Shallcross MA *et al.* Identification of receptor binding residues in the complement protein C5a by site-directed mutagenesis. *Proc Nat Acad Sci* 1989, **86**:292.

Murphy PM. The molecular biology of leukocyte chemoattractant receptors. *Ann Rev Immunol* 1994, **12**: 593.

Oppenheim JJ, Zachariae COC, Mukaida N, Matsushima K. Properties of the novel proinflammatory supergene 'intercrine' cytokine family. *Ann Rev Immunol* 1991, **9**:617.

Picker LJ, Butcher EC. Physiological and molecular mechanisms of lymphocyte homing. *Ann Rev Immunol* 1992, **10**:561.

Proud D, Kaplan AP. Kinin formation: mechanisms and role in inflammatory disorders. *Ann Rev Immunol* 1988, **6**:49.

Shimizu Y, van Seventer GA, Horgan KJ, Shaw S. Roles of adhesion molecules in T cell recognition: fundamental similarities between four integrins on resting human T cells LFA-1, VLA-4, VLA-5, VLA-6 in expression, binding and co-stimulation. *Immunol Rev* 1990, **114**:104.

Shimizu Y, Newman W, Gopal TV, Horgan KJ, Graber N, Beall LD, van Seventer GA, Shaw S. Four molecular pathways of T cell adhesion to endothelial cells: Roles of LFA-1, VCAM-1 and ELAM-1 and changes of pathway hierarchy under different activation conditions. *J Cell Biol* 1991, **113**:1203.

Spertini O, Konsas GS, Munro JM, Griffin JD, Tedder TF. Regulation of leukocyte migration by activation of the leukocyte adhesion molecule-1 LAM-1 selectin. *Nature* 1991, **349**:691.

Springer TA. Adhesion receptors of the immune system. *Nature* 1990, **346**:425.

Springer TA. Traffic signals for lymphocyte recirculation and leukocyte emigration: the multi-step paradigm. *Cell* 1994, **76**:301.

Stamper HB, Woodruff JJ. An *in vitro* model of lymphocyte homing. 1. Characterization of the interaction between thoracic duct lymphocytes and specialized high endothelial venules of lymph nodes. *J Immunol* 1977, **119**:1603.

Staunton DE, Dustin ML, Springer TA. Functional cloning of ICAM-2, a cell adhesion ligand for LFA-1 homologous to ICAM-1. *Nature* 1989, **339**:61.

Staunton DE, Marlin SD, Sratowa C, Dustin ML, Springer TA. Primary structure of ICAM-1 demonstrates interaction between members of the immunoglobulin and integrin supergene families. *Cell* 1988, **52**:925.

Tamatani T, Kuida K, Watanabe T, Koike S, Miyasaka M. Molecular mechanisms underlying lymphocyte recirculation III. Characteristics of LECAM-1 L-selectin dependent pathway in rats. *J Immunol* 1993, **150**:1735.

Tanaka Y, Albelda SM, Horgan KJ, van Seventer GA, Shimizu Y, Newman W, Hallam J, Newman PJ, Buck CA, Shaw S. CD31 expressed on distinctive T cell subsets is a preferential amplifier of beta-1 integrin-mediated adhesion. *J Exp Med* 1992, **176**:245.

Weston SA, Parish CR. Modification of lymphocyte migration by mannans and phosphomannans. Different carbohydrate structures control entry of lymphocytes into spleen and lymph nodes. *J Immunol* 1991, **146**:4180.

Wysocki J, Issekutz TB. Effect of T cell activation on lymphocyte endothelial cell adherence and the role of VLA-4 in the rat. *Cell Immunol* 1992, **140**:420.

15 Cytotoxic Effector Cells

While the humoral immune response, mediated primarily by antibody and complement, plays a major role in host defence (see Chapters 13, 14 and 16), the body also requires a variety of cellular mechanisms to deal effectively with most antigenic challenges. This is particularly true for viral diseases and intracellular bacterial and parasitic infections, as well as for combating tumours. In these diseases, it is necessary to kill infected or neoplastic cells in order to eliminate the infectious agent or prevent growth of a tumour. Of course, humoral and cellular mechanisms usually form an effective collaboration in host defence.

This chapter will discuss both specific and non-specific mechanisms of killing target cells or invading microorganisms and parasites. Both lymphoid and myeloid cell lineages have important roles to play, although antigen specificity is dictated by lymphocytes. The ways in which cells can induce death of the target by cytolysis or apoptosis will also be detailed.

CYTOTOXIC LYMPHOCYTES

In 1960, Govaerts reported the first demonstration of cytotoxic activity by lymphoid cells. In his experiments on the mechanism of kidney allograft rejection in dogs, he noted that thoracic duct lymphocytes from animals which had previously rejected an allograft were able to kill specifically donor kidney epithelial cells *in vitro*. These observations were soon confirmed by many investigators and extended to include killing of syngeneic tumours and virally infected cells. The effector cells involved in this specific killing of target cells were subsequently found to be a subset of T cells, now known as 'cytotoxic T lymphocytes' (Tc).

After initial observations demonstrating the immunological specificity of cytotoxicity, some confusion arose from reports that lymphoid cells from non-immune individuals could kill a variety of target cells in an apparently non-specific manner, particularly following activation with mitogens. Furthermore, normal lymphocytes were also shown to kill cells pre-coated with anti-target cell antibodies. It has since become clear that these cytolytic activities are largely due to a population of non-T, non-B mononuclear cells termed 'natural killer' (NK) cells, so called because they possessed killing capabilities which, unlike Tc, did not need prior activation. NK cells are sometimes referred to as 'large granular lymphocytes' (LGL) because of their prominent azurophilic cytoplasmic granules; many of these cells can also kill antibody-coated target cells (an activity sometimes referred to as 'killer cell' (K cell) activity. Non-specific killing can also be mediated *in vitro* by γδ T cells and by αβ T cells activated with lymphokines such as IL-2. However, the physiological relevance of such killing activity *in vivo* is not clear. The characteristic features of these different cytotoxic lymphocytes are outlined in *Figure 15.1*.

Effector cell types

MHC-RESTRICTED CYTOTOXIC T CELLS
Cytotoxic T lymphocytes are a subpopulation of small lymphocytes which are physiologically important in the killing of allogeneic cells within the grafted tissue. Although other cell types can play a role in limiting viral replication, Tc are critical in clearing most viral infections. Tc can also recognize cells infected with intracellular bacteria such as various strains of mycobacteria and listeria; they can be seen surrounding infected tissue, although they do not seem to provide very effective protection against these pathogens.

Lymphocyte subset		MHC restriction	Receptor(s)	Ligand
Tc αβ-TCR	CD8+	Class I	TCR	MHC Class I + Antigen
	CD4+	Class II	TCR	MHC Class II + Antigen
Tc γδ-TCR		Non-polymorphic Class I + others	TCR	Class I molecules + ?
LGL	NK Activity	–	Ly49 (mouse) p58(man) → NK1.1 (mouse)	MHC Class I ?
	K cell Activity	–	CD16 (FcγRIII) + Antibody	Specific Antigen

Fig. 15.1 The characteristics and specificity of cytotoxic lymphoid cells.

The majority of Tc are CD8$^+$ cells with the αβ TCR. They recognize antigen in association with MHC class I molecules. However, a minority of Tc (probably less than 10%) are CD4$^+$ and recognize antigen associated with MHC class II. These class II-restricted cells can dominate the response to certain viral infections, such as measles. This is clearly dependent upon the ability of the infectious agent to infect class II positive cells but probably also reflects the mode of viral entry into the target cell and subsequent intracellular localization of viral proteins, which will in turn determine the pathways used to process viral antigens for presentation (see Chapter 7). Both types of Tc are derived from a pool of non-lytic precursor virgin T cells which are extremely radiosensitive (implying a high rate of proliferation). Since class II expression is normally limited to professional antigen presenting cells (APCs), class II-restricted CD4$^+$ Tc may be involved in the regulation of immune responses in addition to killing infected or otherwise abnormal cells. What determines whether a CD4$^+$ Tc or a CD4$^+$ Th will be formed from any given precursor cell and at what stage of differentiation such commitment occurs is unknown.

The frequency of precursor cells for any given antigen specificity has been estimated by limiting dilution analyses to be in the range of 0.02–0.2%. Based on cell culture experiments, most of these precursors were thought to require interactions with Th cells, as well as specific antigen, to enable them to differentiate into functionally mature Tc. The primary role of Th cells was seen as the provision of cytokines, as evidenced by the observation that IL-2 and IL-4 can promote antigen-dependent growth and effector differentiation of Tc *in vitro*. However, the importance of Th cells *in vivo* is uncertain, since mice lacking CD4$^+$ cells (either in MHC class II-deficient transgenics or by monoclonal antibody-mediated depletion) develop normal CD8$^+$ Tc. It is possible that under these experimental conditions, CD8$^+$ cells which are able to make their own growth and differentiation factors such as IL-2 are selectively expanded from a minor subpopulation of the initial precursor pool — this is certainly a potential problem when trying to use gene deletions in transgenic mice to answer immunological and other developmental questions. Tc clones propagated *in vitro* can make a variety of cytokines in response to activating stimuli. These include IL-2, IL-3, TNFα and IFNγ cytokines characteristically produced by Th1 cells (see Chapter 8).

Experiments involving the micro-manipulation of individual cells have shown that a single cytotoxic T cell can sequentially kill several target cells. To function in this manner, Tc must be resistant to their own killing mechanisms and able to detach effectively from dying target cells. Hypotheses attempting to explain these capabilities will be discussed later.

NATURAL KILLER CELLS

Natural killer (NK) cells can spontaneously kill certain susceptible target cells in a manner which, unlike Tc, is not triggered by recognition of classical MHC–peptide complexes. Because of their relatively limited specificity repertoire (discussed in detail below), the frequency of any given specificity is high and each cell is armed ready to kill at first contact. These characteristics enable NK cells to act as a first line of defence, playing an important role in natural resistance against cancer and a variety of infectious diseases. They are thought to be particularly important in limiting viral replication during the first days of an infection, while specific Tc are developing from their precursors: patients with rare NK cell defects suffer severe infections with viruses such as cytomegalovirus.

NK cells are found in the LGL subpopulation of lymphocytes, which are present in all vertebrates examined and in humans may represent up to 15% of peripheral blood lymphoid cells. In addition to their large granular appearance, NK cells express CD16 (low affinity Fcγ receptor) and CD56, a member of the NCAM family of adhesion molecules (see Chapter 5). Although these cells do not rearrange or express TCR or mIg molecules, CD3ξ-chains are expressed in association with CD16, CD2 and p58 where they play a role in NK cell activation (see below). By virtue of their CD16 molecules, most NK cells can also mediate target cell killing by antibody-dependent cellular cytotoxicity (ADCC), sometimes referred to as killer cell (K cell) activity. Although K cell activity is expressed by a small percentage of LGLs that appear to lack standard NK cell activity, they are probably NK cells with 'non-standard' target specificities.

Although NK cells can develop normally in the absence of a thymus and in SCID mice which fail to rearrange TCR and Ig genes (and thus lack T and B cells), recent experiments indicate that T cells and NK cells may derive from a common progenitor cell. In the thymus and foetal liver, a small population of immature thymocytes lacking CD3, CD4 or CD8 T cell markers and with unrearranged TCR genes, have been identified which are individually capable of differentiating into either T cells or NK cells depending on their microenvironment — in the thymus they mature into T cells, whereas in extrathymic environments they mature into NK cells (see Chapter 6 for further details). Formal proof of a common T/NK cell precursor, rather than separate lineage-committed cells with the same surface 'immature thymocyte' phenotype, awaits the development of suitable culture conditions for single cell differentiation to T cell and NK cell lineages.

γδ T CELLS

Some human and mouse γδ T cells can kill target cells in an MHC-unrestricted manner. While in some cases this may be due to the development of NK-like activity in CD56$^+$ cells *in vitro*, other cells can be triggered through their γδ TCR. As discussed below, this might represent recognition of non-polymorphic MHC-related molecules and may therefore follow similar rules to activation of MHC-restricted αβ Tc. Indeed, γδ T cells with cytotoxic activity have been shown to express similar cytotoxic granule proteins to Tc. Despite these *in vitro* observations, it is still not clear what role, if any, γδ T cell cytotoxicity may play *in vivo*.

LYMPHOKINE ACTIVATED KILLER CELLS

When lymphocyte populations are cultured with cytokines such as IL-2, cells develop that are capable of killing almost all target cells, including those typically resistant to NK cell activity. This MHC-unrestricted killing is functionally termed LAK (lymphokine activated killer) activity and is selective for tumour cells or cells expressing abnormal surface features; it rarely affects normal cells. Although cytokine-activated NK cells represent the predominant population expressing LAK activity in unseparated lymphocyte cultures, both αβ and γδ T cells can develop this activity too.

As with γδ T cell cytotoxicity, the *in vivo* relevance of LAK activity is not clear: it could simply be an artefactual differentiation response to the high IL-2 concentrations used in culture. Nevertheless, the ability to generate LAK cells *in vitro* has been exploited in the immunotherapy of some forms of cancer. Patients' peripheral or tumour-infiltrating lymphocytes are expanded to very high numbers (10^{11}–10^{12}) with IL-2 and then adoptively transferred back into the same patient. NK cell activity is thought to play an active role in this form of therapy, although the majority of infused cells may not themselves mediate killing of tumour cells, since few seem to localize to the tumour itself.

TARGET CELL RECOGNITION AND EFFECTOR CELL ACTIVATION

Cytotoxic T cells

T cell specificity is determined wholly by the specificity of the TCRαβ receptors. This was confirmed by transferring antigen–MHC specificity to a cell by transfection of *TCRA* and *B* genes. Further confirmation of this is provided by the observation that class I-restricted CD8+ Tc will kill each other, even other members of the same clone, in the presence of their specific antigenic peptides. However, *in vitro* (and most likely *in vivo*) Tc will make non-lethal contact with many surrounding cells, including those bearing antigen. Studies with artificial antigen-presenting particles of various sizes has indicated that Tc activation requires occupancy of a threshold number of TCR complexes (in association with CD4 or CD8 molecules) in a highly localized region of the cell membrane and the lethal hit is selectively targeted to the activating cell. Physiologically, this may be to ensure that cytotoxic T cell responses are not triggered unnecessarily, for example by fragments of dead target cells.

Activation of Tc by their specific target cells is effected by the triggering of complex intracellular signalling pathways as described in detail in Chapter 8 and involves an intimate contact with the target cell, which is mediated by specific receptors and adhesion molecules (*Fig. 15.2*). As with Th cells, adhesive interactions also provide co-stimulatory signals for Tc activation and these signals are more critical for the initial activation of resting Tc precursors than for previously activated Tc. For example, CD28–B7 interaction appears to be involved in the activation of primary cytotoxicity responses in populations of small resting T cells. Interactions between adhesion molecules also play an important role in Tc function *in vivo*. For example, in one series of experiments, the effectiveness of anti-parasite CD8+ Tc on adoptive transfer was shown to correlate with the expression of CD44 and VLA-4 adhesion molecules. However, the relative importance of such adhesive interactions for Tc trafficking and activation is unclear.

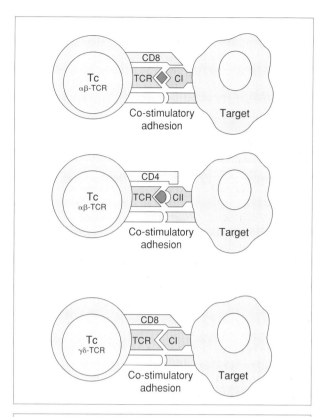

Fig. 15.2 Target cell recognition by cytotoxic T cells. CD8+ and CD4+ T cells which use the αβ TCR recognize their targets by their presentation of MHC plus antigenic peptide. The interactions may be enhanced by co-stimulatory pairs of adhesion molecules on the lymphocyte and target; e.g. CD2/LFA-3, VLA-4/fibronectin, CD28, B7. Cytotoxic T cells with the γδ TCR may recognize non-polymorphic class I molecules such as CD1c using their TCR and other adhesion molecules.

γδ T cells

Some γδ T cell clones are able to kill allospecific targets following specific TCR-mediated recognition. For example, cytotoxic γδ T cells have been described which recognize a relatively restricted set of antigens associated with the CD1c molecule, which has some similarities to MHC class I molecules but is non-polymorphic (*Fig. 15.2*). Similarly, a mouse T cell hybridoma has been described that recognizes its specific antigen in association with Qa-1 class I-like molecules (see Chapter 4). However, these may represent rare exceptions or cross-reactivities of γδ TCR, since γδ T cells appear to develop normally in β2-microglobulin deficient mice which fail to express classical class I molecules or non-polymorphic class I-like molecules such as CD1 and Qa and do not develop CD8+ thymocytes.

NK cells

The nature of the receptors involved in target cell recognition by NK cells has eluded immunologists for a long time. NK cell activity was originally defined as being non-MHC-restricted, since these cells could readily kill tumour cells which lack surface expression of MHC molecules (such as the murine YAC-1 and human K562 target cell lines) and not involving clonally distributed receptors. While it is clear that TCR genes are not involved, since they remain in the germline configuration, recent evidence indicates that, unlike T and B cells, triggering of NK cell-mediated cytotoxicity involves both activating and inhibitory interactions of polymorphic receptors with target cell ligands (*Fig. 15.3*).

INHIBITORY INTERACTIONS
Studies of murine NK cell target specificities showed that several MHC class I-negative cell lines were more susceptible to NK-mediated lysis than class I-positive cells and that resistance could be restored in these cells by transfection of certain class I genes. Further analyses indicated that the efficiency of NK cell killing was inversely correlated with MHC class I expression. The physiological relevance of these observations is highlighted by experiments showing that 'normal' cells from mice lacking class I expression (transgenic knockout mice lacking β_2-microglobulin expression and therefore also lacking MHC class I expression) are sensitive to NK cell-mediated lysis, both *in vitro* and on transfer to normal mice. However, the cells of β_2-microglobulin knockout mice are not sensitive to killing by their own NK cells, suggesting that NK cells have other self–nonself discrimination mechanisms. NK cells in these mice are actually not very effective killers of any target cell, which has lead to the suggestion that class I molecules may play a role in the differentiation of NK cells.

The early studies showing the NK cells' ability to kill effectively MHC-negative target cells led to the conclusion that these cells possessed non-clonally distributed recognition molecules and function. Recent data, however, clearly indicate that NK cell populations derived from a single individual display allospecificity in their target cell killing. Thus, human T cell depleted peripheral blood lymphocyte populations cultured with irradiated allogeneic lymphocytes and IL-2 produced activated NK cell clonal populations which could all kill MHC-negative K562 cells and a subset of clones could kill the allostimulator cells but not third party allogeneic or self target cells. Such analyses of hundreds of clones with a panel of allogeneic blast cells from different people revealed five subgroups of allospecificity, termed groups one to five, with 36% of the clones recognizing at least one target type. It is not yet clear whether only a subset of clones are capable of allorecognition or whether the panel of allospecificities was simply not diverse enough. Susceptibility to any particular NK specificity was found to be a recessive trait; the dominant resistance mapped to the HLA region, thus implying that resistance is correlated with the 'allospecificity'. MHC class I C and B genes were found to provide such protection against NK killing. For example, transfection of murine P815 cells with human HLA-Cw3 rendered them resistant to killing by group 2 NK clones but they remained sensitive to group 1 clones. In contrast, resistance to group 1 clones could be selectively induced by transfection with HLA-Cw4. In the genetic analysis, resistance to lysis by group 2 clones co-segregated with HLA-Cw3

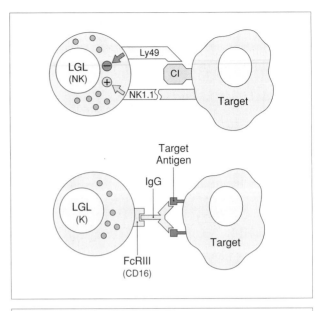

Fig. 15.3 Target cell recognition by large granular lymphocytes (LGLs). When expressing NK cell activity, LGLs interact with targets by a dual recognition system. They are positively stimulated by their NK cell receptors (in the mouse NK1.1) but are inhibited by recognition of MHC class I on the target, recognized by Ly49 in the mouse. LGLs can also recognize targets sensitized with antibody, which they engage using their characteristic Fc receptor, FcγRIII.

as well as with Cw7 and Cw1, which all have Ser 77 and Asn 80 in the peptide binding region of the molecule.

Similarly, Cw4, Cw2, Cw5 and Cw6 which appear involved in resistance to group 1 clones all have Asn 77 and Lys 80 in their peptide binding grooves. Other transfection experiments have indicated that HLA-A2 molecules can also confer resistance to NK cell mediated lysis. Exon-shuffling of different domains of the A2 class I molecule implicated the $\alpha 1 / \alpha 2$ region and mutation analysis showed that a single amino acid substitution, at position 74 in the peptide binding groove, could convert a target cell from a susceptible to a resistant phenotype. Taken together, this and other evidence suggests that NK cell recognition of particular class I-peptide complexes on target cells prevents their activation.

Although masking of other target cell antigens remains a possible explanation for the role of class I molecules, recent information indicates that class I-peptide complexes are specifically recognized by NK cell receptors but, in complete contrast to the TCR of Tc, these deliver a negative signal to the NK cell. Thus, as NK cells traffic throughout the body they may survey tissues for certain class I-self peptide complexes, killing any cell lacking or aberrantly expressing these determinants. From these data, one may propose two possible roles of NK cells in anti-viral defence:

- NK cells may recognize infected cells in the early stages of infection where viral peptides have started to replace host molecules on infected targets.

- Some viruses actively downregulate MHC expression to avoid immune recognition. It is therefore desirable to have a mechanism ensuring that cells failing to express MHC class I are eliminated.

Although the receptors responsible for class I-peptide recognition by NK cells have not been precisely defined, both murine and human candidates have been found. In the mouse, good evidence indicates a role for the Ly-49 cell surface antigen which is expressed by approximately 20% of splenic NK cells as a disulphide-linked homodimer of 44kDa subunits. Analyses at the molecular level indicate that Ly-49 is one member of a family of genes which encode type II integral membrane proteins with an external C-type lectin domain. The functional effects of Ly-49 have so far only been characterized with NK cells from H-2^b mice recognizing a subset of allogeneic target cells. Thus, H-2D^d or D^k target cells are resistant to lysis by Ly-49$^+$ but sensitive to Ly-49$^-$, NK cells from H-2^b spleen cells. The inhibitory effect of Ly-49 is reversed by antibodies to either Ly-49 or the $\alpha1/\alpha2$ domains of H-2D^d and is dominant over activating signals; ADCC by the same cells is also inhibited. Transfection experiments confirmed that the D^d is indeed the protective molecule recognized by Ly-49. Since the different modes of activation involve distinct receptor systems, it is currently believed that upon interaction with the appropriate class I molecule, Ly-49 delivers a negative signal which prevents activation of the cell. Different members of the Ly-49 gene family and, perhaps, allelic variants of each may be involved in recognition of distinct MHC class I molecules. Further analysis of the role of Ly-49 in the mouse has been somewhat hampered by the lack of clonal NK cell populations in this species.

Clonally distributed inhibitory receptors have been characterized on human NK cells through the use of monoclonal antibodies. Antibodies GL183 and EB6 were raised against human (CD3$^-$, CD16$^+$) NK cell clones and found to recognize distinct but overlapping sets of NK cells. Reactivity profiles with these antibodies correlated well with the different groups of clones (defined on the basis of their allospecificities) discussed above. For example, group I clones (which are prevented from lysing targets expressing Cw4 molecules) are GL183$^-$/EB6$^+$, whereas group 2 clones are GL183$^+$/EB6$^+$. Interestingly, in individuals sensitive to group 1 NK cell lysis, NK cells of GL183$^+$/EB6$^+$ phenotype are virtually absent (and the few that are present are unable to lyse autologous cells), providing further evidence for tolerance or clonal deletion of NK cells. These antibodies can selectively overcome the protective effect of appropriate class I molecules, presumably through masking of receptors involved in class I recognition. Immunoprecipitation analyses showed that GL183 and EB6 antibodies recognize distinct but highly homologous 58kDa molecules, termed p58, which are expressed as heterodimers in non-covalent association with both CD3ξ and the γ-chain of FcϵRI. This strongly implies a role for p58 molecules in class I-mediated delivery of negative signals to the NK cell. As with Ly-49 on murine NK cells, signals delivered through p58 molecules are able to inhibit all forms of lysis mediated by NK cells. It is currently unclear whether or not humans have Ly-49 homologues, or mice p58 homologues, although a family of five human NK-specific genes (termed *NKG2*), encoding type II integral membrane proteins with C-type lectin domains, have recently been characterized by subtractive hybridization cloning.

Finally, it is worth noting that, *in vivo*, NK cells can be activated by appropriate target cells despite being in contact with many other normal tissue cells bearing MHC class I molecules. This implies that the inhibitory signals delivered through class I recognition are highly localized so that they do not block activation triggered on contact with specific target cells.

ACTIVATION RECEPTORS

Inhibition of NK cell activation by negative signalling through class I-peptide recognition implies that definable activation receptors must exist on NK cells. Although lysis can be triggered through the CD16 and CD2 molecules on resting NK cells and through CD69 and Ly-6 molecules on activated NK cells, and these pathways can be prevented by appropriate class I recognition, cells lacking these surfaces molecules can still kill susceptible targets. In rodents, other molecules have been described which represent good candidates for NK cell-specific activation receptors but whether or not they are directly responsible for natural killer activity remains to be determined.

NKR-P1 (in rats) and NK1.1 (in mice) are 60kDa disulphide-linked homodimers of a type II integral membrane protein member of the C-lectin superfamily which includes Ly-49 and CD23. Antibodies to these molecules can activate NK cell cytotoxcity and release of serine esterases in a 'redirected lysis' assay. Furthermore, phosphoinositide turnover and increases in intracellular free calcium levels are triggered, which mimic the biochemical signals triggered upon interaction with a suitable target cell. The mouse NK1.1 molecule has been used for some time as a specific NK cell marker, which displays alleleic polymorphism. Screening of cDNA libraries with a rat NKR-P1 probe produced a series of clones representing a murine NKR-P1 family of molecules, one of which was shown by antibody staining and immunoprecipitation to encode the NK1.1 molecule. The nature of the ligands recognized by different NKR-P1 forms is not known, although carbohydrate moieties may play a role since other C-lectin superfamily members (e.g. CD23) are known to bind specific carbohydrates in a calcium-dependent manner.

The difficulty in defining a unique NK cell activation receptor may be explained in part by the existence of polymorphic forms and perhaps by the differential requirements for co-stimulatory signals for activating the cell as with T cells (Chapter 8). Alternatively, multiple receptor–ligand interactions may be involved in NK cell activation by susceptible targets, even though individual receptor types can be shown to trigger lysis experimentally.

THE NKC GENE COMPLEX

Using RFLP analysis in mice, the Ly-49 and NKR-P1 families of genes were found to be closely linked (0.4cM) on mouse chromosome 6 — a region now called the NK gene complex (NKC). It has been estimated that this tight genetic linkage still represents a physical separation of about 500kb, suggesting that more genes involved in NK cell function may be found in this region, producing a clustering of functionally related genes as seen in the MHC (see Chapter 4). One such candidate would be the gene which has been shown to control susceptibility to cytomegalovirus infections in mice. Depletion of NK cells from mice bearing a resistant *Cmv-1* allele results in a marked increase in viral susceptibility, suggesting perhaps that the *Cmv-1* gene is part of the NKC that encodes an NK cell recognition molecule involved in targetting cytomegalovirus infected cells.

Antibody-dependent cellular cytotoxicity (ADCC)

Cells with cytotoxic potential that can bind antibody via Fc receptors (FcR) can mediate ADCC directed to antibody-coated target cells (*Fig. 15.3*). Unlike the other systems discussed above, this is a form of target cell recognition that is shared with granulocytes and macrophages, even though the type of FcR and mode of cytolytic attack may differ. In NK cells, FcR-mediated activation probably triggers the same cytolytic machinery as would be triggered if the target cell were recognized by the NK cell receptor complexes discussed above.

FcR specific for IgG are the major type responsible for the lymphocyte-mediated ADCC. Three distinct IgG-FcR glycoproteins have been characterized, termed FcγRI, II and III. FcγRI (CD64) is of high affinity and is the only one that can bind monomeric IgG. FcγRII (CD32) and III (CD16) are low affinity receptors that bind to the Fc regions of antibodies in immune complexes (see Chapter 2). Cytotoxic lymphocytes express only the CD16 molecule. CD16 exists in two distinct forms (CD16-1 and CD16-2) with identical extracellular amino acid sequence but encoded by separate genes. On neutrophils, CD16-1 is linked to the membrane via a glycosylphosphatidyl inositol (GPI) anchor and, although it can bind immune complexes, it does not appear to activate neutrophil effector function. The CD16-2 form expressed by NK cells, on the other hand, is a transmembrane molecule responsible for triggering ADCC. Both CD16 forms are initially made with transmembrane and cytoplasmic regions but in CD16-1 these are rapidly cleaved at amino acid 203 and replaced with the GPI anchor.

As with T and B cell receptors, CD16 expression and activation on NK cells requires its association with other polypeptide chains which form a signalling complex akin to CD3. Co-transfection experiments in COS-7 cells showed that co-expression of CD16-2 with either CD3ξ or FcεRIγ would lead to surface expression of CD16 complexed with the signalling molecule. Subsequent experiments revealed that CD3ξ is in fact made and used by NK cells in just this manner. Not surprisingly, therefore, triggering of ADCC activity in NK cells interacting with antibody-coated target cells involves similar early signal transduction pathways (including tyrosine phosphorylation and phospholipase C activation) to those initiated through the TCR in T cells and the FcεRI on mast cells.

KILLING — DELIVERY OF THE 'LETHAL HIT'

Following binding and recognition of a cell as a *bona fide* target, activation of the effector cell elicits a complex series of events ultimately leading to delivery of a lethal hit to the target. The nature of these events has been the subject of intense investigation but the current consensus is that most cytotoxic cells can use more than one cytotoxic mechanism, thus helping to ensure that the target cell is killed. The two major pathways involve either the release of lymphocyte granule cytotoxins or receptor-mediated signalling in the target cell.

Granule exocytosis

Studies with cloned, *in vitro* propagated human and murine Tc or human NK cells were instrumental in the initial examination of cytotoxic mechanisms. Membrane-bound cytoplasmic granules, which are characteristic features of NK cells, seen in peripheral blood as large granular lymphocytes, were found in a variety of cloned lymphocyte populations and their presence correlated with the cytotoxic capability of the cell. These granules, characteristic of many cytotoxic effector cells, have been classified into type 1 (dense) and type 2 (vesicular). Subsequently, granules isolated from Tc or NK cell clones (but not from Th) were shown to non-specifically lyse a variety of targets in a Ca^{2+}-dependent manner (*Fig. 15.4*). More recent evidence indicates that type 1 granules are responsible for this. In addition, $F(ab')_2$ fragments of antibodies raised against purified granules were able to block cell-mediated target cell killing. These observations, together with the finding that programming for lysis was Ca^{2+}-dependent, led to the hypothesis that granule exocytosis (a known Ca^{2+}-dependent mechanism) was intimately involved in delivery of the lethal hit.

Support for this model also came from morphological studies of effector cell clones in the process of killing a target cell (*Fig. 15.5*). Immediately following target cell binding (within a few seconds), the cytotoxic cell reorganizes its cytoplasmic constituents, using a kinesin 'motor' to reorientate the Golgi apparatus and granules so that they lie between the nucleus and the target cell contact point. Other cytoplasmic organelles, such as the microtubule organizing centre and associated cytoskeletal proteins, tubulin and actin, also become polarized within the cell. A broadening of the region of membrane contact with the specific target is also seen; this involves interdigitations of the two cell membranes to form a cleft which somewhat resembles a neurological synapse. Similar cytoplasmic reorganizations are also seen during Th cell activation by APCs, (see Chapter 8). Fusions of granules with the effector cell plasma membrane have been observed by electron microscopy and with high resolution cinematographic techniques. Thus this form of lethal hit delivery can be viewed as a polarized secretory process aimed at releasing cytotoxic mediators present in granules to the effector target cell interface. Together, the greatly increased area of surface contact between the cells and the polarization of the secretory process serve to optimize the efficiency of the lethal hit.

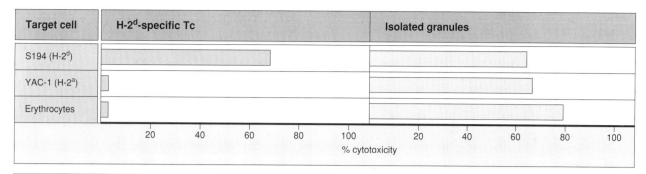

Target cell	H-2^d-specific Tc				Isolated granules				
S194 (H-2^d)									
YAC-1 (H-2^a)									
Erythrocytes									

% cytotoxicity

Fig. 15.4 Granules isolated from cytotoxic cells can non-specifically kill target cells. Killing of three target cell types (S194 and YAC-1 tumour cells and erythrocytes) by a murine H-2^d-specific alloreactive Tc and cytoplasmic granules, purified from these effector cells is shown. Whilst the intact effector cells kill only the specific target, isolated granules can kill all three targets. Similar results have been obtained with NK cell clones, where isolated granules can kill NK-resistant targets (not shown).

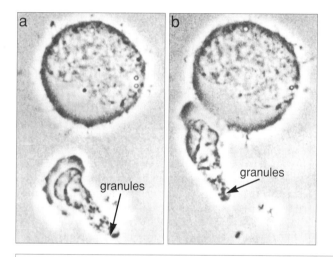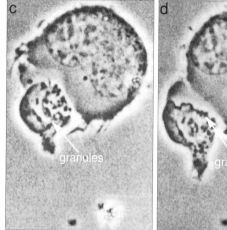

Fig. 15.5 Intracellular reorganizations during effector–target cell interaction. Early events in the interaction of Tc with specific targets were studied with high resolution cinematographic techniques. The figure shows four frames, taken at different times, of a Tc interacting with its target. The location of the granules within the effector cell is indicated in each case. Before contact with the target (a), the effector had granules located in a uropod at the rear and was seen to move randomly by extending pseudopods from the organelle-free, broad leading edge of the cell. Within 2 minutes of contacting the target (b), the Tc had begun to round up and initiate granule reorientation (c). After 10 minutes (d), the granules occupied a position in the zone of contact with the target, where they appear to be in the process of emptying their contents into the intercellular space between the two cells. Courtesy of Dr VH Engelhard.

Some evidence, largely from electron microscopic immunohistochemistry, has suggested that type 2 granules of Tc contain intra-granular vesicles that express surface TCR molecules which could allow directed targeting to the granule to the appropriate MHC–peptide-bearing target cell membranes. A model of granule exocytosis is presented in *Figure 15.6*.

Granule proteins

Granule proteins include perforin, a pore-forming molecule related to C9 and granule-associated enzymes, designated granzymes, fragmentin or cytotoxic cell proteases (CCPs). The relative importance of these components has been debated, although their actions appear complementary.

The incubation of target cells with cytotoxic lymphocytes (or type 1 granules isolated from them) in the presence of Ca^{2+} results in the formation of pores in the target cell membrane. This is mediated by the Ca^{2+}-dependent membrane binding and insertion and polymerization, of the 70kDa molecule perforin. Perforin is structurally related to the complement component C9 which also forms pores (see Chapter 13), although the organization of the two genes is dissimilar. Unlike C9, perforin pore formation does not seem to require other membrane proteins and, unlike the complement system, cell lysis is not inhibited by membrane cofactor protein (CD48) or homologous restriction factor (CD59). Initial studies with purified preparations of perforins suggested that these molecules alone could lyse target cells. However, more recent experiments have shown

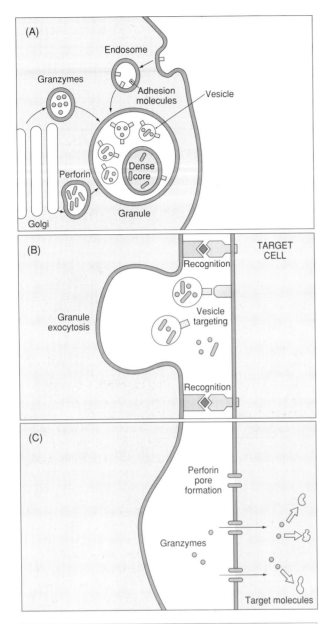

Fig. 15.6 A model of granule exocytosis. (A) The granules of cytotoxic cells consist of a dense core surrounded by vesicles. The organelle has features of lysosomes and secretory granules and has therefore been termed a granulosome. Granzymes and perforin are generated from different areas of the Golgi, relating to their glycosylation and are directed to the granule. The granule also connects with the endosomal system, so that adhesion molecules, including CD8, LFA-1 and the TCR, may be mounted on the surface of the dense core and vesicles. (B) After the cell engages its target (in this example via TCR–MHC–Ag recognition) the granule contents are released into the gap adjoining the target cell. Vesicles may be selectively targeted to the target cell, via their surface adhesion molecules. (C) Polymerization of perforin generates pores on the target cell, which may form channels to allow granzymes to access the cytoplasm of the target. Here they appear to act via endogenous molecules of the target cell.

that the perforin preparations were in fact contaminated with granule serine proteases (granzymes, discussed in some detail below) and that lysis requires both these granule components.

Perforin is constitutively expressed in NK cells, $\gamma\delta$ TCR T cells and in the CD11b$^+$ subset of CD8$^+$ T cells. It may be induced in other T cells by IL-2. The 5' elements on the perforin gene are distinct from those on other IL-2-inducible molecules and from those on the granzymes. Hence the granzyme components and perforin may be differentially regulated. Perforin acts by inserting into the target cell membrane and undergoing irreversible polymerization. Upon complete polymerization, approximately 20 molecules form the assembled membrane channel. These can allow the passage of large molecules and generate transient increases in intracellular free calcium. It is also thought that the perforin pores may allow other mediators to enter the target cell. The relative importance of perforin has been shown in perforin-knockout mice. These animals show poor ability to clear lymphocyte choriomeningitis virus, despite having normal numbers of lymphocytes and NK cells. Within the granules, perforin is thought to be held in an inactive state by chelation of Ca^{2+}, on calreticulin but how the cytotoxic cell protects itself from released perforin is not known.

The granzymes are a group of at least eight serine proteases, designated A–H (*Fig. 15.7*). They contribute towards cytotoxicity but are not essential — there is no correlation between cytotoxic potential and levels of expressed granzymes and cells lacking them can be fully cytotoxic. Stored granzymes have no enzymic activity due to the low pH of the granule, which rises immediately before release. After release granzymes are found co-localized with perforin, which has suggested that they act

Component	Specificity/Function	Expression
Granzyme A	Tryptase	All NK cells Some Tc cells Upregulated by IL-2
Granzyme B	Aspartase DNA degradation	
Granzyme C-H	?	
Perforin	Forms pores in membranes	Activated Tc cells and NK cells
Chondroitin sulphate Proteoglycans	? control of granzymes and perforin	?

Fig. 15.7 Granule components. Perforin and chondroitin sulphate are concentrated in the dense core of the granule and granzymes are known to co-localize with perforin. The cortex of the granule is at pH 5.5 and contains enzymes associated with lysosomes, including α-glycosidase, acid phosphatase and cathepsin-D.

synergistically. The granzymes are not by themselves toxic, which suggests they act on other components of the target cell or with other components of the granule. Granzymes A and B, in association with perforin, can induce DNA degradation and granzyme B is cytostatic for tumour targets. One candidate for this interaction is T cell intracellular antigen (TIA). When hydrolysed and activated by granzymes TIA induces DNA degradation in permeabilized cells.

An alternative radical suggestion is that the granzymes are important in freeing the cytotoxic cell from the target so that it may go on to find new targets.

Fas antigen

Since some cytotoxic T cell killing is independent of Ca^{2+}, it takes place in the absence of granule release. Hence, there is clearly another mechanism for target cell killing which does not involve granule proteins. It has been known that TNF can also kill target cells but over a longer period than taken by cytotoxic T cells. More recently a surface molecule called Fas has been identifed as the potential target of this action. Fas (also called APO-1) is a 48kDa member of the TNF receptor family. It has three extracellular domains and a cytoplasmic tail with homology to TNFR-p55 and another region identified as a 'death domain'. Crosslinking of Fas with antibody induces rapid apoptosis. The molecule is expressed on thymocytes, is lost on maturation and it appears again on mature lymphocytes. MRL-*lpr/lpr* mice lack Fas and their thymocytes are resistant to killing by anti-Fas antibody. There is a good case that Fas is important in the regulation of the size of lymphocyte populations. Since the anti-Fas antibody also induces liver necrosis *in vivo* it is a potential candidate for the target of cytotoxic T cells.

The Fas ligand has been identified from a cDNA expression library. It is a transmembrane protein of 278 amino acid residues homologous to TNF and more weakly to the ligands of CD27, CD30 and CD40. COS cells expressing the Fas ligand were efficient killers of targets expressing Fas. There is no cross-stimulation between the Fas system and TNF. The evidence is therefore accumulating for a family of ligands including the Fas ligand, CD30 ligand and TNF, which can induce apoptosis in selected groups of cells (*Fig. 15.8*). At present it appears that Fas is very important in killing mediated by CD4+ cytotoxic cells but is less important for CD8+ cells.

Target cell death — apoptosis

There are two distinct modes of death of nucleated cells: necrosis and apoptosis (*Fig. 15.9*). Necrosis occurs through an increase in the permeability of the cell membrane. An equilibration of ions across the membrane occurs and cytoplasmic macromolecules exert an unbalanced osmotic pressure so that water is taken up and nuclear chromatin is seen to flocculate. Initially these changes are reversible but they are rapidly followed by irreversible disruption of the integrity of the cell. This mode of cell death is elicited by complement-mediated attack and is also typical of pathological tissue damage,

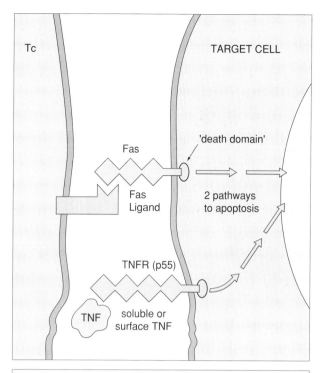

Fig. 15.8 The role of Fas in target cell killing. A ligand on the cytotoxic cell engages Fas on the target. Fas consists of three NGF-receptor family domains, homologous to those in the TNF receptors. Activation of Fas or the TNF receptor can lead to cell death but via different pathways — cell killing by Fas is much more rapid.

as seen with ischaemia and physically or chemically induced death. Necrotic cell death releases cellular components which trigger inflammatory responses. In contrast, apoptosis is an actively regulated process of cell suicide which does not trigger inflammation — a critical feature which allows regulated cell death to play an important role in physiology as well as pathology. For example, apoptosis is involved in the organized removal of cells and tissues, without loss of architecture or scarring, such as the tissue remodelling events of embryological development; apoptosis is also called programmed cell death in processes such as this. It is also the mechanism responsible for the negative selection of immature thymocytes and B cells which occurs in the thymus and germinal centres, respectively (see Chapter 6). Killing by Tc, NK cells or ADCC, whether via granule exocytosis or signalling (Fas-type) mechanisms, ultimately involves the activation of apoptosis in target cells. However, it is clear that this requires signalling to the target cell (e.g. via Fas), since perforin alone or in association with granule enzymes does not induce apoptosis (*Fig. 15.10*).

A cell undergoing apoptosis *in vitro* is seen to round up and shrink in size, with the endoplasmic reticulum dilating and forming vesicles which often fuse with the plasma membrane. This gives a characteristic 'bubbling' appearance in electron micrographs. Unlike the situation

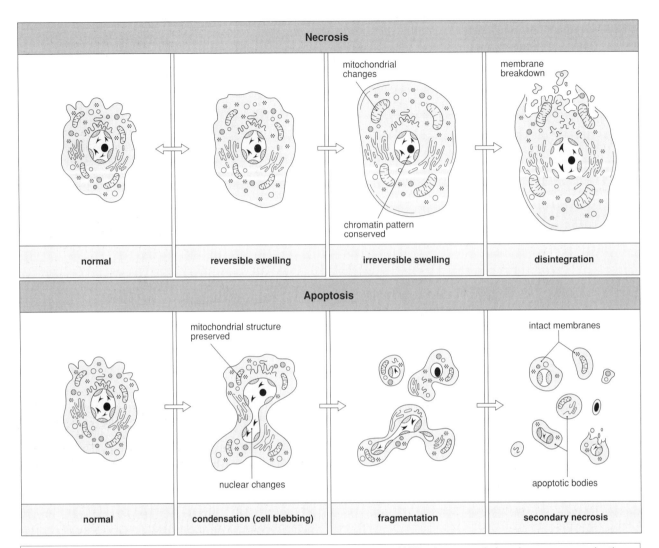

Fig. 15.9 Two mechanisms of cell death, necrosis and apoptosis. Contrasting morphological features of necrosis and apoptosis are illustrated. Both MHC-restricted and unrestricted killing by cytotoxic lymphocytes occurs by the mechanism of apoptosis. In contrast complement-mediated killing results in necrosis.

in necrosis, the chromatin forms dense aggregates and the nuclear membrane invaginates. Convolution of the plasma membrane leads to the cell separating into small membrane-bound segments called 'apoptotic bodies', which retain the ability to exclude vital dyes (such as trypan blue) although the cell is clearly dead. Experimentally, the development of apoptotic bodies appears as blebbing of the cell surface or 'zeiosis'. This maintenance of membrane integrity prevents the release of cytoplasmic constituents and, therefore, the activation of potentially damaging inflammatory responses. However, apoptotic bodies and apoptosing cells are readily phagocytosed by professional phagocytic cells, such as the macrophage, or by other local tissue cells.

A distinctive early feature of apoptosis in many cells is the rapid degradation of chromatin into discrete fragments. These consist of multiples of about 200 base pairs of DNA and produce a ladder-like series of bands on agarose gel electrophoresis. This pattern of cleavage is due to the vulnerability of the DNA between nucleosomes to degradation by endonucleases. In necrosis, such DNA degradation is found only at a late stage. *In vitro* studies of Tc-mediated lysis of the same target cells, even in the presence of added DNAse, have failed to elicit such DNA degradation.

Much research has been carried out on the intracellular mechanisms which transduce the signal for apoptosis. During lymphocyte development, apoptosis may follow activation and involves various kinases and phosphatases. In this case the synthesis of new proteins is required but this is not so with cytotoxicity. Hence apoptosis is an end state of the cell, which may be reached by several pathways. All cells must have available the pathway which allows them to be killed by cytotoxic cells but they potentially have other pathways, depending on their cell type and activation state. Clearly, once the decision is taken to destroy a virally infected target cell, it is advantageous that it is killed as quickly as possible.

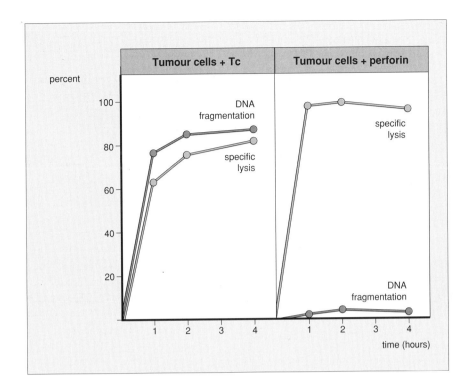

Fig. 15.10 Comparison of target cell killing by Tc and purified perforin. R1.1 tumour cells were incubated with ^{125}I-deoxyuridine (to label DNA) and with ^{51}Cr (to label the cytoplasm). These target cells were allowed to interact with either specific Tc or purified perforin for different amounts of times, before assessing the amount of cell lysis (^{51}Cr release) and DNA degradation (^{125}I release). Intact Tc elicited both cellular lysis and DNA degradation, whereas perforin was able to elicit only lysis. Based on data from Duke *et al*, 1989.

NON-LYMPHOID CYTOTOXIC EFFECTORS

A number of non-lymphoid cells may be cytotoxic to other cells or invading microorganisms, such as bacteria or parasites. Cytotoxicity may may be triggered specifically to a target by ADCC or may involve a range of non-specifically toxic mediators. For example, macrophages and neutrophils both express FcγRI and FcγRII which allows them to mediate killing of tumours by ADCC. In the case of macrophages the effect may be via TNF, since killing is slower than that effected by Tc cells. Both neutrophils and macrophages can use a variety of non-specific cytotoxic mechanisms. These include the production of reactive oxygen intermediates, toxic oxidants and NO, as well as the secreted molecules such as neutrophil defensins, lysosomal enzymes and cytostatic proteins. These have been detailed in Chapter 14.

The other major cell type found in inflammatory lesions is the eosinophil, which is discussed in more depth below. *Figure 15.11* compares the characteristic features of macrophages, neutrophils and eosinophils.

Eosinophils

Eosinophils are derived from bone marrow progenitor cells distinct from the precursors of neutrophils and macrophages. Their differentiation and accumulation in tissues is critically dependent on IL-5, although IL-3 and GM-CSF also contribute. Mature eosinophils are characterized by their granules, which have a crystalloid core which binds the dye eosin. Mature cells express a number of surface markers, none of which are specific to eosinophils. However, they can be distinguished from neutrophils by their expression of CD9, since neutrophils do not express CD9.

Generally, eosinophils are only weakly phagocytic; they ingest some bacteria following activation but are less efficient

	Neutrophils	Eosinophils	Macrophages
Characteristic surface markers	CD16-1$^+$ (CD9$^-$) CD11b$^+$, CD32$^+$ CD66$^+$, CD35$^+$	CD9$^+$ (CD16$^-$) CD11b$^+$, CD32$^+$ CD35$^+$, Fc$_\epsilon$RII$^+$ (CD23)	CD16$^+$, CD32$^+$ CD35$^+$, CD68$^+$ CD11b$^+$
Phagocytic activity	+++	+	+++
Respiratory burst	+++	+++	+++
Enzymes	collagenase elastase myeloperoxidase —	collagenase — eosinophil peroxidase lysophospholipase	collagenase elastase myeloperoxidase —
Killing mechanisms	ADCC respiratory burst defensins	ADCC respiratory burst cationic proteins (MBP, ECP, EDN)	ADCC respiratory burst TNF

Fig. 15.11 Characteristics of neutrophils, eosinophils and macrophages.

than neutrophils at intracellular killing. Their major function appears to be the secretion of various toxic granule constituents, following activation. They are therefore effective for the extracellular killing of microorganisms, particularly large parasites such as schistosomes.

MAJOR BASIC PROTEIN (MBP)

MBP is a major component of eosinophil granules, forming the crystalloid core. Prior to secretion the crystals appear to solubilize. MBP is approximately 11kDa with 117 amino acids. It has been shown to damage, and sometimes kill, parasites but also damages host tissue cells. Because it is highly cationic, some of its protective effects may be due to scavenging negative ions. MBP is also present in granules of other granulocytes but at much lower levels.

EOSINOPHIL CATIONIC PROTEIN (ECP)

ECP is an eosinophil-specific toxin which is very potent at killing many parasites, particularly the schistosomulae of *S. mansoni* — up to 10 times more potent than MBP. The molecule is a ribonuclease although it is not thought to mediate its effects in this way. It is a zinc-containing glycoprotein, synthesized as 22kDa precursors which are processed to 18–19kDa forms for storage. Because of its high charge ECP binds avidly to negatively charged surfaces. It is possible that it forms membrane channels, which allow other mediators access to the target organism.

Eosinophil derived neurotoxin (EDN, also previously called EPX) is also a ribonuclease but with strong neurotoxic activity.

EOSINOPHIL PEROXIDASE (EPO)

EPO is a highly cationic heterodimeric 71–77kDa haemoprotein, consisting of a glycosylated heavy chain (50–58kDa) and a non-glycosylated light chain (14–15kDa). It is distinct from the myeloperoxidase of neutrophils and macrophages. In the presence of H_2O_2, also produced by eosinophils, EPO will oxidize a variety of substrates, including halide ions to produce hypohalite. This may represent the eosinophils most potent killing mechanism for some parasites.

Other mediators

Eosinophils release large amounts of phosphatases following activation, as well as arylsulphatase B and histaminase. Although they can produce collagenase, they differ from neutrophils in not making elastase nor other neutral proteases. They have a high capacity to develop a respiratory burst, generating reactive oxygen intermediates and also produce leukotrienes and other arachidonic acid metabolites. Finally, bipyramidal crystals are often found at sites of eosinophil degranulation. These Charcot–Leyden crystals are composed of lysophospholipase, a myristilated single chain protein containing low levels of carbohydrate. The function of released phospholipase is not known.

Eosinophil activation

Degranulation of eosinophils can be triggered in a number of ways. Binding to IgG-coated parasites via surface FcγRII triggers release of some mediators, including ECP but not EPO. In contrast, triggering via FcεRII leads to the release of EPO but not ECP. Parasite killing may involve contact-dependent degranulation or may simply require deposition of toxins within the local tissue. Degranulation may also be triggered directly *in vitro* by several cytokines, including IL-3, IL-5, GM-CSF, TNF, IFNβ and platelet activating factor (PAF). These mediators also enhance ADCC-mediated degranulation.

Eosinophils are prominent in the inflammatory lesions of a number of diseases, particularly atopic disorders of the gut, skin and respiratory tract, where they are often closely associated with fibrotic reactions. Examples are atopic excema, asthma and inflammatory bowel disease. Although eosinophils may play some regulatory role in these conditions, such as inactivating histamine, their toxic products and cytotoxic mechanisms are a major cause of the tissue damage. For example, in asthma, eosinophil granule proteins are detectable in the blood and lungs following asthmatic attacks. MBP can kill some pneumocytes and tracheal epithelial cells while EPO kills type II pneumocytes. MBP can also induce mast cells to secrete histamine thus exacerbating allergic inflammation.

SUMMARY

Cytotoxicity can be mediated by a number of cell types, including cytotoxic T cells, NK cells and macrophages. The majority of Tc cells express CD8, use an αβ TCR and recognize peptide associated with class I MHC molecules. CD4+, MHC class II-restricted cytotoxic T cells are less prevalent but may come to dominate the cytotoxic response against some viral infection. T cells using the γδ TCR may also be cytotoxic but they are not restricted by conventional polymorphic MHC molecules. NK cells are directed by both positive and negative interactions with their targets. MHC class I delivers a negative signal which may be recognized by Ly-49 in the mouse, while the positive signal is probably recognized by NK1.1. Genes for the receptors of NK cells are apparently clustered in a single region of the genome termed the NKC gene complex. Non-specific lymphokine-activated killers (LAKs) can be induced from both Tc and NK cells following culture with IL-2.

Killing by cytotoxic lymphocytes is mediated by the selective delivery of a lethal hit to the target cell. Several cytotoxic mechanisms may be deployed but the relative importance of each mechanism depends on the cytotoxic cell and the target. In each case, the cytotoxic cell is protected against its own killing mechanisms and can go on to kill new targets.

The granules of cytotoxic lymphoid cells contain perforin and granule enzymes (granzymes). Upon activation, the cytoskeleton of the cytotoxic cell rearranges and the granules are reorientated towards the target before exocytosis. Perforin polymerizes onto the target cell membrane to create holes, resembling the MAC of the complement system. The function of the granzymes is only partly determined. They may enter the target cell via perforin pores to activate endogenous killing mechanisms. Cytotoxic lymphoid cells can also induce rapid apoptosis in target cells. This may be mediated by the Fas molecule which resembles the TNF receptor. Both the Fas ligand and TNF are cytotoxic, although their time courses of action differ. Apoptosis is characterized by pre-lytic degradation of DNA mediated by endogenous endonucleases. It is an end process for cells and may be induced by several pathways.

Macrophages, neutrophils and eosinophils can also kill various target cells either non-specifically through the release of mediators such as TNF or specifically by ADCC. However, the actions of these cells are more commonly directed against invading microorganisms and parasites. Eosinophils contain a number of potent toxic molecules, localized in their specific granules which may be released by exocytosis following contact with a target pathogen. These molecules are effective against many large multicellular parasites but can also cause tissue damage in inflammatory diseases, such as asthma, where eosinophil infiltration is prominent.

FURTHER READING

Berke G. The binding and lysis of target cells by cytotoxic lymphocytes. *Ann Rev Immunol* 1994, **12**:735.

Bleackle RC, Lobe CG, Duggan B, Ehrman N, Fregeau C, Meier M, Letellier M, Havele C, Shaw J, Paetkau V. The isolation of a family of serine protease genes expressed in activated cytotoxic T lymphocytes. *Immunol Rev* 1988, **103**:5.

Duke RC, Persechini PM, Chang S, Liu C-C, Cohen JJ, Young JD-E. Purified perforin induces target cell lysis but not DNA fragmentation. *J Exp Med* 1989, **170**:1451.

Govaerts A. Cellular antibodies in kidney homotransplantation. *J Immunol* 1960, **85**:516.

Hudig D, Ewoldt GR, Woodard SL. Proteases and lymphocyte cytotoxic killing mechanisms. *Curr Opin Immunol* 1993 **5**:90.

Jenne DE, Schopp J. Granzymes, a family of serine proteases released from granules of cytolytic T lymphocytes upon T cell receptor stimulation. *Immunol Rev* 1988, **103**:53.

Klebanoff SJ, Agosti JM, Jörg A, Waltersdorf AM. Comparative toxicity of the horse eosinophil peroxidase H_2O_2 halide system and granule basic proteins. *J Immunol* 1989, **143**:239.

Kupfer A, Singer S, Dennert G. On the mechanism of unidirectional killing in mixtures of two cytotoxic T lymphocytes. Unidirectional polarization of cytoplasmic organellles and membrane-associated cytoskeleton in the effector cell. *J Exp Med* 1986, **163**:489.

Liu C-C, Detmers PA, Jiang S, Young JD-E. Identification and characterization of a membrane-bound cytotoxin of murine cytolytic lymphocytes that is related to tumour necrosis factor. *Proc Natl Acad Sci USA* 1989, **86**:3286.

Ogasawar J, Watanabe-Fukunaga R, Adachi M, Matsuzawa A, Kasugai T, Kitamura Y, Itoh N, Suda T, Nagata S. Lethal effect of the anti-Fas antibody in mice. *Nature* 1993, **364**:806.

Ostergard HL, Clark WR. Evidence for multiple pathways used by cytotoxic T lymphocytes. *J Immunol* 1989, **143**:2120.

Podack ER, Hengartner H, Lichtenheld MG. A central role for perforin in cytolysis? *Ann Rev Immunol* 1991, **9**:129.

Rouvier E, Luciani MF, Golstein P. Fas involvement in Ca^{2+}-independent T cell-mediated cytotoxicity. *J Exp Med* 1993, **177**:195.

Smyth MJ, Ortaldo JR. Mechanisms of cytotoxicity used by human peripheral blood CD4+ and CD8+ T cell subsets: the role of granule exocytosis. *J Immunol* 1993, **151**:740.

Squier MKT, Cohen JJ. Cell-mediated cytotoxic mechanisms. *Curr Opin Immunol* 1994, **6**:447.

Suda T, Takahashi T, Golstein P, Nagata S. Molecular cloning and expression of the Fas ligand, a novel member of the tumour necrosis receptor family. *Cell* 1993, **75**:1169.

Tartaglia LA, Ayers TM, Wong GHW, Goeddel DV. A novel domain within the 55kDa TNF receptor signals cell death. *Cell* 1993, **74**:845.

Thiele DL, Lipsky PE. The role of cell surface recognition structures on human natural killer cells in the initiation of MHC-unrestricted 'promiscuous' killing. *Immunol Today* 1989, **10**:375.

Trapani JA, Kwon BS, Kozak CA, Chintamaneni C, Young JD-E, Dupont B. Genomic organization of the mouse pore-forming protein perforin gene and localization to chromosome 10. Similarities to and differences from C9. *J Exp Med* 1990, **171**:545.

Watanabe-Fukunga R, Brannan CI, Copeland NG, Jenkins NA, Nagata S. Lymphoproliferation disorder in mice explained by defects in Fas antigen that mediates apoptosis. *Nature* 1992, **356**:314.

Yanelli JR, Sullivan JA, Mandell GL, Engelhard VH. Reorientation and fusion of cytotoxic T cell granules after interaction with target cells as determined by high resolution cinematography. *J Immunol* 1986, **136**:377.

Yokoyama WM, Seaman WA. The Ly-49 and NKR-P1 gene families encoding lectin-like receptors on natural killer cells: the NK gene complex. *Ann Rev Immunol* 1993, **11**:613.

16 Immune Response to Pathogens

Since the immune system has evolved to recognize and destroy pathogens, an understanding of the system can only be complete when considered in relation to the pathogens which have evolved along side it. The pathogens we see today are those which can proliferate in spite of immunological defences and likewise natural selection has shaped the immune system so that it can cope with a wide variety of pathogens but is particularly suited to handle those now prevalent. When a new pathogen evolves, it typically causes a high level of mortality; the immune system of the host population is reshaped to select resistant individuals and the disease becomes endemic or dies out. This process occurs over centuries and recorded human history gives examples such as *Pasteurella pestis* and *Mycobacterium tuberculosis* which have followed this pattern. If we did not have our current knowledge of viruses and immunology, the recently evolved AIDS viruses might well follow a similar epidemiological time-course.

Within an individual, and on a much shorter time-scale, pathogens compete with each other and with lymphocytes and effector cells to complete their cycle of infection. It is clear that pathogens have affected both the overall structure of the immune system, as determined in the germline, as well as its day to day activity.

In comparison with the immune response to simple antigens, the reactions which occur to pathogenic microorganisms are extremely complex. Even the simplest viruses express several different antigens and eukaryotic parasites can have several hundred different potential antigens on their surface. Each of these molecules contains several distinct epitopes, sometimes repeated, as in the case of bacterial carbohydrates, and sometimes distinct. Moreover, antigens of microorganisms vary considerably in their accessibility to cells of the immune system. Antigens which normally occur inside a pathogen may become accessible only when the pathogen or an infected cell is killed. Even antigens expressed at the cell surface may present only a limited range of their potential epitopes for antibody binding, depending on their orientation in the membrane. Protective structures, such as bacterial capsules, further limit the effective recognition of epitopes.

It is clear that the immune response to each individual pathogen is a major area of study in its own right. Nevertheless, this chapter aims to bring together some of the unifying principles governing the development of antibody and cell-mediated immune responses to pathogens, by reference to particular examples. A distinction should be drawn at this stage between the overall composition of the immune response, those components of it which are important in the resolution of infection and the components which are responsible for the prevention of reinfection. In many cases, particular

elements of the immune response are critically important; for example, cell-mediated immunity in leprosy. Even when considering a particular effector system, the response directed against some antigens is often much more effective than the responses to others. Sometimes the response may be only marginally beneficial, or even positively detrimental. Detrimental immune responses may be broadly divided into two categories: where the response prevents other elements of the immune system from engaging the pathogen effectively, and where the response induces greater damage to the host than is caused by the organism itself — autoimmunity or hypersensitivity. In other words, immune responses to particular microbial antigens have different degrees of relevance to anti-microbial immunity, depending on the nature of the organism, its pathogenicity and the nature of the immune response it initiates.

Another twist to the story is provided by the organisms themselves. Apart from their basic antigenic complexity, they often deploy strategies to avoid immune recognition or evade immune effector systems. Pathogens which have a stable antigenic structure may avoid immune recognition entirely (e.g. latent *Herpes zoster*) or may localize in areas which are not subject to immune surveillance (e.g. superficial fungi) or they may rely on there being a sufficiently large population of non-immune individuals to allow continuous cycles of acute infection in different subjects (e.g. measles). Many pathogens, however, do not have antigenically stable structures: this is seen as variation in some of the critical surface antigens. Sometimes, variants will arise which replace the previous variant strain globally (e.g. influenza); sometimes, individual microorganisms have the capacity to switch their surface antigens during their own life cycle within a single host (e.g. African trypanosomes). Selective pressure from the host immune system favours modulation of the parasites' surface antigens to allow survival in the host. Consequently, the continuous battle between microorganisms and the immune systems of the host population provides the driving force for evolution of the parasites and the selective pressure for improvement of the immune system. Theoretically, the rapid evolution rate of microorganisms should allow them to evolve quickly in order to evade the body's defences but the enormous flexibility of the immune system, intrinsic in the T cell and B cell antigen receptors, prevents them from gaining the upper hand in most cases.

The strategies of avoiding immune effector mechanisms are as diverse as the pathogens themselves. They include anti-chemotactic agents, anti-phagocytic capsules, resistance to phagocyte microbicidal systems, the release of enzymes and decoy antigens and subversion of the immune system by cytokine analogues or superantigens.

16.1

INTRACELLULAR AND EXTRACELLULAR PATHOGENS

All viruses and many bacteria and protozoa have phases during their life cycle in which they lie dormant or replicate inside host cells and different immune effector systems act against these different stages in the life cycle. In general, systems which act on the extracellular forms are most effective at preventing spread of the pathogen or reinfection, whereas those acting on intracellular forms are important in destroying the source of the infection. For this reason strain-specific antibody is critical in preventing reinfection with influenza virus, even in individuals with effective Tc populations which are capable of destroying infected cells. This distinction between the roles of different effector systems in preventing disease is not so clear cut when one considers bacteria and protozoa, which do not infect cells.

The primary effectors against extracellular pathogens are antibody and complement. Binding of antibody to receptors on the pathogen can prevent it from attaching to its target cell; typical examples are antibodies to the haemagglutinin of influenza or to the gp120 of HIV which binds to CD4 on the target Th cell. Antibody alone, or more effectively in association with complement, opsonizes pathogens for uptake by phagocytes expressing Fc receptors and complement receptors CR1 and CR3. Usually this will lead to intracellular destruction of the pathogen (Chapter 14) but if the phagocyte is unable to destroy it and is a facultative host cell, then antibody may actually promote the spread of infection. Such an eventuality, however, depends on the dynamic balance between the actions of the humoral and cell-mediated immune responses. While the complement lytic pathway is of importance against some extracellular bacteria, it can also act on certain extracellular enveloped viruses, causing membrane disassembly.

Two strategies are available for dealing with intracellular pathogens: either the infected cell directly controls the infection or it is itself destroyed. Various cytokines can enhance the microbicidal capacities of infected cells. Interferons are particularly important in the earliest stages of viral infections, limiting the speed of viral replication and spread by inducing anti-viral proteins. Once the immune system has become activated MHC-mediated presentation of intracellular peptides allows cells to interact with T cells, thereby initiating cytokine release or rendering the cells susceptible to T cell-mediated cytotoxicity. These systems allow recognition of infected cells via peptide fragments derived from the intracellular microbial antigens but, sometimes, intracellular pathogens may express native proteins at the surface of their host cells, making them susceptible to antibody, complement and K cell-mediated attack. For example, erythrocytes parasitized by *P. falciparum* express adhesion proteins at the cell surface which allow them to bind to cerebral endothelium and which are recognized by antibody. Similarly enveloped viruses insert their own (native) proteins into the host cell membrane before budding out.

IMMUNE RECOGNITION OF PATHOGENS

Critical sites

Immune responses directed towards some antigens on a pathogen are more effective than the responses to others in bringing about destruction of the pathogen. Such antigens are termed 'critical sites'. This concept is well illustrated when considering viruses. Viruses have both internal and external protein antigens. The internal antigens are most often associated with the viral nucleic acid, or form part of the internal structure of the virus; some are viral proteins required for the initiation of the infective cycle within the cell (e.g. nucleic acid polymerases). The external antigens include the outer coat or envelope proteins and particularly important are the proteins required for attachment to the host cell (*Fig. 16.1*).

Since attachment to the host cell is the first step in the viral replicative cycle, antibodies directed towards these proteins are most effective in preventing transmission of the virus to new cells. Different viruses attach to their target cells via different surface molecules. For example, the influenza A virus attaches to a number of cell types via the haemagglutinin molecule which is inserted in its envelope. Antibodies directed towards the haemagglutinin are most effective at preventing infection of cells and in preventing reinfection of an individual by the same strain of influenza. In comparison, antibodies to the neuraminidase which is also present in the envelope are less effective in neutralizing viral infectivity and antibodies to the internal M protein are virtually ineffective. For the same reason, the haemagglutinin is most subject to variation in different strains of influenza, the neuraminidase less so and the M protein not at all.

Viruses

ANTIBODY RESPONSES

It is possible to locate the precise antibody binding sites on many viral antigens by a variety of techniques. A direct approach to this problem is to carry out epitope mapping using overlapping peptides of a viral antigen and sera from immune individuals. *Figure 16.2* demonstrates this technique applied to the identification of epitopes of hepatitis delta virus (a defective RNA virus which depends on hepatitis B for some functions). However, there are limitations with this technique: it fails to identify conformational determinants and to distinguish antibodies to critical antigens. For example, although 11 antigenic regions have been identified on the external gD protein of *Herpes simplex*, by monoclonal antibodies, only four of these and the C-terminus have continuous epitopes.

An alternative approach is to use antibodies to select for resistant variant viruses and then to identify which epitopes these antibodies recognize. This is illustrated with respect to human rhinovirus 14. This cold virus is a member of the picornaviruses, which include the causative viruses of polio and foot and mouth disease (FMDV). The structure of these viruses is relatively simple. They consist of a protein capsid containing a strand of RNA associated with an internal protein. Rhinovirus 14 (HRV) has 60 protomers, each consisting of only four proteins: VP1, VP2, VP3 and VP4. VP2 and VP4 are generated by the cleavage of a larger polypeptide, VP0, at the time of virion assembly. VP4 is

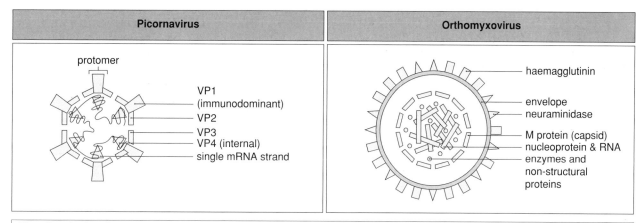

Picornavirus	Orthomyxovirus

Fig. 16.1 Antigenic structure of viruses. The antigens of an enveloped and a non-enveloped virus are illustrated diagrammatically. Picornaviruses have a capsid consisting of only four proteins, VP1–VP4, arranged as 60 protomers, containing a single RNA strand. Neutralizing antibodies bind to the external proteins, particularly VP1, while VP4 which is associated with the RNA is not normally accessible to antibody. Orthomyxoviruses (here exemplified by influenza A) have a core containing nucleocapsid (associated with RNA) and containing several non-structural proteins. This is enclosed in a capsid consisting of the M protein which is in turn surrounded by an envelope derived from the host cell plasma membrane. The envelope contains two viral proteins, the haemagglutinin and neuraminidase. Neutralizing antibodies recognize epitopes on the haemagglutinin, although antibody to the neuraminidase can also contribute to immunity.

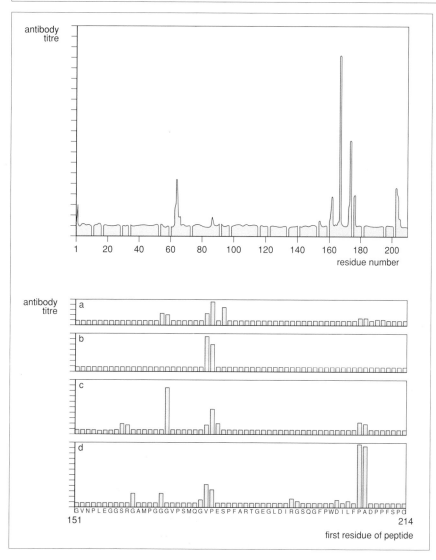

Fig. 16.2 Identification of antigenic regions on hepatitis delta virus antigen. Overlapping hexapeptides, based on the primary sequence of the hepatitis delta virus antigen, were synthesized for use as a solid phase antigen in an enzyme immunoassay. The peptides were reacted with the serum from an individual with high titre antibody to the antigen and reactivity to each peptide measured (top). The antigenic profile shows a region around residue 65 and another between 160 and 205 which react with antibodies. Analysis of the reactivity of four different sera to peptides between residues 151–214 shows that they all react to this region but the precise residues which form the epitopes vary between individuals (bottom). Data from Wang *et al*, 1990.

associated with the RNA on the inside of the capsid and is therefore normally inaccessible to antibody and may be considered a non-critical antigen (*Fig. 16.1*). When cultured with various monoclonal antibodies, mutants arose which survived despite the antibody, thus identifying critical epitopes. Two of these are on VP1, one on VP2 and one on VP3. As might be anticipated from its internal position in

the virion, these neutralizing antibodies do not bind VP4. When the location of the epitopes is seen in relation to the overall virion structure it is immediately apparent that each of the epitopes is on the outside of the capsid. None faces the RNA core (*Fig. 16.3*). Of the two sites on VP1, one of them comprises a single peptide loop, whereas the other depends on two adjoining segments of β-sheet. One can

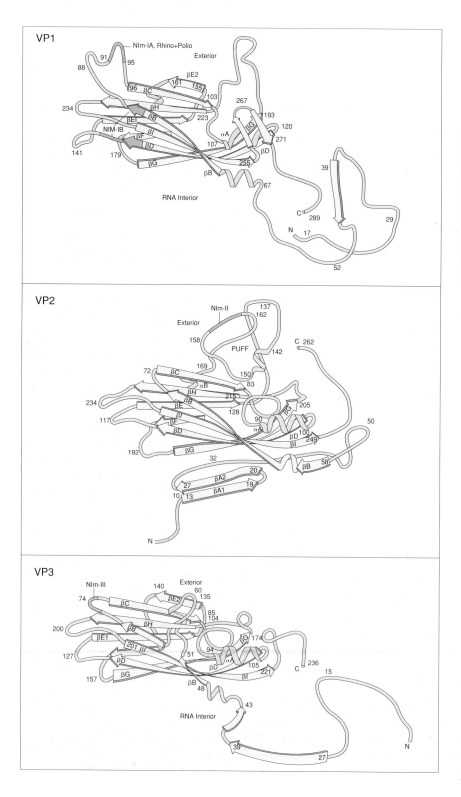

Fig. 16.3 Identification of epitopes on HRV14. The location of epitopes on the three capsid proteins of human rhinovirus 14 is shown. The epitopes referred to as NIm-1A, NIm-1B etc. were identified by the technique of antibody-induced selection of mutants (Rossman *et al*, 1985). Polioviruses have an epitope in an analogous position to NIm-IA, while the neutralizing antibody to foot and mouth disease virus (FMDV) binds elsewhere. Note that each of the epitopes is on an exposed loop on the outside of the virus.

compare which parts of VP1 form epitopes on different picornaviruses, since the overall structure of this protein is very similar for different viruses. Neutralizing antibodies to poliovirus are similar to the anti-HRV antibodies, since they bind to a site around position 93. It is notable that this region forms a prominent external loop of residues in both HRV and polio. By contrast, FMDV lacks the external loop around position 93. Antibodies to the immunodominant determinant of FMDV-VP1 bind to a different external loop corresponding to position 210 on HRV and these antibodies do not neutralize FMDV. Another feature of HRV 14 is interesting. Although there are 60 protomers in the capsid and a corresponding number of binding sites for the target cell, as few as four immunoglobulin molecules can neutralize a virion, suggesting that antibodies do not need to coat the virus completely to prevent infectivity. Either the few antibodies are sufficient to interfere sterically with the viral life cycle, or they can recruit other immune effector systems to destroy the virus. The second possibility appears more likely, since 10–60 times as many Fab antibodies as intact antibody are needed to neutralize the virus.

It is also clear that regions which are antigenic in one species or strain are not necessarily so in another. Relative levels of antibodies against different epitopes are also under Ir gene control, an effect seen in the antibody response to certain epitopes on the measles haemagglutinin, where HLA-Dw2 is associated with high titre responses and HLA-Dw1 with lower titres. In this respect control of the response to viral antigens is similar to that of other antigens.

Theoretically, viruses must retain some constant features on their receptor molecules to allow them to interact with target molecules on the host cell surface; antibodies to these sites should neutralize different strains of a virus. In practice however, the immune response frequently generates strain-specific antibodies to mutable external loops of viruses. It is possible that this is an evolutionary adaptation of viruses allowing them to present highly immunogenic, but mutable, sites for antibody binding. An alternative explanation is that the viruses attach to the cell surface molecules in similar ways to the physiological ligand. Consequently, an antibody directed to the attachment site on the virus might also bind to the physiological ligand and hence not be present due to deletion of self-reactive B cells.

T CELL RECOGNITION OF VIRAL POLYPEPTIDES

Viral peptides have been used extensively to examine how MHC molecules bind and select antigenic peptides. Indeed, the first indication that internal proteins were effectively presented at the cell surface was seen in studies of influenza A, which showed that during a normal infection more cytotoxic T cell clones were generated to the internal matrix (37%) and nucleoprotein antigens (9%) than to the external haemagglutinin (9%). Even mutant membrane antigens such as haemagglutinin lacking a signal sequence are still effectively presented at the cell surface in association with class I molecules of the correct haplotype. These data imply that cytotoxic T cells recognize fragments of any available viral antigen which can associate internally with a class I molecule and be transported to the target cell surface, regardless of the normal situation of the protein. In related experiments, measles

virus matrix protein or nucleoprotein genes were transfected into fibroblasts along with the relevant HLA-DR gene, rendering them susceptible to antigen-specific class II-restricted cytotoxic T cells. This indicates that peptides from different viruses can associate with either class I or class II molecules.

The area of an antigen which is recognized by a T cell can be identified using a series of overlapping peptides which are presented to T cells isolated following immunization with the native antigen — a process analogous to peptide epitope mapping for antibodies. This approach is illustrated in *Figure 16.4* for the haemagglutinin of measles virus. It demonstrates that strains with different MHC haplotype recognize distinct areas of the molecule, but it is also found that strains which respond poorly to the intact antigen can produce proliferative responses to peptides if they are immunized with them directly. Hence, synthetic peptides often do not accurately reflect the spectrum of peptides produced during normal cellular degradation or transport processes. A similar conclusion can be made for presentation by MHC class I molecules. For example, one Tc clone which recognized a matrix protein peptide in association with HLA-Aw69 or HLA-A2 failed to recognize naturally infected cells of the Aw69 haplotype, although they killed infected HLA-A2 cells. This shows that the way in which viral antigens are processed is as important as the MHC molecules available to present them.

The areas of an antigen recognized by T cells differ considerably from those recognized by antibodies. While B cell epitopes are on the most exposed regions of the antigen in areas most subject to variation between viral strains, T cell epitopes are distributed throughout the molecule. Their precise location depends on the MHC haplotype which presents them (*Fig. 16.5*). Moreover, for influenza A the determinants recognized by Tc cells do not usually vary between viral strains.

Presentation of viral peptides follows the general rules of MHC-mediated peptide binding. The cleft on class II molecules accommodates longer peptides than class I molecules (see *Colour figures*). Examination of the structures of viral antigenic peptides occupying the binding site on the same class I molecule (HLA-A2) showed that whereas the anchor residues at P1, P2 and P9 were effectively fixed the orientation of the residues in the centre of the peptides varies greatly, giving the T cells a highly variable area to recognize, where the structure of the MHC-Ag depends mostly on the peptide.

It is interesting that T cells specific for one viral antigen can help B cells specific for another. For example, T cells specific for the M protein can help B cells specific for HA, so that the relative lack of HA-specific T cells may not limit the level of help delivered to HA-specific B cells. This type of help would be difficult to understand, in terms of conventional antigen presentation, where a B cell presents a fragment of an antigen it has specifically endocytosed via its surface Ig. But if an HA-specific B cell takes up intact virus via its surface antibody and then processes it, potentially it will be able to present all of the viral antigens to T cells. Consequently, it may receive help from MHC-restricted Th cells specific for any of the viral antigens — not just from Th cells specific for the haemagglutinin. This is sometimes referred to as intermolecular help.

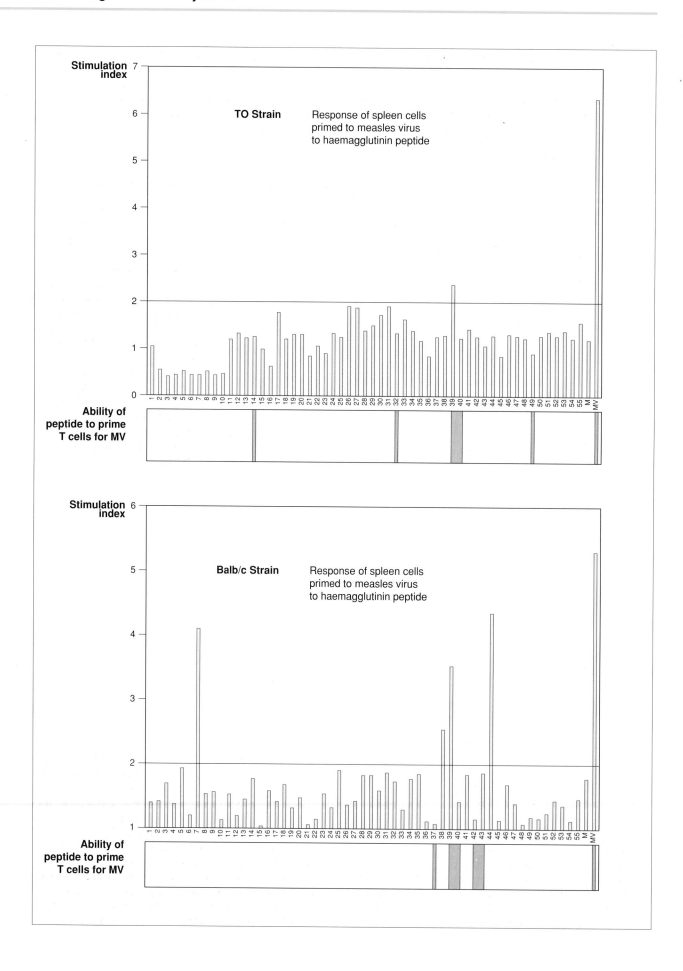

◁

Fig. 16.4 T cell antigenic sites on measles haemagglutinin. Overlapping 15mer peptides of measles haemagglutinin were synthesized and used as antigens in a T cell proliferation assay, with lymphocytes from Balb/c or TO strain mice, primed to the whole virus (MV). Balb/c mice responded to peptides 7, 38, 39 and 44 but TO mice to only peptide 39. When the mice were immunized with peptides rather than the whole virus, approximately half of the peptides primed the animals effectively but only five peptides in each strain primed for T cell responses to the intact antigen. Data from Obeid *et al*, 1993.

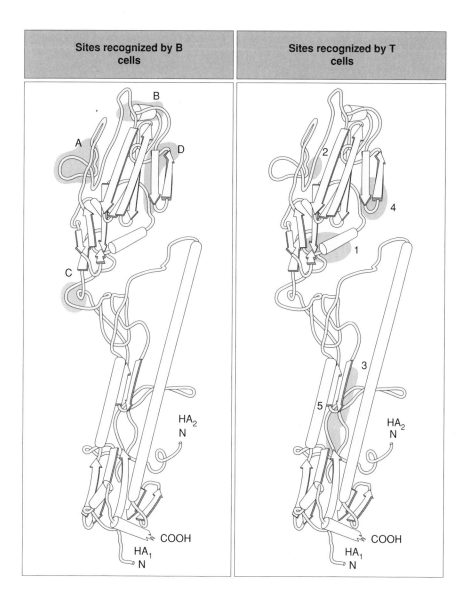

Sites recognized by B cells	Sites recognized by T cells

Fig. 16.5 T and B cell recognition of influenza A haemagglutinin. The structure of the influenza haemagglutinin is shown. Antibody binding sites on the haemagglutinin have been identified by site-induced mutagenesis. There are four such major regions in the head of the molecule (A–D). Other techniques have identified regions which are recognized by T cells. Although these regions depend on MHC haplotype, an example of regions recognized by one individual is shown on the right (1–5). They are distributed throughout the molecule, including the stalk, and may sometimes overlap with B cell epitopes.

Bacteria

In comparison with viruses, bacteria and parasites are much more antigenically complex. Bacterial cell envelopes fall into three major groups: Gram-positive, Gram-negative and mycobacterial. Spirochaetes and corynebacteria have characteristics which span these simple categories. All three groups have an inner cytoplasmic membrane and a peptidoglycan cell wall. Gram-negative organisms have in addition, an outer membrane containing proteins and lipopolysaccharide (LPS), while mycobacteria have an outer glycolipid layer consisting of mycolic acid residues linked to arabinogalactan which is anchored to the cell wall peptidoglycan via phosphate linkages. Many bacterial species also have an outer capsule which is antiphagocytic and makes a major contribution to the virulence of the microorganism. Most bacteria, therefore, provide both carbohydrate and protein antigens for the immune system to grapple with. As with viruses and parasites, those antigens which are of greatest importance in pathogen virulence (and hence in host defence) are also most likely to vary between strains.

The antigenic structure of Gram-positive bacteria is exemplified by *Streptococcus pyogenes* (*Fig. 16.6*). This bacterium often has a capsule consisting of hyaluronic acid which acts as a shield. Hyaluronic acid is a normal constituent of host

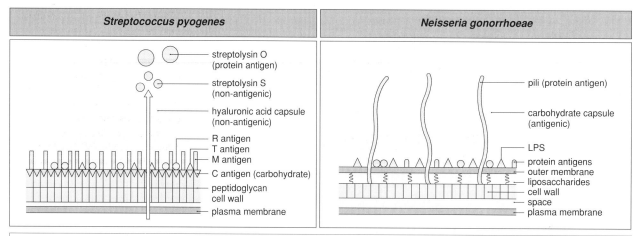

Fig. 16.6 Antigenic structure of bacteria. The surface antigens of a representative Gram-positive (*Streptococcus pyogenes*) and Gram-negative (*Neisseria gonhorroeae*) bacterium are shown. *S. pyogenes* has carbohydrate (C) antigens attached to its peptidoglycan cell wall and an outer set of protein antigens (M, R and T), of which the antibodies to M are most important for immunity. The antiphagocytic capsule of hyaluronic acid is non-antigenic, as is the exotoxin streptolysin S — it is too small to stimulate a response. Antibodies to streptolysin O also occur and can be diagnostic for infection but they do not eliminate the bacterium. *N. gonhorroeae* has an outer membrane containing several antigenic proteins and LPS but the important component of the antibody response is directed to the anti-phagocytic carbohydrate capsule and the pili, required for attachment to epithelial cells.

connective tissue, so the outer capsule of the bacterium is non-antigenic. Attached to the cell wall peptidoglycan are three major protein antigens, M, R and T, as as well as the carbohydrate C antigen. The M protein is the main target for opsonizing antibody. This protein forms the fimbriae which are anti-phagocytic. Anti-bacterial immunity depends almost entirely on anti-M antibodies and, as might be anticipated, there are at least 55 variants of the M protein on different strains of *S. pyogenes*. The C carbohydrate antigen formed of rhamnose and N-acetyl glucosamine units is covalently attached to the cell wall peptidoglycan and also varies between different strains. The antigenic structure of Gram-negative bacteria is illustrated by *Neisseria gonorrhoeae* (*Fig. 16.6*). In contrast to streptococci, the capsule of gonococci is a polysaccharide which is antigenic and type-specific. The outer membrane contains pili formed of type-specific protein antigens. These pili have an anti-phagocytic function, as well as being essential for adherence of the bacteria to host cells in the urinogenital tract. Invasion of epithelial cells follows the attachment. Antibodies to the pili prevent adherence and facilitate bacterial opsonization. The genes for the pili are subject to recombinational events (see below) which produce antigenic variation. Antibodies are also formed to the outer membrane proteins and to LPS. Because the bacterium infects mucosal tissues, specific IgA antibodies to capsule and pili are a major host defence mechanism. However, the organisms' defences include an IgA-specific protease.

From these two examples, it is clear that effective antibodies must be of the right class to activate appropriate effectors and the important antigens are those involved in evasion of immune effector mechanisms, that is, pili, fimbriae and capsular antigens which constitute the major antigens of the outer layer of the bacteria. Often the epitope specificity is important, since it determines whether complement is deposited in a position to damage the outer membrane — serum-resistant strains of enterobacteria have evolved a variety of ways of evading the complement system (Chapter 15). Mycobacteria have an unusual envelope with a surface of esterified mycolic acids. The dominant antigens are carbohydrate-based, phenolic glycolipids, lipoarabinomannans and an arabinogalactan-peptidoglycan complex. There are also numerous protein antigens which can induce an antibody response but although the antibody response to the glycolipids is partly species-specific and may be diagnostically useful, it is largely irrelevant to immunity. This is most obvious in lepromatous leprosy, where the patients have weak cell-mediated immunity, high levels of specific antibody and tissues heavily infected with bacteria.

Although they are antigenically complex, there are some readily identifiable cases where responses to individual antigens are essential for host immunity. The simplest examples are the toxins produced by the causative agents of diphtheria, tetanus and clostridial enteritis. The damage produced directly by the infectious agent in these diseases is slight by comparison with that produced by the secreted toxins. Consequently, protection against these conditions involves immunization to toxoids. Nevertheless, the immune system must still eradicate the primary site of the bacterial infection if the disease is to be resolved. The target antigens for bactericidal antibodies are extremely diverse and include LPS, capsular polysaccharides and other outer membrane proteins. Many of the enterobacteria have a common antigen in their outer membrane which can be the target of antibody-mediated attack. When considering the important target antigens on these bacteria, the prime effector system in bacterial lysis or cytostasis must be considered. Complement-mediated damage to the outer membrane of Gram-negative bacteria is particularly important in resolution of these infections.

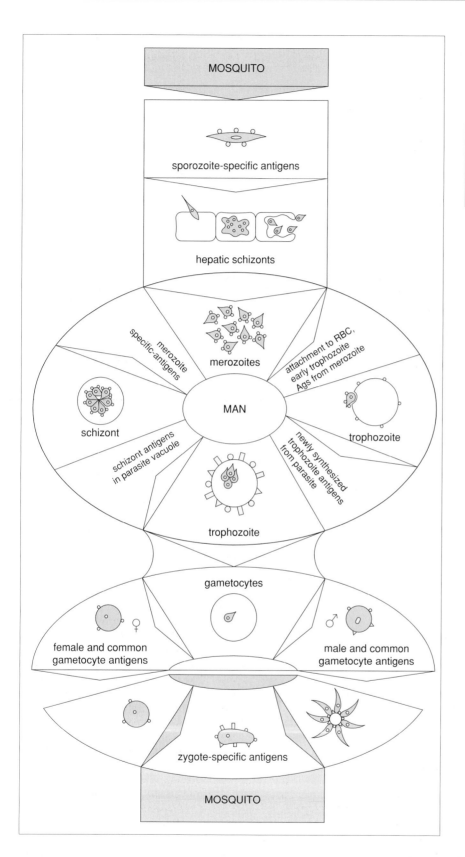

Fig. 16.7 Antigens at different stages of the malarial life cycle. Antibodies to malaria can act at many stages. These include the various asexual blood stage forms, the infected red cells and even the developing gametocytes and zygote following ingestion by the mosquito. Antibodies to all the stages listed have been detected.

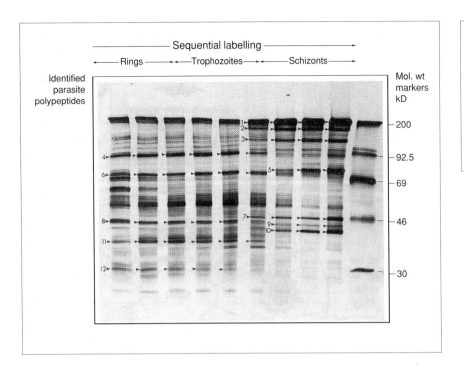

Fig. 16.8 Stage-specific antigens of *P. knowlesii*. SDS PAGE analysis of *P. knowlesii* parasites pulse-labelled at different stages of their life cycle shows that some antigens (e.g. 6) persist for more than one stage, whereas others (e.g. 7) are specific for a single stage of development. Data from Deans, 1984.

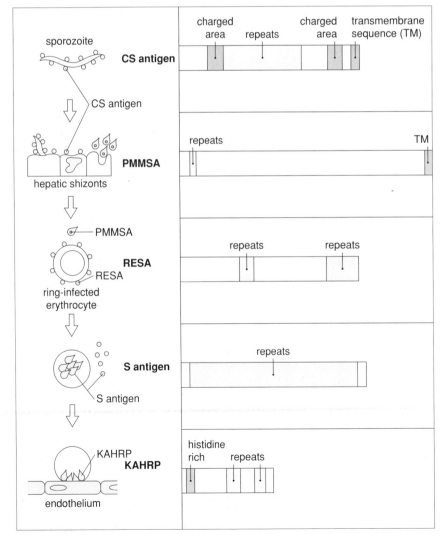

Fig. 16.9 Structures of *P. falciparum* antigens. The gene structures of several malarial antigens have been determined and several are illustrated here. A common feature is the presence of repeated subunits which present a large antigenic load to the host. For example, the CS antigen from *P. falciparum* IMT22 contains 37 repeats of the quadrapeptide NANP and four of NVDP but the numbers of repeats and their lengths vary greatly between strains (and species). The precursor to the merozoite surface antigen (PMMSA) illustrated is from the Wellcome strain, the ring-infected erythrocyte surface antigen (RESA) and S antigens are from strain FC27 and the knob-associated histidine rich protein KAHRP endothelial attachment protein is from strain NF7. Reviewed in Kemp *et al*, 1987.

For this reason, antibodies directed towards proteins in the outer membrane are often most effective. By comparison, antibodies to flagellae or pilae are often ineffective, since these structures are too far from the outer membrane to precipitate classical pathway-mediated attack (see Chapter 15).

Parasites

The wide diversity of parasites makes it impossible to generalize, nevertheless, they are instructive of the problems faced by the immune system; examples will illustrate particular points.

ANTIGENIC COMPLEXITY — PLASMODIA

The antigenic complexity of parasites is exemplified by the four species of *Plasmodium* which produce malaria in man. There are several different stages to the life cycle, each with its own characteristic sets of antigens (*Fig. 16.7*) and antibodies are made to each of these stages. Intracellular stages express both their own antigens and a different set on the surface of the infected cells. Certain antigens may be specific for an individual phase of the life cycle whereas others persist for several phases (*Fig. 16.8*).

Antibodies to antigens expressed at different stages may be equally effective at killing the parasite but can have fundamentally different effects on the outcome of the infection. For example, antibody to the sporozoites, which is already present in the host, could prevent the first stage of infection (the invasion of host liver cells by sporozoites injected by the mosquito). Similarly, antibodies to the merozoite prevent the cycles of reinfection of the red cells, while antibodies to gametocyte-specific antigens can break the cycle of reinfection of the mosquito but are of little help in clearing infection in the original host.

Many of the immunogenic antigens of *Plasmodia* contain short repeated sequences of amino acids (*Fig. 16.9*). These are generally immunodominant and often the repeats are strain-specific. An example is the circumsporozoite (CS) protein which coats the sporozoite. This protein consists of a variable number of tandem repeated sequences of differing immunogenicity which varies structurally between species and, to a lesser extent, between strains. The protein appears to have a role in parasite motility and antibodies to CS protein prevent its telomeric movement across the cell surface. It also mediates highly specific attachment of the sporozoite to hepatocytes in the first few minutes of infection; antibodies to the CS protein also block hepatocyte binding. Unfortunately, antibody binding to the CS protein causes shedding from the cell surface, thus acting as a decoy protein. In *P. vivax* the immunodominant B cell epitope varies between isolates, whereas it is highly conserved in *P. falciparum*. In contrast Th cell epitopes are variable in *P. falciparum* as are those for Tc cells. It has been suggested that this reflects the relative importance of cell-mediated and antibody-mediated immunity for infection with different species of malaria.

The major merozoite antigens are derived from a precursor protein of 195kDa which is processed into three fragments during schizogeny. Two of these are shed as the parasite invades the host cell but one of them remains associated with ring-stage infected erythrocytes. Antibody to these antigens, which are involved in binding to erythrocytes, may be partially protective but monoclonal antibodies raised to different isolates and gene sequencing indicate that both variable and constant epitopes are expressed.

At least 14 different antigens have been identified on the asexual blood stage of *P. falciparum*, differentiated according to molecular weight. In some cases, single antibodies isolate several antigens which have different molecular weights but experiments such as those above indicate that antigen fragmentation is a normal part of the life cycle. Analysis of four of these glycoprotein antigens has shown two of them (GP1 and GP3) to be invariant between eight isolates, while the other two vary. Also present in the blood stage are antigens which are localized in the rhoptry proteins of the paired organelles at the apex of the merozoite. These organelles are internal and are lost during merozoite reinvasion of red cells. Antibody to them is partially able to inhibit red cell invasion but is generally less effective than antibody to the glycophorin binding proteins on the outside of the merozoite, mentioned above.

Antibodies to antigens on the gametes can act in two ways: binding to gametes and zygotes shortly after ingestion by the mosquito, and preventing development of zygotes into ookinetes within the gut of the vector. Antibodies have been identified which act at both these levels, identifying antigens which develop on, and are common to, both male and female gametes. It is rather surprising that the host antibodies can still have some protective action for the human population as a whole, even after ingestion into the vector.

Immunity to malaria develops slowly in an individual and resistance is relative — children are poorly protected, adults more so. Sera of adults in an endemic area recognize a greater number of the local strains and it is thought that the progressive immunity is due to a greater immunological coverage, following exposure to more strains.

In addition to the strain-specific variation, individual clones may undergo programmed variation in a single host. For example, *P. fragile* in its natural host (toque monkey) generates successive waves of parasitaemia, each associated with a new variant of the erythrocyte surface antigens. Since the same programme is followed in different animals, it shows that variation is directed by the genes of the parasite themselves. This is similar to the well-defined programmed variation seen in African trypanosomiasis (see below).

EVASION OF IMMUNE RECOGNITION

Microbial pathogens may evade immune recognition by a variety of strategies including immunological silence, antigenic variation, antigenic disguise and mimicry of host molecules. These forms of evasion are illustrated by particular microorganisms.

Immunological silence

Some viruses can enter a latent state in which transcription of their own proteins is suspended. A classical example is *Herpes simplex*, which may become latent in sensory neurons after a normal lytic cycle of infection in epithelium. The viral

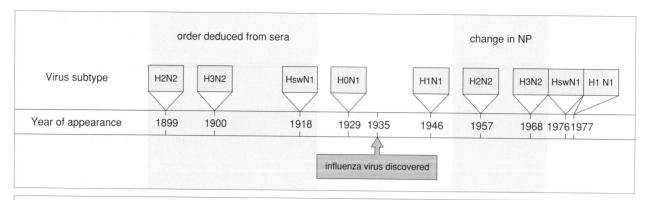

Fig. 16.10 Antigenic shifts in influenza A haemagglutinin and neuraminidase. Since its discovery in 1935, there have been sporadic major changes (shifts) in the surface antigens of influenza virus. The haemagglutinin has changed from type H0 to H1, H2, H3 etc. in successive shifts, during which time the neuraminidase has changed from type N1 to N2 and back again. By looking at the neutralizing antibodies present in the sera of people alive before the discovery of the virus, it has been possible to deduce the type of antigens present on the strains existing then. This suggests that antigenic types can recur, as soon as the overall level of immunity in the population falls below a certain level, so that a new pandemic strain can develop.

genome is detectable in the neurons and two pre-messenger RNAs are transcribed but there is no mRNA and no viral protein is translated. This, and the intrinsically low level of MHC class I expression by neurons, means that Tc cells cannot recognize the infected neuron. In neurons the viral transactivator VP16 which induces expression of immediate early genes in infected epithelial cells is non-functional. Nevertheless the viral genome may become re-activated, usually in circumstances when local immunity is temporarily impaired.

Herpes simplex has another trick available to evade recognition — it interferes with the expression of MHC class I. Within three hours of infection, fibroblasts are resistant to lysis by HSV-specific CD8+ T cells. This is due to a failure to load MHC class I molecules with antigenic peptides in the Golgi. One of the immediate early proteins of HSV is responsible for the block, although its means of action is not known.

A similar defence mechanism is seen with *Leishmania*, which can downregulate expression of MHC molecules on parasitized macrophages.

Antigenic variation

Antigenic variation may occur between different strains of a pathogen; in addition, some pathogens carry multiple variant sets of their critical antigens. In general, viruses and most bacteria do not have enough genetic information for more than one set of surface antigens whereas some protozoa and eukaryotic parasites do change their surface antigens during the life cycle. This may be as a result of different morphological stages in their development, as occurs during the ontogeny of *Plasmodia*, or may include antigen-switching by activation of genes for new surface antigen variants, as is seen in *T. brucei* infection.

One of the most interesting examples of strain variation is seen in influenza A where the HA and neuraminidase (NA) continually undergo slight alterations in their structure as a result of genetic mutation. The new variants that develop cannot be neutralized by antibodies to the previous strain and so the new variants can infect otherwise immune individuals.

The sera induced by later variants are often able to react with a previous variant strain but not vice versa, i.e. last year's antibody does not neutralize this year's virus. This kind of variation is called antigenic drift. Sporadically, a major change of the surface antigens occurs (antigenic shift). This happens by recombination of genetic material between two completely different strains of the virus. The genetic material of the virus is in eight separate RNA strands which readily permits gene reassortment if two different viruses should simultaneously infect the same cell. The shifts which have occurred in the HA and NA molecules during this century are illustrated in *Figure 16.10*. The nucleoprotein also underwent a minor variation in 1946. In the case of influenza, the newly emergent variants tend to displace previous strains completely. This is dissimilar to the situation seen with rhinoviruses, coronaviruses and enterobacteria, where numerous variants coexist in the host population. However, for these viruses and bacteria, a major part of the host immunity is due to specific IgA and this response tends to wane much more rapidly than the IgG-mediated immunity which is effective in preventing reinfection with influenza. Consequently, a single strain of influenza virus cannot regularly reinfect the same host. This, coupled with the virulence of flu epidemics, means that a large proportion of the host population is immune after an outbreak of the disease and, therefore, this type of infection tends to be epidemic rather than endemic.

Some viruses, particularly the lentiviruses, are able to persist in one host for an extended period, even in the face of an immune response. This group of viruses includes visna which infects sheep, the immunodeficiency viruses HIV and SIV, as well as several other animal viruses. Two major features of this group allow them to persist within a single host: the failure of the immune system to produce an adequate response to critical antigens, although there is often a strong response to unimportant target antigens, and antigenic variation during the course of a single infection. In this last respect, it is notable that the viral reverse transcriptase lacks an error correction mechanism and so there is a high level of point mutation

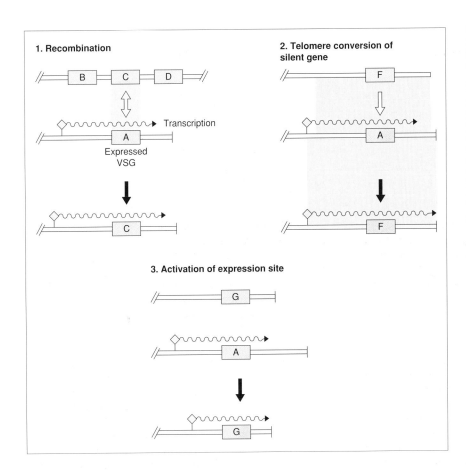

1. Recombination

2. Telomere conversion of silent gene

3. Activation of expression site

Fig. 16.11 Control of variant surface glycoprotein expression. The active gene (A) for the variant surface glycoprotein of *T. brucei* is expressed in a telomeric site. There are up to 1000 additional genes for VSGs held in the genome. These may be activated in one of three ways. 1) A duplicative transposition of a silent non-telomeric gene (C) to replace the currently active gene. 2) The transposition of a silent telomeric gene segment into the active gene site. 3) The activation of a previously silent telomeric site. This follows gene rearrangement in the controlling region of the segment and is accompanied by a close down of the previously active telomeric site.

generated in the DNA which inserts into the host genome. A study using cytotoxic T cells directed against the Gag protein of HIV, isolated from infected individuals, showed that variants of the protein could inhibit the action of the Tc cells. The variants differ by a single amino acid and arise naturally during the course of HIV infections. In effect they can engage the T cell receptor but do not trigger cytotoxicity.

Neisseria use two different mechanisms to vary the subunits of their pili — by DNA transformation or recombination. *Neisseria* take up exogenous homologous DNA from lysed bacteria efficiently and can use it to replace their own pilin gene at a rate of 10^{-3} per cell division. In addition, the bacteria carry an array of silent pilin genes. Low frequency reciprocal recombination between these genes and the active gene leads to the expression of a new variant. In general, antigenic shifts within a host are not driven by the antibody response but the new variants arise spontaneously and are then selected for survival by the pressure of the immune response — Darwinian evolution in miniature.

A remarkable example of antigenic variation within a host is seen with *T. brucei*, the causative agent of sleeping sickness. These protozoal parasites have a surface coat consisting of about seven million identical, closely packed glycoproteins of molecular weight 61kDa, called the variant surface glycoprotein (VSG). As its name suggests, the VSG is expressed in antigenically different forms in different cells. Every organism carries approximately 1000 separate genes encoding different variants of the VSG, although at any one time only one of the variants is expressed. Individuals can

switch from the production of one variant to another, an event which happens at low frequency. This kind of switching is often accompanied by gene rearrangement which brings the new variant gene into proximity of a promoter to allow its expression (*Fig. 16.11*). It was noted that when parasites were transferred to naive hosts the programme of variation is reset. This suggests that particular sets of VSGs are more readily activated than others and that the programme which actually occurs is determined by the favoured switches and the individual's immune response. VSGs are essential for parasite survival in mammals but they are rapidly replaced on the cell surface by a different coat molecule, procyclin, after ingestion by the insect vector.

Analysis of the primary structures of VSGs shows that although they vary widely between strains, they still retain a single overall structure, detectable by X-ray crystallography, which is built around a double core of α-helix. Monoclonal antibodies raised to different purified VSGs recognize at least five separate antigenic domains but only one of these is recognizable on the intact parasite. This is thought to correspond to the outermost domain of the molecule. Notably, the N-terminal region of the VSGs, which is distal to the parasite surface and accessible to antibody on the intact parasite, is also the most variable region of the molecule. The ability to switch VSGs gives the trypanosome a chameleon-like ability to change its surface antigenic appearance. The immune system can successfully eradicate any particular variant by producing variant-specific antibodies, but small numbers of new variants will have arisen which evade the immune response and rapidly replace the previously dominant variant. Since the parasite is always one step ahead of the immune system, the disease is chronic. The importance of antigen switching to survival of this parasite can be judged by the fact that 10% of the organism's genome is devoted to VSGs.

Antigenic disguise and molecular mimicry

A different strategy is adopted by pathogens which evade recognition by mimicking the antigens of the host. Due to the great polymorphism of MHC molecules, it is not possible for an organism to become adapted to every individual in the host population. Some schistosomes have circumvented this problem by disguise. They adopt HLA molecules from their host, incorporating them into their outer tegument to make themselves antigenically invisible.

The ability to produce molecules which resemble those of the host is intrinsic to many different kinds of infection, since the pathogens must often interact with the host. For example, *Mycobacteria* produce a fibronectin-binding protein which facilitates their uptake by macrophages. At the further end of the spectrum, pathogens mimic host antigens merely for the purpose of evading recognition. This is seen particularly with carbohydrate and glycolipid antigens (see below) and may be the root cause of autoimmunity associated with infection.

When we consider the mechanisms for evasion of recognition, it is no coincidence that the most successful vaccination programmes have been directed to pathogens which vary little between strains, have no capacity to vary their surface antigens and do not mutate or recombine their genetic material.

EFFECTOR SYSTEMS

The effectiveness of the response to most pathogens depends on whether an appropriate defence system becomes activated. For example, the neutralizing antibodies to influenza surface proteins prevent reinfection of cells with that strain of virus but do not destroy virally infected cells. In fact, the rate of clearance of virus from the lung of experimentally infected mice is proportional to the level of specific cytotoxic T cell activity and does not relate to antibody levels. This situation is true for many viral infections which have a viraemic phase — antibody prevents transmission between cells, while Tc destroy infected cells.

Cytotoxic T cells are also important in defence against intracellular stages of protozoal parasites. For example, peptide fragments of the CS antigen of *Plasmodia* may be presented by MHC molecules, rendering infected cells susceptible to CD8+ T cell-mediated cytotoxicity.

In some cases, a particular type of antibody response is mandatory for clearance of the pathogen. This is true of many bacterial infections, where specific antibodies to surface antigens are necessary to neutralize the bacterial defences and opsonize the bacteria for phagocytes. It is also true in the immune reaction to schistosomes but in this case specific IgE is essential. Although schistosomulae acquire host MHC class I and class II antigens on their surface shortly after infection of a host, they are impervious to the action of Tc cells. Destruction of the parasite is effected by antibody-dependent cell-mediated cytotoxicity, in which the prime participants are eosinophils, macrophages and, to a lesser extent, platelets. Immune sera can mediate the ADCC but if the sera are depleted of IgE they are inactive. Protective IgE antibodies have been identified which bind to a protein of molecular weight 22–26kDa. Following infection, the schistosomes are susceptible to these mechanisms for 2–3 days, after which time the parasites' defensive mechanisms (primarily antigenic disguise) come into play.

The principle to be seen in these examples is that recognition of a particular antigen is not in itself sufficient to produce an effective immune response. In some cases, a cell-mediated response is appropriate, in others antibody. Antibody class switching gives the immune system the flexibilty to activate different effector systems.

Evasion of effector systems

Many pathogens have strategies for avoiding the effector phases of the immune response, even when they do not evade immune recognition. The most direct strategies are aimed at blunting the effector arm of the immune response. In this group come anti-chemotaxins and enzymes which breakdown antibody or complement. More subtle are the decoy proteins which divert either antibodies or the complement system, as well as the mechanisms which produce immune deviation or immunosuppression.

DECOY PROTEINS

Molecules released by a pathogen can cause antibody or complement to bind away from the cell surface, thus preventing phagocytosis or deposition of complement lytic pathway molecules on the plasma membrane. For example, the VSG of trypanosomes is linked to the parasite surface by a GPI-anchor. C-terminal proteolysis of the VSG causes it to be released as a soluble molecule.

This type of decoy action is also used by malarial sporozoites which express the CS antigen. When sporozoites are treated with immune sera containing anti-CS, they shed a morphologically distinguishable outer layer. This shedding reaction deflects the immunological attack from the sporozoite itself, buying time so that it can reach an hepatocyte. The S antigen of *P. falciparum* is another example of a decoy protein. This molecule appears at the start of schizogeny and is shed by developing merozoites into the vacuole of the schizont; like the CS antigen, it contains repeated epitopes and also shows antigenic variation (see *Fig. 14.10*). Up to 90% of the sequence consists of an 11 amino acid repeat. These repeats are generally highly conserved within the protein, although the sequence varies considerably between strains. These kinds of decoy reactions are well suited to parasites (or stages in their life cycles) which are only briefly in contact with immune defences, whereas antigenic variation is a long-term solution to the problem of evading immunity.

IMMUNE DEVIATION

Sometimes microorganisms can divert the immune response towards reactions, which will allow the pathogen to survive in the host. The role of superantigens in allowing pathogen survival is unresolved. For example, mouse mammary tumour virus expresses a superantigen which can stimulate 5–30% of T cells; this provides an expanded pool of T cells which the virus can then infect. A similar effect is seen with Epstein Barr virus, where the B cell population (target for the virus) becomes expanded in the early stages of the infection. However, these theories do not explain staphylococcal superantigens. Perhaps T cell activation leads to less efficient antibody-mediated responses, or perhaps the effect of stimulating a large number of irrelevant T cells is itself immunosuppressive.

In view of the balance between Th1 and Th2 cells, another way of deviating immune responses is to modulate the cytokines which control their interaction. A clear example of this is the *BCRF-1* gene of EB virus. This produces an analogue of IL-10, thereby diverting the response away from Th1 cells and inflammatory reactions.

IMMUNOSUPPRESSION

Generalized immunosuppression by pathogens is unusual. It does occur where a heavy antigen overload occurs, such as quartan malaria, producing immunopathological reactions including immune complex disease. The problem for the pathogen is that by creating immunosuppression it may leave the host open to infection by other pathogens which may either compete with the first pathogen or kill the host. In either case this is not beneficial for the original pathogen. Nevertheless, there are many examples of localized immunosuppression, often directed towards the inflammatory cytokines IL-1 and TNF. For example, *Vaccinia* virus produces a serine protease inhibitor which blocks the conversion of IL-β precursor into the soluble cytokine. Viral mutants lacking the inhibitor engender a stronger inflammatory reaction *in vivo* and lower viral titres.

An alternative strategy is to block the actions of cytokines which have already been produced. For example, Shope sarcoma virus produces a TNF-binding molecule which blocks its interaction with TNF receptors, again reducing inflammation.

CROSS-REACTIONS OF MICROBIAL AND HOST ANTIGENS

Molecular mimicry may produce a crossreaction between microbial and host antigens triggering a breakdown of self-tolerance following infection with a particular organism. It is sometimes difficult to determine whether an organism does indeed contain a particular cross-reactive antigen or whether the reaction is to host tissue antigen released by pathogen-induced damage. An example of this is the antibodies to cardiolipin which occur in *Treponema pallidum* infection (causative agent of syphilis). These antibodies are also present in leprosy and systemic lupus erythematosus (SLE). Cardiolipin occurs in the envelope of treponemes, which explains the occurrence of the antibody in syphilis but it is not present in *M. leprae*. To explain the presence of this antibody in other infections, one can invoke the adjuvant properties of mycobacteria, acting in association with host

cell damage. In fact, when the specificity of the anti-cardiolipin antibodies, which occur in syphilis and SLE, is analysed it is found that the antibodies of syphilitics have a higher reactivity with phosphatidyl ethanolamine, while the antibodies in SLE react preferentially with phosphatidyl serine. This suggests that the breakdown of self-tolerance in the two groups occurs by different means.

Antigenic crossreaction has also been used to explain the autoimmune reactions which occur to heart muscle and valves, which develop in rheumatic fever after infection with streptococci. Rheumatic fever is an infrequent sequel to streptococcal pharyngitis, ocurring 2–4 weeks after the bacterial infection. It has been explained in terms of crossreaction between the bacterial carbohydrate and a structural protein on heart valves, as well as a crossreaction between an M-associated antigen and cardiac muscle. However, this cannot be the whole story, as it fails to account for the pericarditis (no cross-reactive antigens have been seen in the pericardium), nor does it explain why only a small proportion of infected individuals develop the disease, or why it follows only pharyngitis and not other streptococcal infections. It cannot be a simple matter of breakdown of self-tolerance. Indeed, it is notable that autoimmune reactions occur after many diseases but only in rare instances do they develop into autoimmune disease.

Although many cross-reactive antigens are carbohydrate or glycolipid, producing low affinity antibodies, some microbial proteins can also induce cross-reactive antibodies. A notable example is *Klebsiella*, which has an antigen that structurally resembles HLA-B27. This resemblance is thought to underlie the high relative risk for spondylarthropathies associated with *Klebsiella* and *Yersinia* infections and this MHC haplotype (see *Colour figures*). Another example is seen in the damage which occurs in the late stages of Chagas' disease. This condition is primarily cell-mediated and T cells which recognize a cross-reactive antigen on *T. cruzi* and nervous tissues will reproduce the pathology of Chagas' disease. Recently, a 150kDa surface antigen has been cloned from *T. cruzi* which cross-reacts with a 48kDa antigen found in brain and sciatic nerve and which is a candidate for breaking T cell tolerance in this disease.

SUMMARY

Microorganisms and viruses have large numbers of different antigens but for protective immunity only a number of these are important. These critical antigens are usually located on the outer surface of the pathogen. Viruses must attach to host cells to initiate infection and antibodies to the attachment proteins are often the most effective at preventing infection. The same principle applies to intracellular parasites such as malaria which must attach to a host cell via specific cell-surface proteins. The response to bacteria is complicated by the production of bacterial exotoxins. While it is frequently essential that an adequate response is mounted to these toxins, elimination of the bacteria still depends on the production of antibodies to critical surface antigens.

Recognition of intracellular phases of pathogen life cycles usually depends on T cell-mediated recognition of antigenic peptides presented in association with

MHC molecules. The precise portion of an antigen which is recognized depends on both the processing capability of the infected cell type and the MHC haplotype of the individual. T cells can recognize both internal and external antigens of a pathogen and they do not necessarily have to recognize the same antigen as a B cell to be able to help the B cell produce antibody to the pathogen.

The antigens of microorganisms are not static. Immunity within the host population places them under a continual pressure to change their critical surface antigens, within the limitations of the functions of the molecules concerned. Eukaryotic parasites may carry many different sets of antigens and organisms such as trypanosomes have mechanisms for changing their surface. Genetically simpler pathogens often develop new variants by mutation, recombination or transformation. In some cases, variants coexist within the host population; in others new variants replace the old ones, producing epidemic outbreaks of disease.

In general, those molecules which are of greatest importance for pathogen survival show greatest varibility. These strategies provide a constant challenge to the immune system and an even greater one to immunologists attempting to produce effective vaccines.

Pathogens also interfere with the effector arm of the immune response. The simpler mechanisms deflect the immune response from directly killing the pathogen. These devices include anti-phagocytic proteins, leukocidins, capsules etc. Some pathogens can also deviate the immune response, by interfering with signalling mediated by cytokines or chemotactic agents. Viruses such as *Herpes simplex* can disrupt antigen presentation.

The immune systems which are investigated have evolved in tandem with particular microbial pathogens; it is equally true that the pathogens have been selected by the immune systems of the host population. What is seen today is the result of a dynamic balance between pathogens and their hosts.

FURTHER READING

Alcami A, Smith G. A soluble receptor for interleukin-1β encoded by vaccinia virus: a novel mechanism of virus modulation of the host response to infection. *Cell* 1992, **71**:153.

Bodmer HC, Gotch FM, McMichael AJ. Class I-restricted cytotoxic T cells reveal low responder allele due to processing of viral antigen. *Nature* 1989, **337**:653.

Borst P. Molecular genetics of antigenic variation. *Immunol Today* 1991, **12**:29.

Chen BP, Parham P. Direct binding of influenza peptides to class I HLA molecules. *Nature* 1989, **337**:743.

Clements JE, Gdovin SL, Montelaro RC, Narayan O. Antigenic variation in lentiviral diseases. *Ann Rev Immunol* 1988, **6**:139.

Colonno RJ, Callahan PL, Leippe DM, Rueckert RR, Tomassini JE. Inhibition of rhinovirus attachment by neutralizing monoclonal antibodies and their Fab fragments. *J Virol* 1989, **63**:36.

Cross G. Cellular and genetic aspects of antigenic variation in trypanosomes. *Ann Rev Immunol* 1990, **8**:83.

Deans JA. Protective antigens of blood stage *Plasmodium knowlesi* parasites. *Philos Trans R Soc Lond Biol* 1984, **307**:159.

Fenton B, Clark JT, Wilson CF, McBride JS, Wallikar D. Polymorphism of a 35–48kDa *Plasmodium falciparum* merozoite surface antigen. *Mol Biochem Parasitol* 1989, **34**:79.

Gaylord H, Brennan PJ. Leprosy and the leprosy bacillus. *Ann Rev Microbiol* 1987, **41**:645.

Howard RJ. Antigenic variation of blood stage malaria parasites. *Philos Trans R Soc Lond Biol* 1984, **307**:141.

Jacobson S, Sekaly RP, Jacobson CL, McFarland HF, Long EO. HLA class II-restricted presentation of cytoplasmic measles virus antigens to cytotoxic T cells. *J Virol* 1989, **63**:1756.

Kaufmann SHE. 1993 Immunity to intracellular bacteria. *Ann Revs Immunol* 1989, **11**:129.

Kemp DJ, Coppel RL, Anders RF. Repetitive proteins and genes of malaria. *Ann Rev Microbiol* 1987, **41**:181.

Klenerman P, Rowland-Jones S, McAdam S, Edwards J, Daenke S, Lalloo D, Köppe B, Rosenberg W, Boyd D, Edwards A, Giangrande P, Phillips RE, McMichael AJ. Cytotoxic T cell activity antagonized by naturally occurring HIV-1 Gag variants. *Nature* 1994, **369**:403.

Madden DR, Garboczi DN, Wiley DC. The antigenic identity of peptide-MHC complexes: a comparison of five viral peptides presented by HLA-A2. *Cell* 1993, **75**:693.

Makela MJ. Antibody responses to different antigenic sites on measles virus surface polypeptides in patients with multiple sclerosis. *J Neurol Sci* 1989, **90**:239.

Marrack PC, Kappler JW. The staphylococcal enterotoxins and their relatives. *Science* 1990, **248**:705.

Marrack PC, Kappler J. Subversion of the immune system by pathogens. *Cell* 1994, **76**:323.

Mendis KN, David PH, Carter R. Antigenic polymorphism in malaria: is it an important mechanism for immune evasion? *Immunol Today* 1991, **12**:A34.

Obeid OE, Partidos CD, Steward MW. Identification of helper T cell antigenic sites in mice from the haemagglutinin glycoprotein of measles virus. *J Gen Virol* 1993, **74**:2549.

Pays E. Gene conversion in trypanosome antigenic variation. *Progr Nucl Acids Res Mol Biol* 1985, **32**:1.

Palker TJ, Matthews TJ, Langlois A, Tanner ME, Martin ME, Scearce RM, Kim J, Bersofsky JA, Bolognesi DP, Haynes BF. Polyvalent HIV synthetic immunogen comprized of envelope gp120, T helper cell sites and B cell neutralization epitopes. *J Immunol* 1989, **142**:3612.

Ray CA, Black RA, Kronheim SR, Greenstreet TA, Sleath PR, Salvesen GS, Pickup DJ. Viral inhibition of inflammation: cowpox virus encodes an inhibitor of the interleukin-1β converting enzyme. *Cell* 1992, **69**:597.

Romero P, Marvanski JL, Corradin G, Nussenzweig RS, Nussenzweig V, Zavala F. Cloned cytotoxic T cells recognize an epitope in the circumsporozoite protein and protect against malaria. *Nature* 1989, **341**:323.

Rossman MG, Arnold E, Erichson JW, Frankenberger EA, Griffith JP, Hecht H-J, Johnson JE, Komer G, Luo M, Mosser AG, Rueckert RR, Sherry B, Vriend G. Structure of a human common cold virus and functional relationship to other picornaviruses. *Nature* 1985, **317**:145.

Rothbard JB, Pemberton RM, Bodmer HC, Askonas BA, Taylor WR. Identification of residues necessary for clonally specific recognition of a cytotoxic T cell determinant. *EMBO J* 1989, **8**:2321.

Schrier RD, Gnann JW, Landes R, Lockshin C, Richman D, McCutchan A, Kennedy C, Oldstone MB, Nelson JA. T cell recognition of HIV synthetic peptides in a natural infection. *J Immunol* 1989, **142**:1166.

Smith CA, Davis T, Wignall JM, Din WS, Farrah T, Upton C, McFadden G, Goodwin RG. T2 open reading frame of Shope fibroma virus encodes a soluble form of the TNF receptor. *Biochem Biophys Res Comms* 1991, **176**:335.

Townsend A, Bastin J, Bodmer H, Brownlee G, Davey J, Gotch F, Gould K, Jones I, McMichael A, Rothbard J *et al*. Recognition of influenza virus proteins by cytotoxic T cells. *Philos Trans R Soc London Biol* 1989, **323**:527

Van Voorhis WC, Eisen H. A surface antigen of *Trypanosoma Cruzi* that mimics mammalian nervous tissue. *J Exp Med* 1989, **169**:641.

Wang J-G, Jansen RW, Brown EA, Lemon SM. Immunogenic domains of hepatitis delta virus antigen: peptide mapping of epitopes recognized by human and woodchuck antibodies. *J Virol* 1990, **64**:1108.

Wiley DC, Wilson IA, Skehel JJ. Structural identification of the antibody-binding sites of Hong Kong influenza haemagglutinin, and their involvement in antigenic variation. *Nature* 1981, **289**:373.

York IA, Roop C, Andrews DW, Riddell SR, Graham FL, Johnson DC. A cytosolic herpes simplex virus protein inhibits antigen presentation to CD8[+] T lymphocytes. *Cell* 1994, **77**:525.

17 Therapeutic Manipulation

There are many situations where it would be beneficial to modulate the immune response. For example, in the correction of immune deficiency, or induction of a response to tumours or infectious agents, enhancing the immune response would be a clear goal. In the case of transplantation, autoimmunity or allergy it would be important to devise strategies for preventing or deviating harmful immune responses. There are several stages of the immune response which are attractive targets for the development of therapeutic strategies.

MODULATION OF THE IMMUNE RESPONSE THROUGH THE CYTOKINE OR THE CHEMOKINE NETWORK

As must be clear from Chapter 10 there are several cytokines, chemokines or their receptors which would provide suitable targets for immune intervention. Only a few of these are described below to highlight the potential usefulness of this approach and also some of the drawbacks.

Using IL-12 to potentiate the immune response

One of the most exciting cytokines to emerge recently in the therapeutic arena has been IL-12. This highly potent cytokine (see Chapter 10) which plays a key role in shaping the immune response has enormous therapeutic potential. Its ability to boost Th1 responses and hence cell mediated immune responses makes it a prime agent for vaccine design.

Its ability to modify the course of parasitic and microbial infections is well known. *In vitro* IL-12 has been shown to increase IFNγ and IL-2 production by PBL from HIV infected patients. IL-12 also affects the growth of malaria parasites early in infection and prevents maturation and reduces granuloma formation and immune associated pathology, such as fibrosis, in schistosomiasis. It has been shown to prolong the survival of mice infected with TB and alleviates lung pathology by reducing the bacterial load. Other immunomodulatory responses include the ability to inhibit tumour growth and reduce the number of metastases and in allergic conditions to reduce IgE production and affect eosinophil recruitment. IL-12 is able to render a normally susceptible BALB/c mouse resistant to Leishmaniasis. It is known that control of infection with *L. major* is associated with the development of a Th1 response and that disease progression is associated with the development of a Th2 response against the parasite. Thus BALB/c mice which are susceptible to infection with this parasite are able to control the parasite if anti-IL-4 is administered (see *Fig. 11.12*). A similar end point is obtained if IL-12 is given to BALB/c mice at the time of infection and the associated protection correlates with an increased IFNγ and reduced IL-4 production in response to the parasite (*Fig. 17. 1*).

In the case of infection with *Schistosoma mansoni* a primary cause of pathology is the host granulomatous response to deposited parasite eggs. This response has all the characteristics of a Th2 response as depletion of IFNγ or IL-12 increased the size of the primary granulomas. This also occurred when NK cells were depleted suggesting that this cell type may be a major source of the cytokine in this infection. Injection of IL-12 depressed granuloma formation, prevented the accumulation of eosinophils (*Fig. 17.2*) and additionally when administered at the time of a primary infection gave rise to a long term bias towards a Th1 response. This cytokine may therefore be of great importance in the development of a vaccine which can modulate the pathology arising in Schistosomiasis, a disease affecting 200–250 million people.

The effect of this cytokine in modifying the response to murine tumours has also been encouraging. The studies of Brunda and colleagues showed that *in vivo* administration of IL-12 significantly affected tumour growth and metastases. The cytokine did not have to be given immediately on tumour inoculation but was still effective 14 days after injection of the transformed cells. Although IL-12 increased NK and LAK activity the effect of the cytokine on murine tumour cell survival was thought to be due to an increase in Tc activity as protection was seen in NK deficient beige mice but was not seen in CD8 depleted mice.

This ability of IL-12 to bias the cytokine profile towards that of a Th1 response has obvious implications for the treatment of allergic disorders. There is clear data showing that recombinant IL-12 inhibits class switching to an IgE response.

There may be some situations where this cytokine is however not beneficial. In nematode infections a Th2 response is thought to be beneficial in eliminating the organism. Following infection with *Nippostrongylus brasiliensis* worm survival is regulated by IgE, mucosal mast cells and blood and tissue eosinophils. If IL-12 is administered during the first few days of infection there is an increase in worm survival and fecundity (*Fig. 17.3*) which is mirrored by the depressed production of cytokines IL-3, IL-4, IL-5 and IL-9, an inhibited IgE response to the nematode and a reduced mast cell and eosinophil response.

Another contra-indication which must be borne in mind when considering the use of this agent in vaccine development is that in susceptible individuals it may precipitate those autoimmune conditions dependent on Th1 responses (Chapter 12).

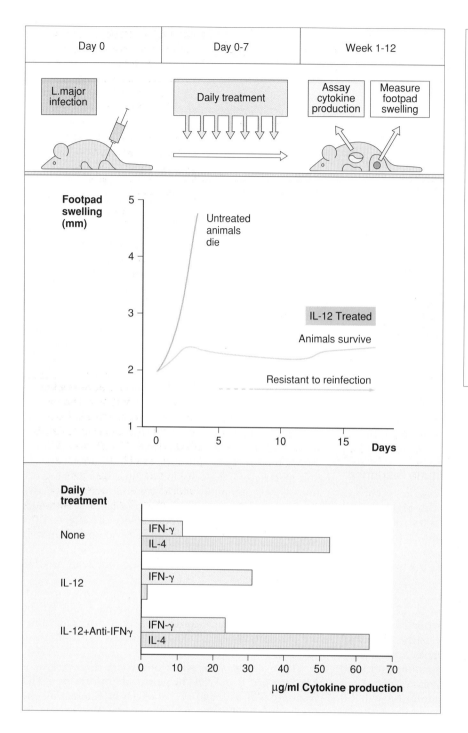

Fig. 17.1 The effect of IL-12 on Leishmaniasis in BALB/c mice. BALB/c mice were infected in the footpad with *L. major* promastigotes and given either no treatment or 0.2µg IL-12 daily for 7 days. The animals which received IL-12 were rechallenged with *L. major* and were still able to control the infection. Mice which are unable to control the infection manifest footpad swelling, develop necrosis and are killed by the infection (upper panel). Data from Sypek *et al*, 1993.

In a similar experimental protocol, the mice were treated with IL-12, with or without anti-IFNγ. Spleen cell production of IFNγ and IL-4 was measured and showed that animals treated with IL-12 are biased towards a Th1 response (lower panel). Data from Heinzel *et al*, 1993.

Blockading the IL-1 response

Interleukin 1 plays an important role in inflammation and thus provides an important target where downmodulation of an inflammatory response is the goal. As seen from Chapter 10 there are several ways of blockading the IL-1 response: neutralizing antibodies to IL-1α and β, soluble IL-1-type I receptors or the IL-1R antagonist (IL-1RA). IL-1RA is able to bind the IL-1 type-1 receptor but does not transduce a signal and is thus a competitive inhibitor. Polymorphisms have been identified in *IL-1A, B* and *IL-1RA* genes and associations between certain alleles and the severity of some inflammatory states such as RA, SLE, psoriasis and ulcerative colitis have been identified. These polymorphisms do not necessarily affect the coding regions but may influence regulation of gene expression.

There have been many experimental studies in which IL-1RA has been successfully used to modulate a pathological state, including improving survival following endotoxin shock, decreasing neutrophil influx in inflammatory responses, prevention of graft versus host disease and a reduction in the incidence and severity of several autoimmune conditions. Clinical trials have also been conducted using IL-1RA in the

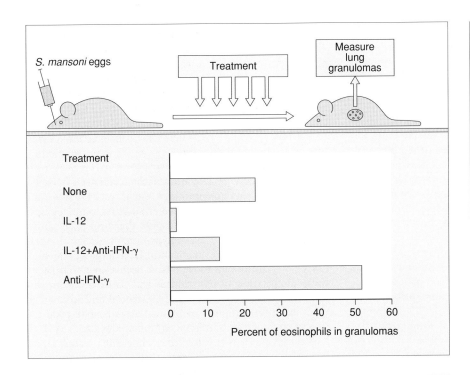

Fig. 17.2 IL-12 depresses the numbers of eosinophils in granulomas. Mice were infected with *S. mansoni* eggs either together with daily administration of IL-12 or saline with or without anti-IFNγ. Granulomas developing in the lung were analysed for the presence of eosinophils. Their presence is characteristic of a Th2 response resulting in IL-4 and IL-5 production. Data from Wynn *et al*, 1994.

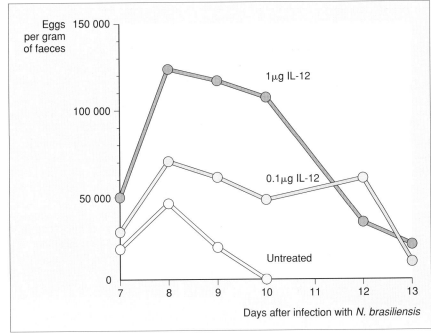

Fig. 17.3 IL-12 depresses the protective immune response against *N. brasiliensis*. Mice were infected with *N. brasiliensis* and given IL-12 daily from d0. Two doses of IL-12 were used, 0.1μg and 1μg. The figure depicts the time course of egg production. Data from Finkelman *et al*, 1994.

treatment of patients with septic shock and have shown significant beneficial effects. It has recently been tested for its efficacy in ameliorating the symptoms of rheumatoid arthritis and again showed significant dose-dependent beneficial effects. It is possible that the ability of IL-1RA to improve these clinical conditions may be related to the ability of this antagonist to downregulate TNF and IL-6 levels (see below). It has been shown in several autoimmune conditions that intravenous administration of high doses of immunoglobulin can be of beneficial effect. It has been suggested that this may be through perturbation of the idiotype network (see

Chapter 11). An alternative explanation explored by Dinarello states that following binding of immunoglobulin to FcγRI receptor, cross-linking induces IL-1RA production.

Neutralizing TNF

TNF, another potent inflammatory cytokine, has been implicated in the pathogenesis of RA as well as cerebral malaria (see Chapter 10). The finding that transgenic expression of TNFα results in the development of chronic arthritis together with the ability of anti-TNFα antibody to prevent collagen induced arthritis suggests that this cytokine might play a pivotal role in immune based joint destruction. Several clinical trials have now been performed to assess the efficacy of TNF-targeted therapy in RA. *In vitro* studies of human synovial cell cultures from RA patients have shown that anti-TNFα not only neutralizes TNFα but also blockades the cytokine cascade by inhibiting the production of other proinflammatory cytokines such as IL-1, IL-6, GM-CSF and the chemokine IL-8. On the basis that TNFα plays a central role in the pathology of the rheumatoid joint, humanized monoclonal anti-TNF antibodies and TNF receptor-Ig conjugates have been administered to RA patients. These agents are showing considerable therapeutic promise in reducing stiffness, pain and the numbers of swollen joints. This clinical improvement has been mirrored by the reduction in the serological parameters of the acute phase response which is elevated in RA patients (*Fig. 17. 4*). There has however been the observation that a small subgroup of RA patients treated with anti-TNF have gone on to develop antibodies to dsDNA and symptoms of SLE. As with IL-12 therapy it presumably must be borne in mind that some perturbations of the cytokine network might unveil new pathological disorders in genetically susceptible individuals.

In animal models a combination of anti-CD4 and anti-TNF antibodies proved to be more potent, suggesting that in man combination therapy might have long-term advantages. It may transpire that the TNFR-Ig fusion protein will provide an agent of longer half life and increased affinity and that, either alone or in combination with T cell-specific reagents, it might provide the best therapeutic approach to the treatment of inflammatory joint disease.

The role of TNFα in cerebral malaria has already been discussed in Chapter 10 and clearly that group of individuals homozygous for the *TNF2* allele which causes higher levels of gene transcription might also benefit from TNF directed therapeutic intervention.

Targeting chemokines

Chemokines play an important role in the extravasation and activation of leukocytes. IL-8 for example increases the number of CD11b/CD18 molecules on neutrophils and enhances their binding to endothelium. This chemokine also causes L-selectin to be shed from the neutrophil thus possibly further facilitating the transition from a rolling cell to a firmly attached cell. The extravasation of leukocytes might also be influenced by chemokines acting as chemoattractants. Reactive oxygen intermediates are released from neutrophils following activation of the respiratory burst by IL-8 while other chemokines such as MIP-1α and RANTES can stimulate the respiratory burst in monocytes. These highly potent molecules are therefore frequently associated with acute as well as chronic inflammatory responses and also play important roles in angiogenesis and fibroplasia. Antibodies to IL-8 have been shown to prevent the accumulation of neutrophils and tissue injury in the lung following ischaemia and reperfusion and to protect from immune complex-mediated alveolitis. The production of chemokines is influenced by cytokines such as IL-4 and IL-10 and it is possible that some disease states may be ameliorated through exploitation of the interplay between cytokines and chemokines.

MODULATION OF THE IMMUNE RESPONSE THROUGH INTERFERENCE WITH KEY STAGES IN LYMPHOCYTE ACTIVATION

T cells are pivotal to the immune response and many therapeutic strategies aimed at downregulating immune responses have been aimed at interfering with T cell activation or the ability of T cells to interact with other cells.

From the previous chapters it is clear that there are several targets on antigen presenting cells or T cells which may be used to manipulate the immune response. These include,

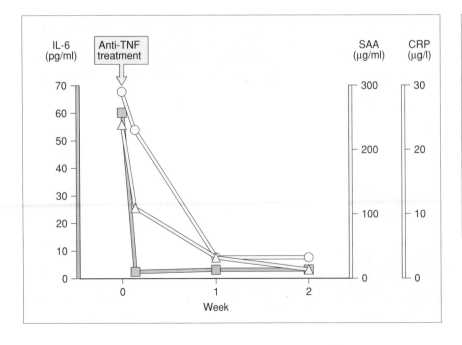

Fig. 17.4 Effect of anti-TNF antibody on the acute phase protein response. The patient received 10mg/kg of an anti-TNF chimaeric monoclonal antibody (mouse Fv / human IgG). IL-6, C reactive protein (CRP) and serum amyloid A (SAA) were measured at different time points after antibody treatment. It can be seen that the TNFα antibody caused a marked reduction in these markers of the acute phase response. Data from Maini *et al*, 1995.

on the APC, MHC molecules, B7 and ICAM-1 and on the T cell, CD2, CD4, CD8, CD28, LFA-1 and VLA-4.

Thus antibodies to class II MHC molecules have been shown to reduce the incidence and severity of a variety of experimentally induced and spontaneously arising auto-immune diseases.

Activation of the naive T cell through the TCR in the absence of engagement of other accessory molecules has been shown to result in T cell unresponsiveness. Non-depleting anti-CD4 antibodies have been extensively employed and shown not only to prevent the induction of experimentally or spontaneously induced autoimmune responses but additionally to prevent primed CD4+ T cells from mediating pathology (Chapters 11 and 12). In those situations such as graft rejection it has been necessary to target both CD4+ T cells and CD8+ T cells with antibodies to prevent graft rejection. Modulation of the CD3-TCR complex through anti-CD3 antibodies has been shown to induce long term remission of insulin dependent diabetes mellitus in NOD mice (*Fig. 17.5*). The interaction between LFA-1 and ICAM-1 has also been targeted with mono-clonal antibodies and shown to be critical for allograft rejection, experimentally induced arthritis and the development of diabetes in NOD mice. Another interaction of great import in T cell activation is that between CD28/CTLA-4 on the T cell and B7.1 and B7.2 on the antigen presenting cell. Interference with this reaction for example by using a soluble immunoglobulin fusion protein of CTLA-4 has been shown to prevent T cell activation. This fusion pro-tein has been shown to prevent allograft rejection and also induction of autoimmunity in NOD mice.

B cells can act as highly effective antigen presenting cells when they are activated but not resting. Presentation by resting B cells may result in T cell non-responsiveness (Chapter 12). The interaction between CD40L (gp39) on the T cell and CD40 on the B cell is of great importance for B cell survival, antibody production (Chapters 9 and 12),

germinal centre formation and the development of memo-ry B cell responses. This interaction is also important for T cell responsiveness. The upregulation of B7.1 and B7.2 on B cells is dependent on CD40–CD40L interaction. Anti-CD40L antibodies have been shown to prevent the T cell mediated rejection of F$_1$ bone marrow by parental mice through induction of T cell tolerance (*Fig. 17.6*). Antibodies to VLA-4 have been shown in animal models to prevent experimental allergic encephalomyelitis (EAE), DTH responses, bronchial asthma, autoimmune diabetes and ulcerative colitis.

It should be remembered that in clinical practice a ther-apy which modifies ongoing inflammatory responses is required. Many of the approaches which have been used experimentally mainly affect the initiation or the early stages of the pathological processes.

INTERFERENCE WITH ADHESION MOLECULES ON ENDOTHELIUM

Inflammatory cells gain access to tissue through adhesion molecules expressed on vascular endothelium and their counter-receptors on the leukocyte. These include the selectins, the vascular mucins, the integrins and molecules such as ICAM-1, ICAM-2, VCAM-1, PECAM-1 and MadCAM-1. Inhibition of the interaction of the leukocytes with the endothelium such that adhesion or transmigration is prevented could ameliorate inflammation. The therapeu-tic approaches which are possible in this regard include the use of monoclonal antibodies or soluble receptor antagonists to blockade competitively the interaction of the leukocyte with endothelium. In many different situations this approach has been of some success. The participation of the LFA-1/ICAM-1 and VLA-4/VCAM-1 adhesion pathways in leukocyte binding to vascular endothelium have made these molecules key targets for therapeutic intervention.

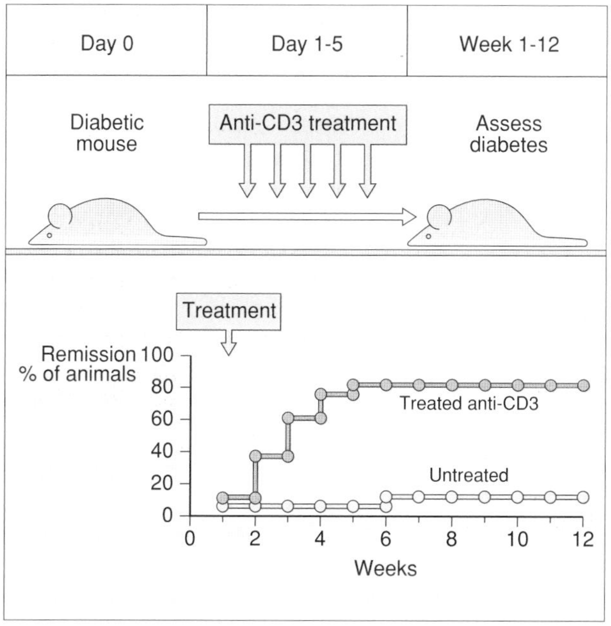

Fig. 17.5 Anti-CD3 antibody can cause remission from IDDM. Overtly diabetic NOD mice were given either hamster anti-CD3 (5µg/day for 5 days) or a control hamster immunoglobulin. Remission from IDDM was defined as a normalization of blood glucose and disappearance of glycosuria. Data from Chatenoud *et al*, 1994.

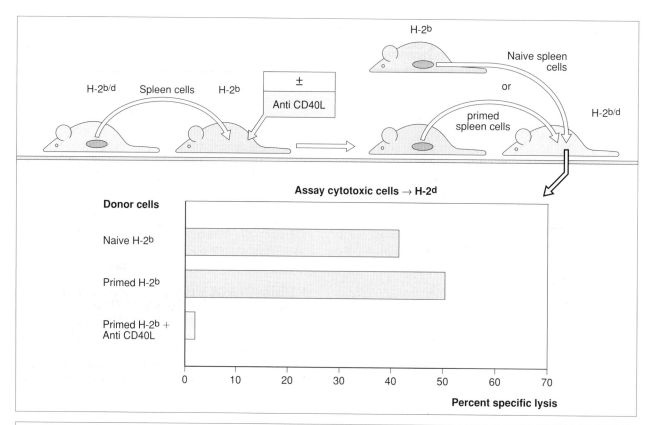

Fig. 17.6 The involvement of CD40/CD40L interaction in the generation of allospecific CTL. (C57BL/6 x DBA/2) F₁ (H-2^(b/d)) spleen cells were transferred into C57BL/6 mice in the presence or absence of anti-gp39 administered on d0 or d3. The recipient mice did not develop alloreactive CTL when injected with anti-gp39 (anti-CD40L). To establish whether CTL tolerance had been established spleen cells from the recipient C57BL/6 mice were transferred into (C57BL/6 x DBA/2) F₁ (H-2^(b/d)) mice. If donor mice had been treated with anti-gp39 no graft versus host disease (GVHD) developed and no alloreactive CTL activity was developed (lower panel, green). In contrast, if the donor mice were not treated or naive C57BL/6 spleen cells were transferred, the recipients developed GVHD and alloreactive CTL (lower panel: grey). The figure depicts the H-2^b anti-H-2^d CTL response. Data from Buhlmann et al, 1995.

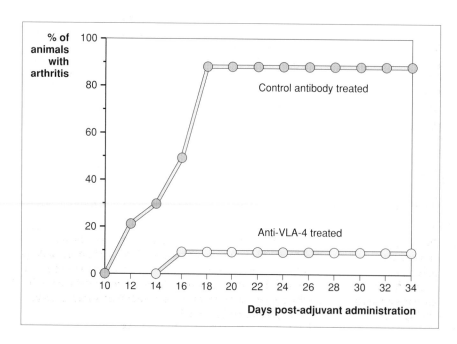

Fig. 17.7 Antibody to α₄ integrin prevents adjuvant-induced arthritis. The anti-α₄ integrin antibody used in this study was not cytotoxic and therefore its activity is thought to be due to blockade of the interaction between the α₄ subunit of VLA-4 and its ligand VCAM-1. Injection of Freund's adjuvant subdermally into the base of the tail of Lewis rats induces arthritis within 3 weeks. On day 10 after injection, adjuvant rats were given an i.p. injection of anti-α₄ integrin or isotype-matched, irrelevant control antibody. Rats given the blocking antibody developed arthritis at a much reduced incidence. Data from Barbadillo et al, 1995.

For example, in animal models of asthma, antibodies to α_4 integrin can prevent eosinophil recruitment and activation and antibodies to E-selectin and ICAM reduce the airway inflammatory response. A monoclonal antibody directed against the rat α_4 integrin of VLA-4 has been shown to block binding to VCAM-1 and additionally to prevent adjuvant induced arthritis in Lewis strain rats (*Fig. 17.7*).

DNA VACCINATION

Intramuscular injection of plasmid vectors encoding viral proteins has been shown to be an exceptionally good way of inducing antibodies and CD8+T cells specific for viral antigens. It is thought that the injected DNA exists as an episome in the muscle cells and that the expressed viral gene encoded

peptides are then efficiently presented on the surface of myoblasts by MHC Class I. *Figure 17.8* shows the ability of injected plasmid DNA encoding the nucleoprotein from influenza virus to generate an effective protective immune response. Even better immune responses can be achieved by co-injecting plasmid encoding cytokine genes such as GM-CSF (*Fig. 17.9*). The ability to generate an effective neutralizing antibody response as well as a CTL response suggests that Th cell activation has occurred. It is unclear whether APC in addition to muscle cells are transfected with the plasmid or whether APC are taking up and re-presenting viral proteins produced by the muscle cells. This approach does not have to be restricted to viral antigens but has also been used to generate efficient immune responses to intracellular microorganisms such as mycobacteria. It may also be possible to use DNA vaccination to boost immune responses to tumours.

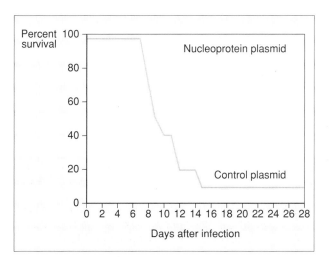

Fig. 17.8 DNA vaccination generates protective immunity to influenza. Mice were immunized three times by intramuscular injection of 100μg plasmid encoding the nucleoprotein of influenza A/PR/8/34 strain or with a control vector at 0, 3 and 6 weeks. At 9 weeks all mice were challenged by lung infection with a lethal dose of influenza. Survival curves are shown. Data from Montgomery *et al*, 1994.

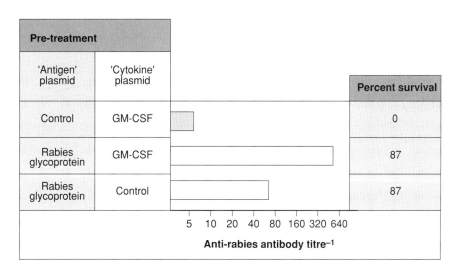

Pre-treatment			Percent survival
'Antigen' plasmid	'Cytokine' plasmid		
Control	GM-CSF		0
Rabies glycoprotein	GM-CSF		87
Rabies glycoprotein	Control		87

Anti-rabies antibody titre⁻¹: 5 10 20 40 80 160 320 640

Fig. 17.9 The effect of GM-CSF on the neutralizing antibody response to rabies virus. The effect of co-injecting plasmids encoding GM-CSF and rabies glycoprotein on the response to rabies virus. Mice were injected on d0 with combinations of plasmids encoding rabies glycoprotein (or control) and/or GM-CSF (or control). Mice were boosted at d14 with the 'antigen' plasmids. At d28 the mice were infected with a lethal dose of rabies virus. Neutralizing serum antibody to rabies was assessed in bleeds taken at 3 weeks and compared with the percent survival rate in each group at 4 weeks. Data from Xiang and Ertl, 1995.

PEPTIDE INDUCED TOLERANCE

Long term epitope-specific tolerance can be induced following neonatal administration of peptide epitopes. Tolerance can also be induced in adults using peptides if the peptide is administered through the appropriate route or if an analogue peptide is used. This is clearly seen in the case of EAE where inhalation or intravenous administration of myelin basic protein (MBP) peptide in high concentration prevented EAE. The various mechanism(s) by which peptide can regulate immune responses *in vivo* have been dealt with in Chapters 11 and 12 and include deviation of the immune response, TCR antagonism, anergy and deletion.

SUMMARY

Numerous strategies are being developed to influence the immune response. In addition to the immunosuppressive regimens involving drugs such as FK506 or Cyclosporin A other approaches are being explored which involve targeting key molecules involved in immune interactions or manipulating the cytokine cascade.

With regard to the potentiation of the immune response, again cytokine manipulation of the immune response is being explored but additionally, DNA vaccination strategies are being used to generate antigen-specific immune responses.

FURTHER READING

Barbadillo C, G-Arroyo A, Salas C, Mulero J, Sanchez-Madrid F, Andreu JL. Anti-integrin immunotherapy in rheumatoid arthritis: protective effect of anti-α_4 antibody in adjuvant arthritis. *Springer Semin Imunopathol* 1995, 16:427.

Blakemore AIF, Tarlow JK, Gordon C, Emery P, Duff GW. Interleukin 1 receptor antagonist gene polymorphism as a disease severity factor in systemic lupus erythematosus. *Arthritis Rheum* 1994, 37:1380.

Brunda MJ, Luistro L, Warrier RR, Wright RB, Hubbard BR, Murphy M, Wolf SF, Gately MK. Antitumor and antimetastatic activity of interleukin 12 against murine tumors. *J Exp Med* 1993, 178:1223.

Buhlmann JE, Foy TM, Aruffo A, Crassi KM, Ledbetter JA, Green WR, Xu JC, Shultz L, Roopesian D, Flavell R, Fast L, Noelle RJ, Durie F. In the absence of CD40 signal, B cells are tolerogenic. *Immunity* 1995, 2:645.

Chatenoud L, Thevet E, Primo J, Bach J-F. Anti-CD3 antibody induced long-term remission of overt autoimmunity in non-obese diabetic mice. *Proc Natl Acad Sci USA* 1994, 92:123.

Cooke A, Wraith DC. Immunotherapy of autoimmune disease. *Curr Opin Imm* 1993, 5:925.

Critchfield JM, Racke MK, Zuniga-Pflucker JC, Cannella B, Raine CS, Goverman J, Lenardo MJ. T cell deletion in high antigen dose therapy of autoimmune encephalomyelitis. *Science* 1994, 263:1139.

Dinarello CA. Is there a role for Interleukin 1 blockade in intravenous immunoglobulin therapy? *Imm Rev* 1994, 139:173.

Finkelman FD, Madden KB, Cheever AW, Katona IM, Morris SC, Gately MK, Hubbard BR, Gause WC, Urban JF. Effects of Inter-leukin 12 on immune responses·and host protection in mice infected with intestinal nematode parasites. *J Exp Med* 1994, 179:1563.

Furie MB, Randolph GJ. Chemokines and tissue injury. *Am J Pathol* 1995, 146:1287.

Heinzel FP, Schoenhaut DS, Rerko RM, Rosser LE, Gately MK. Recombinant Interleukin 12 cures mice infected with *Leishmania major*. *J Exp Med* 1993, 177:1505.

Hollenbaugh D, Ochs HD, Noelle RJ, Ledbetter JA, Aruffo A. The role of CD40 and its ligand in the regulation of the immune response. *Imm Rev* 1994, 138:23.

Maini RN, Elliott MJ, Brennan FM, Williams RO, Qiu Chu C, Paleolog E, Charles PJ, Taylor PC, Feldmann M. Monoclonal anti-TNFα antibody as a probe of pathogenesis and therapy of rheumatoid disease. *Imm Rev* 1995, 144:195.

Metzler B, Wraith DC. Inhibition of experimental autoimmune encephalomyelitis by inhalation but not oral administration of the encephalitogenic peptide: influence of MHC binding affinity. *Int Immunol* 1993, 5:1159.

Miescher PA, Spiegelberg HL, Izui S. Therapeutic implications of α_4 integrins. *Springer Sem Immunopathol* 1995, 16:357.

Montgomery DL, Shiver JW, Leander KR, Perry HC, Friedman A, Martinez D, Ulmer JB, Donelly JJ, Liu MA. Heterologoues and homologous protection against influenza A by DNA vaccination: optimization of DNA vectors. *DNA Cell Biol* 1993, 12:777.

Morris SC, Madden KB, Adamovicz JJ, Gause WC, Hubbard BR, Gately MK, Finkelman FD. Effects of IL-12 on *in vivo* cytokine gene expression and Ig isotype selection. *J Immunol* 1994, 152:1047.

Sypek JP, Chung CL, Mayor SEH, Subramanyam JM, Goldman SJ, Sieburth DS, Wolf SF, Schaub RG. Resolution of cutaneous Leishmaniasis: Interleukin 12 initiates a protective T helper type 1 immune response. *J Exp Med* 1993, 177:1797.

Wynn TA, Eltoum I, Oswald IP, Cheever AW, Sher A. Endogenous Interleukin 12 (IL-12) regulates granuloma formation induced by eggs of *Schistosoma mansoni* and exogenous IL-12 both inhibits and prophylactically immunizes against egg pathology. *J Exp Med* 1994, 179:1551.

Xiang Z, Ertl HCJ. Manipulation of the immune response to a plasmid-encoded viral antigen by co-inoculation with plasmids expressing cytokines. *Immunity* 1995, 2:129.

Linkage: The condition where two genes are both present in close proximity on a single chromosome and are usually inherited together.

Linkage disequillibrium: A condition where two genes are found together in a population at a greater frequency than that predicted simply by the product of their individual gene frequencies.

LMP: Originally low molecular weight polypeptide. Proteasome component LMP2 and LMP7, encoded in the MHC class II region.

Low zone tolerance: Sub-immunogenic doses of T dependent antigens which can tolerize T cells.

LPR (lymphoproliferation gene): A gene found in MRL mice which is involved in the generation of autoimmune phenomena.

LPS (lipopolysaccharide): A product of some Gram-negative bacterial cell walls, which can act as a B cell mitogen.

Ly antigens: Two series of mouse lymphocyte cell surface markes. Ly1 (CD5) is present on T helper cells, but also some immature lymphocytes and B cells. Ly2 (CD8) is present on cytotoxic T cells. Others do not yet have a CD designation. Lyb5 identifies a subset of B cells which recognize type II T-indpendent antigens.

Lymph node: Secondary lymphoid organs.

Lymphokines: A generic term for molecules other than antibodies which are involved in signalling between cells of the immune system and are produced by lymphocytes (cf. interleukins).

Lymphotoxin: Cytokine produced by activated T cell.

Lytic pathway: The complement pathway effected by components C5–C9, which is responsible for lysis of sensitized cell plasma membranes.

MAC (membrane attack complex): The assembled terminal complement components C5b–C9 of the lytic pathway, which becomes inserted into cell membranes.

Macrophage: Large phagocytic cells.

MAF (macrophage arming factor): Factor released by activated T cells which cause macrophage activation, of which IFNγ, is a major component.

MALT (mucosa-associated lymphoid tissue): Generic term for lymphoid tissue associated with the mucosa of the gastrointestinal tract, bronchial tree etc.

Mast cell: Large cells present near blood vessels, particularly that store histamine. Responsible for local hypersensitivity responses and allergic reaction.

MHC (major histocompatibility complex): A genetic region found in all mammals whose products are primarily responsible for the rapid rejection of grafts between individuals, and which function is signalling between lymphocytes and cells expressing antigen.

MHC restriction: A characteristic of many immune reactions, in which cells cooperate most effectively with other cells sharing an MHC haplotype.

Microglial cells: Phagocytic cells of the brain, which are probably derived from the monocyte lineage and can present antigen.

MIF (migration inhibition factor): A group of peptides produced by lymphocytes, which are capable of inhibiting macrophage migration.

Minor histocompatibility antigens: Antigens that can lead to graft rejection in addition to the major or MHC antigens. Most are thought to be peptides of polymorphic proteins bound to MHC molecules.

Mitogen: Substances that cause cells, particularly lymphocytes, to undergo cell division.

MLR/MLC (mixed lymphocyte reaction/culture): Assay system for T cell recognitiion of allogenic cells, in which response is measured by proliferation in the presence of the stimulating cells.

MOG: Myelin oligodendrocyte glycoprotein. Component of myelin, the gene for which is in the class I region of the MHC.

Monoclonal: Derived from a single clone; for example, monoclonal antibodies which are produced by a single clone and are homogeneous.

Monocytes: Macrophage precursor cells.

Mononuclear phagocyte system: The group of fixed and mobile phagocytic cells derived from bone marrow stem cells, and previously called the reticuloendothelial system.

MRL.lpr: A spontaneously autoimmune strain of mouse which has been used as a model of rheumatoid arthritis.

Myeloma: A lymphoma produced from cells of the B cell lineage.

Naive lymphocytes: Cells that have not seen their antigen yet so have not been stimulated.

Necrosis: Cell death resulting from irreversible damage to the plasma membrane.

Network theory: A proposal, first put forward by Jerne and since developed, which states that T cells and B cells mutually interregulate by recognizing idiotopes on the antigen receptors.

Neutrophil chemotatic factor: A protein mediator of chemotaxis released by mast cells, now termed IL-8.

NIP (4-hydroxy, 5-iodo, 3-nitrophenylacetyl): A commonly used hapten.

NK (natural killer) cell: A group of lymphocytes which have the intrinsic ability to recognize and destroy some virally infected cells and some tumour cells.

Non-repsonder: Refers to strains of animals which fail to make an immune response to antigens that are immunogenic in others.

NP (hydroxy, 3-nitrophenlacetyl): A hapten which partially cross-reacts with NIP.

Nude mouse: A genetically athymic mouse. It also carries a closely linked gene producing a defect in hair production.

Null cells: Blood lymphocytes which fail to express B cell or T cell surface markers.

Nurse cells: The *in vitro* form of thymic epithelial cells, which are closely surrounded by developing T cells and are thought to be involved in thymic education.

NZB, NZB/W: Two spontaneously autommimmune strains of mouse. The NZB is used as a model of autoimmune haemolytic anaemia. The (NZB × NZW)F1 (NZB/W) develops autoantibodies to DNA and devlops a nephritis resembling that seen in systemic lupus erythematosus.

Obese chicken: Strain of chicken which develops autoimmune thyroiditis.

Oncogene: Mutations resulting in alterations of protein sequence or mode of expression of a gene resulting in predisposition to tumour formation.

Open reading frame: DNA sequences could theoretically be translated in any of three reading frames. The open reading frame is one without stop codons.

Opsonization: A process by which phagocytosis is facilitated by the deposition of opsonins (e.g. antibody and C3b) on the antigen.

PAF (platelet activating factor): A factor released by granulocytes, particularly basophils, and other cells which causes platelet aggregation and has chemotactic and inflammatory effects.

PALS (periarteriolar lymphatic sheath): The accumulations of lymphoid tissue constituting the white pulp of the spleen.

Parallel sets: This refers to different antibodies which share idiotopes but have different antigen-binding specificity, and may be regulated concomitantly through the idiotypic interactions.

Paratope: The part of an antibody molecule which makes contact with the antigenic determinant (epitope).

Passenger cells: Cells in a graft which migrate into the recipient lymphoid tissue and are particularly effective at producing allogenic sensitization.

Pathogen: An organism which causes disease.

PC (phosphoryl choline): A commonly used hapten whch is also found on the surface of a number of microorganisms.

PCR: Polymerase chain reaction.

Perforin: Pore-forming protein (PFP) released by cytotoxic T cells and NK cells which polymerizes to form pores in the target cell membrane.

Peyer's patches: Small clumps of lymphocytes in the small intestine.

PFC (plaque forming cell): An antibody-producing cell detected *in vitro* by its ability to lyse antigen-sensitized erythrocytes in the presence of complement.

PHA (phytohaemagglutinin): A mitogen for T cells.

Phagocytosis: The process by which cells engulf material and enclose it within a vacuole (phagosome) in the cytoplasm.

Phagosome, phagolysosome: The membrane-bound vacuole formed by phagocytosis and containing the phagocytosed material. After fusion of lysosomes with the phagosome, it is referred to as a phagolysosome.

Pinocytosis: The process by which liquids or very small particles are taken into the cell.

Plasma cell: An antibody-producing B cell, which has reached the end of its differentiation pathway.

Pokeweed mitogen (PWM): A mitogen for B cells.

Polyclonal: A term which describes the products of a number of different cell types (cf. monoclonal).

Polymorphism: Variability at a locus. Polymorphic alleles are present in a population at a minimum frequency. An alteration in a gene of a single individual is a mutation.

Prednisolone: Immunosuppressive steroid.

Primary lymphoid tissues: Lymphoid organs in which lymphocytes complete their initial maturation steps, including the fetal liver, adult bone marrow and thymus, and the Bursa of Fabricius in birds.

Primary response: The immune responses (cellular or humoral) seen following an initial encounter with a particular antigen.

Primary transcript: Direct transcripts of genomic DNA, before excision of introns to produce mRNA.

Prime: To give an initial sensitization to antigen.

Private specificities: Epitopes unique to a particular MHC haplotype.

Privileged sites: Tissues in which graft rejection reactions are very weak or absent following implantation of allogenic tissue.

Properdin pathway: Original designation of the alternative pathway of complement activation, named after the molecule properdin (factor P) which stabilizes the alternative pathway C3 convertase.

Prostaglandins: Pharmacologically active derivatives of arachidonic acid. Different prostaglandins are capable of modulating cell mobility and immune responses.

Proteasome: Multisubunit barrel structure in the cytoplasm and nucleus of the cell responsible for non-lysosomal protein breakdown. Plays a role in antigen processing.

Protein-A: A cell wall component of certain strains of staphylococci, which binds to a site in the Fc region of most IgG istotypes.

Pseudoalleles: Tandem variants of a gene; they do not occupy a homologous position of the chromosome (e.g. C4).

Pseudogenes: Genes which have homologous structures to other genes but which are incapable of being expressed (e.g. Jk3 in the mouse).

Public specificities: Epitopes common to MHC molecules of several different haplotypes.

Qa **genes:** A mouse gene locus adjacent to the classical MHC locus, which encodes types IV MHC molecules.

Radioimmunoassay: A number of different, sensitive techniques for measuring antigen or antibody titres, using radiolabelled reagents.

RAG-1/RAG-2: Recombination activating gene. The RAG products are essential for receptor gene rearrangement and mutations result in immunodeficiency.

Receptor: A cell surface molecule which binds specifically to particular proteins or peptides in the fluid phase.

Recombinant strain: A strain of animal in which a genetic cross-over has occurred at a defined chromosomal location.

Recombination: A process by which genetic information is rearranged during meiosis. This process also occurs during the somatic rearrangements of DNA which occur in the formation of genes encoding antibody and T cell receptor molecules.

Recurrent idiotype: An idiotype present in the immune response of different animals or strains to a particular antigen.

Respiratory burst: Increase in oxidative metabolism of phagocytes following uptake of opsonized particles.

Reticuloendothelial system: A diffuse system of phagocytic cells derived from the bone marrow stem cell which are associated with the connective tissue framework of the liver, spleen, lymph nodes and other serous cavities.

RFLP (restriction fragment length polymorphism): A technique which examines microheterogeneity within DNA sequences from different individuals. It is based on the ability of DNA restriction enzymes to recognize (and cleave) at particular base sequences, present in one individual, but not another.

Rosetting: A technique for identifying or isolating cells by mixing them with particles or cells to which they bind (e.g. sheep erythrocytes to human T cells). The rosettes consist of a central cell surrounded by bound cells.

SDS-PAGE: Polyacrylamide gel electrophoresis in detergent sodium dodecyl sulphate. Proteins unfold in this detergent and their migration is in proportion to their MW.

Secondary response: The immune response which follows a second or subsequent encounter with a particular antigen.

Secretory component: A polypeptide produced by cells of some secretory epithelia, which is involved in transporting secreted polymeric IgA across the cell and protecting it from digestion in the gastrointestinal tract.

Selectins: Adhesion molecules containing a lectin-like domain, including ELAM, MEL-14 and GMP-140.

Self tolerance: The idea that, although the immune system recognizes the body's own proteins, it does not react again them.

Site-directed mutagenesis: A technique in which amino acid residues at particular binding sites or enzymatically active residues are changed by introducing point mutations into the encoding DNA.

SLE (systemic lupus erythematosus): An autoimmune disease of humans, usually involving anti-nuclear antibodies.

Somatic mutation: A process which occurs during B cell maturation and affects the antibody gene region. It permits refinement of antibody specificity.

Superantigen: An antigen which is particularly effective in causing selection of T cell populatons, during thyymic ontogeny, including molecules such as Staphylococcal enterotoxin A and B which can act as mitogens for particular families of T cells.

Suppressor T cells: T cells that down-regulate immune responses. Their mode of action is controversial.

Synergism: Cooperative interaction.

T cell bypass: The theory that autoimmunity develops because self tolerance at the T cell level is bypassed.

T dependent/T indpendent antigens: T dependent antigens require immune recognition by both T and B cells to produce an immune response. T independent antigens can directly stimulate B cells to produce specific antibody.

T15: An idiotype associated with antiphosphoryl choline antibodies, named after the TEPC 15 myeloma prototype sequence.

TAC: The human IL-2 receptor α-chain (CD25).

Tachyphylaxis: The process by which subsequent doses of a pharmacological reagent produce decreasing effects.

TAP: Transporter associated with antigen processing.

Targeting sequences: Amino acid sequences in proteins involved in their specfic localization to appropriate cytoplasmic, membrane or nuclear compartments.

TCR (T cell antigen receptor): The receptor of T cells consists of a heterodimer (αβ or γδ) which recognizes antigen/MHC and is specific for a particular clone of T cells. This is associated with a group of monomorphic polypeptides which make up the CD3 complex.

Th1, Th2 cells: Subsets of mouse T cell clones defined by their capabilities in producing different sets of cytokines.

Thy1: A cell surface antigen of mouse with allotypic variants.

Thymic epithelial cells: Thymic antigen-presenting cells, expressing high levels of class II MHC antigens, thought to be important in the development of T cell immune recognition.

Thymic hormones: A group of molecules, including thymosin, thymulin, thymopoietin and thymostimulin, produced by the thymus, which help to maintain T cell function and development in secondary lymphoid tissues.

Ti: The antigen specific (idiotypic) portion of the T cell receptor i.e. the αβ or γδ heterodimers as distinct from the entire complex with the CD3 molecules.

***TLA* locus:** A mouse gene locus adjacent to the classical MHC locus, which encodes type IV MHC molecules.

TNF (tumour necrosis factor): Two cytokines, whose genes are closely linked in the MHC.

Tolerance: A state of specific immunological uresponsiveness.

Transfection: Direct insertion of exogenous genetic mateiral (usually DNA) into a recipient cell.

Transformation: Morphological changes in a lymphocyte associated with the onset of division. Also used to denote the change to the autonomously dividing state of a cancer cell.

Transgenic: An animal or strain containing an exogenous gene(s).

Triggering of mast cells: Stimulation of mast cell degranulation, effected by crosslinking of surface bound IgE, direct triggering by C3a and C5a, or by drugs.

Ubiquitin: A protein coupled to denatured or otherwise abnormal cytoplasmic proteins, involved in signalling proteolysis.

V domains: The N-terminal domains of antibody heavy and light chains and the α and β chains of the T cell receptor which vary between different clones and form the antigen-binding site.

***V* genes:** Sets of genes whch encode the major portion of the V domains of antigen binding molecules (Ig and the TCR). They become recombined with *D* and/or *J* segments during lymphocyte ontogeny.

Vasoactive amines: Products such as histamine and 5-hydroxytryptamine released by basophils, mast cells and platelets which act on the endothelium and smooth muscle of the local vasculature.

VEAs (very early antigens): Early activation markers on T cells.

Veiled cells: Cells found in lymph which develop into dendritic cells in the T cell areas of secondary lymphoid tissues.

VLAs (very late antigens): The adhesion molecules of the β₁-integrin family.

White pulp: The lymphoid component of spleen, consisting of periarteriolar sheaths of lymphocytes and antigen-presenting cells.

Xenogeneic: Referring to interspecies antigenic differences (cf. heterologous).

Appendix

CD	identity/function	mol. wt (× 10³)	T cell	B cell	NK/non-lineage	monocyte	macrophage	granulocyte	platelet	Langerhans cell/dendritic cell	stem cell
CD1a		49	Thy								
CD1b		45	Thy							LC	
CD1c		43	Thy							DC	
CD2	LFA-3 receptor	50									
CD2R		50	★								
CD3	TCR subunit (γ,δ,ε,ζ,η)	25,20,19,16,22									
CD4	MHC class II receptor	55									
CD5		67									
CD6		100									
CD7		40			●				●		
CD8	MHC class I receptor	36/32									
CD9		24		pre-B							
CD10	CALLA, neutral endopeptidase	100		pre-B							Lymph
CD11a	LFA-1 (α chain)	180									
CD11b	CR3 (α chain)	165									
CD11c	CR4 (α chain)	150									
CDw12		90–120							●		
CD13	Aminopeptidase N	150									
CD14	LPS-binding protein	55					●			●(LC)	
CD15	sLe^X					●					
CD16	FcγRIIIA/FcγRIIIB	50–65									
CD16b	FcγRIIIB	48									
CDw17	Lactosylceramide										
CD18	(β chain of CD11)	95									
CD19		95									
CD20	ion channel?	37/35									
CD21	CR2	140		Mat						FDC	
CD22		135									
CD23	FcεRII	45–50		Mat, ★		★	E				
CD24		41/38									
CD25	IL-2 receptor (β)	55	★	★	★						
CD26	Dipeptidylpeptidase IV	120	★								
CD27		55									
CD28		44		★							
CD29	VLA (β chain)	130									
CD30		120	★	★							
CD31	PECAM-1	140									
CD32	FcγRII	40									
CD33		67									BM
CD34		105–120									BM
CD35	CR1	160–260									
CD36		90			●						
CD37		40–52	●	Mat			●				
CD38		45	Thy, ★	PC							Lymph
CD39		70–100		Mat		●				FDC	
CD40		50								FDC	
CD41		120/25									
CD42a	GPIX	23									
CD42b	GPIB–α	135,23									
CD42c	GPIB–β	22									
CD42d	GP V	85									
CD43	Leukosialin	95									
CD44		80–95									
CD45	Leucocyte common antigen(LCA) T200										

CD markers

CD	identity/function	mol. wt (×10³)	T cell	B cell	NK/non-lineage	monocyte	macrophage	granulocyte	platelet	Langerhans cell/dendritic cell	stem cell
CD45RA	Restricted LCA	220			●			●			
CD45RB	Restricted LCA	190/205/220									
CD45RO	Restricted LCA	190									
CD46	MCP(membrane cofactor protein)	66/56									
CD47		47–52									
CD48		41									
CD49a	VLA-1 $\alpha_1$integrin	210	★								
CD49b	VLA-2 $\alpha_2$integrin	160	+	+	+	+	+	+			
CD49c	VLA-3 $\alpha_3$integrin	125									
CD49d	VLA-4 $\alpha_4$integrin	150,80,70	+	+		+				LC	
CD49e	VLA-5 $\alpha_5$integrin	135,25									
CD49f	VLA-6 $\alpha_6$integrin	120,25	●						+		
CD50	ICAM-3	124	+	+	+	+	+	+			
CD51	Vitronectin receptor α	120/24									
CDw52	Campath-1	21–28									
CD53		32–40									BM
CD54	ICAM-1										
CD55	DAF(Decay accelerating factor)	70									
CD56	NKH1 = NCAM	220/135	●								
CD57		110			●						
CD58	LFA-3	40–65									
CD59	TAP, protectin	18–20									
CDw60	NeuAc–NeuAc–Gal										
CD61	Vitronectin receptor β	105									
CD62P	P-selectin	150							+		
CD62E	E-selectin	115									
CD62L	L-selectin	75-80	+			+		+			
CD63		53	●	●				●			
CD64	FcγRI	70									
CDw65	Ceramide dodecasaccharide										
CD66a	BGP	180–200						+			
CD66b	Previously CD67	95-100						+			
CD66c	NCA	90-95						+			
CD66d	CGMI	30						+			
CD66e	Carcinoembryonic antigen (CEA)	180-200						+			
CD68		110									
CD69		32/28	★	★							
CD70	CD27-ligand	55,75.95,110.170	★	★							
CD71	Transferrin receptor	95	★	★	★	★					
CD72		43/39									
CD73	Ecto-5'-nucleotidase	69									
CD74	MHC class II invariant chain	41/35/33									
CDw75	α 2,6 sialyltransferase	53		Mat							
CD76				Mat							
CD77	Globotriaosylceramide										
CDw78											
CD79a	Igα	33,40		+							
CD79b	Igβ	33,40		+							
CD80	B7,BBI	60		+							

This table shows the recognized CD markers of haemopoietic cells and their distribution. Thy = thymocytes; DC = dendritic cells; LC = Langerhans' cells; N = neutrophils; E = eosinophils; GC = germinal centre B cell; FDC = follicular dendritic cell; PC = plasma cell; BM = bone-marrow cell. A filled rectangle or + = cell population present; a half-filled rectangle = subpopulation. ● = subject to further analysis; ★ = activated cells only; Rest = resting cells only; Lymph = lymphoid cells; Mat = mature cells only.

designation	identity	cells which express marker
CD81	TAPA-1	B cells
CD82		B cells
CD83		B cells
CDw84		B cells
CD85		B cells
CD86		B cells
CD87		Myeloid cells
CD88	C5a receptor	Monocytes/Neutrophils
CD89	Fcα receptor	Myeloid cells
CDw90	Thy –1.	T Cells - Monocytes
CD91	α2 -macroglobulin receptor	Myeloid cells
CDw92		Myeloid cells
CD93		Myeloid cells
CD94		NK Cells
CD95	APO-1 Fas	Activated Tc cells
CD96	TACTILE	Activated cells
CD97		Activated cells
CD98		T cells
CD99		T cells
CD100		T cells
CDw101		T cells
CD102	ICAM-2	Endothelium
CD103		
CD104	ß4 - integrin	Lymphocytes
CD105	Endoglin	Endothelium
CD106	VCAM-1	Activated Endothelium
CD107a	LAMP-1	Platelet
CD107b	LAMP-2	Platelet
CDw108		Endothelium
CDw109		
CD115	M-CSF receptor	Monocytes/Macrophages
CDw116	GM-CSF receptor	Myeloid precursors
CD117	cKIT	
CDw119	IFNα receptor	
CD120a	TNF receptor (55 KDa)	
CD120b	TNF receptor (75 KDa)	
CDw121a	IL-1 receptor (Type 1)	
CDw121b	IL-1 receptor (Type 2)	
CD122	IL-2 receptor (ß) (75 KDa)	
CDW124	IL-4 receptor	
CD126	IL-6 receptor	
CDw127	IL-7 receptor	
CDw128	IL-8 receptor	
CDw130	IL-6 receptor - gp 130 S1g	

cytokine receptors

Index

Index

Index